Textbook of Endodontology

KU-242-438

QM Library

23 1400061 8

WITHDRAWN
FROM STOCK
QMUL LIBRARY

Textbook of Endodontology

Second Edition

Edited by

Gunnar Bergenholtz
Preben Hørsted-Bindslev
Claes Reit

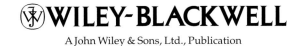

WILEY-BLACKWELL

A John Wiley & Sons, Ltd., Publication

This edition first published 2010
© 2003 Blackwell Munksgaard
© 2010 Blackwell Publishing Ltd

Blackwell Publishing was acquired by John Wiley & Sons in February 2007. Blackwell's publishing programme has been merged with Wiley's global Scientific, Technical, and Medical business to form Wiley-Blackwell.

First edition published 2003
Second edition 2010

Registered office
John Wiley & Sons Ltd, The Atrium, Southern Gate, Chichester, West Sussex, PO19 8SQ, United Kingdom

Editorial offices
9600 Garsington Road, Oxford, OX4 2DQ, United Kingdom
2121 State Avenue, Ames, Iowa 50014-8300, USA

For details of our global editorial offices, for customer services and for information about how to apply for permission to reuse the copyright material in this book please see our website at www.wiley.com/wiley-blackwell.

The right of the author to be identified as the author of this work has been asserted in accordance with the Copyright, Designs and Patents Act 1988.

All rights reserved. No part of this publication may be reproduced, stored in a retrieval system, or transmitted, in any form or by any means, electronic, mechanical, photocopying, recording or otherwise, except as permitted by the UK Copyright, Designs and Patents Act 1988, without the prior permission of the publisher.

Wiley also publishes its books in a variety of electronic formats. Some content that appears in print may not be available in electronic books.

Designations used by companies to distinguish their products are often claimed as trademarks. All brand names and product names used in this book are trade names, service marks, trademarks or registered trademarks of their respective owners. The publisher is not associated with any product or vendor mentioned in this book. This publication is designed to provide accurate and authoritative information in regard to the subject matter covered. It is sold on the understanding that the publisher is not engaged in rendering professional services. If professional advice or other expert assistance is required, the services of a competent professional should be sought.

Library of Congress Cataloging-in-Publication Data
Textbook of endodontology/edited by Gunnar Bergenholtz, Preben Hørsted-Bindslev, Claes Reit. — 2nd ed.
      p. ; cm.
   Includes bibliographical references and index.
   ISBN 978-1-4051-7095-6 (hardback: alk. paper) 1. Endodontics. I. Bergenholtz, Gunnar.
      II. Hørsted-Bindslev, Preben. III. Reit, Claes.
   [DNLM: 1. Dental Pulp Diseases—therapy. 2. Periapical Diseases—therapy. WU 230 T355 2010]
   RK351.T49 2003
   617.6'342—dc22

                                                                              2009024733

A catalogue record for this book is available from the British Library.

Set in 9.5/12.5pt Palatino by Gray Publishing, Tunbridge Wells, Kent
Illustrations by Jens Lund Kirkegaard
Printed and bound in Singapore by Fabulous Printers Pte Ltd

3   2012

QM LIBRARY (WHITECHAPEL)

Contents

List of Contributors   xi
Preface   xiii

1   Introduction to endodontology   1
Claes Reit, Gunnar Bergenholtz and Preben Hørsted-Bindslev

Endodontology   1
The dawn of modern endodontology   2
The objective of endodontic treatment   3
Clinical problems and solutions   3
The diagnostic dilemma   5
The tools of treatment   6
Extraction and dental implant?   6
References   6

Part 1   The Vital Pulp

2   The dentin–pulp complex: structures, functions and responses to adverse influences   11
Leif Olgart and Gunnar Bergenholtz

Introduction   11
Constituents and normal functions of the dentin–pulp complex   11
Basal maintenance   18
Appropriate responses of the healthy pulp to non-destructive stimuli   19
Responses to external threats   19
Effects of potentially destructive stimuli   23
References   30

3   Dentinal and pulpal pain   33
Matti Närhi

Introduction   33
Classification of nerve fibers   33
Morphology of intradental sensory innervation   33
Function of intradental sensory nerves under normal conditions   36
Sensitivity of dentin: hydrodynamic mechanism in pulpal A-fiber activation   37
Responses of intradental nerves to tissue injury and inflammation   39
Local control of pulpal nociceptor activation   42
Dentin hypersensitivity   42
Pain symptoms and pulpal diagnosis   43
References   44

4   Treatment of vital pulp conditions   47
Preben Hørsted-Bindslev and Gunnar Bergenholtz

Introduction   47
Clinical scenarios   47
Treatment options   48
Factors influencing choice of treatment   50
Management of exposed pulps by direct pulp capping/partial pulpotomy   52
Pulpectomy   59

Emergency treatment   65
References   69

5   Endodontics in primary teeth   73
Ingegerd Mejàre

Introduction   73
The normal pulp   73
Pulpal inflammation in the primary tooth   73
Wound dressings – characteristics, modes of action and reported clinical success rates   75
Objectives of pulp treatment   79
Operative treatment procedures   79
Indications and contraindications for pulp treatment in primary teeth   85
Future directions   85
References   88

Part 2   The Necrotic Pulp

6   The microbiology of the necrotic pulp   95
Gunnel Svensäter, Luis Chávez de Paz and Else Theilade

Introduction   95
Evidence for the essential role of microorganisms in apical periodontitis   95
Routes of microbial entry to the pulpal space   96
Modes of colonization   97
Ecological determinants for microbial growth in root canals   98
Methods for studying the root canal microflora   103
Composition of the endodontic microflora   106
Association of signs and symptoms with specific bacteria   109
Concluding remarks   110
References   110

7   Apical periodontitis   113
Zvi Metzger, Itzhak Abramovitz and Gunnar Bergenholtz

Introduction   113
The nature of apical periodontitis   113
Interactions with the infecting microbiota   118
Clinical manifestations and diagnostic terminology   123
References   126

8   Systemic complications of endodontic infections   128
Nils Skaug and Vidar Bakken

Introduction   128
Acute periapical infections as the origin of metastatic infections   128
Chronic periapical infections as the origin of metastatic infections   135
References   138

9   Treatment of the necrotic pulp   140
Paul Wesselink and Gunnar Bergenholtz

Introduction   140
Objectives and general treatment strategies   140
Scheme for a routine procedure in root canal therapy   143
Considerations in complex cases   152

Effects of root canal therapy on the intracanal microbiota   153
Management of symptomatic lesions   153
References   156

Part 3   Endodontic Treatment Procedures

10   The surgical microcope   **163**
Pierre Machtou

Introduction   163
Components   163
Ergonomics and working techniques   164
Microinstrumentation   167
Critical steps   167
Concluding remarks   168
References   168

11   Root canal instrumentation   **169**
Lars Bergmans and Paul Lambrechts

Introduction   169
Principles of root canal instrumentation   169
Root canal system anatomy   170
Procedural steps   174
Endodontic instruments   180
Instrumentation techniques   183
Limitations of root canal instrumentation   186
Preventing procedural mishaps   188
References   190

12   Root canal filling materials   **193**
Gottfried Schmalz and Preben Hørsted-Bindslev

Introduction   193
Requirements   194
Gutta-percha cones   198
Sealers   202
Materials for retrograde fillings (root-end fillings) and replantation   214
Mandibular nerve injuries   215
References   216

13   Root filling techniques   **219**
Paul Wesselink

Introduction   219
Specific objectives   219
Selecting a root canal filling material   219
Root filling techniques for gutta-percha   221
Root filling techniques employing gutta-percha and sealer   224
Procedures prior to root canal filling   229
Assessing root filling quality   229
Filling of the pulp chamber and coronal restoration   230
Conclusions and recommendations   231
References   231

Part 4   Diagnostic Considerations and Clinical Decision Making

14   Diagnosis of pulpal and periapical disease   **235**
Claes Reit and Kerstin Petersson

    Introduction   235
    Evaluation of diagnostic information   235
    Diagnostic strategy   237
    Clinical manifestations of pulpal and periapical inflammation   238
    Collecting diagnostic information   238
    Diagnostic classification   247
    References   253

15   Diagnosis and management of endodontic complications after trauma   **255**
John Whitworth

    Introduction   255
    Common dental injuries   255
    Dental trauma and its consequences   258
    General considerations in the management of dental trauma   267
    Diagnostic quandaries – to remove or review the pulp after trauma?   273
    Pulp regeneration – the dawn of a new era?   274
    References   274

16   The multidimensional nature of pain   **277**
Ilana Eli and Peter Svensson

    Introduction   277
    Neurobiological factors affecting the pain experience   278
    Psychological factors affecting the pain experience   280
    Gender and pain   282
    Special populations   284
    Management and treatment of pain   285
    Concluding remarks   287
    References   287

17   Clinical epidemiology   **290**
Claes Reit and Lise-Lotte Kirkevang

    Introduction   290
    Clinical epidemiology   290
    Diagnosis   292
    Cause   292
    Prevalence, frequency and incidence   293
    Risk for apical periodontitis   295
    Treatment   296
    Prognosis   296
    Longevity of root filled teeth   297
    Back to the case   298
    References   298

18   Endodontic decision making   **301**
Claes Reit

    The outcome of endodontic treatment   301
    Factors influencing treatment outcome   302
    Prevalence of endodontic "failures"   304

Variation in the management of periapical lesions in endodontically treated teeth   304
Clinical decision making: descriptive projects   305
Endodontic retreatment decision making: a normative approach   306
Concluding remarks   311
References   311

Part 5   The Root Filled Tooth

19   The root filled tooth in prosthodontic reconstruction   317
Eckehard Kostka

Introduction   317
Problems associated with root filled teeth as abutments   317
Core build-ups   322
Clinical techniques   325
Prosthodontic reconstruction   327
References   332

20   Non-surgical retreatment   335
Pierre Machtou and Claes Reit

Introduction   335
Indications   335
Access to the root canal   335
Access to the apical area   339
Instrumentation of the root canal   342
Antimicrobial treatment   344
Preventive retreatment   346
Prognosis   346
References   346

21   Surgical endodontics   348
Peter Velvart

Introduction   348
General outline of the procedure   349
Pain control after surgery   361
Bone healing   362
Prognosis   362
References   364

Failures after surgical endodontics   366
Thomas von Arx

Index   371

List of Contributors

Editors

Gunnar Bergenholtz Institute of Odontology, The Sahlgrenska Academy at University of Gothenburg, Sweden

Preben Hørsted-Bindslev School of Dentistry, Faculty of Health Sciences, Aarhus University, Denmark

Claes Reit Institute of Odontology, The Sahlgrenska Academy at University of Gothenburg, Sweden

Contributors

Itzhak Abramovitz Hebrew University and Hadassa Faculty of Dental Medicine, Hebrew University, Jerusalem, Israel

Thomas von Arx School of Dental Medicine, University of Berne, Switzerland

Vidar Bakken Faculty of Medicine and Dentistry, University of Bergen, Norway

Lars Bergmans School of Dentistry, University of Leuven, Belgium

Luis Chávez de Paz Faculty of Odontology, Malmö University, Sweden

Ilana Eli The Maurice and Gabriela Goldschleger School of Dental Medicine, Tel Aviv University, Israel

Lise-Lotte Kirkevang School of Dentistry, Faculty of Health Sciences, Aarhus University, Denmark

Eckehard Kostka School of Dental Medicine, Charité, Medical Faculty of the Berlin Humboldt University, Germany

Paul Lambrechts School of Dentistry, University of Leuven, Belgium

Pierre Machtou Denis Diderot School of Dentistry, Paris 7 University, France

Ingegerd Mejàre Faculty of Odontology, Malmö University, Sweden

Zvi Metzger The Maurice and Gabriela Goldschleger School of Dental Medicine, Tel Aviv University, Israel

Matti Närhi Faculty of Medicine, University of Kuopio, Finland

Leif Olgart Karolinska Institute, Stockholm, Sweden

Kerstin Petersson Faculty of Odontology, Malmö University, Sweden

Gottfried Schmalz School of Dentistry, University of Regensburg, Germany

Nils Skaug	deceased
Gunnel Svensäter	Faculty of Odontology, Malmö University, Sweden
Peter Svensson	School of Dentistry, Faculty of Health Sciences, Aarhus University, Denmark
Else Theilade	School of Dentistry, Faculty of Health Sciences, Aarhus University, Denmark
Peter Velvart	Private practice, Zürich, Switzerland
Paul Wesselink	Academic Center for Dentistry Amsterdam (ACTA), The Netherlands
John Whitworth	School of Dental Science, Newcastle University, UK

Preface

The *Textbook of Endodontology* is intended to serve the educational needs of dental students, as well as of dental practitioners seeking updates on endodontic theories and techniques. The primary aim has been to provide an understanding of the biological processes involved in pulpal and periapical pathologies and how that knowledge impinges on clinical management, and to present that information in an easily accessible form. Therefore, we have supplemented the core text with numerous figures and photographs, as well as with boxes highlighting key facts, important clinical procedures and key research. Case studies are given at the end of some chapters in order to further illustrate topics described in the text. In these various ways, the book provides information both at a foundation level, and at a more detailed level for the graduating student and practitioner.

The key information boxes are color coded as an easy-to-use navigational aid for readers. Core concepts are colored pink, while advanced concepts are purple. Clinical procedures are coded green and key literature boxes are blue.

Although not designed to provide a comprehensive review of the literature, this book is also intended to stimulate the reader to delve into the research that forms our current knowledge base in endodontology. To aid the reader, a selective reference list is provided and comments have been added to especially weighty or useful references. Important and interesting investigations are presented in the core and advanced concept boxes, and we hope that these features will encourage the student to carry on with his or her own exploration of the subject area.

This is the second edition of the book, which features three new chapters reflecting the use of the surgical microscope, diagnosis and management of endodontic complications subsequent to dental trauma, and endodontic epidemiology. The dedicated support of our co-authors – 23 highly respected clinicians and scientists – who, in addition to the editors, have contributed to this book, is greatly appreciated. We thank them all sincerely for their time, effort and endurance during the editing process.

Gunnar Bergenholtz
Preben Hørsted-Bindslev
Claes Reit

Chapter 1
Introduction to endodontology

Claes Reit, Gunnar Bergenholtz and Preben Hørsted-Bindslev

Endodontology

The word "endodontology" is derived from the Greek language and can be translated as "the knowledge of what is inside the tooth". Thus, endodontology concerns structures and processes within the pulp chamber. But what about "knowledge"? What does it actually mean to "know" things? Most people would probably say that knowledge has something to do with truth and providing reasons for things. It is often believed that dental and medical knowledge is simply scientific knowledge – science is based on research and deals with how things are constructed and work. But as practicing dentists we also need other types of knowledge. Although it is important to know about tooth anatomy and how to produce good root canal preparations for example, we must also develop good judgment and ability to make the "right" clinical decisions. There are at least three different forms of knowledge that the dental practitioner requires and, in a tradition that goes all the way back to Aristotle, we will refer to the Greek terms for these forms: *episteme*, *techne* and *phronesis* (1).

Episteme

Episteme is the word for theoretical–scientific knowledge. The opposite is *doxa*, which refers to "belief" or "opinion". There is a massive body of epistemic knowledge within endodontology, for example on the biology of the pulp, the microorganisms that inhabit root canals, the procedures and materials used in the clinical practice of endodontology (endodontics) and the outcome of endodontic therapies. Science produces "facts". It must be understood that modern science is an industry and is affected by many factors, both internal and external. Although this is not the place to discuss the philosophy of science, the concept of "truth" and the growth of scientific knowledge is not unproblematic. There has been substantial contemporary philosophical discussion reflecting on epistemic knowledge, and the interested reader is referred to one of the many good introductory texts that are available (3).

The results of science are presented in lectures, articles and textbooks. So from a student's point of view the learning situation is rather straightforward, provided that the subject is structured well and ample time given for reading and reflection. This book, in large part, is composed of epistemic knowledge.

Techne

The first person to challenge the deeply intrenched theoretical concept of knowledge was the British philosopher Gilbert Ryle. In his book *The Concept of Mind* (10) he introduces "knowing-how" and distinguishes it from "knowing-that". "Knowing-how" is practical in nature and concerns skills and the performance of certain actions. This concept of knowledge implies the ability not only to do things, but also to understand what you are doing. To say that you have practical knowledge, it is not enough to produce things out of mere routine or habit. You have to "know" what you are doing and be able to argue about it. Practice must be combined with reflection. The idea that there is a tacit or silent dimension of knowledge has had a great impact on the contemporary discussion. Michael Polanyi, for example, said that "We know more than we can tell" (9). When trying to explain how we master practical things such as riding a bicycle or recognizing a face, it is not possible to articulate verbally all the knowledge that we have. Certain important aspects are "tacit". Likewise, it is not sufficient to teach students about root canal preparation simply by asking them to read a book or presenting the subject matter in a lecture. It has to be *demonstrated*. Knowledge is very often transmitted by the act of doing.

A substantial body of endodontic knowledge must be characterized as *techne*. It is not possible to learn all about the procedures in endodontology by studying a textbook. Observing a good clinical instructor, watching other dentists at work, performing the procedures oneself and reflecting on what has been learned are all important.

Phronesis

According to Aristotle, *phronesis* is the ability to think about practical matters. This can be translated as "practical wisdom" (5) and is concerned with why we might decide to act in one way rather than in another. When thinking about the "right" action or making the "right" decision we enter the territory of moral philosophy. The person who has practical wisdom has good moral judgment. Modern ethical thinking has been influenced significantly by ideas that originated during the enlightenment. Morality is concerned with human actions and there are certain principles that can separate "right" from "wrong" decisions. Jeremy Bentham (2) and the utilitarians launched the utility principle and Immanuel Kant (6) invented the categorical imperative, each creating a tradition with great impact on today's medical ethics and decision making.

Aristotle, on the other hand, believed that there are no explicit principles to guide us. He understood practical wisdom as a combination of understanding and experience and the ability to read individual situations correctly. He thought that *phronesis* could be learnt from one's own experience and by imitating others who had already mastered the task. He stressed the cultivation of certain character traits and the habit of acting wisely.

The clinical situation demands that the dentist exercises practical wisdom, "*to do the right thing at the right moment*". In order to develop *phronesis*, theoretical studies of moral theory and decision-making principles might be helpful. Neoaristotelians such as Martha Nussbaum (8) have suggested that reading literature should be part of any academic curriculum, the idea being that it increases our knowledge and understanding of other people. However, the essence of *phronesis* has to be learnt from practice.

Concepts of endodontology

From the above it can be concluded that endodontology encompasses not only theoretical thinking but also the practical skills of a craftsperson and the practical thinking needed for clinical and moral judgment. Unfortunately, through the years, undue prestige has been given to theoretical–scientific thinking and this has hindered the development of a rational discussion of the other types of knowledge. The serious student of endodontology has to investigate all three aspects, but, as argued above, there are limits to what can be communicated within the covers of a textbook.

The dawn of modern endodontology

It all started with a speech at the McGill University in Montreal. In the morning of October 3, 1910, Dr William Hunter gave a talk entitled "The role of sepsis and antisepsis in medicine". Hunter said that:

> "In my clinical experience septic infection is without exception the most prevalent infection operating in medicine, and a most important and prevalent cause and complication of many medical diseases. Its ill-effects are widespread and extend to all systems of the body. The relation between these effects and the sepsis that causes them is constantly overlooked, because the existence of the sepsis is itself overlooked. For the chief seat of that sepsis is the mouth; and the sepsis itself, when noted, is erroneously regarded as the result of various conditions of ill-health with which it is associated – not, as it really is, an important cause or complication.
>
> "Gold fillings, gold caps, gold bridges, gold crowns, fixed dentures, built in, on, and around diseased teeth, form a veritable mausoleum of gold over a mass of sepsis to which there is no parallel in the whole realm of medicine or surgery. The whole constitutes a perfect gold trap of sepsis."

The cited text was published in the *Lancet* in 1911. But Hunter's words rapidly spread and were intensively discussed among laymen and given banner headlines in the newspapers. Essentially, Hunter proposed that microorganisms from a dental focus of infection can spread to other body compartments and cause serious systemic disease. The fear that illnesses and even those of chronic or of unknown origin were caused by oral infections, brought thousands of people to the waiting rooms of dentists with demands to have their teeth removed. As a result of the focal infection theory teeth were extracted in enormous numbers.

Although not directly stated by Hunter, teeth with necrotic pulps were seen as one of the main causes of "focal infection". Laboratory studies had disclosed the presence of bacteria in the dead pulp tissue. In the 1920s, dental radiography came into general use and radiolucent patches around the apices of teeth with necrotic pulps indicating an inflammatory bone lesion were possible to detect. If such teeth were extracted and cultured, microorganisms were often recovered from the attached soft tissue. It became virtually incontestable that pulpally diseased teeth should be removed.

Reflecting on this period in the history of dentistry, Grossman (4) wrote: "The focal infection theory promulgated by William Hunter in 1910 gave dentistry in general, and root canal treatment in particular, a black eye from which it didn't recover for about 30 years." However, in hindsight, this period can also be regarded as the dawn of modern endodontology. Researchers started to question and oppose the clinical consequences of the focal infection theory. Microbiologists began mapping out the microflora of infected root canals. Pathologists investigated the reaction patterns of the pulp and peri-apical tissues and came to understand the protective power of the host defense mechanisms. Clinicians invented aseptic methods to treat the root canal, and radiography made it possible to confine the procedures to within the root canal space. It was further demonstrated that root canal infections could be combated successfully and it became obvious that root canal infections were not such a serious threat to the human organism as once believed. Pulpally compromised teeth could therefore be spared and endodontic treatment became a necessary skill of the modern dentist.

The objective of endodontic treatment

The consequences of inflammatory lesions in the pulp and periapical tissue (Fig. 1.1) have tormented human-kind for thousands of years. Historically, therefore, the main task of endodontic treatment has been to cure toothache due to inflammatory lesions in the pulp (pulpitis) and the periapical tissue (apical periodontitis). For a long period of time a commonly used method to remedy painful pulps was to cauterize the tissue with a red-hot wire or with chemicals such as acid. In 1836, arsenic was introduced to devitalize the pulp, a method that would be used for well over 100 years. Procedures to remove the pulp without toxic chemicals were introduced in the early part of the 19th century and small, hooked instruments were used. The advent of local anesthesia at the beginning of the 20th century made pulpectomy a painless procedure.

Signs of root canal infection, such as abscesses with fistulae, were also dealt with historically using highly toxic chemicals. These substances were introduced to the root canal, and forced through the foramen into the fistula. Often the treatment was more damaging than the disease condition itself, and the tooth and parts of the surrounding bone were often lost in the process.

While relief of pain is still a primary goal of endodontic treatment, patients also may want to exclude the compromised tooth, as both a general and local health hazard. This means that intra- as well as extraradicular infections should be eradicated and that materials implanted in the root canal should be innocuous and not cause adverse tissue reactions or systemic complications. Using modern endodontic treatment procedures, these treatment objectives can be attained in the large majority of cases.

Clinical problems and solutions

The vital pulp

Under normal, physiological conditions the pulp is well protected from injury and injurious elements in the oral cavity by the outer hard tissue encasement of the tooth and an intact periodontium (Fig. 1.2). When the integrity of these tissue barriers is breached for any reason, microorganisms and the substances they produce may gain access to the pulp and adversely affect its healthy condition. The most common microbial challenge of the pulp derives from caries. Even in its early stages substances from caries-causing bacteria may enter the pulp along the exposed dentinal tubules. Like any connective tissue, the pulp responds to this with inflammation. Inflammation has an important aim to neutralize and eliminate the noxious agents. It also organizes subsequent repair of the damaged tissue. Thus, the pulp may react in a manner that allows it to sustain the irritation and remain in a functional state. Yet, when caries has extended to the vicinity of the pulp, the response may take a destructive course and result in severe pain and death (necrosis) of the tissue.

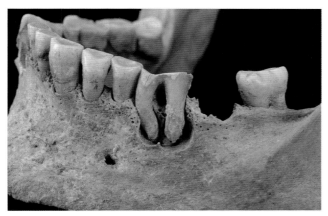

Fig. 1.1   A medieval skull found in Denmark showing teeth with serious attrition. In the first left molar the pulp chamber is exposed and the alveolar bone is resorbed around the root apices, indicating a once-present periapical inflammation due to necrosis of the pulp followed by root canal infection.

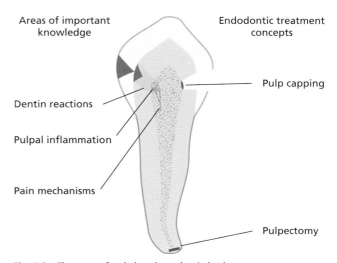

Fig. 1.2   The scope of endodontology: the vital pulp.

An inflamed or injured pulp may have to be removed and replaced with a root filling – a procedure termed pulpectomy. This measure is undertaken especially in cases when the condition of the pulp is such that an inflammatory breakdown is deemed imminent. A manifest infection may otherwise develop in the root canal system.

A pulpectomy procedure is carried out under local anesthesia and with the use of specially designed root canal instruments. These instruments remove the diseased pulp and prepare the canal system so that it can be filled properly. The purpose of the filling is to prevent microbial growth and multiplication in the pulpal chamber. Thus, pulpectomy is a measure primarily aimed at preventing the development of a manifest root canal infection and painful sequelae.

Pulpectomy may also be carried out any time a pulp is directly exposed to the oral environment. This may occur after clinical excavation of caries or after a traumatic insult or iatrogenic injury. If the exposure is fresh and the pulp judged not to be seriously inflamed it may not have to be removed. If the open wound is treated with a proper dressing and protected from the oral environment by *pulp capping*, healing and repair of the wound

are possible. For common terminologies used to specify the endodontic disease conditions and their treatments, see Core concept 1.1.

The necrotic pulp

As mentioned above, injury to the pulp may lead to necrosis of the tissue (Fig. 1.3). The necrotic pulp is defenseless against microbial invasion and will allow microorganisms indigenous to the oral cavity to reach the pulp chamber, either along an open direct exposure or through uncovered dentinal tubules or cracks in the enamel and dentin. Lateral canals exposed as a result of progressive marginal periodontitis may also serve as pathways for bacteria to reach the pulp. The specific environment in the root canal, characterized by the degrading pulp tissue and lack of oxygen, will favor a microbiota dominated by proteolytic, anaerobic bacteria. These microorganisms may organize themselves in clusters and in microbial communities attached to the root canal walls as well as inside the dentinal tubules of the root. In these positions microorganisms stay protected from host defense mechanisms and can therefore multiply rapidly to large numbers. Microorganisms attempt to

Core concept 1.1	Common terms and expressions used for endodontic disease conditions and treatment procedures
Pulpitis	Inflammation of the dental pulp. *Symptomatic* and *asymptomatic pulpitis*, as well as *irreversible* and *reversible pulpitis*, are commonly used terms to specify lesions with and without painful symptoms. The terms *total* and *partial pulpitis* are also in use.
Pulp necrosis	Pulp death. Pulp chamber is devoid of a functional pulp tissue. Necrosis can be more or less complete, i.e. partial or total.
Apical periodontitis	Inflammatory reaction of the tissues surrounding the root apex of a tooth. *Symptomatic/asymptomatic apical periodontitis* and *acute/chronic apical periodontitis*, respectively, are applied to indicate lesions with and without overt clinical symptoms such as pain, swelling and tenderness. *Dental* or *apical granuloma* is a histological term for an established lesion. *Apical, periapical* and *periradicular* are interchangeable terms to state the location of the process at or near the root tip.
Pulp capping	Treatment procedure aimed at preserving a dental pulp that has been exposed to the oral environment.
Partial pulpotomy	Treatment procedure by which the most (often inflamed) superficial portion (1–2 mm) of the coronal pulp is surgically removed with the aim of preserving the remaining tissue.
Pulpotomy	Treatment procedure by which the entire coronal pulp tissue is surgically removed with the aim of preserving the remaining tissue. The term pulpotomy is also used to describe a pain-relieving procedure in an emergency treatment of symptomatic pulpitis.
Pulpectomy	Treatment procedure by which pulp tissue (often inflamed) is surgically removed and replaced with a root filling.
Root canal treatment (RCT)	Treatment of teeth with necrotic pulps where root canals are often infected.
Non-surgical retreatment	Treatment of root filled teeth with clinical and/or radiographic signs of root canal infection, where root fillings are removed, canals disinfected and refilled. May also be carried out to improve the technical quality of previous root fillings.
Surgical retreatment	Treatment procedure by which the root apex of a tooth is surgically accessed to manage a root canal infection that has not been successfully treated by RCT. *Retrograde endodontics* or *surgical endodontics* are other terms for this procedure.

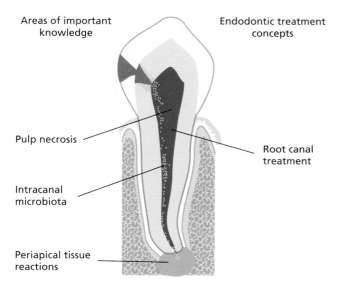

Areas of important knowledge / Endodontic treatment concepts

Pulp necrosis

Intracanal microbiota

Periapical tissue reactions

Root canal treatment

Fig. 1.3   The scope of endodontology: the necrotic pulp.

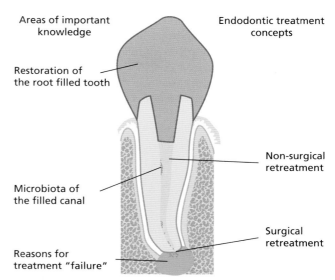

Areas of important knowledge / Endodontic treatment concepts

Restoration of the root filled tooth

Microbiota of the filled canal

Reasons for treatment "failure"

Non-surgical retreatment

Surgical retreatment

Fig. 1.4   The scope of endodontology: the root filled tooth.

invade the periodontal tissues via the apical foramen or any other portal of exit from the root canal, and may do so before the host defense has been effectively organized. Once established, however, organisms will normally be held back but not eliminated from the root canal space. A chronic inflammatory lesion will ensue, normally around the root tip, and remain for as long as no treatment is initiated.

The periapical tissue reaction is often visible in a radiograph as a localized radiolucency because the adjacent bone has been resorbed in the course of the inflammatory process. The condition may or may not be associated with pain, tooth tenderness and various degrees of swelling.

Treatment of the necrotic pulp is by *root canal treatment* (RCT) and is aimed to combat the intracanal infection. The canal is cleaned with files in order to remove microbes as well as their growth substrate. Owing to the complex anatomy of the root, instruments cannot reach all parts of the canal system and therefore antimicrobial substances are added to disinfect the canal. In order to avoid reinfection and to prevent surviving microbes from growing, the canal is then sealed with a root filling.

The root filled tooth

Pulpectomy and RCT do not always lead to a successful clinical outcome. For example, a tooth may continue to be tender or periapical inflammation may persist. Such treatment "failures" are often associated with defective root fillings, which allow organisms from the initial microbiota to survive in the root canal or new bacteria to enter via leakage along the margins of the coronal restoration (Fig. 1.4).

The root canal in such cases may be retreated using either a non-surgical or a surgical approach. In *non-surgical retreatment* the root filling is removed and the canal is reinstrumented. Antimicrobial substances are applied to kill the microbes and the space is refilled. Crowns, bridges and posts may mean that it is sometimes not feasible to reach the root canal in a conventional way. In such cases, a *surgical retreatment* may be attempted. A mucoperiosteal flap is then raised and entrance to the apical part of the root made through the bone. Surgical retreatment often involves cutting of the root tip, instrumentation of the apical root portion and placement of a filling at the apical end.

The diagnostic dilemma

The disease processes in the pulp and periapical tissues take place in a concealed body compartment that normally is not available for direct inspection. Instead, the clinician has to rely on indirect information to assess the condition of the tissue and reach a diagnosis. The reliance on indirect signs and symptoms entails the risk of making false-positive and false-negative diagnoses. For example, the patient's report of pain has been found to be an inaccurate sign because there is no exact relationship between the amount of tissue damage and level of pain encountered. Furthermore most inflammatory episodes within the pulp or periapical bone pass by without symptoms. Another factor is that the discriminatory ability of the intrapulpal nerves is not perfect, which means that if a patient has toothache due to pulpitis there is a high risk that he or she may "point out the wrong tooth". Nevertheless a patient's experience of pain and especially its character serve as important indicators of an endodontic disease condition. Along with pulp vitality testing and radiographic examination, the disease history is a prime source of diagnostic data. Yet, to avoid erroneous diagnoses all data have to be interpreted with utmost care and with in-depth knowledge of possible errors and the factors that influence diagnostic accuracy.

The tools of treatment

To many dentists, RCT can best be described by using Winston Churchill's words on golf: "An impossible game with impossible tools". The complexity of root canal anatomy, the relative stiffness of root canal instruments, being unable, often, to visualize the area properly, and the lack of space in the mouth provide substantial challenges to the skill and patience of the dentist. Intracanal work is exceptionally demanding; this is clearly demonstrated by numerous radiographically based epidemiological surveys, which repeatedly report that many root fillings do not meet acceptable technical standards. Because clinical outcome is strongly related to the quality of treatment, the high frequency of substandard performances is a subject of great concern to the profession.

The last 10–15 years have seen a tremendous technological development that facilitates endodontic treatment and enhances the potential to increase its overall standard (7). For example, the advent of super-flexible nickel–titanium alloy has made it possible to fabricate instruments that are highly flexible and can follow the anatomy of the root canal and therefore produce good quality canal preparations. Furthermore, systems have been developed that allow the instruments to be maneuvered by machine rather than by hand, improving fine-scale manipulation and decreasing operator fatigue.

The surgical microscope has brought light and vision into the pulp chamber. Working under high magnification, it is now far easier to remove mineralizations, locate small root canal orifices and control intracanal procedures than with the naked eye or with loupes. However, high-quality microscopes are expensive and, thus far, the technology has found limited adoption by dentists other than those specialized in endodontics.

In the midst of this technological boom it must not be forgotten that endodontics is primarily about controlling infection. While the intracanal work is aimed to eliminate infectious elements and give space for the subsequent root filling, this effort would be futile if measures were not undertaken to prevent oral contaminants from entering the root canal space during the procedure. Luckily, there are few medical treatments that can be carried out as aseptically as endodontic therapy. Shielding the tooth with a rubber dam is the oldest and still the most effective way to ensure that the operation field remains

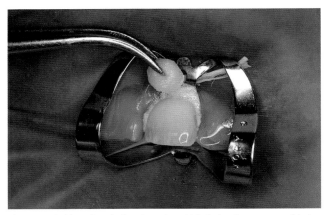

Fig. 1.5 Rubber dam isolated tooth, which is in the process of being disinfected.

sterile (Fig. 1.5). This measure also facilitates the procedure and is critically important to the clinical success of endodontic therapy.

Extraction and dental implant?

Extraction and placement of dental implants to replace endodontically compromised teeth has gained popularity in recent years. Such a measure can certainly be a valuable option in cases of severely damaged teeth that either have a hopeless prognosis or cannot be provided with a proper restoration. Yet, dental implants must not be overused or misused because an endodontic treatment, for example, may appear complicated. Clearly endodontic therapy represents a very realistic opportunity to restore most teeth with diseased pulps to a healthy state. Indeed endodontic therapy has reached a level of sophistication today that dentists, with proper knowledge and training, can carry out the procedures with a high rate of success. Epidemiological data have furthermore shown that endodontically treated teeth maintain a functional place in the oral cavity for long periods of time (11).

References

1. Aristotle (Iruin T, ed.). *Nicomachean Ethics*. London: Hackett Publishing, 1988.
2. Bentham J. *Introduction to the Principles of Morals and Legislation (1789)* (Burns JH, Hart DLA, eds). London: Methuen, 1982.
3. Chalmers AF. *What is this Thing called Science?* Buckingham: Open University, 1999.
4. Grossman LI. Endodontics 1776–1996: a bicentennial history against the background of general dentistry. *J. Am. Dent. Assoc.* 1976; 93: 78–87.
5. Hughes GJ. *Aristotle on Ethics*. London: Routledge, 2001.

6. Kant I. *Foundations of the Metaphysics of Morals (1785).* Indianapolis: Bobbs–Merrill, 1959.

7. Molander A, Caplan D, Bergenholtz G, Reit C. Improved root-filling quality among general dental practitioners educated in nickel titanium rotary instrumentation. *Int. Endod. J.* 2007; 40: 254–60.

8. Nussbaum M. *Poetic Justice. The Literary Imagination and Public Life.* Boston: Beacon Press, 1995.

9. Polanyi M. *Personal Knowledge: Towards a Postcritical Philosophy.* London: Routledge, 1958.

10. Ryle G. *The Concept of Mind.* London: Penguin, 1949.

11. Salehrabi R, Rotstein I. Endodontic treatment outcomes in a large patient population in the USA: an epidemiological study. *J. Endod.* 2004; 30: 846–50.

Part 1
The Vital Pulp

Chapter 2

The dentin–pulp complex: structures, functions and responses to adverse influences

Leif Olgart and Gunnar Bergenholtz

Introduction

The extent to which the dental pulp will sustain impairment in the clinical setting depends on its potential to oppose bacterial challenges and withstand injury by various forms of trauma. To understand the biological events that operate and most often prevent the pulp from suffering a permanent breakdown, the specific biological functions of both dentin and pulp under pathophysiological conditions will be addressed in this chapter. These two tissue components of the tooth form a functional unit that often is referred to as the *dentin–pulp complex* (Fig. 2.1).

Constituents and normal functions of the dentin–pulp complex

Dentin and dentinal tubules

Dentin provides elasticity and strength to the tooth that enable it to withstand loading forces by mastication and trauma. Dentin also elicits important defense functions aimed at preserving the integrity of the pulp tissue.

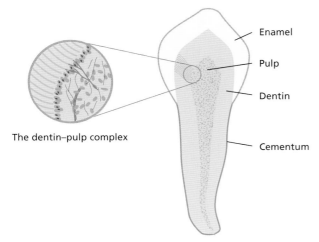

The dentin–pulp complex

Fig. 2.1 The soft tissue of the pulp is surrounded by dentin and enamel or cementum. Inset depicts the interface zone between dentin and pulp.

Under normal, healthy conditions, when dentin is covered by enamel and cementum, fluid in the dentinal tubules can contract or expand to impinge on the cells in the pulp in response to thermal stimuli applied on the tooth surface. Hence, dentin of the intact tooth can transform external stimuli into an appropriate message to cells and nerves in the pulp – a feature that is useful clinically to test its vital functions (see Chapter 14). A sensory transducer function triggered by elastic deformation is also in effect to detect overload resulting in reflex withdrawal and sharp transient pain.

When enamel and cementum are damaged for any reason, the exposed dentinal tubules serve as pathways to the pulp for entry of potentially noxious elements in the oral environment including bacterial macromolecules, which may provoke inflammation (4). The deeper the injury the more tubules become involved (Fig. 2.2). In the periphery there are about 20 000 tubules per square millimeter, each having a diameter of 0.5 µm. At the pulpal ends the tubular apertures occupy a greater surface area because the tubules converge centrally and become wider (2.5–3 µm) (20). Thus, at the inner surface of dentin there are more than 50 000 tubules per square millimeter. In root dentin, especially towards the apex, the tubules become more widely spaced. Also, in the pulpal portion of root dentin they are thinner and have a smaller diameter (ca. 1.5 µm). There are extensive branches between the tubules that allow intercommunication.

Movement of particulate matter and macromolecules by way of the dentinal tubules may occur not only from the external environment to the pulp but also in the opposite direction. Hence, following injury which has resulted in disruption of the tight junctions that normally hold the odontoblasts together (71), fluid in the pulp may enter the tubules and bring plasma proteins with antimicrobial properties (41).

The potential for elements to permeate the dentinal tubules is normally greatly restricted by a variety of tissue structures, including collagen fibers and cellular processes. The odontoblasts normally extend cytoplasmic processes into the tubules. Controversy exists, however,

11

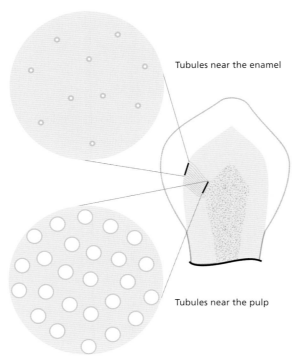

Tubules near the enamel

Tubules near the pulp

Fig. 2.2   Density of dentinal tubules in various portions of the crown region in teeth. It has been estimated that the surface area taken by cross cut tubules is ca. 2–3% in the periphery. Near the pulp the dentinal tubules assume ca. 25% of the surface area (61).

as to how far. While some believe that these processes extend all the way to the enamel or cementum junctions others contend that only the innermost part (0.5–1 mm) of dentin is filled (15). A large number of the tubules also contain nerve terminals. Furthermore, cells belonging to the immunosurveillance system of the pulp extend dendrites into the tubules of the predentin layer (52). Consequently, the space available in the tubules for the transport of particulate matter and macromolecules is normally much smaller than the tubular space *per se* (61) (Fig. 2.3). This is especially true at their pulpal ends.

The odontoblast – a multifunctional cell

The most recognized function of the odontoblasts is to form and maintain dentin. Like many other tissue-supporting cells, odontoblasts also contribute to host defense. By lining the periphery of the pulp with cellular extensions into dentin they are, thus, in the unique position of being the first cell to encounter and react to noxious elements entering dentin from the oral environment (Fig. 2.4). Upon challenge the odontoblasts generate and release a multitude of molecules that can help to defeat invading microorganisms. The response also gives rise to activation of specific receptors present on adjacent cells, vessels, nerves and on the odontoblast itself (Advanced concept 2.1). Thus, the odontoblasts, together with local resident defense cells and blood-borne invading cells, have a broad repertoire of response patterns and play important roles in activating both innate and adaptive immune responses of the pulp (for reviews see Refs 23, 24) (Fig. 2.5).

Dentin formation

The original odontoblasts, here also termed primary odontoblasts, produce dentin both during tooth development and after completion of root formation. The fact that intratubular cellular processes stay behind makes dentin tubular in nature. Owing to the continued function of the odontoblasts, the pulpal space gradually narrows over time and in old individuals it may become so small that endodontic treatment is difficult.

The odontoblasts may also produce new dentin at an increased rate in response to mild stimuli: e.g. during initial precavitated stages of enamel caries (10); by slowly progressing caries in general (9); or following a shallow preparation for restorative purposes. This type of new dentin has been termed reactionary dentin (67) (see also Core concept 2.1).

Dentin   Predentin   Pulp

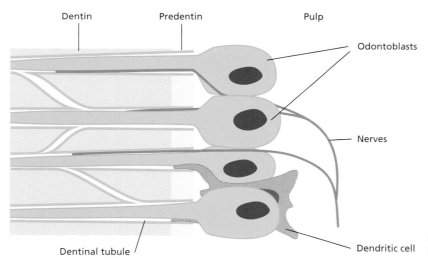

Odontoblasts

Nerves

Dentinal tubule

Dendritic cell

Fig. 2.3   Cellular extensions of odontoblasts, nerves and cells of the immune system (dendritic cells) occupy the pulpal ends of the dentinal tubules.

Odontoblasts are supplied with a multitude of receptors, which enable them to sense and respond to microbial elements and thereby alert the immune system. Thus, several members of the Toll receptor family have been identified on odontoblasts (19, 23). Upon activation of such receptors production of proinflammatory cytokines and chemokines is initiated; these, in turn, recruit immune cells. Recent observations suggest that odontoblasts are more potent attractants than pulpal fibroblasts in this respect (67). Odontoblasts may also release antimicrobial peptides with the capability of direct killing both Gram-positive and Gram-negative bacteria (18). Odontoblasts furthermore respond to proinflammatory cytokines secreted by adjacent resident cells and invading immune cells. Specific substances that regulate vascular permeability and angiogenesis are also released upon microbial challenges (70). Consequently, the strategic peripheral position of the odontoblast and its varied spectrum of response patterns make the cell a prime mover of the pulp's defense to both externally and internally derived adverse influences.

Primary dentin: dentin formed by primary odontoblasts.

Reparative dentin: dentin formed in response to injury by either primary or secondary odontoblasts (repairing odontoblasts). Equivalent terms commonly used are *irregular secondary dentin*, *irritation dentin* and *tertiary dentin*.

Note that primary dentin and secondary dentin are terms sometimes used to designate dentin formed by primary odontoblasts before and after termination of root development, respectively. Consequently, the term tertiary dentin has emerged to denote dentin formed in response to irritation or injury. The current text makes no such distinction.

Dentinal repair

Following injury or irritation (e.g. by a restorative procedure or rapidly progressing caries), the primary odontoblasts may die. Because these cells are postmitotic cells, they are unable to regenerate by cell division. New dentin may nevertheless be formed. Such dentinal repair appears to occur through the activity of so-called repairing odontoblasts or *secondary odontoblasts*. The precursor of these cells is thought to be a population of postnatal

stem cells that are present in the pulp tissue proper (22). Following their recruitment and upregulation, a mineralizing matrix is laid down on the dentinal wall. Repair by secondary odontoblasts is also possible against an appropriate wound-healing agent applied to treat direct exposure of the pulp (see Chapter 4). Hence, a new generation of odontoblast-like cells, capable of making new dentin locally, can evolve in the pulp upon injury.

Secondary odontoblasts produce dentin at a rate that is dependent on the extent and duration of the injury. The development of this hard tissue leads to an increase in dentin thickness (Figs 2.6 and 2.7).

It should be noted that dentin formed by secondary odontoblasts is more irregular and amorphous and contains fewer dentinal tubules than primary dentin (11). These tubules will not necessarily be in direct line with the tubules of the primary dentin (Fig. 2.8). Consequently, a complex of primary and reparative dentin becomes less permeable to externally derived matter. It also follows that such dentin is less sensitive to thermal, osmotic and evaporative stimuli (12; see also Chapter 3). The quality of the new hard tissue is not always as good as that of primary dentin. When it is formed rapidly, e.g. following an ischemic injury by dental trauma, it may become highly porous and contain areas filled with soft tissue. Although the pulpal space in radiographs may appear

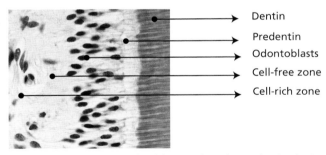

Dentin

Predentin

Odontoblasts

Cell-free zone

Cell-rich zone

Fig. 2.4 Tissue section stained with hematoxylin and eosin showing dentin, predentin and pulp tissue proper with odontoblasts lining the periphery.

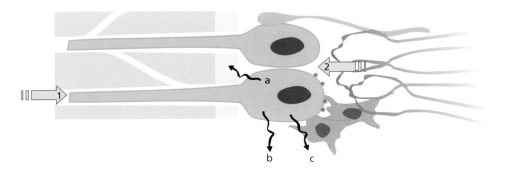

Fig. 2.5 The odontoblast has many functions which change during tooth development, maturation and injury of teeth. (a) *Sensor*: 1. affected from outside by antigens, mechanical forces, thermal gradients; 2. bombarded from inside by circulating hormones, paracrine and autocrine substances. (b) *Secretory cell*: a. for dentin lay down, b. for maintenance, c. for immune defense. (c) *Pain mediator*: acting as a transducer between external stimuli and pulpal sensory nerves.

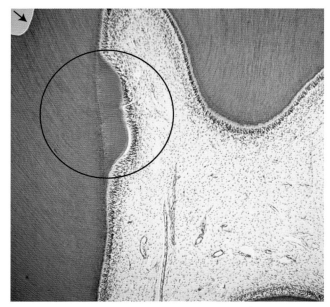

Fig. 2.6 Microphotograph showing hard tissue repair following a cavity preparation (arrow). The circle indicates bulk of new dentin being formed.

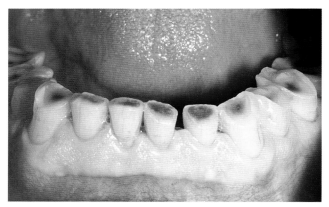

Fig. 2.7 Clinical photograph of anterior lower teeth showing extensive loss of tooth structure due to tooth wear. Reparative dentin formed in the pulp has prevented direct exposure of the tissue to the oral environment.

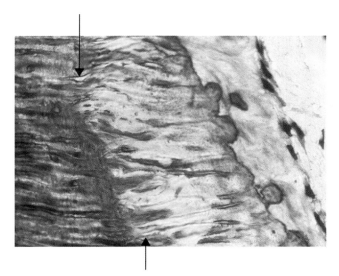

Fig. 2.8 Tissue section of an interface zone between primary dentin and reparative dentin as indicated by arrows. Note that the dentinal tubules are less numerous in the secondary dentin than in the primary dentin to the left. Also, few of the tubules are in direct line with those of the primary dentin, thus making the entire complex less permeable. Pulpal tissue and nuclei of pulp cells are to the right. (Courtesy of Dr Lars Bjørndal and with permission of Caries Research, Karger.)

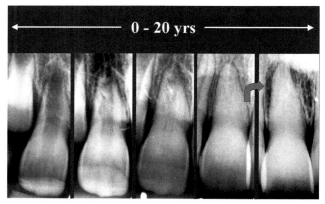

Fig. 2.9 Series of radiographs of a tooth in a patient who suffered a luxation injury at a young age. Hard tissue is successively deposited in the pulp. Arrow indicates change in status between the 15-year and 20-year follow-up radiographs. In the radiograph to the right, a periapical radiolucency is seen, suggesting pulpal infection. (From Robertson *et al.* (65) with permission of the *Journal of Endodontics*.)

completely obliterated, these areas are large enough to give room for bacterial growth and multiplication in case of an ensuing infectious exposure (Fig. 2.9). Similarly, hard-tissue repair of pulpal wounds may occasionally show gross defects, which makes it highly permeable to bacteria and bacterial elements. Therefore, hard-tissue deposition in the pulp, although adding to the defense potential of the tissue in certain instances, should be viewed as a scar tissue.

Nerves

Pulpal nerves monitor painful sensations. By virtue of their peptide content they also play important functions in inflammatory events and subsequent tissue repair (Fig. 2.10). In addition, they control dentin formation (Fig. 2.10).

There are two types of nerve fiber that mediate the sensation of pain: A-fibers conduct rapid and sharp pain sensations and belong to the myelinated group, whereas C-fibers are involved in dull aching pain and are thinner and unmyelinated. The A-fibers, mainly of the A-delta type, are preferentially located in the periphery of the pulp, where they are in close association with the odontoblasts and extend fibers to many but not all dentinal tubules. The C-fibers typically terminate in the pulp

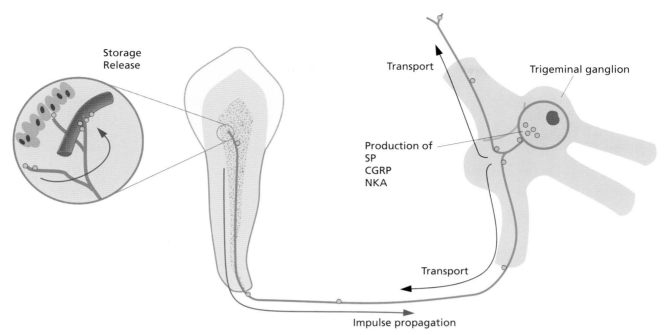

Fig. 2.10   A large portion of the sensory fibers, including C-fibers and some A-delta fibers, contain vasoactive neuropeptides such as calcitonin gene-related peptide (CGRP), substance P (SP) and neurokinin A (NKA). The neuropeptides are produced in the trigeminal cell bodies and are transported via axonal flow to the nerve terminals in the pulp, where they are stored. In addition to their effect on pulpal blood flow and vessel permeability, SP and CGRP exert stimulatory effects on the growth of pulpal cells, such as fibroblasts and repairing odontoblasts. They are also active in the recruitment of immunocompetent cells in response to bacterial exposures.

tissue proper, either as free nerve endings or as branches around blood vessels (56). The nature of A- and C-fibers and their respective roles in pain transmission are described in Chapter 4.

Nerves belonging to the autonomic nervous system, such as sympathetic vasoconstrictor fibers, are also present (48). They enter the pulp together with blood vessels and sensory axons. Histochemically, they can be traced in the pulp via their content of noradrenaline and neuropeptide Y. Upon release, these substances result in contraction of the smooth-muscle sphincters in arteries and small arterioles apical to and within the pulp (58).

Both sensory and sympathetic nerves stimulate dentin formation as evidenced by reduced dentin formation in the absence of sensory nerves and after sympathectomy, respectively (32). Sensory and sympathetic nerves also interact in pulpal inflammation. For example, an intact innervation is significant for recruitment and activation of cells of the immune system (see Key literature 2.1).

As yet, there is little evidence that parasympathetic vasodilator blood flow control plays an important role in the local function and defense of the pulp.

Vascular supply

Current knowledge of the vascular architecture of the pulp has been influenced greatly by the use of the microvascular resin cast method (Fig. 2.11) (68). This technique

Key literature 2.1

Based on experimental studies Haug and Heyeraas (25) suggested that immune responses are subjected to modulation by the sympathetic nervous system (SNS) in dental tissues. The SNS was shown to inhibit the production of proinflammatory cytokines, while stimulating the production of anti-inflammatory cytokines. In rat dental tissues, it was found that the SNS is significant for recruitment of inflammatory cells such as CD 43+ granulocytes. Sympathetic nerves appeared to have an inhibitory effect on osteoclasts, odontoclasts, and on IL-1alpha production. The SNS stimulated reparative dentin production, since reparative dentin formation was reduced after sympathectomy. Sprouting of sympathetic nerve fibers occurs in chronically inflamed dental pulp, and neural imbalance caused by unilateral sympathectomy recruits immunoglobulin-producing cells to the rat dental pulp. In conclusion, this article presents evidence in support of interactions between the sympathetic nervous system and cells producing hard tissue, and pulpal inflammation.

allows resin to fill up even the smallest capillaries of the pulp. A vascular cast is then obtained, which, following corrosion of surrounding tissue structures, can be examined in the scanning electron microscope.

In all developmental stages the crown pulp shows a larger vascular network than the root pulp. In more central portions of the pulp the vascular network is less dense than in peripheral pulp. Anastomosis between

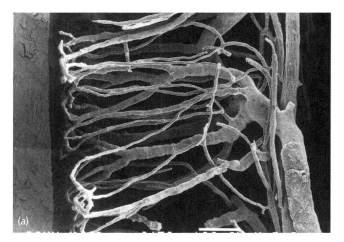
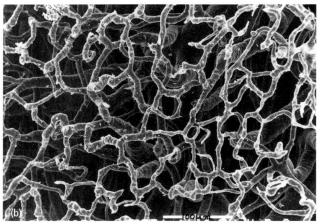
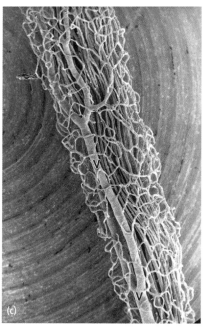
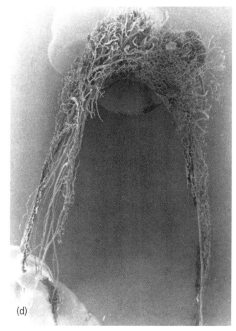

Fig. 2.11   Series of microphotographs of the vascular network in the pulp of teeth. (a) In the young tooth of dogs there is a dense terminal capillary network in the pulp–dentin border zone. (b) The superficial capillary network in the odontoblast region in a view perpendicular to the pulpal surface. (c) Blood vessels in the distal root canal of a mature dog premolar. The superficial capillaries drain directly into large venules (V). In the mature tooth, continuous dentin formation and narrowing of the pulp cavity lead to remodeling of the vascular tree. (d) The vascular network of an adult human tooth. With a narrow apical foramen, the number of arterioles is reduced to 5–8 and venules to 2–3 (40). The number of main vessels, arterioles and venules in the central pulp is also reduced and the typical hairpin loops of the terminal capillary network become less pronounced. The detailed vascular architecture of the pulp is similar in cat, dog and human teeth. (Courtesy of Dr K. Takahashi.)

incoming and outgoing blood vessels has been observed in the central pulp of adult animal teeth (40) and seems to be more frequent in the apical pulp than in the crown pulp (38). Shunt connections between supplying and draining pulpal vessels have also been found just outside the apical foramen in the periodontal ligament (69). It is reasonable to assume that these shunts provide control of blood perfusion through the pulpal tissue. Hence, in the case of a local inflammatory event causing increased resistance to pulpal blood flow, arteriovenous shunts may come into play and redirect incoming blood.

Lymphatics

Both morphological and functional studies in animals show the existence of lymphatic vessels in the pulp (8, 26). These vessels are important to adjust for increased colloid osmotic pressures exerted by proteins and macro-molecules accumulating extracellularly in inflamed areas. Another important function is to serve as pathways to the regional lymph nodes for antigen-presenting cells.

Immune defense

The dentin–pulp complex is uniquely organized to offset microbial threats from caries and other breaches of the outer hard tissue encasement of the tooth to the oral environment. While permeable to bacterial elements by virtue of the dentinal tubules, dentin nonetheless carries out an important filter function of significance to the pulp's immune defense. Primarily two mechanisms account for this effect: (i) the peripherally directed flow of dentinal fluid, and (ii) the absorbance of bacteria and bacterial macromolecules to the inner walls of the tubules (63). Thereby, dentin is able to temper exposures of noxious elements to the pulp, allowing it to adapt and organize an effective immune defense response.

Constituents making up the innate immune defense of the pulp include resident tissue cells, *viz.* odontoblasts and immune cells, nerves and vessels (Fig. 2.12). The basal set up of immune cells is limited to antigen-presenting cells (APCs), macrophages and T-lymphocytes (T-cells) of the memory type (23). Neither B-cells nor mast cells are residents of the normal pulp and will not appear in the tissue unless there is an inflammatory event.

APCs in the normal pulp are of two types. One has a pronounced dendritic configuration and belongs to the family of dendritic cells (DCs). The other is of the monocyte/macrophage lineage. Both constitutively carry class II MHC molecules on their cell surface. This molecule, found on all cells capable of antigen presentation, is a gene product of the major histocompatibility complex (MHC) and acts as a stimulatory molecule in T-cell activation both locally and in the regional lymph nodes.

The DCs in the pulp are strategically positioned in the periphery of the tissue, where foreign antigens are most likely to enter (Figs 2.12 and 2.13). Here, they compete for available space with the odontoblasts and make contact with these cells via their cytoplasmatic processes (52). Pulpal DCs are also in close proximity with nerve tissue elements and blood vessels in the paraodontoblastic region, suggesting interactive potentials (53, 54).

The primary function of DCs is to alert the immune system for an effective subsequent elimination, and not to directly combat invading microorganisms. In peripheral sites, like the pulp, they occur in an immature

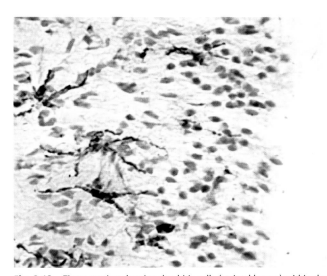

Fig. 2.13 Tissue section showing dendritic cells (stained brown) within the odontoblastic and subodontoblastic layer. Immunohistochemical staining was carried out with OX6-antibody, which is a marker for class II MHC molecules.

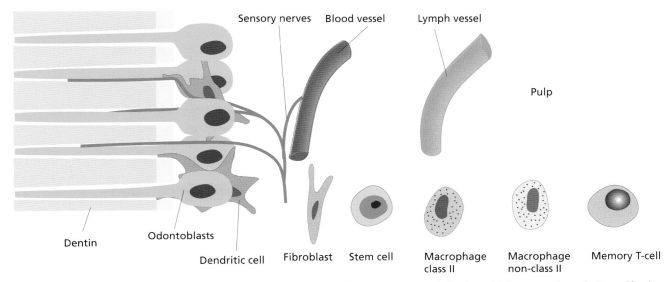

Fig. 2.12 Constituents of primary significance in the defense of the pulp against foreign substances, including bacterial elements, make up the innate "first line of defense".

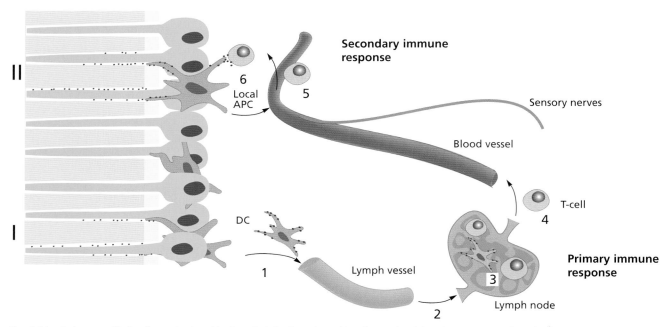

Fig. 2.14 Antigen-specific T-cells are developed in the pulp following primary (I) and secondary (II) antigen exposures along dentinal tubules. Dendritic cells (1 in figure) capture protein antigen for processing to peptide fragments and carry (2) and present peptide fragments in the context of the class II molecules on their cell surface to naïve T-cells in the regional lymph nodes (3: primary immune response). Following clonal expansion, these cells enter the circulation (4 in figure). Following their patrolling of tissues as memory T-cells, they may participate in secondary immune responses at local sites, e.g. in the pulp (5 in figure), if exposed to the appropriate antigen by local APC (6 in figure). This route constitutes adaptive pathogen-specific immunity.

state. Maturation to become professional APCs (capable of activating T-cells that have not been exposed to antigen before, so-called naïve T-cells) comes from capturing incoming foreign antigens. Upon exposure they usually start migrating to the regional lymph nodes. Once there, fragments of the antigen bound to the class II MHC molecule will be shown to the appropriate naïve T-cells that become activated in a primary immune response (Fig. 2.14). DCs are particularly effective in microbial sensing, capturing and processing foreign antigens and are thus a key initiator of the adaptive immune response.

The class II molecule-expressing macrophages are distributed in a remarkably high number in the pulp and seem to form a dense network together with pulpal DCs (33, 34). Like other connective tissues, macrophages in the pulp are heterogeneous in terms of phenotype and function. While there are those serving in local antigen presentation, there is also a large population of non-class II molecule-expressing, resident macrophages (histiocytes), primarily located perivascularly with primary functions in phagocytosis.

Basal maintenance

Blood flow

It is assumed that odontoblasts and nerve endings, especially during tooth development, have a high energy demand. This may also be true in mature teeth. Hence, although there is limited collateral circulation, the peripheral pulp is well vascularized (see Fig. 2.11) The blood flow through the young adult pulp during resting conditions is relatively high compared with that of other oral tissues (50). In the adult dog, blood flow per 100 g of tissue is ca. 40 ml/min in teeth with a fully formed apex. By comparison, in the gingiva it is ca. 30 ml/min. The dense capillary network in peripheral pulp also allows filtration of fluid from the blood vessels, thereby supplying the dentinal tubules with fluid. In old teeth blood perfusion becomes successively lower.

Local control

The level of the resting blood flow in the pulp is to a great extent controlled by the neuropeptides substance P (SP) and calcitonin gene-related peptide (CGRP). Both CGRP and SP maintain a continuous relaxation of feeding arterioles (7). This continuous influence on the blood supply to the pulp depends on a basal release of the peptides without apparent nerve activation.

Nitric oxide (NO) – a short-lived gas molecule that is produced enzymatically in the endothelial cell lining of vessels – also serves to maintain a physiological blood perfusion of the pulp (37). It has a powerful vasodilator action and, unlike neuropeptides, causes relaxation of the draining venules in the pulp under physiological conditions (7) (see Advanced concept 2.2).

Advanced concept 2.2   Mechanisms regulating pulpal blood flow

The physiological regulation of blood flow and tissue pressures in the pulp has been studied in some detail in animal teeth. For example, treatment with antagonists to neuropeptides, or axotomy leading to degeneration of the sensory innervation, almost halves the pulpal blood flow and reduces the interstitial fluid pressure in the pulp. Pharmacological blocking of nitric oxide (NO) production also reduces blood flow but, at the same time, increases tissue pressure. Thus, when the physiological action of NO is intact, flow resistance in draining vessels is low (dilated vessels), allowing appropriate blood flow, volume and tissue pressure in the pulp (8). The constitutive NO-producing enzyme (eNOS) is activated by normal pulse-dependent shear stress in pulpal vessels (37).

Advanced concept 2.3   Spreading of vascular reactions

A transient increase in pulpal blood flow is produced by electrical or noxious stimulation of adjacent tissues and teeth, as demonstrated in anesthetized animals (57). Thus pinching or insertion of an injection needle in the vestibular oral mucosa and delivery of a short train of electrical impulses to the lip or adjacent teeth give rise to a blood flow increase several minutes in duration. This phenomenon demonstrates the extensive branching of sensory nerves in and around teeth and their wide receptive fields, implying that spreading of neurogenic vascular reactions may take place between different oral tissues within the same nerve territory.

Remote control

The regulatory control of pulpal blood flow also involves autonomic nerves. This remote system influences blood circulation in the pulp as well as in adjacent tissues within the same innervation territory.

Although parasympathetic vasodilator nerves do not seem to play a significant role, there is firm evidence for sympathetic vasoconstrictor control in the dental pulp. The system does not seem to be active tonically and may not support local moment-to-moment demands of the tissue. However, physical and mental stresses trigger sympathetic vasoconstriction in the oral region, including the pulp, as part of the general fight-and-flight reaction (58).

In general terms, both the sympathetic and the parasympathetic systems operate at the general or segmental levels and tend to ignore the needs of an individual tissue such as the pulp. Therefore, the locally active mechanisms, such as the blood flow control, most favorably meet the nutritional demands of the healthy pulp. Suitable adjustment of blood flow in the pulp is mainly the result of a balance between the locally governed relaxing factors and a certain myogenic constrictive tone of the vessels.

Appropriate responses of the healthy pulp to non-destructive stimuli

Functionally, the unique dentin–odontoblast unit acts as a transducer of various external stimuli of moderate intensity. This enables the tissue constituents of the peripheral pulp to be alerted appropriately. Thus, in the intact healthy tooth, a limited cold stimulus or elastic deformation of dentin due to a sudden heavy load on the tooth is transformed to minute and rapid movements of the dentinal fluid (14). Such movements excite adjacent nerves, resulting in a rapid reflex withdrawal reaction, which is immediately followed by a brief, sharp pain, alerting the individual to further withdrawal. This is an important alarm system protecting the tooth from overload leading to crown or root fractures by mastication forces, for example (59).

In parallel there is a transient increase in blood perfusion in the pulp (49). This is part of an instant local defense reaction and is brought about by the fine terminal branches of sensory nerves supplying both cells in the odontoblast region and small feeding arterioles deeper in the pulp. Excitation of the most terminal branches in the peripheral area of the pulp results in a reflex propagation of impulses in adjacent nerve terminals belonging to the same nerves (axon reflex) (59). Because these nerves contain vasodilating neuropeptides, it takes only a few seconds for a short-lasting (<10 min) increase in blood perfusion of the pulp. CGRP is the dominating mediator of this response. As a result of the transient increase in local blood volume, pulpal tissue pressure increases (see Advanced concept 2.3).

Collectively, the reflex withdrawal, the pain and the local blood flow increase are judged as being appropriate and essential responses for the protection and maintenance of the normal function of the pulp.

Responses to external threats

During the lifespan of a tooth a variety of external insults may challenge the healthy condition of the encased pulp. Mechanical, thermal and chemical injuries, as well as elements of microbial origin, are threats that may cause damage to the pulp. Often, however, the pulp can mobilize effective responses resulting in survival with only transient consequences.

General response pattern

Episodes of sustained and repeated irritation of the intact tooth or an exposed dentin surface cause extended pulpal reaction and mobilize elements in a proinflammatory response. The predisposition of the pulp to react with more complex but transient cascades of events is shared by most peripheral tissues and is an important function to maintain and regain health. As far as the pulp is concerned, there are some unique features that affect its ability to sustain injury:

- The encasement within rigid hard-tissue walls restricts edema formation and expansion. In other words, the pulpal tissue is confined to a *low-compliance system*.
- The lack of collateral blood supply in one-rooted teeth limits the supply and drainage of blood.

Both of these factors have implications for the way in which inflammatory responses develop in the pulp and may, on severe challenge, be contributory to pulp tissue breakdown.

Restorative procedures

Restorative procedures undertaken in dentistry to manage caries, fractures and losses of teeth cannot normally be undertaken without generating damage to the pulp. It is primarily the cutting procedure that causes pulpal irritation by releasing frictional heat from the use of rotary instruments. Because the thermal conductivity of dentin is low, it is mostly dehydrating effects that are damaging. Critical to this effect is insufficient water irrigation (Fig. 2.15). Direct heat injury does not normally occur unless the procedure is carried out close to the pulp. Also, the frequent beating of the tooth structure by

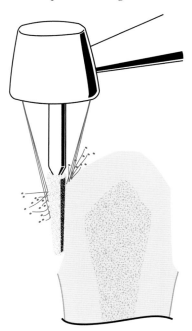

Fig. 2.15 Preparing teeth for restorations generates frictional heat, which causes dehydration and tissue damage to the pulp. Such injury is lessened by proper water irrigation during the cutting procedure.

improperly centered instruments may cause traumatic effects. All these injuries produce neurovascular responses of a nature similar to those described above.

Preparation trauma with rotary instruments is likely to injure the odontoblast layer (71). Owing to dehydration of the tubular content, odontoblasts may even be sucked into the dentinal tubules. This particular effect is termed *odontoblast aspiration* and can be observed in tissue sections by the presence of their nuclear profiles within the dentinal tubules.

Injury by preparation trauma to the odontoblast layer opens up pathways for a peripherally directed flow of tissue fluid along the tubules. The fluid flow is possible owing to the higher tissue pressure in the pulp than externally. Under normal conditions it is 5–10 mmHg higher in the pulp (26). This corresponds fairly well with the local blood pressure. Under inflammation, the pulp tissue pressure increases. By contrast, it may be reduced during flight-and-fight reactions, apprehension and by the use of anesthetic solution containing vasoconstrictor (60).

Protective roles of the dentinal fluid

Provided that anesthesia with a vasoconstrictor is not used and as long as a dentin exposure remains open, there will be a slow continuous outward flow of fluid along the dentinal tubules ($0.4\,\mu l/min/cm^2$) (Fig. 2.16). It has been estimated that the individual tubule can be emptied and refilled ten times a day (12).

Both the continuous and the stimulus-induced dentinal fluid flow may serve to limit invasive threats. Following exposure of dentin to the oral environment, bacterial elements may enter the pulp along the tubules by diffusion. However, a peripheral flow of dentinal fluid both dilutes and opposes such an inward transport of elements (Fig. 2.17). Thus, freshly exposed dentin subjected to a painful stimulus has some capacity to flush the tubules, whereby diffusion of harmful agents is counteracted (1, 73). It needs to be recognized, however, that the peripheral flow of fluid cannot completely prevent the inward diffusion of bacterial elements (3, 5). Also, under periods of negative tissue pressure noxious agents on the surface of dentin, by virtue of the fluid, may be drawn into the pulp and aggravate a pulpal lesion.

Nevertheless, the protective effect of the fluid is likely to be enhanced during pulpal inflammation and may contribute to the process of pulpal healing and repair seen following bacterial exposure of dentin (4, 47, 75). Along with the increase of plasma proteins in the extravascular tissue compartment, the content of plasma proteins will also increase in the dentinal fluid (41). This means that a variety of antimicrobial elements, such as immunoglobulin and complement factors, is carried into

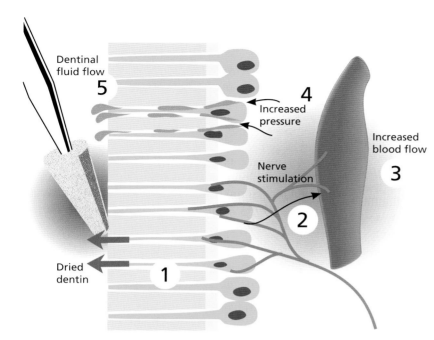

Fig. 2.16   When exposed dentin is dried (1 in figure) or subjected to a painful stimulus, such as a blast of compressed air or scraping with an explorer, the outward movement of the dentinal fluid is rapidly accelerated. This results in nerve stimulation (2 in figure) and a nerve-mediated increase of pulpal blood flow (3 in figure). Consequently, many vessels, which during resting conditions were only partly blood-filled, now fill up and increase the volume of filled blood vessels in the pulp. This in turn requires room for expansion (4 in figure). Because the space for the encapsulated pulp is restricted, the instant fill-up of vessels prompts an increase in the interstitial tissue pressure (27). The resultant force enhances the outward filtration of dentinal fluid (5 in figure) (49).

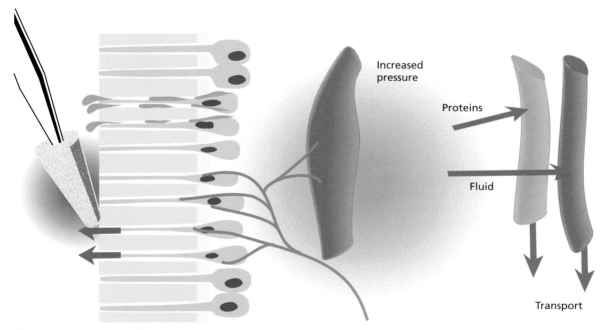

Fig. 2.17   Preparation of dentin for restoration causes an increased pulpal blood flow that results in accumulation of fluid and macromolecules outside the leaking vessels. In turn, this will cause a sustained increase in intrapulpal pressure, which may be double that in the normal pulp (32). The fluid pressure promptly causes an enhanced outward dentinal fluid flow in exposed dentin. The interstitial fluid accumulation is, however, limited by the counteracting pressure increase and by removal of the proteins via lymph vessels. The surplus fluid is slowly transported away by absorption via intact venules in adjacent tissue compartments (27). Adjacent lymph and blood vessels also contribute to the clearance of noxious substances.

the tubules and may bind to bacteria and bacterial macromolecules. Such binding is likely to impede further penetration to the pulp. The increased concentration of plasma proteins also affects the viscosity of the fluid and makes it less pervious. Thus, several factors associated with the dentinal fluid may aid in limiting threats that may follow exposure of dentin to the oral environment.

QM LIBRARY (WHITECHAPEL)

Blood flow changes

Preparation of dentin by rotary instruments results instantaneously in increased pulpal blood flow (Fig. 2.15). Activation of the peptide-containing sensory nerve arrangement, described above, mediates this response (see Core concept 2.2).

In deep-cavity or crown preparations, a direct effect of moderate heat on pulpal cells and vessels also augments pulpal blood flow. Excessive generation of heat represents an inappropriate operative procedure and cannot be abated by the local protective mechanisms, thus potentially causing serious damage to the tissue. For this reason, it is essential that a proper water-cooling system is in effect when cutting teeth with rotary instruments.

Preparation in vital dentin usually makes the use of local anesthetics necessary. As a result, the appropriate nerve-mediated vascular responses to the preparation trauma will be attenuated for a while. This is not regarded as a serious problem because intrapulpal nerves are only blocked for a few minutes after injection. However, when a vasoconstrictor (adrenaline/epinephrine) is used, there will be a long-lasting period of reduction of basal blood flow. Infiltration anesthesia in the upper front tooth region may lower blood perfusion of the pulp in adjacent teeth by 70–80% for <1 hour (60). These changes are not as prominent with a mandibular block but the pulp is likely to be vulnerable to the clinical procedures directed to the tooth structure. It is therefore advisable to avoid catecholamine vasoconstrictors when preparing for restorations in teeth with vital pulp.

Migration of inflammatory cells

A local injury to the pulp activates the migration of inflammatory cells. Following injury, a variety of substances is released from resident cells that prompts neutrophils and mononuclear leukocytes (monocytes and T- and B-lymphocytes) to leave the vasculature. If there is no or little bacterial involvement in conjunction with the injury, e.g. after a preparation trauma, the infiltration of neutrophils will be limited and these cells will soon disappear. By contrast, on a concomitant bacterial exposure, for example along the margins of a poorly sealed restoration, neutrophils may accumulate in large numbers and enter the pulpal ends of the dentinal tubules (Fig. 2.18). In such a position they are likely to contribute to pulpal protection by blocking both the diffusion of bacterial macromolecules and the penetration of bacterial organisms (4).

Peripheral blood monocytes also infiltrate the site of injury. Once in the tissue, monocytes become activated and turn into macrophages that will exert a multitude of important functions including:

- bacterial killing;
- cleansing of cellular debris;
- antigen presentation;
- stimulation of tissue repair by angiogenesis and fibroblast proliferation.

For further information on mediators of pulpal inflammation see Advanced concept 2.4.

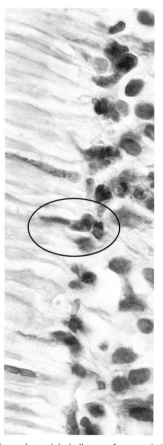

Fig. 2.18 Following a bacterial challenge of exposed dentin, neutrophils may enter the tubules of the affected dentin at their pulpal ends (encircled) and prevent the dissemination of bacterial elements to the pulp. (From Bergenholtz and Lindhe (5).)

Core concept 2.2   Neurovascular responses

- Neurovascular reactions, including vasodilation and increased vessel permeability in response to external, relatively innocuous stimuli, are proinflammatory events.
- The response is reversible in the normal pulp and serves to support the tissue in overcoming potential threats.
- The response is significant because:
  - challenged cells are dependent on optimal nutrition
  - clearance of harmful products from the affected tissue compartment is augmented
  - a moderate increase in tissue pressure tends to limit invasion of noxious elements along patent dentinal tubules by increasing the peripheral flow of dentinal fluid.

Advanced concept 2.4   Mediators of pulpal inflammation

In concert, numerous locally produced mediators of inflammation, including eicosanoids, cytokines and neuropeptides, support the inflammatory process and the subsequent repair phase. Both CGRP and SP exert chemotactic attraction on leukocytes, induce expression of adhesion molecules on vessel walls necessary for the exit of these cells to the tissue and modulate T-lymphocyte activity (34, 62).

In many animal models, increased plasticity of pulpal innervation has been observed. Within 48 hours after experimental exposure of the pulp to the oral environment, neuropeptides, including SP and CGRP, are increased in the nerve terminals close to the inflammatory zone. In addition, there is extensive branching and sprouting of the peptide-containing nerve terminals in the border zone of the inflammatory process (39). This outgrowth of peptide-containing nerves is part of an acute defense response that is fully developed within 48 hours after injury and lasts for as long as the irritation persists. These local phenomena are governed by the trigeminal cell bodies via peripheral influences. The activating signal is conveyed by a neurotrophin: nerve growth factor (NGF). This substance is normally formed at a low level in pulpal fibroblasts and serves to maintain the integrity of the peripheral nerve endings (46) and to accelerate tissue repair (45). Consequently, the increased local innervation and increased levels of neuropeptides support the mobilization and activation of cells necessary for an optimal defense and repair response.

Effects of potentially destructive stimuli

In the clinical environment a variety of potentially destructive elements, primarily of a bacterial nature, can endanger the vital function of the pulp. Also, dental procedures and various forms of accidental trauma may cause injury leading to pulpal breakdown (see Chapter 15).

Caries

Caries is a major cause of painful events and inflammatory injuries of the pulp. In the process of destroying the tooth structure, various substances are produced that evoke inflammatory lesions upon reaching the pulp. The pulp is usually able to endure the bacterial exposure, especially when caries is confined to the primary dentin only. By contrast, once into reparative dentin or the pulp tissue proper, severe inflammatory involvement usually occurs (43, 64) that may jeopardize the continued vital function of the tissue.

Caries is defined as *initial* as long as the process has not resulted in macroscopic destruction of the enamel (cavitation). In reality, dentin is often involved early on (11). Progression of caries tends to be intermittent, with periods of rapid destruction interspersed with periods where caries advances slowly. Sometimes it may be stopped temporarily or permanently (arrested caries)

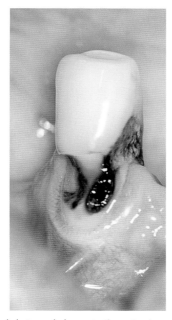

Fig. 2.19 Clinical photograph demonstrating extensive caries in the cervical region of a lower canine. Part of the lesion seems to be arrested, as indicated by the pigmented, leather-like appearance at the buccal aspect. At the mesial surface there is plaque accumulation and the lesion is soft to probing, indicating progression.

(Fig. 2.19). The character of the carious lesion in these respects influences the degree of inflammatory involvement of the pulp.

Responses to caries confined to primary dentin

Inflammatory tissue changes as well as repair phenomena can be seen in the pulp at all stages of an active carious lesion. In fact, tissue responses have been observed even at very early stages, before any surface breakdown, when caries is confined to the enamel only (10, 11, 13).

The extent of the response depends on the quantity of bacterial irritants that reach the pulp at a given point. It is also a function of distance. Consequently, while still in the periphery, bacteria will release substances that will have to travel much further than in a lesion close to the pulp. However, the distance factor is generally of lesser significance when reactive processes in terms of intratubular mineralizations (*dentinal sclerosis*) have emerged. Dentinal sclerosis makes the involved dentinal tubules more or less impermeable. It is caused by increased secretion of peritubular dentin that becomes highly mineralized and by reprecipitation of mineral crystals that were dissolved by acids in the carious lesion (11). These precipitations will occur within a limited area pulpally to the advancing demineralizing front (Fig. 2.20). Sclerotic dentin has a transparent and glass-like appearance. Upon advancement of the caries process, the mineral deposits will become dissolved and new precipitates may appear

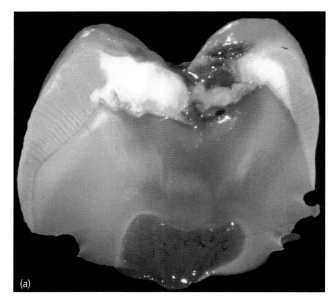

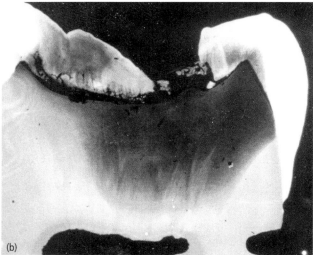

Fig. 2.20 (a) Central part of an active carious lesion in a molar. (b) Microradiograph shows radiopacities within the demineralized dentin, which, towards the pulpal aspect, is bordered by a rim of hypermineralized dentin (dentinal sclerosis). (Courtesy of Dr L. Bjørndal with permission of *Caries Research*, Karger.)

in tubules closer to the pulp. Hence, a carious lesion in dentin is a dynamic process that includes events of breakdown and remineralization in different parts of the dentin body where caries is advancing (Fig. 2.20).[1]

It is important to understand that, even during its initial exposure of dentin, caries evokes inflammatory responses in the pulp, i.e. long before bacteria in the pro-

cess have reached the pulp tissue itself. Support for this view has been gained from experimental studies in humans and animals where known components of bacteria (in dental plaque) were applied to freshly prepared dentin cavities (3, 5). Within hours, and in association with the pulpal ends of the exposed dentin, an acute inflammatory response developed in the pulp. The result of these experiments suggests that dentinal tubules are indeed permeable to bacterial elements and supports the view that even a small initial carious lesion is able to provoke an inflammatory pulpal lesion (13).

During growth and cell death of microorganisms in the caries process, elements are liberated that may initiate pulpal responses by different mechanisms. These include:

• Penetration of bacterial components, which act as antigens and initiators of the immune response.
• Release of inflammatory mediators from pulpal cells, including odontoblasts (see above).

The peripherally located odontoblasts and dendritic cells are both capable of activating a variety of effector mechanisms of innate and adapative immunity. The highly motile dendritic cells, after obtaining protein fragments, will move to regional lymph nodes and initiate a primary immune response upon which antigen-specific T-lymphocytes are recruited (see Fig. 2.14). By virtue of carrying Toll receptors, pulpal nerves are also activated by bacterial cell wall elements such as LPS and teichoic acid (74).

Neutrophils will not normally infiltrate the pulp during early dentinal caries. Instead, the inflammatory infiltrate is most often composed of macrophages, T-cells and plasma cells. These mononuclear cell infiltrates can be seen either in clusters or dispersed in the pulp tissue proper underneath the carious lesion.

The number of APCs is also increased (35), represented by an accumulation of dendritic cells and class II molecule-expressing macrophages (Fig. 2.21). These cells participate in the secondary immune response taking place in the pulp and are likely to enhance the defense and repair capacity of the tissue.

Although the inflammatory reaction may be pronounced in rapidly progressing caries in a young tooth, where the distance to the pulp is short, it is less distinct in a mature tooth where caries is progressing slowly. In fact, in the latter case the inflammatory activity is limited and sometimes the only evidence of bacterial irritation is the emergence of a small rim of reparative dentin (9). The number of class II molecule-expressing cells is also decreased, suggesting that the influx of bacterial substances in these lesions is reduced or inhibited (35). The fact that the tissue change becomes so limited on slowly advancing caries is likely to be explained by the previously described reactive processes taking place in

---

1 NB: Dentinal sclerosis can occur in the absence of caries. It is a common change associated with aging and develops successively in a coronal direction from the apical region of the tooth, as individuals grow older. It may also develop at the peripheral ends of the tubules subsequent to their oral exposure by abrasion and cervical erosion. After a period of time, mineral salts are deposited, which will reduce the sensitivity of the involved dentin.

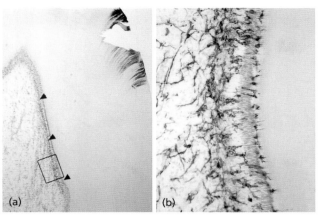

Fig. 2.21 (a) Numerous class II molecule-expressing cells (stained brown) accumulated underneath a superficial carious lesion, extending into the dentin of a human tooth (dark stain, upper right). (b) Extension of dendrites into the tubules. (Courtesy of Dr T. Okiji.)

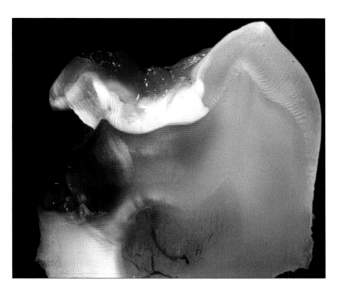

Fig. 2.22 Section through a tooth with a far-reaching carious lesion. Note the large blood-filled vessels in the pulp tissue. (Courtesy of Dr Lars Bjørndal.)

dentin. Thus, it is possible that the modifying factor explaining differences in pulpal responses between rapidly and slowly progressing lesions is the extent to which intratubular mineralizations were deposited to block or reduce the permeability of the affected dentin (11). The formation of reparative dentin also contributes to reduced dentin permeability. Yet, in the periphery of a carious lesion new dentinal tubules become involved and, associated with these, inflammatory/immunological reactions and subsequent repair phenomena continue to emerge in the pulp.

In teeth where caries has progressed over long periods of time, pulps may display intrapulpal mineralizations and increased fibrosis at the expense of the neurovascular supply. Tissue changes of this nature render the pulp tissue less cellular and, thus, less likely to resist repeated injury.

Response to deep caries

Once the carious lesion with its bacterial front has penetrated the primary dentin and progressed into reparative dentin and/or to the pulp tissue proper, a massive mobilization of the inflammatory defense will take place (43, 64) (Fig. 2.22). A most conspicuous feature is the aggregation of neutrophils. Often a local abscess develops (Fig. 2.23). Clinically, upon excavation of caries, a droplet of pus may sometimes appear at the exposure site.

Although short-lived in an acute inflammatory lesion, neutrophils release tissue-destructive elements, including oxygen radicals, lysosomal enzymes and excessive amounts of nitric oxide. These agents contribute to degradation of the pulpal tissue (see Advanced concept 2.5). There will also be renewed and intense immunological activity, as expressed by an accumulation of immune cells (35). Collectively, this means that the microbial load on the pulp has increased dramatically and the vital

---

Advanced concept 2.5   Nitric oxide in the pulpal response to a carious exposure

In acute pulpal inflammatory lesions the formation of nitric oxide (NO) is dramatically increased (44). Endotoxins from Gram-negative bacteria and cytokines, such as interleukin-1, tumor necrosis factor and interferon-gamma, are typical activators triggering a rapid production of NO-producing enzymes. This occurs both in immune cells and in vascular endothelium in areas close to and around an inflammatory site (51). NO is regarded as a central component in innate immunity aimed at eliminating invading microorganisms. Hence, NO can increase the blood flow and relax the draining vessels, thereby supporting appropriate outflow and pressure adjustment (7). In addition, NO may exert antibacterial activity and has an inhibitory effect on neutrophil infiltration in the acute phase of inflammation (42). In fact, the final destruction of microorganisms phagocytosed by macrophages is due to NO (28). These immune cells produce large amounts of NO. Thus, NO may assist in modifying the acute pulpal inflammatory response (36).

Massive and long-lasting NO formation may have destructive effects. It can react with oxygen free radicals produced during the inflammatory process to form the stable product, peroxynitrite. Peroxynitrite is a strong oxidant that causes tissue injury (2). Thus, although NO supports the defense response in moderate tissue inflammation, in severe reactions such as that upon caries exposure of the pulp, it may become severely toxic and contribute to the breakdown of the tissue.

---

functions of the pulp at this stage are clearly threatened (Fig. 2.24). Nevertheless, in spite of the massive bacterial attack and the intense inflammatory response, the pulp may retain vital functions for an extended period of time, although the end result is likely to be pulpal necrosis.

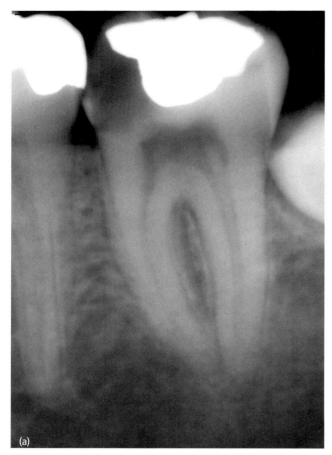

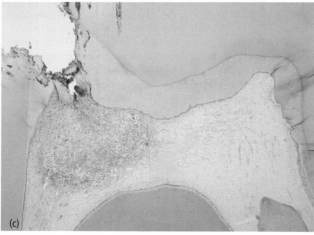

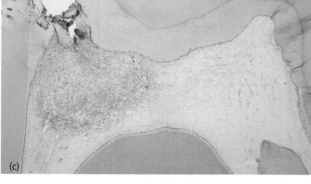

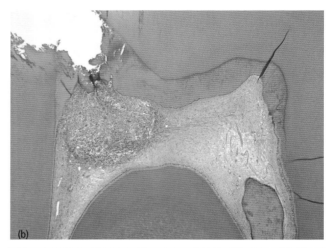

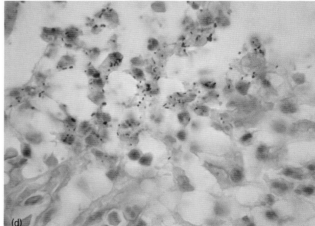

Fig. 2.23 (a) Radiograph of a second lower molar in a 30-year-old man with deep caries at the mesial aspect of the tooth. (b) Microphotograph showing a localized abscess with the remainder of the pulp displaying normal tissue structures. (c) Section stained to visualize bacterial organisms in blue at the caries exposure site. (d) Numerous bacterial profiles are seen in the abscess area, under combat by neutrophilic granulocytes. (Courtesy of Dr Domenico Ricucci.)

Neurovascular events

Besides the accumulation of neutrophils and immunocompetent cells near the carious lesion, the inflammatory response also involves extensive neurovascular reactions. These responses consist of branching and sprouting of neuropeptide-containing nerve terminals, increased pulpal blood flow, increased vascular permeability and extravasation of fluid and plasma proteins. In the process, severe painful symptoms may or may not appear (see Chapter 3). The locally increased tissue pressure as a result of vascular leakage may lead to stasis and local ischemia, thus contributing to the risk of pulpal necrosis.

The earlier assumption that increased pulpal tissue pressure, as a dominant factor, would compress thin-walled venules in a vicious circle resulting in a dramatic reduction of pulpal blood flow and possibly pulpal necrosis (strangulation theory) is misleading and has

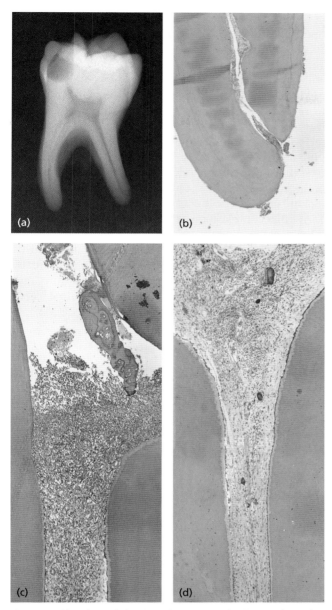

Fig. 2.24 (a) Radiograph showing a deep, mesioocclusal carious lesion that has advanced to the pulp in a lower molar. Histological examination of the pulp in the extracted tooth reveals partial pulpal breakdown at the breakthrough of the carious lesion. (b) The apical pulp displays a normal appearance. (c) An intense inflammatory infiltrate extends into the orifice of the mesial root canal. (d) The pulp tissue of the distal root canal shows less leukocyte infiltration with an intact odontoblast cell layer. (Courtesy of Dr Domenico Ricucci.)

found no support (72). Thus, the clearance of excess fluid and proteins via blood and lymph vessels (27) in the vicinity of the lesion zone, as described above, gives the pulp relief and may allow it to survive for a period of time.

A summary of the tissue changes in the pulp as a response to caries can be found in Core concept 2.3.

Core concept 2.3   Tissue changes in the pulp to caries

Caries confined to dentin

- During its course towards the pulp, caries completely destroys dentin and transforms it into a mushy mass of decomposed tissue containing an abundance of bacterial elements that can provoke inflammatory changes in the pulp. Yet, owing to reactive processes in dentin (plasma protein depositions and dentinal sclerosis) and immune responses of the pulp, the vital function of the tissue is seldom endangered as long as caries is confined to primary dentin.
- The inflammatory involvement with superficial and medium–deep caries in dentin is normally limited to the peripheral portions of the pulp. Inflammatory cells, primarily mononuclear leukocytes (macrophages, plasma cells and T- and B-lymphocytes), infiltrate the tissue but to a limited degree. Signs of repair (e.g. the formation of reparative dentin) are often, but not always, a prominent feature.
- Pulps in teeth with longstanding and/or slowly progressing caries may display increased fibrosis, reduced nervous and vascular supply and intrapulpal mineralizations resulting in reduced defense competence.

Direct exposure

- Next to the bacterial front there is accumulation of neutrophils and tissue destruction.
- In adjoining areas there is:
    - immune cell activation and accumulation of macrophages
    - branching and sprouting of neuropeptide-containing nerve terminals
    - intense vascular activity and localized increased tissue pressure.

Total necrosis of the pulp may develop after a period of time.

Response of the periapical tissue

The inflammatory response of the pulp to an open exposure by caries is often confined to the site of breakthrough, with the apical portion of the pulp remaining uninflamed. The lesion in certain cases may be more widespread and involve the periapical tissue adjacent to apical foramina. These changes include early mobilization of APCs (55), edema formation and some bone resorption, which may be visible radiographically.

Pulp polyp

In young individuals when the pulp chamber is wide, caries may initiate a proliferative response and cause what is termed a *pulp polyp* (Fig. 2.25). A prerequisite for this condition is that the roof of the pulpal chamber has been totally destroyed. The tissue proliferation is an expression of the reparative phase of the pulpal response and is made possible by the fact that the process no longer occurs within a closed system. Pulpal polyps may

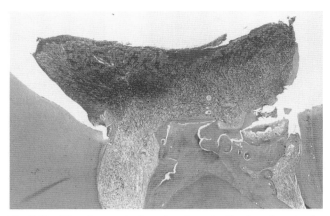

Fig. 2.25 Microphotograph of a pulp polyp extending from the pulp of a young tooth broken down by caries. Note the dense inflammatory infiltrate in the proliferating tissue. (Courtesy of Dr Domenico Ricucci.)

become epithelialized upon making contact with the gingival tissue.

Dental treatment procedures

While the primary objective of dental treatment procedures is to eliminate infectious agents in the treatment of caries and periodontal disease and to restore tooth function and esthetics, these procedures can seldom be carried out without causing injury to the pulp. In the short term, most irritation is survivable. It is only following advanced disease and the use of inappropriate procedures that the risk of severe injury is imminent. On a long-term basis scar tissue formation, in the form of reparative dentin, increased fibrosis and intrapulpal mineralization, may lower the pulp's defense potential and lead to breakdown in response to new injuries (6).

The threats to the pulp in conjunction with dental procedures relate to:

- The damage inflicted in conjunction with the use of rotary instruments.
- Leakage of bacterial elements from the oral environment along margins of restorations that show poor adaptation to the remaining tooth structure.
- Toxic effects of medicaments and components of materials used to restore cavities and cement crowns and inlays.

It is reasonable to assume that preparation trauma, bacterial influences and material toxicities in combination are more detrimental to the pulp than each of these factors alone (4).

Preparation trauma

A cutting procedure by rotary instruments will not normally cause damage to an extent that the vital function of the pulp is jeopardized. As remarked above, preparation for restoration close to the pulp, however, generates substantial frictional heat which can cause a significant and detrimental temperature increase in the pulp. Repair will usually ensue, but the formation of reparative dentin can be extensive and thereby render the pulp vulnerable to repeated injury. In fact, clinical follow-ups of teeth restored with cast restorations (full crowns and teeth included as abutments in bridgeworks) have shown that pulpal necrosis may occur with an increasing frequency over time (6, 16). Often one will find the coronal portion of the pulp in such teeth obliterated by reparative dentin, making endodontic therapy difficult.

Another complication of cavity and crown preparation is internal bleeding. In rare instances it may be so extensive that pulpal necrosis occurs almost instantaneously. The tooth structure of such teeth may turn red initially and later a gray color. In patients treated with anticoagulants (warfarin) the risk of a sustained intrapulpal bleeding should be recognized.

Bacterial leakage

Bacteria and bacterial elements in the oral environment may penetrate margins of dental restorations and seriously affect the healthy condition of the pulp. The term *bacterial leakage* (synonym: *microleakage*) is used to imply this form of pulpal irritation.

Research in recent years has indeed demonstrated that bacterial leakage in restoration margins is a major threat to the vital functions of the pulp subsequent to restorative therapies (4, 61). In particular in deep and extensive exposures of dentin, the infectious load on the pulp can be substantial (Fig. 2.26).

In principle, the inflammatory events of the pulp in response to these bacterial exposures are similar to those detailed for caries. Some distinct differences should be recognized. Polymorphonuclear leukocytes (PMNs) play an important role in the initial responses owing to the more sudden and extensive bacterial exposure than that in the relatively slowly progressing carious lesion. These cells accumulate in areas of the pulp adjacent to the involved dentinal tubules. The presence of bacterial elements also prompts neutrophils to migrate into the tubules. This is probably a most significant defense factor that, in addition to the protective effects of the dentinal fluid (described above), helps to block further penetration of bacteria and bacterial products into the pulp. Collectively, these mechanisms are likely to explain why pulpal repair and healing are still possible even when a restoration does not completely seal its margin (4) (Key literature 2.2).

Contrary to caries, occlusion of dentinal tubules by mineral deposits seldom occurs underneath fillings. Thus, dentin in areas unaffected by caries may remain

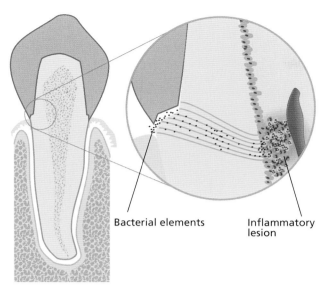

Fig. 2.26 In contraction gaps or after incomplete coverage of dentin following restorative procedures, bacterial elements in the oral cavity may gain access to pulp along the exposed dentinal tubules. This is regarded as a serious threat to the pulp because it may induce painful symptoms and inflammatory lesions in the pulp.

Key literature 2.2

Lundy and Stanley (47), in an experimental study in humans, prepared small but deep dentin cavities in teeth scheduled for extraction. The cavities were left unrestored to the oral environment for various periods of time to observe and correlate pulp tissue responses to the degree of occurring painful symptoms. The initial response of the pulp after 1–2 days consisted of severe infiltrates of neutrophils. By contrast, at subsequent observations there was no breakdown of the pulps even if the remaining dentin wall to the pulp was thin. Instead, reduced inflammation and evidence of repair were seen as early as 9 days after dentin exposure. Weeks and months after the initiation of oral exposure, normal pulpal tissue and the formation of reparative dentin were seen in the large majority of specimens. On testing for sensitivity, teeth became increasingly painful over the first few days. These symptoms subsequently subsided, along with recovery of the pulp. Findings confirm the potential of the pulp to withstand bacterial challenges when there is still a wall of dentin separating the pulp from the oral environment. Both reduced or blocked dentin permeability and inflammatory and immunological responses in the pulp are mechanisms that are likely to impede further bacterial irritation.

---

permeable and sensitive unless reparative dentin has been formed in the pulp.

Effects of restorative materials

In addition to the trauma from preparing teeth for restoration and the subsequent leakage of bacterial elements, release of constituents of restorative materials may have an adverse influence on the pulp. For years the toxicity of restorative materials was regarded a major cause of pulpal inflammation and breakdown in restorative procedures. However, research in recent years has shown that toxic components in restorative materials are a lesser threat to the pulp than previously anticipated (4). This has been best demonstrated in experimental studies where dental materials in common use (amalgam, zinc phosphate cement, resin composites) were applied directly on pulpal tissue and where the surface of the restoration was sealed bacteria-tight (17). These experiments demonstrated that the pulp around sealed restorations resumed a healthy state. By contrast, restorations without a bacteria-tight surface seal allowed bacterial penetration to the pulp–restoration interface resulting in a severe inflammatory lesion.

The risk of severe pulpal complication is even less when a dentin barrier remains. Dentin seems to serve as a detoxifying tissue, in that highly toxic materials are absorbed to the inner walls of the dentinal tubules (29). Dentin furthermore buffers the effects of acids and bases (30). It needs to be recognized that experiments *in vitro* and *in vivo* have demonstrated that the hydrophilic resin primer 2-hydroxyethyl methacrylate (HEMA) and the bonding resin monomer, triethylene glycol dimethacrylate (TEGDMA), used in modern restorative procedures, readily penetrate thin dentin walls upon topical application (21, 31). Several adverse effects are possible, including pulpal cell injury and allergic reactions in susceptible patients, but these have not been confirmed to be prevalent. Therefore, the threat to the pulp in conjunction with modern restorative procedures does not seem to be as much related to the materials *per se* as it is to the improper seal that may result (Core concept 2.4).

Dental trauma

Accidental trauma resulting in fractures and luxations of teeth causes injuries that put the vital functions of the

---

Core concept 2.4   **Pulpal response to bacterial leakage at tooth/restoration interfaces**

- Leakage of bacteria and bacterial products in tooth/restoration interfaces induces inflammatory lesions in the pulp across the dentin.
- Although these responses do not normally lead to pulpal breakdown, they may cause painful symptoms and pulpal scars.
- Clinicians are cautioned not to leave dentin exposures unprotected or with poorly fitted permanent or temporary restorations.
- There is a vast difference in the infectious load on the pulp when a large area of dentin is uncovered, e.g. in a full crown preparation in comparison to a small and shallow cavity preparation. On such exposures protective measures are particularly important.

pulp at risk in a number of ways. Chapter 15 gives a detailed account of the specific effects on the pulp of the various forms of dental trauma that may occur.

References

1. Abou Hashieh I, Franquin JC, Cosset A, Dejou J, Camps J. Relationship between dentine hydraulic conductance and the cytotoxicity of four dentine bonding resins *in vitro*. *J. Dent.* 1998; 26: 473–7.
2. Beckman JS, Koppenol WH. Nitric oxide, superoxide, and peroxynitrite: the good, the bad, and ugly. *Am. J. Physiol.* 1996; 271: C1424–37.
3. Bergenholtz G. Effect of bacterial products on inflammatory reactions in the dental pulp. *Scand. J. Dent. Res.* 1977; 85: 122–9.
4. Bergenholtz G. Evidence for bacterial causation of adverse pulpal responses in resin-based dental restorations. *Crit. Rev. Oral Biol. Med.* 2000; 11: 467–80.
    Review paper for further reading on the effects of microbial elements on the pulp in restorative procedures.
5. Bergenholtz G, Lindhe J. Effect of soluble plaque factors on inflammatory reactions in the dental pulp. *Scand. J. Dent. Res.* 1975; 83: 153–8.
6. Bergenholtz G, Nyman S. Endodontic complications following periodontal and prosthetic treatment of patients with advanced periodontal disease. *J. Periodontol.* 1984; 55: 63–8.
7. Berggren E, Heyeraas K. The role of sensory neuropeptides and nitric oxide on pulpal blood flow and tissue pressure in the ferret. *J. Dent. Res.* 1999; 78: 1535–43.
8. Bishop M, Malhotra M. An investigation of lymphatic vessels in the feline dental pulp. *Am. J. Anat.* 1990; 187: 247–53.
9. Bjørndal L, Darvann T. A light microscopic study of odontoblastic and non-odontoblastic cells involved in tertiary dentinogenesis on well-defined cavitated carious lesions. *Caries Res.* 1999; 33: 50–60.
    Histology and microradiographic techniques were used to study the events taking place in dentin and pulp on both advanced and slowly progressing carious lesions.
10. Bjørndal L, Darvann T, Thylstrup A. A quantitative light microscopic study of the odontoblast and subodontoblastic reactions to active and arrested enamel caries without cavitation. *Caries Res.* 1998; 32: 59–69.
11. Bjørndal L, Mjör I. Dental caries: characteristics of lesions and pulpal reactions. In: *Pulp–Dentin Biology in Restorative Dentistry*. New Malden: Quintessence Publishing Co., 2002; 55–75.
12. Brännström M. *Dentine and Pulp in Restorative Dentistry*. London: Wolfe Medical, 1982.
13. Brännström M, Lind P-O. Pulpal response to early dental caries. *J. Dent. Res.* 1965; 44: 1045–50.
    In this study, clusters of mononuclear leukocytes and small areas of reparative dentine were observed in the pulp of young premolars underneath initial carious lesions.
14. Brännström M, Lindén L-Å, Åström A. The hydrodynamics of the dental tubule and of pulp fluid. A discussion of its significance in relation to dentinal sensitivity. *Caries Res.* 1967; 1: 310–17.
15. Byers MR, Sugaya A. Odontoblast processes in dentin revealed by fluorescent Di-I. *J. Histochem. Cytochem.* 1995; 43: 159–68.
16. Cheung, GS, Lai SC, Ng RP. Fate of vital pulps beneath a metal–ceramic crown or a bridge retainer. *Int. Endod. J.* 2005; 38: 521–30.
17. Cox CF, Keall CL, Keall HJ, Ostro E, Bergenholtz G. Biocompatibility of surfaced sealed dental materials against exposed pulps. *J. Prosthet. Dent.* 1987; 57: 1–8.
18. Dommisch H, Winter J, Açil Y, Dunsche A, Tiemann M, Jepsen S. Human beta-defensin (hBD-1, -2) expression in dental pulp. *Oral Microbiol. Immunol.* 2005; 20: 163–6.
19. Durand SH, Flacher V, Roméas A, Carrouel F, Colomb E, Vincent C, et al. Lipoteichoic acid increases TLR and functional chemokine expression while reducing dentin formation in *in vitro* differentiated human odontoblasts *J. Immunol.* 2006; 176: 2880–7.
20. Garberoglio R, Brännström M. Scanning electron microscopic investigation of human dentinal tubules. *Arch. Oral Biol.* 1976; 21: 355–62.
21. Gerzina TM, Hume WR. Diffusion of monomers from bonding resin–resin composite combinations through dentine *in vitro*. *J. Dent.* 1996; 24: 125–8.
22. Gronthos S, Mankani M, Brahim J, Robey PG, Shi S. Postnatal human dental pulp stem cells (DPSCs) *in vitro* and *in vivo*. *Proc. Natl. Acad. Sci. USA* 2000; 97: 13625–30.
    Study presenting the first evidence of the existence of postnatal human stem cells in the dental pulp.
23. Hahn CL, Liewehr FR. Innate immune responses of the dental pulp to caries. *J. Endod.* 2007; 33: 643–51.
24. Hahn CL, Liewehr FR. Update on the adaptive immune response of the dental pulp. *J. Endod.* 2007; 33: 773–81.
25. Haug SR, Heyeraas KJ. Modulation of dental inflammation by the sympathetic nervous system. *J. Dent. Res.* 2006; 85: 488–95.
26. Heyeraas KJ. Pulpal hemodynamics and interstitial fluid pressure: balance of transmicrovascular fluid transport. *J. Endod.* 1989; 15: 468–72.
27. Heyeraas KJ, Kvinnsland I. Tissue pressure and blood flow in pulpal inflammation. *Proc. Finn. Dent. Soc.* 1992; 88 (Suppl. 1): 393–401.
28. Hibbs JB Jr, Taintor RR, Vavrin Z, Rachlin EM. Nitric oxide: a cytotoxic activated macrophage effector molecule (published erratum appears in *Biochem. Biophys. Res. Commun.* 1989; 158: 624). *Biochem. Biophys. Res. Commun.* 1988; 157: 87–94.
29. Hume WR. An analysis of the release and the diffusion through dentin of eugenol from zinc oxide–eugenol mixtures. *J. Dent. Res.* 1984; 63: 881–4.
30. Hume WR. Influence of dentine on the pulpward release of eugenol or acids from restorative materials. *J. Oral Rehabil.* 1994; 21: 469–73.
31. Hume WR, Gerzina TM. Bioavailability of components of resin based materials which are applied to teeth. *Crit. Rev. Oral Biol. Med.* 1996; 7: 172–9.
    The potential hazards for the pulp when using composite resin materials as dental restorative material are detailed in this review paper.

32. Jacobsen EB, Heyeraas KJ. Effect of capsaicin treatment or inferior alveolar nerve resection on dentine formation and calcitonin gene-related peptide- and substance P-immunoreactive nerve fibres in rat molar pulp. *Arch. Oral Biol.* 1996; 41: 1121–31.

33. Jontell M, Bergenholtz G. Accessory cells in the immune defense of the dental pulp. *Proc. Finn. Dent. Soc.* 1992; 88: 345–55.

34. Jontell M, Okiji T, Dahlgren U, Bergenholtz G. Immune defense mechanisms of the dental pulp. *Crit. Rev. Oral Biol. Med.* 1998; 9: 179–200.

35. Kamal AM, Okiji T, Kawashima N, Suda H. Defense responses of dentine/pulp complex to experimentally induced caries in rat molars: an immunohistochemical study on kinetics of pulpal Ia antigen-expressing cells and macrophages. *J. Endod.* 1997; 23: 115–20.

   Studies on pulpal responses to dental caries primarily rely on observations in extracted human teeth, while few experimental studies are available. In this experimental study in rats the immune response of the pulp to induced caries was explored.

36. Kawashima N, Nakano-Kawanishi H, Suzuki N, Takagi M, Suda H. Effect of NOS inhibitor on cytokine and COX2 expression in rat pulpitis. *J. Dent. Res.* 2005; 84: 762–7.

37. Kerezoudis NP, Olgart L, Edwall L. Differential effects of nitric oxide synthesis inhibition on basal blood flow and antidromic vasodilation in rat oral tissues. *Eur. J. Pharmacol.* 1993; 14: 209–19.

38. Kim S, Dörscher-Kim JE, Liu M, Grayson A. Functional alterations in pulpal microcirculation in response to various dental procedures and materials. *Proc. Finn. Dent. Soc.* 1992; 88 (Suppl. 1): 65–71.

39. Kimberly CL, Byers MR. Inflammation of rat molar pulp and periodontium causes increased calcitonin gene-related peptide and axonal sprouting. *Anat. Rec.* 1988; 222: 289–300.

40. Kishi Y, Takahashi K. Change of vascular architecture of dental pulp with growth. In: *Dynamic Aspects of Dental Pulp* (Inoki R, Kudo T, Olgart L, eds). New York: Chapman and Hall, 1990; 97–129.

41. Knutsson G, Jontell M, Bergenholtz G. Determination of plasma proteins in dentinal fluid from cavities prepared in healthy young human teeth. *Arch. Oral Biol.* 1994; 39: 185–90.

42. Kubes P, Suzuki M, Granger DN. Nitric oxide: an endogenous modulator of leukocyte adhesion. *Proc. Natl. Acad. Sci. USA* 1991; 88: 4651–5.

43. Langeland K. Tissue response to dental caries. *Endod. Dent. Traumatol.* 1987; 3: 149–71.

44. Law A, Baumgardner K, Meller S, Gebhart G. Localization and changes in NADPH-diaphorase reactivity and nitric oxide synthase immunoreactivity in rat pulp following tooth preparation. *J. Dent. Res.* 1999; 78: 1585–95.

45. Lawman MJ, Boyle MD, Gee AP, Young M. Nerve growth factor accelerates the early cellular events associated with wound healing. *Exp. Mol. Pathol.* 1985; 43: 274–81.

46. Lewin GR, Mendell LM. Nerve growth factor and nociception. *Trends Neurosci.* 1993; 16: 353–9.

47. Lundy T, Stanley H. Correlation of pulpal histopathology and clinical symptoms in human teeth subjected to experimental irritation. *Oral Surg.* 1969; 27: 187–201.

48. Luthman J, Luthman D, Hökfelt T. Occurrence and distribution of different neurochemical markers in the human dental pulp. *Arch. Oral Biol.* 1992; 37: 193–208.

49. Matthews B, Vongsavan N. Interactions between neural and hydrodynamic mechanisms in dentine and pulp. *Arch. Oral Biol.* 1994; 39 (Suppl.): 87–95S.

50. Meyer MW. Pulpal blood flow: use of radio-labelled microspheres. *Int. Endod. J.* 1993; 26: 6–7.

51. Moncada S, Palmer RM, Higgs EA. Nitric oxide: physiology, pathophysiology, and pharmacology. *Pharmacol. Rev.* 1991; 43: 109–42.

52. Ohshima H, Maeda T, Takano Y. The distribution and ultrastructure of class II MHC-positive cells in human dental pulp. *Cell Tissue Res.* 1999; 295: 151—8.

53. Okiji T, Jontell M, Belichenko P, Bergenholtz G, Dahlström A. Perivascular dendritic cells of the human dental pulp. *Acta Physiol. Scand.* 1997; 159: 163–9.

54. Okiji T, Jontell M, Belichenko P, Dahlgren U, Bergenholtz G, Dahlström A. Structural and functional association between substance P- and calcitonin gene-related peptide-immunoreactive nerves and accessory cells in the rat dental pulp. *J. Dent. Res.* 1997; 76: 1818–24.

55. Okiji T, Kawashima N, Kosaka T, Kobayashi C, Suda H. Distribution of Ia antigen-expressing nonlymphoid cells in various stages of induced periapical lesions in rat molars. *J. Endod.* 1994; 20: 27–31.

56. Olgart L. Local mechanisms in dental pain. In: *Mechanisms of Pain and Analgesic Compounds* (Beers RF Jr, Borrett EG, eds). New York: Raven Press, 1979; 285–94.

57. Olgart L. Neurogenic components of pulpal inflammation. In: *Proceedings of the International Conference on Dentine/Pulp Complex 1995*, Chiba, Japan (Shimono M, Maeda T, Suda H, Takahashi K, eds). Tokyo: Quintessence Publishing, 1979; 169–75.

58. Olgart L. Neural control of pulpal blood flow. *Crit. Rev. Oral Biol. Med.* 1996; 7: 159–71.

   Review paper describing mechanisms governing pulpal hemodynamics.

59. Olgart L, Edwall L, Gazelius B. Involvement of afferent nerves in pulpal blood-flow reactions in response to clinical and experimental procedures in the cat. *Arch. Oral Biol.* 1991; 36: 575–81.

60. Olgart L, Gazelius B. Effects of adrenaline and felypressin (octapressin) on blood flow and sensory nerve activity in the tooth. *Acta Odontol. Scand.* 1977; 35: 69–75.

61. Pashley DH. Dynamics of the pulpo-dentine complex. *Crit. Rev. Oral Biol. Med.* 1996; 7: 104–33.

   Comprehensive review on functions and responses of the dentin–pulp complex to injurious elements.

62. Payan BG, Brewster DR, Goetzl EJ. Specific stimulation of human T lymphocytes by substance P. *J. Immunol.* 1983; 133: 3260–5.

63. Pissiotis E, Spångberg LS. Dentin permeability to bacterial proteins *in vitro*. *J. Endod.* 1994; 20: 118–22.

64. Reeves R, Stanley HR. The relationship of bacterial penetration and pulpal pathosis in carious teeth. *Oral Surg.* 1966; 22: 59–65.

65. Robertson A, Andreasen FM, Bergenholtz G, Andreasen JO, Norén JG. Incidence of pulp necrosis subsequent to pulp

canal obliteration from trauma of permanent incisors. *J. Endod.* 1996; 22: 557–60.

66. Smith AJ, Cassidy N, Perry H, Begue-Kirn C, Ruch JV, Lesot H. Reactionary dentinogenesis. *Int. J. Dev. Biol.* 1995; 39: 273–80.

67. Staquet MJ, Durand SH, Colomb E, Roméas A, Vincent C, Bleicher F, *et al.* Different roles of odontoblasts and fibroblasts in immunity. *J. Dent. Res.* 2008; 87: 256–6.

68. Takahashi K, Kishi Y, Kim S. A scanning electron microscope study of the blood vessels of dog pulp using corrosion resin casts. *J. Endod.* 1982; 8: 131–5.

69. Takahashi K, Sakai S. Regulation mechanisms of pulpal blood flow outside the dental pulp. In: *Dentine/Pulp Complex* (Shimono M, Takahashi K, eds). Tokyo: Quintessence Publishing, 1996; 158–61.

70. Telles PD, Hanks CT, Machado MA, Nör JE. Lipoteichoic acid up-regulates VEGF expression in macrophages and pulp cells. *J. Dent. Res.* 2003; 82: 466–70.

71. Turner DF, Marfurt CF, Sattelberg C. Demonstration of physiological barrier between pulpal odontoblasts and its perturbation following routine restorative procedures: a horseradish peroxidase tracing study in the rat. *J. Dent. Res.* 1989; 68: 12162–8.

72. Van Hassel HJ. Physiology of the human dental pulp. *Oral Surg. Oral Med. Oral Pathol.* 1971; 32: 126–34.

73. Vongsavan N, Matthews B. The permeability of cat dentine *in vivo* and *in vitro*. *Arch. Oral Biol.* 1991; 36: 641–6.

74. Wadachi R, Hargreaves KM. Trigeminal nociceptors express TLR-4 and CD14: a mechanism for pain due to infection. *J. Dent. Res.* 2006; 85: 49–53.

75. Warfvinge J, Bergenholtz G. Healing capacity of human and monkey dental pulps following experimentally induced pulpitis. *Endod. Dent. Traumatol.* 1986; 2: 256–62.

Chapter 3
Dentinal and pulpal pain

Matti Närhi

Introduction

The dental pulp is exceptionally richly innervated by trigeminal afferent axons (7, 10) that seem to subserve mostly, if not exclusively, nociceptive function (30, 39, 43). Accordingly, they respond to stimuli that induce or threaten to induce injury to the pulp tissue, and their activation may induce defensive, withdrawal-type reflexes in the masticatory muscles (37, 43, 49). The pain responses induced by external stimuli can be extremely intense. The dense innervation of the pulp and dentin gives a morphological basis for the high sensitivity of these tissues. In addition to the afferent sensory nerves, the dental pulp is innervated by autonomic sympathetic efferents that play a role in the regulation of the blood flow in the pulp (47) and, in addition, may have regulatory functions in pulpal inflammation (24, 54). The existence and functional significance of parasympathetic innervation are still controversial (47).

Classification of nerve fibers

Nerves can be divided into different groups according to axon size and structure, which determine the conduction velocities of the individual fibers (22) (Table 3.1). In the nervous system the different-sized fibers are distributed in a functionally meaningful manner, namely thick

myelinated fibers in those nerve tracts where fast conduction is demanded and fine-caliber fibers in those tracts where the speed of conduction is not as critical. For example, the efferent Aα-motoneurons, which transmit nerve impulses to the skeletal muscles, have thick myelinated axons and conduction velocities of up to 120 m/s (22). The afferent Aβ-type sensory axons (with conduction velocities of 30–70 m/s) transmit touch and pressure sensations and, usually, their receptors respond to light mechanical forces, i.e. they have low stimulation thresholds (22).

Pain is conducted by two different sets of neurons: thin myelinated Aδ-fibers with conduction velocities of 5–30 m/s and neurons with unmyelinated axons with conduction velocities of 0.5–2.5 m/s. Because of this organization, the sensation perceived in response to noxious stimulation consists of two discrete and different components: first sharp and rather well-localized pain mediated by Aδ-fibers and then delayed, dull pain that is mediated by C-fibers and can radiate to a wide area surrounding the affected tissue (39). The poor localization of the C-fiber pain is due to more extensive convergence of the afferent C-fibers, compared to A-fibers, to the second-order neurons in the brain stem (22). Under experimental conditions, the temporal discrimination and the quality differences of the two pain components can be demonstrated clearly in response to stimulation of extremities (39). The same dichotomy in the quality of pain can be shown when stimulating teeth (30), although temporal discrimination is not as obvious because of the short distance between the brain and the site of stimulation.

Morphology of intradental sensory innervation

The sensory neurons of the dental pulp have their cell bodies in the trigeminal ganglion (7, 10). The teeth of the upper jaw are innervated by neurons of the maxillary and those of the lower jaw by neurons of the mandibular division of the trigeminal nerve. The pulpal axons are located in the alveolar branches of the nerve and finally

Table 3.1 Examples of different nerve fiber types, their functions, diameters and conduction velocities.

Fiber type	Function	Diameter (μm)	Conduction velocity (m/s)
Aα	Motoneurons Muscle afferents	12–20	70–120
Aβ	Mediation of touch and pressure sensations	5–12	30–70
Aδ	Mediation of pain, temperature and touch	2–5	5–30
C	Mostly mediation of pain	0.4–1.2	0.5–2.5

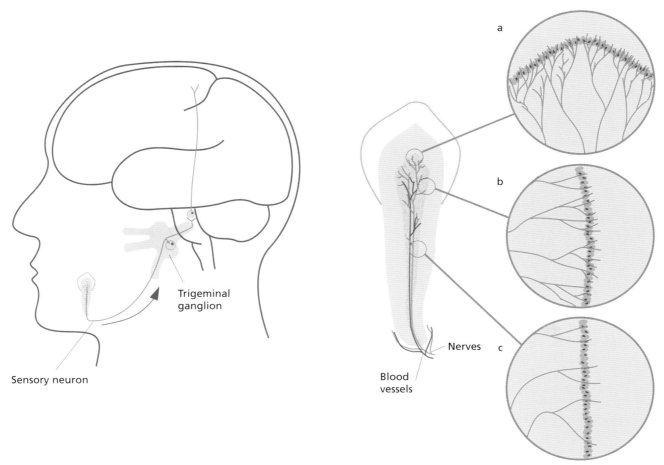

Fig. 3.1   Schematic drawing presenting the innervation of the dental pulp. Several branches from the alveolar nerve enter the apical area of the tooth. Some nerve bundles innervate the periodontal tissues. Multiple bundles enter the pulp in close proximity to the blood vessels through the apical foramen; they branch further on their way to the tooth crown. Most of the intradental axons have their terminals in the pulp/dentin border of the coronal pulp, which is the most densely innervated area in the tissue (a). There are fewer nerve endings in the cervical area (b) and the pulp/dentin border in the root pulp is sparsely innervated (c).

enter the pulp through the apical foramen or multiple foramina of the root apex in close proximity to the intradental blood vessels (Fig. 3.1).

Several hundred axons per tooth enter the pulp at the root apex; for premolars, this number is close to a thousand (7, 26, 29). The nerve fibers enter the tooth pulp in multiple bundles that contain both myelinated and unmyelinated axons (Fig. 3.2) (7, 26, 29). The majority of the axons (70–80%) are unmyelinated (7, 26, 29).

In species as varied as human, cat, dog, monkey and ferret, it appears that there are no gross differences in intradental innervation (7, 10). Rat molars also have similar innervation but in the incisors, which are continuously erupting, the innervation is sparse and of a different structure. For example, these teeth lack dentinal nerve fibers (7, 10).

Only a small proportion of the pulpal afferents terminate in the root. Most of the nerve bundles extend to the coronal pulp, branching on their way (Fig. 3.1). The terminal branch endings are located mostly in the pulp/

dentin border area of the coronal pulp (Fig. 3.3). A dense network of fine nerve filaments, known as the nerve plexus of Raschkow, is formed close to the odontoblasts. Several nerve terminals also enter the odontoblast layer and many of them extend into the dentinal tubules (7, 10) (Fig. 3.3). Both morphological and functional studies indicate that the fine nerve filaments in the dentinal tubules are mostly terminals of the myelinated intradental axons (7, 10, 40, 43). Some of the axons also terminate in the deeper parts of the pulp, often in close proximity to the pulpal blood vessels, and they may have a significant role in the mediation of pulpal blood flow responses to external irritation, as well as in pulp tissue inflammation and repair (9, 10, 47, 48; see also Chapter 2).

The terminal branching of the pulpal nerve fibers is extensive (7). Individual myelinated axons may innervate more than 100 dentinal tubules. Accordingly, innervation of the pulp/dentin border is extremely dense. Both myelinated and unmyelinated fibers terminate as free nerve endings. These are the receptors or nociceptors,

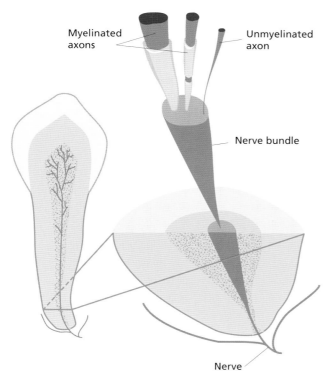

Fig. 3.2   A schematic drawing showing a nerve bundle entering the pulp chamber in the apical area of the tooth. The nerve bundle contains both unmyelinated and myelinated axons of variable sizes.

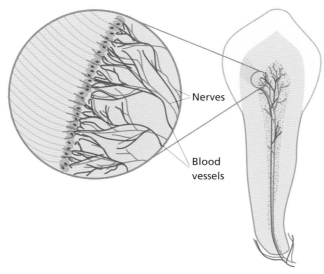

Fig. 3.3   Innervation of the pulp/dentin border in the coronal pulp. The nerve fibers entering the area form a dense network known as the plexus of Raschkow. The fibers form free nerve endings in the peripheral pulp and in the odontoblast layer. Many nerve terminals are also located in the dentinal tubules. Some fibers branch to innervate the adjacent blood vessels (see text for details).

which respond to various external stimuli in normal teeth and to the environmental changes and various inflammatory mediators that occur under pathological conditions.

As in other tissues, the sensory nerves of the dental pulp contain neuropeptides such as substance P and calcitonin gene-related peptide (CGRP) (8–12). Several different neuropeptides have been identified in various parts of the nervous system (18, 34) that act as neuro-mediators or modulators and have significant regulatory effects on impulse transmission in the central nervous system. Many of them have also been shown to function in peripheral tissues as, for example, mediator substances in the effector organs of the autonomic sympathetic and parasympathetic nerves (34). The sensory neuropeptides in the afferent nerves play an important role in the initial stages of the inflammatory process (neurogenic inflammation) following injury in the peripheral tissues (47, 48) and also seem to regulate the later stages of inflammation and repair (8–12).

The location of the nerve terminals in dentin is limited to the inner 150–200 μm of the tubules (7, 10). The outer layers of dentin are not innervated. It should also be noted that innervation of the dentin is densest in the coronal part, especially in the pulp tips under the cusps, where about 50% of the tubules have been shown to contain nerve fibers (7). Many tubules contain several nerve endings (7, 28). Considering the structural dimensions of dentin it can be estimated that approximately 15 000–20 000 nerve endings/mm^2 exist in the pulp/dentin border area at the pulp tip. Innervation of the pulp/dentin border becomes less dense towards the cervical areas and the number of innervated tubules becomes considerably lower (7, 10). In addition, the distance that the nerve fibers penetrate into the tubules is much shorter than in the coronal areas. In the root, the innervation of the peripheral pulp and dentin is sparse (7). In this respect the structural organization of intradental innervation seems to be poorly correlated to the sensitivity of different dentin areas in the clinical situation, namely, that exposed cervical dentin seems to be especially sensitive. However, this obvious discrepancy can be due to differences in the time the dentin has been exposed and in the responses of the pulp–dentin complex to irritation in the coronal dentin compared with the cervical dentin (see section on dentin hypersensitivity below). The variation in dentinal innervation in different parts of the tooth may explain the different types of pain response induced in the coronal versus the root dentin in human teeth (32).

Some afferent nerve fibers may branch to innervate both the dental pulp and the adjacent tissues or multiple teeth. Such organization may, to some extent, contribute to the poor localization of dental pain and may also allow neurogenic vasodilation and inflammatory reactions to occur in an area of tissue wider than that affected by the original insult. Correspondingly, within the dental pulp the terminal branching of the nerve fibers may contribute to the spread of the inflammatory reactions (44).

Function of intradental sensory nerves under normal conditions

Knowledge of the function of intradental nerves is mostly based on electrophysiological recordings performed on experimental animals (40, 43, 44, 46). Comparison of the nerve responses to the sensations induced from human teeth with the same stimuli, as well as to the clinical cases of dental pain, has given insight to the contribution of the different intradental nerve fiber groups to different dental pain sensations. The apparently similar structure and function of the innervation in the different species examined (human, monkey, dog, cat and ferret) gives a reasonable basis for such comparisons (Advanced concept 3.1).

As already mentioned, the pulp and dentin are innervated by two different groups of afferents: A- and C-fibers (30, 40, 43). The functional classification is based on the conduction velocities of the axons and corresponds to the morphological findings showing the existence of both myelinated and unmyelinated nerve fibers in the pulp (7, 26,29).

Intradental A- and C-fibers are functionally different (10, 30, 43, 44). The A-fibers respond to various "hydrodynamic" stimuli applied to dentin, such as drilling, probing, air-drying and hypertonic chemical solutions (40, 42, 43). There seems to be a common mechanism of nerve fiber activation in response to the different stimuli. This hydrodynamic mechanism will be described and discussed in detail later in this chapter. The pulpal C-fibers are polymodal, which means that they respond to several different stimuli when they reach the pulp proper (30, 40, 43). The fibers have high thresholds and are activated by intense thermal (heat and cold) and mechanical stimulation (30, 40, 43). They also respond to such inflammatory mediators as bradykinin and histamine (40, 43), which are both formed and/or released in response to tissue injury and associated inflammatory reactions. Thus, the results from the electrophysiological studies indicate that intradental A-fibers are responsible for the sensitivity of dentin and may give the first warning signals whenever dentin is exposed, whereas the C-fibers may be activated mostly under pathological conditions.

Discrete receptive fields of the intradental nerve fibers can be located in either the pulp or dentin (30, 40, 44, 62). The receptive fields of C-fibers are found in the pulp proper and the pulp tissue has to be exposed for their activation. Also, some A-fibers, mostly slowly conducting, have their receptive fields in the pulp and thus cannot be activated by dentinal stimulation (44, 62). On the other hand, the receptive fields of those A-fibers that are activated by hydrodynamic stimulation of dentin can be located by probing the exposed dentin surface (44, 62). In normal teeth the receptive fields are usually small spots a few millimeters in diameter (Fig. 3.4). Some fibers may have two or even three separate receptive fields that can be located at a considerable distance from each other, in the coronal dentin and cervical area in some cases (62). Typically, the receptive fields of individual fibers overlap extensively, meaning that stimulation of a small area in dentin or pulp can activate multiple nerve fibers; this is an important factor, considering the intensity of the pain responses induced by external stimulation. These functional findings are in accordance with the structure of innervation of the pulp/dentin border area, with the extensive and overlapping terminal branching of the individual axons (see above) (Fig. 3.4).

The intradental C-fibers are activated by a direct effect of the applied stimuli on the nerve endings (30, 40, 43). For example, in thermal stimulation the response latencies are rather long and nerve firing does not begin until the temperature within the pulp has changed by several

---

Advanced concept 3.1   Electrophysiological methods for the recording of pulp nerve activity

Two different methods have been applied in the electrophysiological recordings of pulp nerve function. Recording from dentin is performed by placing the electrodes in dentinal cavities (51). This method allows the discrimination of the action potentials of faster-conducting A-fibers. The activity of the C-fibers cannot be recorded and classification of the individual nerve fibers with respect to their conduction velocities and electrical thresholds is not possible. The recordings were initially performed on cat canine teeth (51). It is important to note that the method has been applied to human teeth as well and those experiments have shown that intradental nerve activity is related to pain sensations perceived by the subjects in response to the external stimuli applied, showing that pulpal nerves are able to conduct nociceptive information (16). In the cat teeth the recordings from dentin have shown that pulpal A-fibers respond to mechanical and osmotic stimulation of dentin (46) and are activated or sensitized by certain inflammatory mediators and heat injury (1, 45, 48). It was also shown that the activity of the intradental A-fibers is greatly affected by changes in the pulpal blood flow.

In single-fiber recordings the individual fibers innervating the examined teeth are dissected from the alveolar nerve and are identified by electrical stimulation of the tooth crown (40). The method has been used in dog, cat and ferret teeth and it allows detailed functional classification of the examined nerve fibers with respect to their electrical thresholds, conduction velocities, receptive fields (the area in the dentin or pulp where an individual fiber can be activated) and sensitivity to a variety of stimuli applied to the dental hard tissues or to the pulp (40, 43).

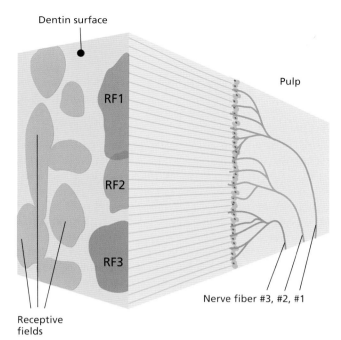

Dentin surface

RF1

RF2

RF3

Receptive
fields

Pulp

Nerve fiber #3, #2, #1

Fig. 3.4 Schematic drawing showing the receptive fields of ten individual pulp nerve fibers on the exposed dentin surface. The receptive fields are of variable shape and overlapping, and in a normal tooth are rather small. The terminal branching of three nerve fibers (fibers 1, 2 and 3) in the pulp/dentin border on the right side of the figure and the corresponding receptive fields (RF1, RF2 and RF3) on the dentin surface are shown as examples. The RF of each individual fiber corresponds to the area in the pulp/dentin border innervated by the particular axon and connected to the receptive field on the dentin surface by the dentinal tubules.

degrees centigrade (30, 40). Similarly, activation of the most slowly conducting Aδ-fibers seems to result from a direct effect of the stimuli on the nerve endings (44, 62). It also seems that the pulpal C-fibers and slowly conducting Aδ-fibers are "silent" in normal healthy teeth and may become active only in cases of pulp injury and inflammation. On the contrary, the A-fibers (mostly faster conducting) responsible for the sensitivity of dentin respond readily whenever dentin is exposed. The nerve activation is immediate or of a very short latency compared with C-fibers, which is in accordance with their activation mechanism (see below).

Comparison of the above-described nerve responses to the pain sensations induced from human teeth under similar stimulation conditions has revealed how different intradental nerve fiber groups may contribute to the different dental pain conditions. For example, "hydrodynamic" stimuli, which activate only pulpal A-fibers, induce sharp pain when applied to dentin in human subjects (42, 43). Intense thermal stimulation of human teeth has been shown to induce an initial sharp pain sensation followed by delayed dull and lingering pain if the stimulation is continued (30). Similar stimulation of the cat canine tooth induces a brief, short latency firing

of intradental A-fibers followed by a long latency activation of C-fibers (30, 40, 43). Consequently algogenic (pain-producing) agents, which activate selectively either A- or C-fibers in experimental animals (40, 43), induce sharp or dull and lingering pain in human subjects (2). Altogether, the above results indicate that intradental A-fibers mediate the sharp dental pain sensations and are responsible for dentin sensitivity, whereas C-fibers mediate the dull pulpal pain or toothache connected with pulpitis.

In spite of the type of stimulus applied to a tooth, pain is the only sensation induced in response to activation of the pulpal sensory nerves, according to most studies. The only exception is low-intensity electrical stimulation (39, 43), which can induce so-called prepain sensations that probably result from low-level (liminal) activity in the pulpal nociceptive afferents. Considering any clinical situations when an electric pulp tester is used, it is important to note that the initial sensation at threshold level is usually not painful. When the stimulus intensity is increased, the sensation becomes painful and any other stimulus applied to the tooth induces pain, although its quality may vary in response to different stimuli. The variation is due to differences in the nerve response patterns and the activation of different types of nerve fibers (35).

Sensitivity of dentin: hydrodynamic mechanism in pulpal A-fiber activation

The "hydrodynamic hypothesis" explaining the sensitivity of dentin was first presented by Gysi (23) in 1900. Today it is widely accepted that the sensitivity of dentin is based on hydrodynamic activation of the intradental A-fibers (Fig. 3.5). This concept is supported by a considerable amount of *in vitro* and *in vivo* data from both human and animal experiments (5, 6, 40, 42, 44). It was shown in the early 1960s and in a number of later studies that stimuli inducing pain, when applied to human dentin, are able to induce fluid flow in dentinal tubules *in vitro* (5, 6). The strong capillary forces in the fine tubules cause the hydrodynamic fluid flow. In general, desiccating or evaporative stimuli are the most effective because the capillary force contributes to the outward movements of the tubule contents. It is much more difficult to induce inward fluid flow (6, 50). Moreover, the nerve fibers seem to be more sensitive to outward than inward fluid movements (59). The fluid flow causes mechanical distortion of the tissue in the pulp/dentin border area where most of the nerve endings are located (Figs 3.1 and 3.3–3.5). Accordingly, with all hydrodynamic stimuli the final factor inducing activation of the nerve endings or receptors is a mechanical effect. The results from single pulp nerve recordings showing that

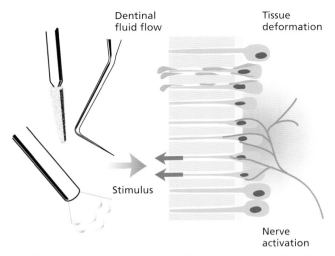

Fig. 3.5   The hydrodynamic mechanism of pulp nerve activation. Any stimulus capable of removing fluid from the outer ends of the dentinal tubules activates hydrodynamic fluid movement. The lost fluid is replaced by an immediate outward flow due to the high capillary forces in the dentinal tubules. The fluid flow causes mechanical distortion of the tissue with the nerve endings in the pulp/dentin border.

individual nerve fibers respond to several different hydrodynamic stimuli are in line with this concept (40, 43, 44).

The fluid flow in the dentinal tubules must be rapid enough to induce sufficient mechanical effect for activation of the nerve endings in the pulp/dentin border. Although there is continuous, slow outward flow in the tubules of exposed dentin due to the high capillary and tissue fluid pressure in the pulp, such a flow is not sufficient to cause nerve activation (50, 58, 59). As already mentioned, stimuli that are able to remove fluid from the tubule apertures, e.g. evaporative or desiccating, are the most effective in activating the pulpal nociceptors because the capillary forces contribute to their effect, resulting in an immediate rapid outward flow (5, 6).

Thermal stimulation is also able to induce hydrodynamic nerve activation because temperature changes cause volume changes in the dentin and tubule contents. However, the temperature change must be rapid enough to cause sufficient fluid flow for nerve activation. In general, cold is more effective than heat because it induces outward fluid movement (6, 59). If intense enough, thermal stimulation (both heat and cold) is able to induce hydrodynamic nerve activation in an intact tooth without any dentin exposure (30). In cases of pulpal inflammation, the intradental nociceptors may become sensitized and activated by a direct effect of heat or cold (43, 44), resulting in a significant increase in the thermal sensitivity of the affected teeth.

Various hypertonic solutions can induce pain when applied to human dentin and activate intradental nerves in experimental animals (3, 5, 43). This action is based on their ability to extract fluid from the dentinal tubules,

owing to their high osmotic pressure, resulting in activation of the capillary forces and fluid movement (5, 6). Several studies have shown that the capability of hypertonic solutions to induce pain in human teeth (3, 5, 6) and to activate intradental nerves in experimental animals (43) is related to their osmotic pressure rather than to the chemical composition of the applied solution. Such results give further support to the view that the intradental nerves are activated by the hydrodynamic mechanism.

The experimental induction of pain with hypertonic solutions corresponds to a clinical situation: when a patient complains of dental pain in connection with eating sweets (which form a saturated sucrose solution when mixed with the saliva on the tooth surface), this indicates that dentin with patent tubules is exposed in a tooth or teeth. The exposure can be found on visible occlusal or cervical surfaces but also in the margins of leaky fillings.

A major characteristic of sensitive human dentin is that the dentinal tubules are patent (5, 6, 41, 42). The hydraulic conductance of dentin and the amount and speed of the dentinal fluid flow are, to a great extent, dependent on the dentin having open or blocked tubules (6, 50). In practice, this means that all exposed dentin is not sensitive. For the induction of hydrodynamic fluid flow by capillary forces, removal of fluid from the tubule apertures is essential. Blocking of the tubule openings prevents or reduces the removal of dentinal fluid by the applied hydrodynamic stimuli and thus reduces dentin sensitivity (42).

The effect of the condition of dentin on its sensitivity has been shown in a number of human and animal experiments. For example, after drilling, the dentin surface is covered with a smear layer (drilling debris) and the tubule openings are blocked by the smear plugs. Etching of the exposed surface with acid is able to remove the smear and open the tubules, thus increasing the sensitivity of the dentin to a great extent (5, 6, 40, 42, 43). Blocking of the dentinal tubules, e.g. with oxalates or resins, reduces or abolishes the pulp nerve responses in experimental animals (40, 42, 43) and desensitizes dentin in human subjects (6, 42). It has also been reported that a significant positive correlation exists between the density of the open dentinal tubules and the intensity of the pain responses induced from exposed cervical dentin surfaces (41). In addition to the surface condition, changes occurring deeper in dentin, such as intratubular mineralization and secondary or irritation dentin formation in the pulp, may affect the hydraulic conductance of dentin and thus its sensitivity (6, 50).

The results of the studies listed above give strong but still only indirect evidence supporting the idea that the sensitivity of dentin and intradental A-fiber activation are based on the hydrodynamic mechanism. In fact,

Vongsavan and Matthews (58, 59) have shown a direct relationship between the measured dentinal fluid flow and intradental nerve activity in response to hydrostatic pressure changes in cat teeth.

Other suggested mechanisms of pulp nerve activation include the possibility of direct activation of the nociceptors when dentin is stimulated. However, such a mechanism does not fit with the findings regarding the response properties of intradental nerve fibers and sensory responses in human subjects, showing that algogenic agents are unable to induce nerve activity or pain when applied to peripheral dentin (40, 45). Moreover, as described earlier, neuroanatomical studies have shown that peripheral dentin is not innervated (7). The possible role of the odontoblasts in pain impulse transmission has been discussed and studied but the evidence supporting such a view is vague (see Advanced concept 3.2).

It can be concluded that the sensitivity of dentin is based on hydrodynamic activation of intradental A-fibers and, because patent dentinal tubules are the most important factor for nerve activation, blocking of the tubules would be the method of choice to abolish or prevent dentinal pain symptoms.

Advanced concept 3.2   Odontoblasts as receptor cells?

The possible function of odontoblasts – with their cell processes in the dentinal tubules – as receptor cells has been discussed for a long time (4, 36, 40). It has been suggested that these cells have membrane properties like those of excitable cells and thus would be able to respond to external stimulation by creating a receptor or generator potential (36). This potential would then cause propagation of action potentials, which would be transmitted further in the nerve fibers. However, evidence supporting the idea of receptor cell function of the odontoblasts is controversial. Although the membrane properties with the characteristics of the ion channels and consequent electrical responses of the cells possess some properties similar to neuronal satellite cells (15), their electrophysiological responses do not resemble those of sensory receptors (15, 36). Moreover, morphological studies have been unable to identify any cell contacts between odontoblasts and the adjacent nerve fibers, which would be typical for synaptic connections or electric coupling of the two cells (7, 10, 36). According to morphological studies, the odontoblast process is limited to the inner third or half of the dentinal tubule (7, 28) and thus might not contribute to the sensitivity of peripheral dentin. Also, studies on human teeth and electrophysiological recordings on experimental animals have indicated that dentin can remain sensitive and intradental nerve fibers are activated even when the odontoblast layer has been destroyed (5, 6, 27). In conclusion, on the basis of the currently available evidence, the proposed receptor cell function of odontoblasts seems improbable. However, odontoblasts may have important functions as supporting cells for the fine nerve terminals and in the regulation of environmental conditions, including the composition of dentinal and tissue fluid around nerve endings (10). Such environmental changes may modify the sensitivity of intradental nociceptors.

Responses of intradental nerves to tissue injury and inflammation

In normal intact teeth quite intense external stimuli are needed for the induction of any activity in the pulpal nociceptors. They stay mostly "silent" because their thresholds to various stimuli are high and they are also well protected by the dental hard tissues. As a result, hot or cold foods and drinks do not cause any significant discomfort or pain in a healthy dentition. When dentin is exposed, activation of the hydrodynamic forces can intensify the effects of the external stimuli to a great extent. This allows activation of the intradental A-fibers, mediating sharp dentinal pain. The intensity of the pain is most often still mild or, at greatest, moderate and considerably well localized. Such initial pain responses after dentin exposure can be regarded as a warning signal indicating that dentin is exposed and there are patent dentinal tubules that form a connection between the pulp and the dentin surface. In addition, the protective or withdrawal reflexes induced by the pulpal A-fiber activation in the jaw muscles can modify the masticatory function and contribute to the prevention of excess tooth wear or, in some extreme cases, even cracking of the tooth crown (37, 41, 49).

In inflamed teeth, external stimuli that are not painful in healthy dentition can induce extremely intense pain responses. For example, patients with pulpitis often complain that temperature changes caused by hot or cold foods or drinks induce pain. Also, spontaneous pain without any obvious external irritation may be present. Such symptoms indicate that the pulpal nociceptors have been sensitized, which means that their thresholds to heat, cold and other stimuli are decreased. Also, the silent nociceptors, which do not respond in healthy teeth, may be activated as indicated by the animal experiments (43, 44). The sensitization can be induced by a number of inflammatory mediators that are released and/or formed in the pulp as a result of the insult (40, 43, 44, 46). Owing to the environmental changes and the activation of different mediators, intradental A- and C-fibers may be affected differentially during the progress of the inflammation (40, 43, 44), which may explain the changes in the type of pain symptoms found in clinical cases of pulpitis.

Peripheral neural changes affecting pain responses in inflamed teeth

As in other tissues, injury to the pulp results in an inflammatory reaction, which is an initial promoter of the healing and repair processes. Stimulation of exposed dentin is able to induce injury, which includes dislocation of the odontoblasts into the dentinal tubules as shown in histological studies (5, 6, 27). Also, nerve endings located in the tubules or adjacent to the odontoblasts become damaged (10, 33). Such morphological changes are prominent after dehydrating stimuli and clearly show the efficacy of the hydrodynamic link in the mediation of the stimulation effects from the dentin surface to the pulp. Thus, even a light stimulus such as an air blast can, in fact, be noxious to the pulp owing to the amplifying effect of the capillary and hydrodynamic forces. In spite of the morphological changes with destruction of the odontoblast layer and dentinal nerve endings, the exposed dentin surface remains sensitive in human subjects (5, 6, 33) and intradental nerve fibers in experimental animals maintain their responsiveness to dentinal stimulation (27). Thus, dentin sensitivity is not dependent on the existence of intact odontoblasts or nerve endings in the dentinal tubules.

Neurogenic vasodilation and inflammation

Whenever an insult causes activation of the intradental nociceptors, the initial reaction in the pulp tissue is neurogenic vasodilation mediated by the terminals of the afferent nerve fibers (Fig. 3.6). The propagated action potentials are conducted over the entire cell membrane of the neuron. As a result of ortodromic conduction the impulses reach the trigeminal nuclei and then higher brain centers, including the cortex, to evoke a pain sensation. Antidromic transmission along the collateral terminal branches of the axons results in the release of CGRP and substance P, which induce vasodilation and an increase in the permeability of the blood vessel walls. Because the responses are evoked by the propagated nerve impulses, they are induced immediately by external irritation. Thus, this initial component of the inflammatory reaction is dependent on afferent nerve fibers and is called neurogenic inflammation.

The extensive branching of the pulpal afferents also allows a spread of the neurogenic effects in a wider area of the pulp than was originally stimulated. It is also possible that activation of axons innervating the pulp and the surrounding structures may result in a spread of the neurogenic inflammatory reactions between the adjacent tissues in rather early stages of inflammation (47, 48).

Inflammatory mediators

As outlined in Chapter 2, many different mediators are activated at different stages during the inflammatory reaction and tissue repair, originating from numerous sources, e.g. various tissue components of the pulp, migrating inflammatory cells and the circulating blood. These mediators have important effects in the regulation of the inflammatory reaction and tissue repair. The neurogenic factors interact closely with other mediators (48), e.g. sensory neuropeptides can induce the release of histamine. Autonomic nerves also seem to be involved and it has been suggested that sympathetic nerve endings form contacts with the afferent nociceptive terminals to prevent the release of sensory neuropeptides by a preterminal inhibitory effect (48). The sympathetic nerves may also sprout in carious or inflamed teeth and their other mediator neuropeptide Y (NPY) is also able to prevent CGRP release from the nociceptive sensory nerve endings (17, 20, 54) and, in this way, inhibit the inflammatory reaction.

After heat injury, intradental nerves are sensitized and show ongoing firing and increased responses to thermal stimulation (1). The fact that the induced activation is inhibited by anti-inflammatory drugs indicates that the sensitization is mediated by prostaglandins (1). Serotonin has been shown to sensitize pulpal A-fibers (43, 45). After local application of serotonin into deep dentinal cavities, the responses of A-fibers to hydrodynamic stimulation of dentin are enhanced and they show ongoing activity (43). Bradykinin and histamine activate pulpal C-fibers (40, 43). The differential sensitivity of the intradental

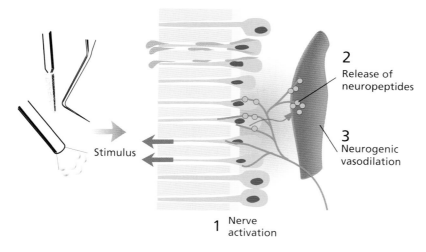

2
Release of
neuropeptides

3
Neurogenic
vasodilation

Stimulus

1 Nerve
activation

Fig. 3.6 Schematic drawing presenting the induction of neurogenic vasodilation and inflammation in the pulp/dentin border. Activation of the nociceptors by external stimulation results in nerve impulse conduction along all collateral endings of the same axon. Some of the endings are located adjacent to the blood vessels. In response to their activation, the terminals release sensory neuropeptides, which induce vasodilation and increase the permeability of the vessel wall.

A- and C-fibers to various inflammatory mediators may give an explanation of the changes in the type and intensity of the pain symptoms during the progress of pulpal inflammation. The conditions in the pulp tissue, such as alterations in the blood flow and consequently the amount of available oxygen, may also play a role. In general, the unmyelinated C-fibers are more resistant than the myelinated A-fibers to reduced oxygen pressure (18), and single-fiber recordings in cats suggest a similar difference in the intradental nerves (43). Moreover, lowered pH may favor activation of C-fibers via sensitization of TRPV1 receptors (21) and, in fact, recent electrophysiological recordings indicate that C-fibers get more active while the A-fiber activity is reduced in inflamed teeth of experimental animals (38).

Morphological versus functional changes of pulpal nerves in inflammation

In addition to nerve impulse transmission there is another, slower type of signaling between the nerve terminals in the peripheral tissues and the soma of the neuron via axonal transport. This process is bidirectional, including both antero- and retrograde transportation of various cytochemical signaling agents. It allows transmission of information regarding the conditions of the tissues around the nerve endings to the soma of the neuron (10). An injury to the nerve terminals and other tissue components in the pulp results in metabolic activation of the neurons in the trigeminal ganglion. As a result, various signaling molecules, receptors, mediators and modulators are synthesized and transported to the nerve endings in the injured tissue, where they take part in regulation of the inflammatory process and tissue repair (8, 10). Also, profound morphological changes take place in the peripheral nerve terminals (12). These changes are regulated by growth factors and other signaling molecules activated during the process (8, 10). It should also be noted that the action potential firing and the transport of signal molecules into the central nervous system result in discrete cytochemical changes in the second-order neurons of the brain stem (13), which may be related to central sensitization with an increased nociceptive impulse transmission in the trigeminal pain pathways.

The sensory neuropeptides, CGRP and substance P, present in the afferent nerves of normal healthy tissues (8–12) seem to be confined to the fine-caliber pain-mediating afferents (10, 18). It is also indicated that the neuropeptides are predominantly located in the unmyelinated C-fibers and that some small Aδ-fibers are CGRP immunoreactive (31, 35, 48).

Morphological changes shown to take place in response to injury and inflammation in the intradental nerve endings include an increase in their neuropeptide content and sprouting of the nerve terminals (8, 9). As already mentioned, the sensory neuropeptides are able to induce vasodilation and an increase in the permeability of the vessel walls (47, 48). Such vascular reactions are an essential part of the inflammatory reaction and are necessary to satisfy the nutritional needs related to the increased metabolic activity in connection with tissue repair and healing. The above-described structural neural responses are probably important for tissue repair because they allow more effective regulatory function of the nerve terminals in the healing process (11, 12; Key literature 3.1). Also, the time course of the morphological changes in the nerve terminals indicates that they are an essential part of the tissue responses. They are obvious within a couple of days after the insult in the rat molars and they disappear concomitantly with tissue repair and resolution of the insult in reversible cases (8, 9).

The experimental findings regarding the functional correlates of the morphological changes in the pulpal nociceptors described above are limited. Considering the extent of the changes, they may have important effects on the tooth sensitivity. Electrophysiological studies indicate that the receptive fields of single intradental nerve fibers in inflamed dog teeth are wider than in uninflamed controls (44) (Fig. 3.7). Such a change correlates with the morphological findings showing sprouting of the axon terminals (8, 9). Along with the expansion, overlap of the receptive fields of single afferents in dentin is increased, resulting in an increase in the number of fibers activated by stimulation of any particular area in dentin (Fig. 3.7). Accordingly, such changes may contribute to increased dentin sensitivity in inflamed teeth (42, 44).

Electrophysiological experiments have shown that in inflamed teeth the proportion of A-fibers that respond to dentinal stimulation is increased significantly (44), especially in slowly conducting A-δ fibers (44). Many of these fibers are "silent" under normal conditions but seem to become active as a result of the inflammatory reaction (44). The change may be caused by sprouting and consequent formation of new nerve endings and also by sensitization of the original nerve terminals by the

Key literature 3.1

Byers and Taylor (12) (see also: Byers, Suzuki and Maeda; 11) compared the responses after pulp exposure in denervated and normally innervated rat molars and found that the absence of sensory nerves affected the tissue response significantly. Six days after occlusal pulp exposure, the denervated teeth showed more advanced pulp necrosis and less remaining vascular, vital pulp tissue compared with the control teeth with normal sensory innervation. The results indicate that the existence of intact sensory innervation with its responses to tissue injury may be important for regulation of the inflammatory response and consequently for tissue defense and repair reactions in the pulp.

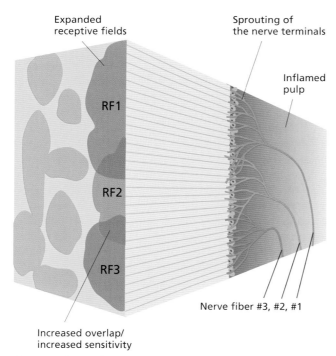

Expanded receptive fields

Sprouting of the nerve terminals

Inflamed pulp

RF1

RF2

RF3

Nerve fiber #3, #2, #1

Increased overlap/ increased sensitivity

Fig. 3.7 Schematic drawing showing receptive fields of the same intradental nerve fibers as presented in Fig. 3.4. Terminal sprouting of three fibers (fibers 1, 2 and 3) in the pulp/dentin border is shown on the right and consequently the receptive fields (RF1, RF2 and RF3) on the dentin surface have expanded and show increased overlap (cf. Fig. 3.4).

inflammatory mediators. Activation of the "silent" nociceptors may significantly increase the sensitivity of the affected teeth.

Local control of pulpal nociceptor activation

A puzzling clinical finding is that pulpitis may often result in total pulp necrosis without any symptoms. Recent studies have revealed a number of local mediators in the peripheral tissues that regulate the inflammatory process and consequently the sensitivity of the nociceptors (48, 56). In the dental pulp, for example, peripheral endogenous opioids, somatostatin and noradrenaline have been suggested to possess such effects (10, 19, 44, 48). As already mentioned another mediator of the sympathetic fibers seems to inhibit the release of CGRP and, thus, may slow down the inflammatory reaction and nociceptor activation (17, 20, 54). It is indicated that the release of the mediators is closely linked to specific steps in the inflammatory process and is regulated by a negative feedback loop (48). The inhibitory factors may be needed to attenuate the inflammatory reaction and at the same time they inhibit the activation of the pulpal nociceptors. In addition, environmental changes

due to alterations in local blood flow are able to modify the responsiveness of the intradental nerves (43, 46).

In addition to the described local factors in the pulp tissue itself, a large number of chemical agents released from carious lesions in decayed teeth and diffusing from the dentin surface through patent tubules may modulate nerve activity (46). Thus, numerous local mechanisms may affect the activation of the intradental nerves and contribute to the wide variability of pulpitis symptoms.

Dentin hypersensitivity

Dentin hypersensitivity is a pain condition that develops following exposure of dentin surfaces. The condition is most often located in the cervical area of the tooth (6, 42, 50) and can be a considerable clinical problem. Typically, patients complain of a sharp or shooting pain that is induced by cold foods or drinks, tooth cleaning or even a light touch of the exposed dentin surface (42, 50, 61). The pain symptoms can be extremely intense, continue for years and thus have great impact on the patient's everyday life. The condition and main features of sensitive dentin, as well as the hydrodynamic nerve activation mechanism as the basis for dentin sensitivity, have been described in detail in an earlier section on dentin sensitivity. The following text will focus on the factors that may prolong the condition, especially the role of inflammatory mechanisms and neural effects.

In favorable cases the repair reactions of the pulp–dentin complex in response to dentin exposure usually lead to a gradual tubule block by intratubular mineralization and/or irritation dentin formation to protect the pulp, leading to natural desensitization of dentin. However, sometimes the dentinal tubules may stay open and the sensitivity of dentin is maintained (6, 42, 50). Such variation in the local responses in dentin is poorly understood. It may be due to a compromised defense capability of the pulp tissue or to intense and continuous external irritation. Possible differences in the repair reactions in the coronal versus cervical pulp–dentin complex may explain why persistent symptoms of dentin hypersensitivity are often found in the cervical and root areas but rarely in the coronal dentin (42, 50). In this respect the structure of the intradental innervation is interesting, showing a dense network of nerve endings in the crown (7); the afferent nerves may play an important role in the repair and defense reactions of the pulp and dentinal mineralization (11, 12, 25). Also, the time course of the dentin exposure may be significant. Gingival recession in the cervical area may cause much faster exposure compared with that caused by attrition on the occlusal or incisal tooth surfaces and thus not allow sufficient time for favorable repair reactions to take place in the pulp. If the dentinal tubules remain open, it may result in an inflammatory reaction in the pulp (6) and a more or less persistent pain condition.

The method of choice in the treatment of dentinal pain would be blocking of the patent tubules. The action mechanism of a number of products marketed for hypersensitive dentin is based on this principle but in some cases dentin sensitivity may remain even when the tubules have been blocked completely (42). This may be an indication of pulpal inflammation and consequent sensitization of the intradental nociceptors. Thus, the products used in the clinic for the treatment of dentin hypersensitivity may, in some cases, have diagnostic value in the discrimination of inflamed teeth.

Exposed dentin with patent tubules is sensitive if the underlying pulp is vital. The definition "hypersensitive dentin" would implicate that dentin can be more sensitive than normal and it is tempting to state this, considering how extremely intense the dentinal pain responses sometimes can be (42). In fact, the electrophysiological and morphological studies presented above give support to this concept. Namely, local application of serotonin in healthy teeth can increase the sensitivity of intradental A-fibers to dentinal stimulation (42, 43). Moreover, morphological and functional changes showing sprouting of the pulp nerve terminals (8–12), expansion of the receptive fields of pulpal A-fibers (10, 44) and activation of "silent" nociceptors (44) may contribute to an increase in dentin sensitivity in inflamed teeth. Accordingly, in teeth with hypersensitive dentin, pulpal inflammatory reactions may play a significant role in the development and maintenance of the pain symptoms. It should be noted, however, that the above neural changes are reversible. They can be resolved if the pulpal irritation can be abolished and consequently the inflammatory reaction attenuated (8, 9). Thus, effective tubule block may contribute to the reduction of dentin sensitivity both directly, by reducing the hydraulic conductance, and indirectly, by allowing resolution of the pulpal neural changes induced by inflammation.

Central nervous system mechanisms

Both structural and functional changes in the central nervous system take place following peripheral nociceptor activation in response to tissue injury and inflammation. These changes become more prominent in long-lasting pain and may result in persistent alterations in those parts of the pain pathways that participate in the regulation of pain impulse transmission from the periphery to the higher centers of the brain. Results from psychophysiological studies and neurophysiological experiments indicate that central regulation is also important in various dental pain conditions.

The human experiments of Sigurdsson and Maixner (55) showed that radiation of the pain in pulpitis is via secondary hyperalgesia due to central sensitization. By conditioning painful stimulation of the arm, the secondary hyperalgesia could be abolished and the primary source of the pain more accurately localized.

Electrophysiological studies have shown that noxious stimulation of teeth results in discrete cytochemical responses in the second-order neurons of the trigeminal brain stem nuclei mediating orofacial pain (12, 13). These morphological changes are obvious within a few hours after stimulation of the peripheral nociceptors and may represent the first signs of initial sensitization of the central pain pathways. Injuries to the dental nerves caused by tooth extractions and pulpotomies have been shown to induce long-lasting functional changes in the trigeminal brain stem neurons (53). The neurons show increased spontaneous activity and expansion of their peripheral receptive fields, indicating that they have formed connections to peripheral neurons that do not normally activate them.

In summary, it is indicated that inflammation and injury in the peripheral tissues may result in changes in impulse transmission in the central pain pathways. It is not known exactly to what extent the central mechanisms play a role in dental pain conditions but they may be significant, especially in cases of long-lasting pain.

Pain symptoms and pulpal diagnosis

At its worst, pulpitis can cause extremely intense pain. On the other hand, it is a common clinical finding that a large number of teeth develop total pulp necrosis without being painful and with no symptoms (6). As described above, local mechanisms affecting nociceptor activation in the pulp (10, 44, 48) and regulation of the impulse transmission in the central nervous system (55) have significant modulatory effects on the development of pain in pulpitis. The poor correlation between the pain symptoms and the actual condition of the pulp in inflamed teeth has been established in histopathological studies (6, 52). From a diagnostic point of view, the great variation of symptomology in pulpal inflammation is important to note (see Chapters 4 and 14).

The nerve fibers in the pulp may maintain their structural identity even in advanced pulpitis where there is considerable destruction of the other components of the pulp tissue (57). It is not known if the remaining axons are capable of impulse transmission under such conditions but clinical experience shows that pain can be evoked in connection with endodontic treatment of teeth where most of the pulp tissue is necrotic. Comparison of the electrical thresholds of single intradental nerve fibers and those of human teeth also indicates that activation of only a few intradental axons is sufficient to evoke pre-pain or pain sensations in human teeth (39, 43). With pulp diagnosis such results are significant because they indicate that a few surviving nerve fibers in a pulp with advanced tissue necrosis may give a positive sensory response to dental stimulation. Thus, evoked sensations in response to electrical stimulation with a pulp tester do not necessarily mean that the pulp is healthy. In fact, dentin can be sensitive in spite of considerable tissue damage in the underlying pulp tissue (6). All these findings indicate that the correlation between the dental sensory responses and the condition of the pulp tissue is poor. Accordingly, it should be noted that pain symptoms are not a reliable basis for pulp diagnostics.

In inflammatory lesions, mediators such as histamine and bradykinin activate C-fibers (40, 43). After reduction of the pulpal blood flow by periapical adrenaline injections they maintain their functional capacity better than A-fibers (35), where the impulse conduction is blocked, probably because of hypoxia in the pulp tissue. This means that during the progress of pulpitis, pulpal C-fibers may maintain their capability for nerve impulse conduction longer than A-fibers. In fact, they can become even more active in the advanced stages of pulpal inflammation owing to their susceptibility to inflammatory mediators and lowered pH (21). The functional properties of the two pulp nerve fiber groups may explain the changes in the quality of pain symptoms during pulpitis: from rather sharp or shooting and quite well localized, to dull and lingering. Thus, the type and duration of symptoms in patients with pulpal inflammation are of diagnostic value and may give some indication of the pulp's condition. However, it must be underlined again that the correlation between the symptoms and histopathological changes in pulpitis is poor and determination of the type and extent of the inflammatory changes on the basis of the symptomology is inaccurate.

References

1. Ahlberg KF. Dose dependent inhibition of sensory nerve activity in the feline dental pulp by antiinflammatory drugs. *Acta Physiol. Scand.* 1978; 102: 434–40.
2. Ahlquist ML, Franzen OG, Edwall LGA, Fors UG, Haegerstam GAT. Quality of pain sensations following local application of algogenic agents on the exposed human tooth pulp: a psychophysiological and electrophysiological study. In: *Advances in Pain Research and Therapy* (Fields HL, ed), vol. 9. New York: Raven Press, 1985; 351–9.
3. Anderson DJ. Chemical and osmotic excitants of pain in human dentine. In: *Sensory Mechanisms in Dentine* (Anderson DJ, ed.). Oxford: Pergamon Press, 1963; 88–93.
4. Avery JK, Rapp R. An investigation of the mechanism of neural impulse transmission in human teeth. *Oral Surg.* 1959; 12: 190–98.
5. Brännström M. A hydrodynamic mechanism in the transmission of pain-producing stimuli through the dentine. In: *Sensory Mechanisms in Dentine* (Anderson DJ, ed.). Oxford: Pergamon Press, 1963; 73–9.
6. Brännström M. *Dentine and Pulp in Restorative Dentistry.* Nacka, Sweden: Dental Therapeutics AB, 1981.
   This book gives an extensive description of different aspects regarding the responses of the pulp–dentin complex to clinical procedures. Dentine sensitivity and dental pain in general are discussed in detail in relation to pulp tissue reactions and pulp diagnosis.
7. Byers MR. Dental sensory receptors. *Int. Rev. Neurobiol.* 1984; 25: 39–94.
   This is a review paper describing the structure of the dental innervation. The morphology of both pulpal and periodontal nerves and receptors is presented and discussed in relation to the functional aspects.
8. Byers MR. Effect of inflammation on dental sensory nerves and vice versa. *Proc. Finn. Dent. Soc.* 1992; 88 (Suppl. 1): 459–506.
9. Byers MR. Neuropeptide immunoreactivity in dental sensory nerves: variation related to primary odontoblast function and survival. In: *Dentine/Pulp Complex* (Shimono M, Maeda T, Suda H, Takahashi K, eds). Tokyo: Quintessence, 1996; 124–9.
10. Byers MR, Närhi M. Dental injury models: experimental tools for understanding neuroinflammatory interactions and polymodal nociceptor function. *Crit. Rev. Oral Biol. Med.* 1999; 10: 4–39.
    This paper presents a comprehensive review on morphological and functional aspects of dental nociceptors. In particular, neural responses to injury and inflammation are covered. The activation mechanisms and afferent functions of the intradental nerves in the mediation of nociceptive information to the brain are presented. The role of the nociceptors in regulation of the inflammatory and repair reactions in the pulp tissue is also described. In addition, the use of intradental nerve stimulation as a pain model and the application of the dental injury models to study the polymodal nociceptor function and neurogenic inflammatory reactions are discussed.
11. Byers MR, Suzuki H, Maeda T. Dental neuroplasticity, neuro-pulpal interactions, and nerve regeneration. *Microsc. Res. Tech.* 2003; 60: 503–15.
12. Byers MR, Taylor PE. Effect of sensory denervation on the response of rat molar pulp to exposure injury. *J. Dent. Res.* 1993; 72: 613–18.
13. Chattipakorn SC, Light AR, Willcockson HH, Närhi M, Maixner W. The effect of fentanyl on *c-fos* expression in the trigeminal brain stem complex produced by pulpal heat stimulation in the ferret. *Pain* 1999; 82: 207–15.
14. Coimbra F, Coimbra A. Dental noxious input reaches the subnucleus caudalis of the trigeminal complex in the rat, as shown by c-fos expression upon thermal or mechanical stimulation. *Neurosci. Lett.* 1994; 173: 201–4.
15. Davidson RM. Neural form of voltage-dependent sodium current in human cultured dental pulp cells. *Arch. Oral Biol.* 1994; 39: 613–20.
16. Edwall L, Olgart L. A new technique for recording of intradental sensory nerve activity in man. *Pain* 1977; 3: 121–6.
    This is the first report on intradental nerve recording in human subjects. The action potentials were recorded from dentin. The nerve responses to dental stimulation were related to pain

responses reported by the subjects. The results show that intradental nerves are able to conduct nociceptive information.

17. El Karim IA, Lamey PJ, Linden GJ, Awawadeh LA, Lundy FT. Caries-induced changes in the expression of pulpal neuropeptide Y. *Eur. J. Oral Sci.* 2006; 114: 133–7.

18. Franco-Cereceda A, Henke H, Lundberg JM, Petermann JB, Hökfelt T, Fischer JA. Calcitonin gene-related peptide (CGRP) in capsaicin-sensitive substance P-immunoreactive sensory neurons in animals and man: distribution and release by capsaicin. *Peptides* 1987; 8: 399–410.

19. Fristad I, Bergreen E, Haug SR. Delta opioid receptors in small and medium-sized trigeminal neurons. *Arch. Oral Biol.* 2006; 51: 273–81.

20. Gibbs JL, Hargreaves KM. Neuropeptide Y Y1 receptor effects on pulpal nociceptors. *J. Dent Res.* 2008; 87: 948–52.

21. Goodis HE, Poon A, Hargreaves KM. Tissue pH and temperature regulate pulpal nociceptors. *J. Dent. Res.* 2006; 85: 1046–9.

22. Guyton AC, Hall JE. *Textbook of Medical Physiology.* Philadelphia, PA: Elsevier–Saunders, 2006.

23. Gysi A. An attempt to explain the sensitiveness of dentine. *Br. J. Dent. Sci.* 1900; 43: 865–8.

24. Haug SR, Heyeraas KJ. Modulation of dental inflammation by the sympathetic nervous system. *J. Dent. Res.* 2006; 85: 488–95.

25. Heyeraas KJ, Haug SR, Bukoski RD, Awumey EM. Identification of Ca^{2+}-sensing receptor in rat trigeminal ganglia, sensory axons and tooth dental pulp. *Calcif. Tisue Int.* 2008; 82: 57–65.

26. Hirvonen TJ. A quantitative electron-microscopic analysis of the axons at the apex of the canine tooth pulp in the dog. *Acta Anat.* 1987; 128: 134–9.

27. Hirvonen T, Närhi M. The effect of dentinal stimulation on pulp nerve function and pulp morphology in the dog. *J. Dent. Res.* 1986; 65: 1290–3.

28. Holland GR. Odontoblasts and nerves; just friends. *Proc. Finn. Dent. Soc.* 1986; 82: 179–89.

29. Holland GR, Robinson PP. The number and size of axons at the apex of the cat's canine tooth. *Anat. Rec.* 1983; 205: 215–22.

30. Jyväsjärvi E, Kniffki K-D. Cold stimulation of teeth: a comparison between the responses of cat intradental A and C fibres and human sensation. *J. Physiol.* 1987; 391: 193–207.

31. Lawson SN. Peptides and cutaneous polymodal nociceptor neurones. *Prog. Brain Res.* 1996; 113: 369–86.

32. Lilja J. Sensory differences between crown and root dentin in human teeth. *Acta Odontol. Scand.* 1980; 38: 285–91.

33. Lilja J, Nordenvall K-J, Brännström M. Dentine sensitivity, odontoblasts and nerves under desiccated or infected experimental cavities. *Swed. Dent. J.* 1982; 6: 93–103.

34. Lundberg JM. Peptidergic control of the autonomic regulation system in the orofacial region. *Proc. Finn. Dent. Soc.* 1989; 85: 239–50.

35. Maggi CA, Meli A. The sensory-efferent function of capsaicin-sensitive sensory neurons. *Gen. Pharmacol.* 1988; 19: 1–43.

36. Magloire H, Vinard H, Joffre A. Electrophysiological properties of human dental pulp cells. *J. Biol. Bucc.* 1979; 7: 251–62.

37. Matthews B, Baxter J, Watts S. Sensory and reflex responses to tooth pulp stimulation in man. *Brain Res.* 1976; 113: 83–94.

38. Modaresi J, Dianat O, Soluti A. Effect of pulpal inflammation on nerve impulse quality with or without anesthesia. *J. Endod.* 2008; 34: 438–41.

39. Mumford JM, Bowsher D. Pain and prothopatic sensibility. A review with particular reference to teeth. *Pain* 1976; 2: 223–43.

40. Närhi MVO. The characteristics of intradental sensory units and their responses to stimulation. *J. Dent. Res.* 1985; 64: 564–71.

41. Närhi M, Kontturi-Närhi V. Sensitivity and surface condition of dentin – a SEM-replica study (abstract). *J. Dent Res.* 1994; 73: 122.

42. Närhi M, Kontturi-Närhi V, Hirvonen T, Ngassapa D. Neurophysiological mechanisms of dentin hypersensitivity. *Proc. Finn. Dent. Soc.* 1992; 88 (Suppl. 1): 15–22.

43. Närhi M, Jyväsjärvi E, Virtanen A, Huopaniemi T, Ngassapa D, Hirvonen T. Role of intradental A- and C-type nerve fibres in dental pain mechanisms. *Proc. Finn. Dent. Soc.* 1992; 88 (Suppl. 1): 507–16.

44. Närhi M, Yamamoto H, Ngassapa D. Function of intradental nociceptors in normal and inflamed teeth. In: *Dentine/ Pulp Complex* (Shimono M, Maeda T, Suda H, Takahashi K, eds). Tokyo: Quintessence Publishing, 1996; 136–40.

45. Olgart L. Excitation of intradental sensory units by pharmacological agents. *Acta Physiol. Scand.* 1974; 92: 48–55.

46. Olgart L. The role of local factors in dentin and pulp in intradental pain mechanisms. *J. Dent. Res.* 1985; 64: 572–8.

47. Olgart L. Neural control of pulpal blood flow. *Crit. Rev. Oral Biol. Med.* 1996; 7: 159–71.

48. Olgart L. Neurogenic components of pulp inflammation. In: *Dentine/Pulp Complex* (Shimono M, Maeda T, Suda H, Takahashi K, eds). Tokyo: Quintessence Publishing, 1996; 169–75.

    The afferent nociceptive nerve fibers also have important efferent function in neurogenic regulation of inflammatory and repair reactions in their target tissues. This review paper describes these inflammatory mechanisms, including the mediators involved.

49. Olgart L, Gazelius B, Sundström F. Intradental nerve activity and jaw-opening reflex in response to mechanical deformation of cat teeth. *Acta Physiol. Scand.* 1988; 133: 399–406.

50. Pashley DH. Mechanisms of dentine sensitivity. *Dent. Clin. North Am.* 1990; 34: 449–73.

51. Scott D Jr, Tempel TR. A study in the excitation of dental pulp nerve fibres. In: *Sensory Mechanisms in Dentine* (Anderson DJ, ed.). Oxford: Pergamon Press, 1963; 27–46.

52. Seltzer S, Bender IB, Ziontz M. The dynamics of pulp inflammation: correlations between diagnostic data and actual histopathological findings in the pulp. *Oral Surg. Oral Med. Oral Pathol.* 1963; 16: 969–77.

    In the early 1960s the research group of Dr Seltzer and Dr Bender showed a definite poor correlation between the clinical pain symptoms and the actual histopathological condition of the pulp. The present paper is one of their significant series of studies regarding pulp diagnostics.

53. Sessle BJ. The neurobiology of facial and dental pain: present knowledge, future directions. *J. Dent. Res.* 1987; 66: 962–81.

54. Shimeno Y, Sugawara Y, Iikubo M, Shoji N, Sasano T. Sympathetic nerve fibers sprout into rat odontoblast layer but not into dentinal tubules in response to cavity preparation. *Neurosci. Lett.* 2008; 435: 73–7.

55. Sigurdsson A, Maixner W. Effects of experimental clinical noxious counterirritants on pain perception. *Pain* 1994; 57: 265–75.

56. Stein C. Peripheral mechanisms of opioid analgesia. *Anesth. Analg.* 1993; 76: 182–91.

   It has been thought that opioids, e.g. morphine, have only central effects. This paper presents evidence that they can inhibit nociceptor activation in the peripheral tissues.

57. Torneck CD. Changes in the fine structure of human dental pulp subsequent to caries exposure. *J. Oral Pathol.* 1977; 6: 82–95.

58. Vongsavan N, Matthews B. The relationship between fluid flow in dentine and the discharge of intradental nerves. *Arch. Oral Biol.* 1994; 39: 140S.

59. Vongsavan N, Matthews B. The relationship between the discharge of intradental nerves and the rate of fluid flow through dentine in the cat. *Arch. Oral Biol.* 2007; 52: 640–7.

60. Wells JE, Bingham V, Rowland KC, Hatton J. Expression of Nav1.9 channels in human dental pulp and trigeminal ganglion. *J. Endod.* 2007; 33: 1172–6.

61. West NX. Dentine hypersensitivity. *Monogr. Oral Sci.* 2006; 20: 173–89.

62. Yamamoto H, Narhi M. Function of nerve fibres innervating different parts of dentine. *Arch. Oral Biol.* 1994; 39: 141S.

Chapter 4
Treatment of vital pulp conditions

Preben Hørsted-Bindslev and Gunnar Bergenholtz

Introduction

A multitude of harmful elements, alone or in combination, may cause adverse reactions in the dental pulp under clinical conditions (Fig. 4.1; see also Chapter 2). If not properly managed they may result in:

- painful pulpitis;
- pulp tissue breakdown (pulp necrosis);
- root canal infection, leading to periapical inflammatory lesion (apical periodontitis).

These effects are the result of inflammation and associated tissue destruction. Tissue destruction *per se* is a basic feature of inflammation in general and is a means by which the host carries out an effective defense against foreign matter, including bacteria and bacterial elements. However, as far as the pulp is concerned it can be devastating and result in total breakdown of the tissue.

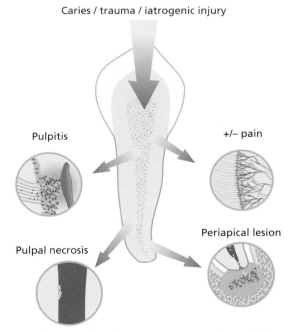

Caries / trauma / iatrogenic injury

Pulpitis

+/– pain

Periapical lesion

Pulpal necrosis

Fig. 4.1 Adverse pulpal reactions to caries, trauma or iatrogenic injury.

Infection and inflammation in the periapical tissue (see Chapter 7) frequently follow such an event, termed pulp necrosis. Vital pulp therapy involves clinical procedures aimed at:

- relieving painful symptoms of pulpitis;
- preventing the development of a destructive course of pulpal inflammation and subsequent infection of the root canal space.

In this chapter the rationales for the clinical procedures employed and the techniques and the materials applied to attain these objectives are described.

Clinical scenarios

Any direct exposure of the pulp to the oral environment involves the risk of destructive inflammatory breakdown (Fig. 4.2). It should be noted that a pulpal wound has little self-healing capacity unless properly treated. In contrast to the skin and mucosal tissues, where cuts or wounds normally heal within a short period of time, the pulp has no epithelia that can bridge the defect. This means that even a small exposure may present the bacterial flora of the oral cavity with the potential to cause a destructive and irreversible (non-healing) inflammatory condition.

Exposure of the pulp may result from caries, fracture, crack and inadvertent deep cavity and crown preparation. Although caries progresses at a fairly slow pace, the other injuries cause a sudden and immediate exposure of the tissue. This is significant from a therapeutic point of view. For example, after a longstanding exposure to caries the pulp may already be in a compromised state such that healing and repair are not possible, making it necessary for radical removal. On the other hand, on a recent fracture or deep cavity and crown preparation, a fairly healthy pulpal tissue is often challenged and the potential for a conservative tissue-saving procedure is more promising. This is especially true if the injury is treated without delay. If an exposure by crack, fracture or deep cavity is left untreated or undiagnosed, an acute

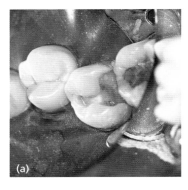
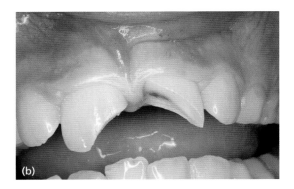
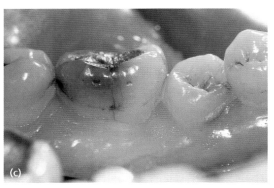
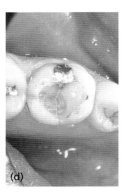

Fig. 4.2 Examples of clinical conditions requiring vital pulp therapy: (a) pulpal tissue directly exposed during excavation of caries; (b) pulpal tissue directly exposed by trauma; (c) non-exposed pulp but tooth presents with pain and there is a crack line on the lingual surface; (d) following removal of the filling, the crack continues through the pulpal wall.

inflammatory reaction ensues, which may result in a non-healing lesion.

Pulpal inflammatory lesions of a destructive nature may also appear without direct exposure of the tissue to the oral environment. Such cases can be seen in conjunction with a restorative treatment, which often is carried out within a fairly short period of time (weeks, months) prior to the onset of the symptoms. The cause may be related to the injury induced in the pulp by the restorative procedure and leakage of bacterial elements through gaps along the margins of the restoration (see Chapter 2).

Inflammatory changes of the pulp may occur with or without pain. The pain symptoms vary and, in their end stages, prior to pulpal breakdown, can be excruciating, requiring immediate attention. Symptoms suggestive of a more or less severe pulpal inflammatory involvement are summarized in Core concept 4.1.

Treatment options

In cases where the pulp has become directly exposed to the oral environment, the clinician may consider one of two treatment strategies. One approach is conservative and aims to preserve the pulp and re-establish non-painful and healthy conditions in the long term (Figs 4.3 and 4.4). The other is a procedure whereby the entire tissue is radically removed and replaced with a root canal filling (Fig. 4.5).

> **Core concept 4.1   Pain symptoms commonly associated with a pulpal inflammatory lesion**
>
> - Increased sensitivity elicited by exposure to cold drinks, food and air or touch of an exposed dentin surface may be early signs of pulpal inflammation. These symptoms are usually not suggestive of an advanced lesion. In the context of a recent restorative or periodontal treatment, such symptoms may emerge shortly after the procedure but often subside along with recovery of the tissue.
> - Short, intermittent periods of lingering pain (seconds to minutes) by exposure to cold drinks, food and air may be signs of a pulpal inflammatory lesion in progress. Nevertheless, such symptoms may prevail for long periods of time (months, years) without resulting in pulp necrosis.
> - Longstanding (hours) severe pain, spontaneous or intermittently provoked by external stimuli, including hot food and drinks, is an alarming sign suggestive of an irreversible (non-healing) pulp condition.

Prior to a definitive treatment, a preoperative emergency treatment may have to be carried out. Such a treatment is usually called for to alleviate a severely painful tooth or to maintain an accidental pulpal exposure.

Vital pulp treatments include:

- *Stepwise excavation*, which refers to a procedure whereby caries is excavated in a stepwise fashion in order to prevent iatrogenic pulpal exposure. This procedure may be used in situations of deep caries

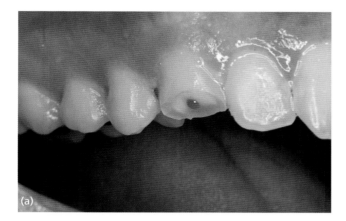

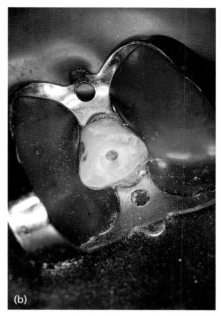

Fig. 4.3 (a) Clinical photograph of a pulp exposed to the oral cavity following a crown fracture by trauma. Pulp has been exposed for approximately 1 day. (b) The superficial portion of the pulp has been removed to prepare the site for a partial pulpotomy procedure.

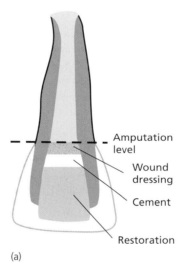

- - - Amputation level

Wound dressing

Cement

Restoration

(a)

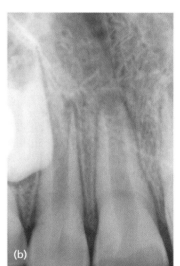

Fig. 4.4 Pulpotomy is a partial removal of pulpal tissue, also termed pulp amputation. (a) The tissue is normally cut level with the root canal orifices in two- and multirooted teeth. In teeth with one root canal, tissue may be removed to the level of the cementoenamel junction. (b–d) Radiographs of a treated upper incisor: (b) coronal fracture in tooth 11 with incomplete root formation; (c) deposit of calcium hydroxide after removal of coronal pulp; (d) root filling after completion of the root. In general, the pulpotomized tooth is followed radiographically and a root filling is not normally required. (Courtesy of Dr M. Cvek.)

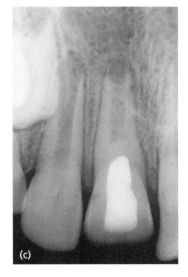

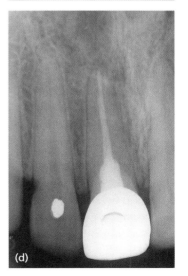

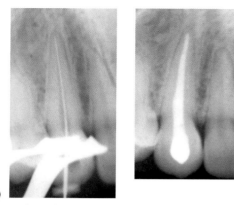

(a)

(b)

Fig. 4.5 Radiographs showing: (a) an instrument in the root canal of an upper canine in conjunction with a pulpectomy procedure; (b) the instrumented canal that has been filled.

without signs of irreversible inflammatory changes in the pulp (see Chapter 5).

- *Indirect pulp capping* is a term used for a procedure where residual caries is permanently left in the cavity (see Chapter 5).
- *Direct pulp capping/partial pulpotomy.* These procedures are aimed at maintaining the pulp after it has become exposed to the oral environment (Fig. 4.3a). The open exposure is sealed off by the use of an appropriate wound dressing. The purpose of the seal is to prevent access of bacterial organisms in the oral cavity and to promote soft-tissue healing and hard-tissue repair of the exposed area. In pulp capping there is no removal of pulpal tissue, whereas in a partial pulpotomy some pulpal tissue is removed at the exposure site to a depth of ca. 1–2 mm (Fig. 4.3b). This measure is carried out to clean the wound of infected tissue and to prepare a space for the wound dressing so that it can be applied securely (for a detailed description of the technique, see further below and Chapter 5).
- *Pulpotomy* is a term used for partial removal of diseased pulp tissue. The procedure is often carried out in teeth with incomplete root formation, and for this reason pulpectomy cannot be performed. Pulp is normally cut level with the canal orifices in two- and multirooted teeth and to the level of the cemento-enamel junction in teeth with a single root canal (Fig. 4.4). The remaining pulp tissue is covered with wound dressing. The aim of this procedure is to maintain the pulp of the root portion vital and functioning so that root development can be completed (see also Chapter 5). The term apexogenesis is sometimes used for this procedure. In fully developed teeth, pulpotomy is often carried out as a temporary measure on an emergency basis until time is available for pulpectomy.
- *Pulpectomy* is an invasive procedure where the pulp tissue is removed until 1–2 mm from the anatomical

apex by root canal instruments and subsequently replaced with a root filling (Fig. 4.5). A more detailed description of this treatment is given below.

Factors influencing choice of treatment

It is a most difficult task for a clinician to advocate the proper treatment when a pulp is exposed or when clinical signs and symptoms suggest inflammatory involvement. A conservative measure saves effort, time and money, whereas a pulpectomy, especially in the posterior tooth region, is often a technically demanding and time-consuming procedure. This is why direct pulp capping has enjoyed some popularity over the years for the management of pulp exposures: it is non-invasive, easy to carry out and normally does not require an elaborate dental restoration afterwards. Nevertheless, a pulpectomy is the treatment of choice when the prognosis for pulpal survival is deemed questionable. If the pulp is assumed to be in an irreversible condition, a pulpectomy is always to be preferred in a fully developed tooth. The treatment is predictable and eliminates the risk for subsequent inflammatory breakdown of the tissue and associated infections and painful events. If a tooth is incompletely developed, pulpectomy is precarious and pulpotomy serves as the alternative treatment (Fig. 4.4; Core concept 4.2).

In young individuals with incompletely developed roots, preservation of as much pulp tissue as possible is essential. This allows for continued development of the tooth structure. A pulpectomy, by eliminating the soft tissue of the pulp, prevents further growth and leaves a weakened tooth that is vulnerable to fracture. Cvek (19) reported that there is a close linear relationship between the degree of root closure in teeth where the pulp is lost

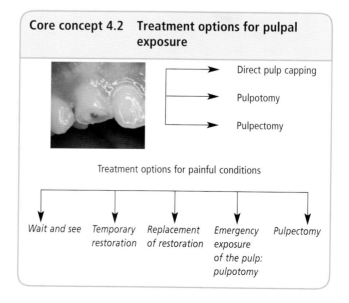

Core concept 4.2   Treatment options for pulpal exposure

→ Direct pulp capping

→ Pulpotomy

→ Pulpectomy

Treatment options for painful conditions

Wait and see | Temporary restoration | Replacement of restoration | Emergency exposure of the pulp: pulpotomy | Pulpectomy

and the rate of intra-alveolar fracture over time. In very immature roots the frequency of fracture was as high as 80% within 3–4 years after root canal therapy.

Pulpectomy not only eliminates the pulp but requires the sacrifice of hard tissue as well. Often the loss has to be larger than that initiated by the injury itself. This is because the treatment requires access to the root canal system and sufficient removal of the canal walls to allow proper filling. Inevitably this will reduce the resistance of the tooth to fracture by mastication forces (74). It also means that after completion of the procedure a rather extensive restoration is needed (see Chapter 19).

In conclusion, the time, effort, sacrifice of tooth structure and costs for a pulpectomy are greater than those for a pulp capping or partial pulpotomy procedure. Yet, critical to the choice of therapy is how the case presents itself and how that is deemed to affect the potential for pulpal survival upon a conservative tissue-saving measure. Therefore, the decision to carry out an invasive procedure or not must be based on a careful analysis of the clinical information that can be gained from the disease history and clinical examination of the patient.

Assessment of the preoperative condition of the pulp

Diagnostic criteria of an irreversibly injured pulp are by no means clear-cut. In fact, there are no objective means available, at present, by which the true condition of the pulp can be decided by, for example, a blood or tissue sample. Two conditions are used to guide the clinician:

1. The presence and character of painful symptoms.
2. The presence and type of pulp exposure.

Core concept 4.1 summarizes the typical pain symptoms associated with pulpal inflammation. Although lingering pain, provoked by external stimuli, is often used to suggest an irreversible condition, studies have failed to find a strong correlation of such a symptom complex with the true condition of the pulp (6, 75). In these studies pulps were examined histologically after recording pain history and extraction of the teeth. It was found that report of severe pain was not necessarily associated with an advanced inflammatory breakdown of the pulp, and vice versa. Hence, a rather severe pulp condition could have appeared without being accompanied by pain. Conversely, severe pulpal pain was sometimes present on rather modest tissue changes. Consequently, comparative studies have shown pain to be a rather weak predictor of the condition of the pulp, whether reversibly or irreversibly inflamed.

Nevertheless, the existence of a history of pain and the character of the pain presentation are crucial clinical manifestations because the mere presence of pain prompts a therapeutic decision. If combined with deep

> ### Key literature 4.1
>
> In his classical clinical study Nyborg (56) prospectively followed a series of 225 cases that had been pulp capped due to exposure in conjunction with excavation of caries. The follow-up period varied from 10 months to 13 years. At recalls, teeth were examined both clinically and radiographically for evidence of pulpal breakdown (painful symptoms and/or signs of apical periodontitis). Eighty-one teeth were assessed histologically. Of the teeth that were asymptomatic at the time of treatment, the success rate was substantially higher (85%) than if patients had experienced pain prior to capping. Of the latter category, only 9 of 20 teeth were deemed to have a healthy pulp at the final follow-up. The study revealed that many teeth that were clinically without signs of pulpal pathology displayed severe inflammatory changes on histological examination.

caries, cracked tooth, fracture or recent restorative procedure, a progressing inflammatory lesion may be imminent and an invasive therapy by pulpectomy would be required. This view is supported by the observation that pulp capping of carious exposures was less successful in patients displaying painful symptoms than in patients without pain at the time of treatment (56) (Key literature 4.1).

A typical scenario suggestive of a progressing inflammatory condition of the pulp is when a tooth first becomes increasingly more sensitive to cold air or cold drinks and food products, which subsequently turns into shorter or longer periods of lingering pain elicited by the same stimuli. The intermittent character of the pain experience is a truly characteristic feature and helps in the differential diagnosis from other painful conditions (see also Chapters 3 and 14). In the most severe cases, excruciating pain may linger for hours. Pain may occur spontaneously or be provoked by hot or cold drinks and food. In the end stages, prior to complete breakdown of the pulp, patients may find that cold water alleviates the symptoms. The report of severe pain may be the only presenting symptom. Tenderness to percussion of the offending tooth and even of the neighboring teeth may or may not be observed in the final stages of pulpal inflammation.

Pulpal inflammatory lesions may cause the radiographic presentation of loss of lamina dura, small periapical radiolucency and/or periapical sclerosis (Fig. 4.6). These findings in themselves are not necessarily indicative of an irreversible condition but can be helpful in identifying the offending tooth in a painful case.

In conclusion, clinical and radiographic signs are less than decisive diagnostic measures to determine the spread of pulpal inflammation in a given case, and yet they are the only signs currently available for diagnosis in clinical practice. The decision to carry out an invasive procedure often has to be taken on the basis of the

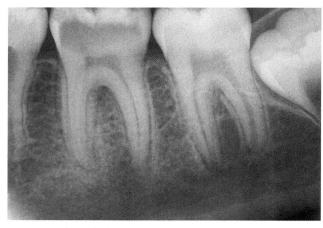

Fig. 4.6 Radiograph showing extensive caries in the crown of tooth 36. Although inflamed, the pulp is still vital and functioning. Apically there are widened periodontal membrane spaces at both roots and bone sclerosis is associated with the mesial root.

existence and the character of the pain symptoms (Core concept 4.3).

Management of exposed pulps by direct pulp capping/partial pulpotomy

Objective

Pulp capping and partial pulpotomy are procedures to consider when there is no history of lingering pain to external stimuli and when the pulp has been:

- accidentally exposed to the oral environment by cavity preparation and traumatic injury;
- exposed in conjunction with excavation of caries or hemisection in periodontal therapy.

Core concept 4.3

- A pulpectomy procedure should be carried out when a pulpal condition is deemed irreversible.
- A pulp capping/partial pulpotomy procedure may be carried out when an exposed pulp is healthy or deemed reversibly inflamed.
- Under clinical conditions the cut-off point between irreversibly inflamed and reversibly inflamed is often hard to identify.

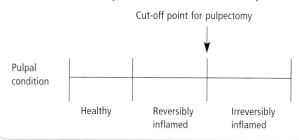

Cut-off point for pulpectomy

Pulpal condition

Healthy   Reversibly inflamed   Irreversibly inflamed

Ultimately the procedures aim to preserve the vital functions of the pulp. Although not necessary for a successful outcome, it is considered advantageous that wound healing results in hard-tissue repair of the open exposure to enhance pulpal protection from secondary harmful events (Fig. 4.7).

Historical perspectives

In 1883 Hunter (37) claimed that "Even though the pulp may be suppurating and the pus welling up in volumes, I shall save it" and he pressed a mixture of sparrow droppings onto the exposed pulp and achieved success "fully equal to 98 per cent".

Since Hunter so drastically introduced pulp capping, the treatment procedure has been vigorously disputed in the dental profession and is still a matter of controversy. The discussion often has been polarized, both as to when to do it, if at all, and as to what capping material should be preferred (10). The radicals have claimed that the long-term outcome of the treatment is unpredictable and is doomed to failure, therefore the more invasive pulpotomy or pulpectomy must be carried out when the pulp is exposed. The conservatives, on the other hand, hold that success can be achieved, even in teeth following large and longstanding carious exposures; they contend that pulp capping/partial pulpotomy is indeed worthwhile because if it fails then root canal therapy can be carried out.

The reason for the dispute has been the *de facto* uncertainty, already described, about the preoperative and postoperative diagnosis of the pulpal condition. Both are due to insufficient clinical measures to evaluate the true status of the pulp. Because major inflammatory changes may be present without concomitant clinical symptoms, a pulp-capped tooth may survive for years without presenting clinical symptoms, even though there is extensive inflammatory breakdown (51, 56) (see also Key literature 4.2). A further reason has been a mediocre understanding of the healing potential of the pulp. Inflammation in the pulp is a dynamic process and for

---

Key literature 4.2

Cvek (16) followed a series of 60 young teeth that were treated with partial pulpotomy subsequent to pulp exposure by trauma for up to 5 years. Fifty-eight (97%) cappings were deemed successful, i.e. teeth were comfortable and without clinical or radiographic signs of necrosis and root canal infection. A further indication of preserved pulp vitality was completion of root development in teeth with incomplete root closure. In the study there was no difference in success rate, regardless of the time the pulp had been exposed to the oral environment (some teeth had received treatment first after several weeks), the size of exposure or the stage of root closure.

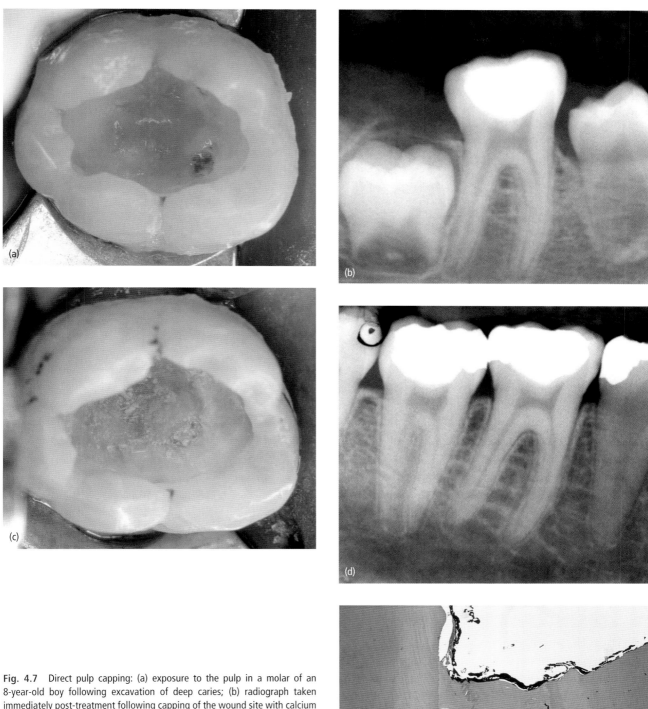

Fig. 4.7 Direct pulp capping: (a) exposure to the pulp in a molar of an 8-year-old boy following excavation of deep caries; (b) radiograph taken immediately post-treatment following capping of the wound site with calcium hydroxide. Note the incomplete closure of the roots; (c) hard-tissue repair of the exposure site seen following a re-entry 1 year and 7 months after treatment; (d) radiograph taken 7 years after treatment showing complete root closure and normal periapical structures indicating a successful outcome of the treatment (courtesy of Dr D. Ricucci); (e) histological section showing hard-tissue formation 90 days following experimental pulp capping with a calcium hydroxide cement. Pulpal tissue has a normal appearance.

previously unaffected pulp that is housed in a large pulp chamber, especially in the young patient, the healing potential is substantial. Even after exposure to the oral environment for a period of time, healing is possible (16). Contrary to previous beliefs, inflammatory changes in one part of the pulp will not inevitably lead to pulp necrosis and may heal if the proper measures are taken to sustain and optimize the healing potential.

Factors of importance for a successful outcome

As indicated above, healing and repair of an exposed pulp depend initially on the preoperative condition of the tissue. Consequently, if inflammation has reached an irreversible state, no treatment can remedy the condition and a failure will show up as pulp necrosis. This may or may not be preceded by painful events. Factors recognized as important for the long-term survival of the pulp to capping/partial pulpotomy are discussed below.

Type of injury

An accidental pulp exposure through intact dentin occurring during cavity and crown preparation has the greatest potential for a successful outcome. In this situation the pulp may be healthy and the bacterial contamination limited, therefore the immediate condition for healing is optimal.

In a traumatic injury, where the pulp has been exposed by a blow or fall, the healing conditions are favorable even though the wound may have been exposed to the oral environment for a period of time. Both clinical observations and experimental studies in animals (12, 16, 17, 35) have demonstrated that bacterial contamination of the wound site over a short period is negligible (Key literature 4.2). Following proper disinfection and debridement, healing and hard-tissue repair are possible in such cases (16, 26, 50).

In exposures by caries, on the other hand, there may be a massive penetration of bacterial organisms to the tissue. This has usually resulted in a localized acute inflammation of the pulp, often as an abscess (see Chapter 2). The healing potential of such lesions is therefore unpredictable. The procedure of caries excavation, in addition, may exacerbate the lesion by forcing infected dentin chips into the wound. Nevertheless, capping of carious exposures may occasionally be considered if symptoms of pulpitis are absent. It is generally agreed that the most favorable prognosis exists when perforation is made during the very final excavation of the deepest part of the carious lesion and when there is only a small exposure. On such careful case selections an overall 5-year survival rate of 80% was found in 510 cases analyzed by Hørsted et al. (40) and there was no difference in outcome between carious and non-carious expo-

sures. This finding is in accordance with the 93% success rate after 2 years reported for direct capping or partial pulpotomy carried out in carious molars of children and teenagers (11, 23, 50, 66, 88). Yet, others have reported very bleak results of capping caries exposures. In one study only 37% of the treated pulps had survived at the 5-year check-up and as little as 13% survived for 10 years (5).

Age

Although not consistently observed (5, 7), it seems reasonable that the prognosis for capping and partial pulpotomy would be better in young than in old individuals (40, 88). The fact that the pulp of young teeth is rich in cells and blood vessels makes it prone to react favorably to microbiological and traumatic challenges. On the other hand, in an aged tooth and/or tooth exposed to previous injury the pulp is often poor in cells, fiber-rich and partly mineralized. Therefore it is likely to be more vulnerable and less able to survive a capping procedure. The size of the pulpal space in an old tooth is also much smaller, thus providing a greater risk for pulpal breakdown upon destructive stimuli (8). In the study by Hørsted et al. (40), pulpal survival 5 years after pulp capping was 70% for 50–80-year-olds but 85% for 30–50-year-olds and 92% for 10–30-year-olds.

Size and location of the pulp exposure

It was long held that cappings should be considered only when there is exposure of an occlusal or incisal portion of the pulp, because capping of a more cervical exposure was thought to be less successful owing to possible circulatory disturbances and necrosis of the coronally located portion of the tissue. Later, it was shown that cervical exposures may heal without compromising the rest of the pulp provided that a gentle treatment procedure is applied (12, 13, 62).

The high success rate in clinical and radiographic follow-up studies after partial pulpotomy (16, 26, 50) has further put to question the relevance of exposure size as a significant parameter. It was once believed that cappings should be reserved only for pinpoint exposures. Current knowledge suggests that the total volume of the pulp tissue in relation to the size of the exposure is more pertinent.

Clinical procedure

The procedure of pulp capping/partial pulpotomy is simple. Success essentially depends on the extent to which the wound site can be maintained free of infection in both the short and the long term (Clinical procedure 4.1).

Clinical procedure 4.1   Pulp capping

(1) Remove any blood clot with a sharp excavator in the case of timelag between exposure and treatment.

(2) Establish hemostasis by applying gentle pressure on the wound with a cotton pellet moistened with chlorhexidine, sterile saline or analgesic solution. Renew the cotton pellet if necessary and wait for complete hemostasis.

(3) Gently apply capping material to the wound without firm pressure.

(4) Cover the wound dressing with a hard-setting cement such as a glass ionomer cement.

(5) Restore and seal the cavity with a restoration.

(6) After 1 week, evaluate the presence or absence of symptoms.

(7) After 6 months, evaluate:

- symptoms
- reactions to thermal stimuli – absent, short, prolonged
- sensitivity to electric pulp testing – positive/negative
- periapical radiographic changes
- radiographically verified 'bridge' formation.

Based on the findings, continue recalls or do root canal treatment.

(8) Repeat (7) at yearly intervals.

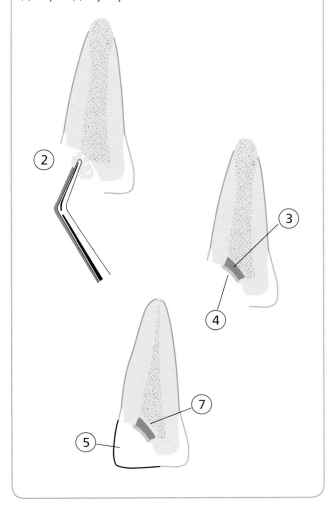

Pulp capping is regarded as appropriate for immediate minor exposures, whereas partial pulpotomy is more apt for wounds that have been exposed to microbial challenges for a period of time, including major carious exposures. The recommendation is based on the results of experimental studies showing that after accidental exposure the infection remains superficial over the first 24 hours (12, 17, 36). Over longer periods, infection usually has involved deeper areas of the pulp and therefore partial pulpotomy is advisable in these situations.

A partial pulpotomy offers the advantage that it removes the superficial and potentially infected layer of the pulp. Some surrounding dentin is removed as well, which creates a well-defined space for placement of the capping material (see Fig. 4.3b). The preparation should be carried out 1–2 mm deep with an end-cutting diamond bur in an air turbine under copious water irrigation in order to reduce the trauma on the tissue (see also Chapter 5). The operation is normally simple in a traumatized incisor but more demanding in a molar where, owing to the generally large wound cavity, bleeding may be difficult to stop.

A most critical step in pulp capping and pulpotomy procedures is to stop bleeding and to eliminate major blood clots prior to placement of the wound dressing. Blood clots serve as bacterial substrate and may support the growth of contaminating oral microorganisms. If bleeding cannot be controlled properly, pulpectomy should be carried out. Another important consideration is to apply a gentle technique to avoid dilaceration and displacement of capping material to the deep portions of the pulp (38) (Fig. 4.8).

Integrity of the permanent restoration

Results of clinical studies and experiments in laboratory animals suggest that the integrity of the permanent restoration is of vital importance for the successful outcome of these procedures (7, 13, 40, 56). Even though the wound dressing may enhance hard-tissue repair of the exposure, the hard tissue often becomes porous and allows bacterial organisms to penetrate if they gain access to it (Fig. 4.9). In their experimental study, Cox *et al.* (13) observed that inflammatory pulpal lesions were frequent underneath repaired wounds and that these lesions correlated with the concomitant presence of bacteria in the newly formed hard tissue. The organisms conceivably originated from the oral environment after penetrating spaces at the margins of the permanent restoration. Deteriorating surface restoration leading to bacterial leakage is the likely reason for the increasing failure rate of pulp cappings observed in clinical follow-ups carried out over long periods of time (Fig. 4.10; Core concept 4.4) (5, 40).

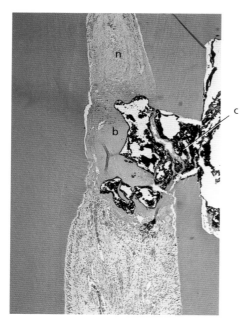

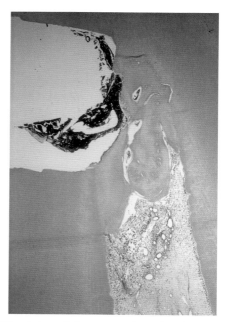

Fig. 4.8   Histological section of a pulpal exposure capped with calcium hydroxide cement. The capping material (c) has been pushed into the pulp, a major bleed occurred (b) and the incisal pulp tissue became necrotic (n). The treatment most likely failed because a gentle procedure was not used.

Fig. 4.9   Microphotograph from an experimental study carried out by Cox *et al.* (13), showing an inflammatory lesion underneath hard-tissue repair 13 months after pulp capping. The porous nature of the hard tissue being formed is obvious.

Capping materials and healing patterns

Calcium hydroxide

Since the 1930s calcium hydroxide water slurry and commercial hard-set compounds based on calcium hydroxide have been the prime materials for conservative treatment of pulpal wounds by pulp capping or pulpotomy. Calcium hydroxide suspensions and pastes are charac-terized by their inherent high pH. When applied to an exposed pulp, calcium hydroxide water slurry (pH 12.5) cauterizes the tissue and causes superficial necrosis. Such a treatment is detrimental to the pulp but only to a minor extent. Indeed, experience has shown that, in compari-son with many other compounds, healing is predictable with this material (Fig. 4.11). It was even originally believed that the necrotic zone was a prerequisite for

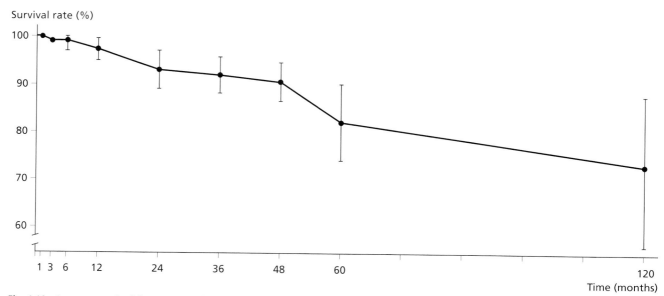

Fig. 4.10   In a retrospective follow-up study of pulp cappings in 510 teeth by Hørsted *et al.* (40) it was found that, although the overall survival rate at 5 years was as high as 82%, the number of surviving pulps declined over time.

Core concept 4.4

In selecting cases for pulp capping/partial pulpotomy, consider the factual conditions that prevail, i.e. whether they act in favor of or against a successful outcome.

Critical factors are:

- Age of patient
- Degree of hemostasis that can be obtained
- The potential to provide a permanent restoration of long-term integrity.

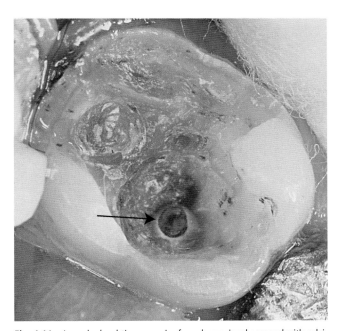

Fig. 4.11 Irregular hard-tissue repair of a pulp previously capped with calcium hydroxide (→). A crevice can be probed along the rim of the exposure, which may indicate that the hard tissue has been formed below a superficial layer of necrotic tissue.

hard-tissue repair to be organized. Later studies have demonstrated that this is not necessarily so and that hard-tissue repair can develop in a less alkaline environment without a distinct zone of necrosis (24, 77, 80).

Hard-tissue repair of pulpal wounds is not unique to calcium hydroxide but can occur with a number of other materials (14, 18) and with a variety of biologically active matrices and molecules (53, 61, 83). Although the position of calcium hydroxide is challenged by new both bioactive and non-biologic materials (see further below), calcium hydroxide, on the basis of solid clinical documentation, is still a material of choice.

Wound healing patterns

The sequence of events in the healing process following treatment of a pulpal wound has been described in numerous experimental studies in both humans and laboratory animals (24, 72, 87). In these studies healthy pulps were treated with calcium hydroxide as wound dressing:

- One day after capping with a caustic material such as calcium hydroxide there will be a superficial layer of tissue necrosis and inflammatory cell infiltrates (72, 87). At lower pH no necrosis develops and there will be only signs of bleeding and slight infiltrates of leukocytes (24).
- During the first few days thereafter, blood clots are resolved and the tissue is in a process of reorganization.
- The inflammatory reaction is gradually reduced and a collagen-rich matrix is formed in close relation to the necrotic zone or directly adjacent to the capping material.
- In the following week, mineralization of the amorphous tissue starts (Fig. 4.12).

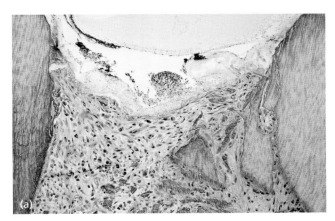
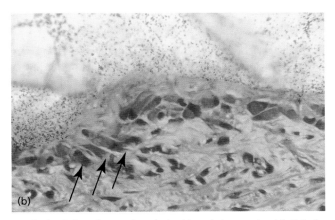

Fig. 4.12 Microphotographs from the study by Fitzgerald (24) showing tissue reorganization 5 days after capping of a healthy pulp in a monkey (a). Note the displacement of dentin chips. Unless infected these chips do not impair but rather support the repair process and also become enclosed in it. Nine days after capping, new odontoblasts have appeared at the wound site and started to lay down a mineralizing matrix (arrows in b). (Courtesy of Dr M. Fitzgerald.)

The first mineralized tissue that may form is irregular in nature and contains many cell inclusions. Subsequently a more dentin-like tissue with tubules is formed.

Repair by hard tissue of a pulpal wound is a multifactorial process involving a wide range of cells, extracellular molecules and physicochemical interactions (28, 83). Although the exact mechanism by which hard-tissue repair of a pulpal exposure is initiated is not fully understood, it is clear that secondary odontoblasts are crucial in the process (45, 87) (see Chapter 2). These cells are recruited from ectomesenchymal cells (stem cells) located in the pulp. Following a series of DNA replications, these cells migrate to the site of injury and differentiate into elongated and polarized odontoblast-like cells (25).

The new hard tissue laid down will not necessarily be homogeneous. In fact, it will frequently contain cell inclusions and tunnel defects (13, 38), rendering it permeable to bacteria and bacterial elements in the oral cavity (Fig. 4.9). For this reason the formed hard tissue is often less able than primary dentin to protect the pulp from such elements and there will always be a risk for pulpal infection from possible surface seal breakdown. "Dentin bridge", the often-used term for the hard-tissue repair process, is thus inaccurate.

Other materials for capping

Materials other than calcium hydroxide may also allow hard-tissue repair of pulpal wounds. This has given some strength to the theory that proper protection of the wound during the healing phase may be just as important as the choice of a specific capping material. Accordingly, dentin bonding systems have been advocated for direct pulp cappings because the formation of a hybrid layer and subsequent restoration with resin composite was believed to result in leakage-free restoratives. Some animal studies, primarily in non-human primates, have shown promising results with dentin formation covering the exposure site similar to the results with calcium hydroxide (15, 48). Histological studies in humans, however, have failed to confirm these findings and less or only sparse hard tissue was found after direct pulp capping with these materials compared with calcium hydroxide (3, 21, 41, 63, 73). On the contrary, pulpal inflammation, foreign body reactions and necrosis have been reported despite absence of infection (2, 21, 29, 41). Because of degradation of the resin bond, adhesive restorations are not leakage proof after some period in the oral cavity (20, 31). Therefore lack of hard-tissue repair of the exposure will allow a later infection of the pulp tissue. Even though the "bridge" may be permeable to some extent it gives better protection against a massive attack of microorganisms than no hard-tissue barrier. If bacterial leakage could be permanently prevented, hard-

tissue formation at the exposure site would of course not be necessary.

In a search for materials superior to calcium hydroxide in stimulation of the pulp tissue cells to form a more solid "bridge", interest has focused on the use of hydroxyapatite, tricalcium phosphate and mineral trioxide aggregate as potential capping materials (34, 64). However, if hard tissue subjacent to hydroxyapatite occurs, it has been described as irregular and incomplete and the use of tricalcium phosphate seems to be most effective if calcium hydroxide is added (44, 79).

Mineral trioxide aggregate (MTA) has gained considerable interest in recent years (84). The material consists mainly of refined Portland cement with bismuth added for radiopacity. It sets slowly to a hard cement after mixing with water (see Chapter 12). The pH is comparable to the pH of calcium hydroxide and thus the wound healing events would be similar to those of calcium hydroxide (see above). There is mounting histological evidence in humans of a hard tissue producing effect similar or superior to that seen with calcium hydroxide (4, 43, 55). An advantage of this material in comparison with calcium hydroxide is that it sets hard and will not be readily dissolved in tissue fluid or saliva. Both materials have an initial bacteriocidal effect due to the high pH.

A direct application of bioactive molecules significant for the terminal differentiation of odontoblasts has been proposed as an alternative way to achieve healing of pulpal wounds (70, 83) rather than the indirect effect of caustic materials such as calcium hydroxide and MTA. Although promising in animal experiments, considerable research and development will need to be carried out before bioactive molecules find clinical applications (9).

In conclusion, solid experimental and clinical documentation accumulated over many years supports the use of calcium hydroxide in pulp capping and pulpotomy procedures. Predictable repair and healing of pulpal wounds can be expected provided the treatment is undertaken on the basis of careful case selection and by the use of a proper technique (see Core concept 4.4).

The increasing number of concurrent results with MTA suggests that this cement may overtake calcium hydroxide as the preferred material for pulp capping and partial pulpotomy. It is not unreasonable to assume that both these non-biological agents will be replaced in the future by methods which aim not only to preserve the pulp but also to stimulate pulp–dentin regeneration. However, much developmental work has yet to be conducted before stem cells and bioactive proteins, for example, find clinical application.

Postoperative recall

Because of the inherent risk for pulp infection and necrosis, direct pulp capping/partial pulpotomy should be followed up clinically and radiographically. The post-operative control can be seen as a two-phase procedure: the initial phase entails an evaluation of whether healing and asymptomatic conditions have been attained; and the subsequent phase refers to the continued follow-up on a yearly basis. The latter is prompted by the prevailing risk of pulp necrosis and subsequent root canal infection that may occur several years after treatment.

During the first weeks, minor sensations of spontaneous pain of short duration may occur. Such symptoms are expected to disappear. However, if symptoms get worse, the development of an irreversible inflammatory condition is to be suspected and pulpotomy or pulpectomy should be considered.

A 6-month recall is considered appropriate for the first follow-up. Then, if possible, cases should be followed up annually. Core concept 4.5 outlines the examinations to be undertaken. Treatment is considered successful if there is no history of spontaneous pain, a positive reaction to electrical pulp testing (EPT) and normal periapical structures in radiographs. Incompletely developed teeth showing continued root closure are also a positive sign of healing even if EPT is negative. Apposition of hard-tissue repair at the exposure site may or may not be seen radiographically. The restoration integrity should be checked for deficient margins, because marginal fractures or bulk fractures facilitate penetration of microorganisms to the wound site.

Pulpectomy

Pulpectomy is primarily carried out to prevent the development of a destructive course of pulpal inflammation, which may result in root canal infection and associated painful events (Fig. 4.13). This means that pulpectomy may be considered in any permanent tooth where there are clinical signs indicating irreversible inflammatory changes in the pulp. A prerequisite is that root development is complete. Hence, the treatment may be per-

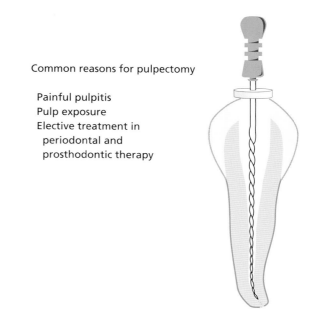

Common reasons for pulpectomy

Painful pulpitis
Pulp exposure
Elective treatment in
    periodontal and
    prosthodontic therapy

Fig. 4.13   Common reasons for pulpectomy.

formed regardless of whether the tissue is directly exposed to the oral environment or not. Pulpectomy is also the treatment of choice for any direct exposure of the tissue, when the prognosis for direct pulp capping or partial pulpotomy is deemed questionable. Moreover, pulpectomy may be carried out following hemisection in periodontal therapy, and when retentive measures are needed in prosthodontic therapy. In these latter situations, the treatment is elective, which means that it is not prompted by a disease condition of the tissue.

Objective

Pulpectomy seeks to establish a condition where the tooth, following completion of treatment and after a follow-up period, is without clinical and radiographic signs of root canal infection (Fig. 4.14). In addition, the filling of the canal should be of such a quality that bacteria and bacterial elements in the oral environment are unable to penetrate the pulpal chamber and cause a periapical inflammatory lesion. The expectation is that such a healing result lasts permanently and for the duration of the patient's life. This objective is clearly attainable provided that treatment is carried out properly and with due consideration of the potential risk of bacterial contamination both during and after the procedure. It needs to be understood that although the treatment on many occasions involves removal of diseased and, to some extent, infected tissue, most of the tissue is not infected. This is particularly true for the apical portion of the pulp. An important objective of the treatment is therefore to maintain the sterile conditions of the root canal.

Core concept 4.5

Procedure for clinical follow-up of pulp capping/partial pulpotomy should include checks of:

- History of spontaneous pain or lingering pain on temperature change
- Reaction to electric pulp tester
- Status of the restoration
- Periapical condition
- Radiographic evidence of hard-tissue repair.

Note that inflammatory changes and pulp necrosis may be present, despite hard-tissue formation, in an otherwise asymptomatic tooth.

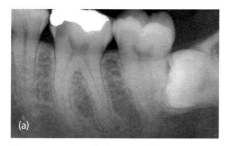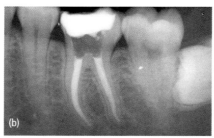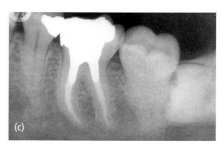

Fig. 4.14 Series of radiographs demonstrating a successful outcome of a pulpectomy in a lower molar: (a) deep caries mesially in tooth 36; (b) the final dense fill of the canal to proper length; (c) radiograph taken 4 years after completion of treatment. Tooth is asymptomatic and there are no radiographic signs of peri-apical inflammation indicating root canal infection. (Courtesy of Dr A. Gesi.)

Critical procedural steps

Pulpectomy involves three principal steps:

1. Removal of the pulp tissue in its entirety.
2. Shaping of the root canal.
3. Filling the root canal space thus obtained.

The tissue is removed by specially designed instruments that can be used to clean and widen the root canal space, both by hand and by rotary instrumentation. The various instruments and techniques are comprehensively described in Chapter 11 and will not be dealt with here. The technique for filling instrumented root canals is presented in Chapter 13.

In order to achieve a predictable and successful outcome of pulpectomy, the following critical measures are considered in some detail:

- anesthesia;
- aseptic technique;
- access to and preparation of the root canal space;
- location and management of the apical wound.

Anesthesia

Pulpectomy is a highly painful procedure that should not be carried out without proper anesthesia. Routine procedures, including local infiltration or regional blocks, are to be followed and are usually sufficient. However, pulp anesthesia sometimes fails and one may find that the tissue can still be very sensitive and cannot be touched without causing intense pain, even if the injection has been given properly. This complication is more common in mandibular posterior teeth than in maxillary teeth, where infiltration anesthetics normally are effective (65). It is a common clinical finding, especially in patients with painful pulpitis, that complete anesthesia can be difficult to achieve. Provided that the injection is given adequately and at the proper dosages, several mechanisms can be held responsible:

1. Afferent nerve fibers deriving from inflamed tissue sites may have changed resting potentials and low-

ered excitability thresholds, which not only are restricted locally but extend throughout the affected nerve. Anesthetic agent is therefore unable to prevent total impulse transmission (52, 85).
2. Patients under stress and anxiety have a lowered pain threshold.
3. Accessory innervation, e.g. nervus mylohyoideus, may send branches to mandibular molars. The frequency has been estimated to be approximately 20% (78).

In the case of insufficient pulp anesthesia, one or several supplementary measures may be undertaken:

1. Repeat injection and wait another 5–10 min.
2. If not effective, combine regional block anesthesia with infiltration. For example, on mandibular blocks combine with infiltration at the bottom of the mouth distally to the tooth, to numb a potential extra nerve supply of nervus mylohyoideus. The needle must be placed close to the mandibular cortex. Combine infiltration of the maxillary incisor with a deposit deep into the nasopalatine duct to catch nerve branches.
3. If still not effective, supplement with so-called periodontal ligament injection or intraosseous injection (Clinical procedure 4.2).
4. As a final, desperate move one may be forced to give an injection directly into the pulp (intrapulpal injection) (Clinical procedure 4.2). It is important that such a measure is carried out only in full compliance with the patient. In an apprehensive or severely anxious patient the procedure should be avoided. It is then advisable to postpone treatment and reschedule the patient with a prescription for premedication. Different regimens may be practiced, including a combination of oral administration of non-steroidal anti-inflammatory drugs and benzodiazipine in proper dosages. After treatment the patient should be accompanied.

Formerly, when pain control could not be obtained in these extreme situations, pulpal devitalization was used. The procedure involved application of a highly tissue

Clinical procedure 4.2

In the most headstrong cases where pulpal anesthesia is difficult to obtain, supplemental anesthesia of different modes may be attempted.

Intraligamentary injection
- Place short needle in the gingival sulcus, mesial or distal to the tooth.
- Advance into the periodontal ligament until resistance is met.
- Slowly inject 0.2 ml of anesthetic solution, which will penetrate the cancellous bone to the pulp.

This technique should not be used in teeth with marginal periodontitis.

Intraosseous injection
- Use infiltration anesthesia of soft tissue covering root apex and cortical bone.
- Perforate the periapical cortical bone with a solid needle driven by a contra-angle handpiece.
- Insert a short needle in the drilled canal.
- Inject 0.5 ml of non-vasopressor-containing, fast-penetrating anesthetic, e.g. articain (49, 54).

Intrapulpal injection
- Apply a cotton pellet saturated in anesthetic to the pulpal floor.
- Remove anesthetized dentin with a slow-speed handpiece. Repeat anesthesia of dentin if necessary.
- Make a small perforation of the pulp, aiming at a snug fit of the needle in the perforation.
- Inject 0.5 ml of anesthetic into the pulp under firm pressure.
- Repeat procedure, if necessary, for each root canal following removal of the coronal pulp.

toxic agent, e.g. formaldehyde, onto the exposed pulp. Such a material would fix the tissue and render it necrotic within 1 week. Thereupon an endodontic procedure could be carried out. This method is not used nowadays because of the strong risk of leakage along the temporary filling to the marginal periodontium, where serious tissue destruction can result (see Case study 1).

Aseptic technique

Asepsis relates to measures undertaken during surgical operations to prevent the access of extraneous microorganisms to a given wound site. In endodontic therapies, including pulpectomy, potential sources of bacterial contamination of the pulpal chamber are from:

- infected debris;
- saliva and gingival exudate;
- non-sterile instruments.

Hence, asepsis in endodontics involves procedures aimed at controlling these sources of infection.

Initially, prior to any attempt to enter root canals with instruments to extirpate the tissue, caries should be removed totally by careful excavation. Otherwise, there is an obvious risk that during canal instrumentation infected dentin is brought to the apical portion of the canal where it may induce and maintain an inflammatory lesion. Similarly, the tooth should be cleaned of any calculus and dental plaque. A defective filling is another source of bacterial contamination and should be eliminated and replaced before the initiation of treatment (Fig. 4.15).

Proper asepsis in endodontics cannot be attained without the use of a rubber dam. Apart from providing an aseptic field of operation, a rubber dam facilitates the procedure and prevents instruments being dropped, which may be swallowed or aspirated into the lungs. Also, a rubber dam prevents leakage to the oral environment of tissue-irritating medicaments used during the treatment.

On intact teeth or teeth with only minor loss of tooth substance, a rubber dam normally can be applied without much effort. However, teeth with substantial substance loss may require different build-ups, including the placement of orthodontic or copper bands. Other measures to optimize rubber dam application include gingivectomy and a crown-lengthening procedure.

Following the placement of a rubber dam it should be tested for leakage. This is best done with hydrogen peroxide (30%), which is carefully applied to the margins

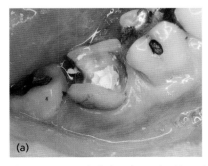 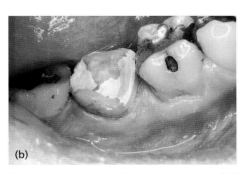 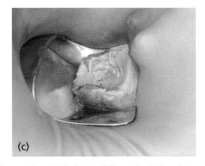

Fig. 4.15 Proper isolation of a tooth with a rubber dam is an absolute prerequisite to obtain an aseptic field of operation. (a) Defective fillings should be eliminated and (b) replaced with, for example, a glass ionomer cement or any other restorative that can prevent leakage of saliva and gingival exudate to the root canal during the procedure. (c) Rubber dam and clamp.

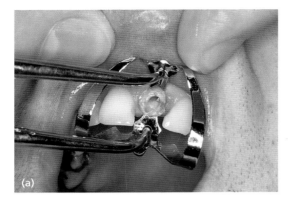

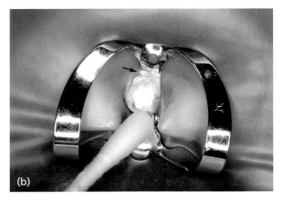

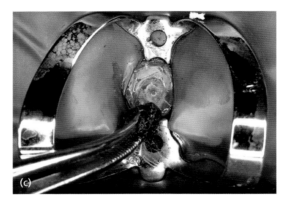

Fig. 4.16 Clinical photographs showing rubber dam application on upper incisor: (a) proper clamp is tested; (b) swab with hydrogen peroxide (30%) shows foaming action that needs attention (→); (c) disinfection with iodine tincture.

of the rubber dam. Leakage of saliva or gingival exudate will show up as an intense foaming action (Fig. 4.16a, b).

To control leakage, the dam may be tightened to the tooth structure by dental tape. The technique is to bring the tape through the tooth contacts and tie it underneath the clamp. Also, various forms of sealing agents may be used for the purpose of excluding oral fluid contamination. Finally the dam, the tooth and the pulpal wound should be disinfected with either an iodine tincture solution (5–10%) or chlorhexidine in alcohol (Fig. 4.16c).

An important step in the aseptic chain is to use sterile instruments. Instruments for root canal preparation are best maintained in boxes, which can be autoclaved. During the operation, care should be exercised to avoid contamination of the part of the instrument that goes into the canal by, for example, finger touch or other non-sterile item.

Access to and preparation of the root canal space

Technically, pulpectomy can be quite a demanding microsurgical operation. This is particularly true in posterior, multirooted teeth, where proper access to the root canal system may be difficult to attain. Pulpectomy also may be difficult in narrow and severely curved root canals. Complications that may result include:

- overlooked root canals;
- incomplete elimination of pulpal tissue;
- lateral and apical overinstrumentation;
- incomplete filling of the root canal space.

Procedural errors of this nature reduce the likelihood of a successful outcome if microbes are brought into the pulp chamber in conjunction with or after the procedure. Therefore proper access to all root canals and their thorough biomechanical instrumentation are critical. For a detailed account of the procedures associated with opening and instrumenting teeth for endodontic therapy, the reader is referred to Chapter 11.

To be completed successfully, a pulpectomy also requires sufficient time. It must not be rushed because of the imminent risk of leaving tissue elements behind (Fig. 4.17). In other words, a pulpectomy should be completed in one and the same sitting and the canal then be enlarged so that it can receive either a temporary or permanent root filling.

Location and management of the apical wound

Clinical, radiographic and histological studies have shown that containing instrumentation and root filling within 1–2 mm from the anatomical apex provide the best conditions for healing, while apical overinstrumentation and overfilling negatively affect the result (67). Radiographic follow-up studies have also shown that leaving more than about 3 mm of the apical pulp reduces the chance of successful outcome (46, 47). Several points

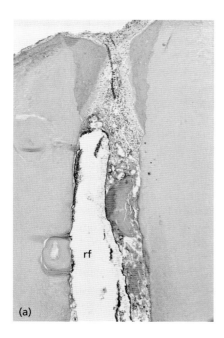 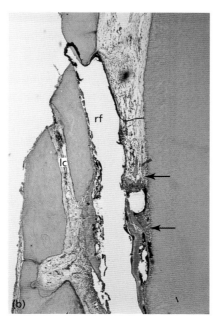

Fig. 4.17 It is important to recognize that non-instrumented tissue in overlooked canals and tissue remnants left on canal walls, in fins and in other canal irregularities, serve as potential sites for bacterial growth after pulpectomy. In addition, tissue remnants prevent the establishment of a proper root filling that can seal off the instrumented canal. (a) Demineralized section of upper incisor. Root filling material (rf) is seen occupying the left part of the canal, and a mud of dentinal shavings and tissue remnants in the right part. Some inflammatory cells are located in the residual pulp tissue. (b) Demineralized section of upper incisor. The root filling (rf) does not follow the main canal. Remnants of root filling material and pulpal tissue are present in a lateral canal (lc). Inflammatory cells and dentinal shavings are seen lateral to the root filled main canal (←).

are strong arguments for the view that pulpectomy should be performed slightly short of the anatomical apex:

- The apical region of the root canal is reasonably well vascularized by virtue of its close relationship to the periapical tissue and to ramifications of the canal in the apical root structure. This provides sufficient conditions for healing, as opposed to a more coronal level of the root canal that is normally without collateral blood circulation (58).
- As the pulpal tissue and dentin in the apical portion most often are not diseased or infected, removal of the tissue here and antimicrobial treatment are unnecessary.
- Instrumentation through the apical foramen may damage the root structure to the extent that a proper seal of the apical portion of the canal is jeopardized. Often an overinstrumented canal results in overfilling and a poor seal, to the detriment of a successful outcome. Root filling materials, in addition, are not inert and overfilling may cause tissue injury, inflammation and foreign body reaction in the apical region (see Chapter 12).

Consequently the apical wound level should ideally be placed slightly short of the apical foramen, where the canal is at its narrowest point. At this site many canals are almost circular and the wound surface can be kept to a minimum, leaving fair conditions for healing of the wound. This point is often termed the apical constriction (see Chapter 11). However, studies of the anatomy of the root apex have shown that the level of the apical constriction varies, although it is most often within 1 mm short of the apical foramen (22). In addition, the apical

foramen often exists at a distance from the anatomical apex. These are further reasons to place the apical wound at a safety distance of about 1–2 mm from the anatomical apex.

Placing an instrument in the canal to the assumed correct length and assessing the remaining distance to the anatomical apex in a radiograph determine the proper level. This procedure is termed working-length determination by the use of a trial file. Working-length determination can also be carried out electronically (see Chapter 11).

Confining the wound level to a distance of 1–2 mm from the apex favors a shaping technique that is aimed at creating a step in the canal against which the root filling can be condensed. Accordingly, the chance of a tight fit between the filling and the canal walls increases, and the risk of overinstrumentation and displacement of the root filling material into the periapical tissue and bone decreases.

Permanent or temporary root filling?

Provided that the extirpation procedure can be completed without complications, an immediate permanent canal filling is appropriate if there is sufficient time available for the filling procedure (Key literature 4.3). If not, or if there is bleeding that is difficult to stop or concern about the technical outcome of the procedure in general, a temporary root filling is advocated. Leaving the canal unfilled is inappropriate because it may facilitate the growth of contaminating microorganisms. Calcium hydroxide is then the material of choice. The rationale for its use is that:

Key literature 4.3

In a randomized controlled clinical study by Gesi *et al.* (27) the outcome of pulpectomy following completion of the treatment in one session was compared with a two treatment session over 1 week employing calcium hydroxide as an intracanal dressing (27). The subjects (*n* = 256) were followed for up to 3 years and assessed for clinical as well as radiographic signs of emerging root canal infection. Failures of this nature were at a low rate (7%) and evenly distributed between the two treatment groups. Notable is also that postoperative pain, recorded 1 week after permanent filling, was significantly associated with overfilling with no difference between the treatment groups. The study confirmed that pulpectomy can be highly successful if attention is given to proper asepsis, careful instrumentation and adequate filling of the instrumented canal space.

- It fills up the canal space and prevents the multiplication of any contaminating bacterial organisms.
- It helps to stop bleeding.
- It necrotizes any tissue remnants on the canal walls, which, upon a subsequent sitting, can be eliminated by instrumentation and the use of NaOCl irrigation (32).
- It favors the formation of hard tissue at the apical end of the root canal and at any cut lateral canals (76) (Fig. 4.18).

Wound healing after pulpectomy

The healing pattern following pulpectomy is characterized by an initial inflammatory reaction in the apical tissue due to the trauma induced by the cutting procedure. The residual pulp is often lacerated and may even be lost in the process (57). If, by accident, the root canal instrument has been pushed through the apical foramen during working-length determination or instrumentation of the canal, the apical termination of the preparation should still be confined to 1–2mm from the anatomical apex to reduce the risk of periapical surplus of root filling material. In the absence of wound infection, reorganization soon occurs. This involves replacement of the injured tissue by connective tissue derived from the periapical

region (39, 59). In the process, some internal or external root resorption may develop that is repaired later on (Key literature 4.4).

Patients may experience some tenderness immediately following pulpectomy. These symptoms disappear in a few days' time, along with recovery of the apical tissue.

Materials used to fill root canals may compromise the normal healing pattern, owing to their irritating capacity, and result in a longstanding inflammatory lesion. In particular, this is the case when root filling material is extruded into the residual pulp and the periapical tissue, or into uninstrumented apical ramifications (27, 68). Inflammatory cells accumulate close to the root filling material and remain for as long as toxic components are released. Eventually the material will be lined off by fibrous connective tissue. These lesions usually go on unnoticed without causing much discomfort to the patient. On overfills extending into the periapical tissue, a radiolucent area can sometimes be found to circumscribe the material, thus reflecting the tissue irritation that is going on. The process of phagocytosis may eliminate the excess root filling material and occasionally also material inside the canal (see Chapter 12). Hence, the responses to root filling material may remain for years and prevent complete healing. A slight excess of root filling material does not cause extensive lesions: a bacterial etiology should be suspected for more extensive lesions.

It is not uncommon for dentin chips removed from the canal walls during instrumentation to be displaced into or packed against the residual pulp (Fig. 4.19). Unless infected, this is usually regarded as beneficial because dentin chips:

- separate the root filling material from the apical tissue;
- are instrumental in building up a hard-tissue barrier (81).

It should be emphasized that neither the packed dentin chips nor the apposition of hard tissue onto displaced dentin chips is impermeable to bacteria and bacterial elements (71), therefore further treatment, e.g. a later access to the canal to prepare for a post space, must be performed under aseptic conditions.

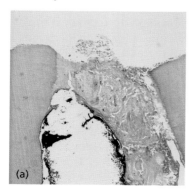 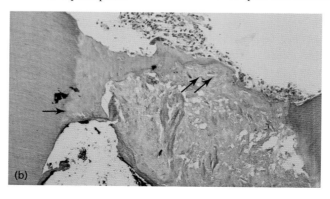

Fig. 4.18 Microphotographs showing apical hard-tissue repair in tooth subjected to pulpectomy and filling with a calcium hydroxide-containing cement 3 months earlier. (b) High magnification shows hard-tissue formation in relation to the root filling material (single arrow) and dentinal shavings (double arrow).

Key literature 4.4

In an experimental study, deliberate apical overinstrumentation was performed by Hørsted and Nygaard-Östby (39) in 20 maxillary incisors and canines scheduled for extraction. The pulps were clinically healthy. The apical pulp tissue was removed and the indicator file was taken through the apical foramen (a).

To study the character of the subsequent tissue response, final shaping, filing and root filling were made substantially short of the radiographic foramen (b). After extracting the teeth 6–10 months later, histological examination revealed a cell-rich well-vascularized connective tissue within the apical part of the canal. This tissue bordered the root filling material and harbored only a few inflammatory cells. Hard tissue was deposited on the canal walls in areas of previous internal root resorption (c).

The authors concluded that unintentional removal of the entire vital pulp to the periodontal membrane does not necessitate subsequent filling of the entire canal provided that strict asepsis is maintained during the treatment. Thus, if unintentional overinstrumentation is experienced, the root canal instrument should be withdrawn and further shaping and filing should be restricted to the original working length in order to facilitate a tight fit of the root filling and avoid surplus root filling material. The potential for revascularization and regeneration of tissue in the root canal system as demonstrated in this and other studies has recently gained renewed interest. Research is in progress to develop methods by which pulps in teeth with pulp necrosis can be regenerated (30, 53).

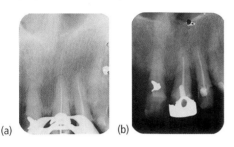

(a)   (b)

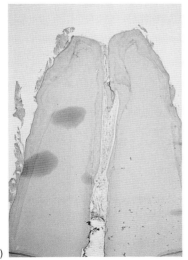

(c)

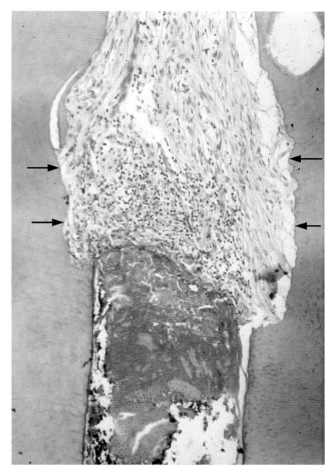

Fig. 4.19   Dentin chips removed from the canal walls during instrumentation are packed against the apical pulp tissue. About 2 months following root filling there is a slight inflammatory reaction of the tissue close to the dentin chips and resorption of the canal walls (→), but normal appearance of fibrous tissue and canal lumen further apically.

Emergency treatment

Emergency treatment is primarily carried out to give relief from painful symptoms. It may also be driven by an unforeseen complication that is not associated with pain but that requires temporary treatment until a definitive treatment can be conducted. As for teeth with vital pulps, emergency treatment may occur due to:

- painful pulpitis;
- pulp exposure because of caries, iatrogenic injury or trauma in an otherwise non-painful tooth;
- mid-treatment or post-treatment pain subsequent to pulpectomy.

Time often sets limits for what is possible to achieve. Time constraints may be due to unscheduled appointments in between regularly scheduled patients in the clinic, or because a complication occurred at the end of a scheduled treatment session. This means that an emergency treatment, by its very nature, is often a compromise. Nevertheless, the operation has to be carried out and should be directed to either alleviate or prevent the development of a painful condition or any other adverse sequelae. This part of the chapter describes procedures that may be undertaken to meet such objectives as far as the vital pulp is concerned.

Painful pulpitis

In an emergency situation one may be faced with patients in different degrees of pain and thus of different urgency for treatment. Although severely discomforting to the patient, there may just be an enhanced sensitivity to thermal, osmotic and tactile stimuli, which disappears upon removal of the pain stimulus. In yet other cases the condition is severe and lingering and the urgency for treatment is high (see Core concept 4.1).

Also, the cause may vary. Most often teeth in pain are associated with a deep carious lesion or restoration penetrating either to the vicinity of or straight to the pulp. There may also be a cracked or fractured tooth, where either large areas of dentin or a frank exposure of the pulp have emerged. Patients who fairly recently have been exposed to periodontal therapy may also present with episodic bursts of more or less lingering pain to external stimuli, indicating painful pulpitis.

Identifying the offending tooth is an important primary task and yet it may represent a most demanding diagnostic challenge (see also Chapter 14). The primary reason is that symptoms other than the patient's report of pain are rarely present. This means that if there is not an overt deep carious lesion, which is the most common cause of painful pulpitis, the clinician may be faced with the dilemma of assessing which one of several teeth is affected (Case study 2).

Management principles

Patients with pulpal pain may require a pulpectomy procedure but this decision should be taken only after careful consideration of the causes and the extent to which the pain condition can be alleviated by a more conservative approach. Determining the urgency for one or another mode of treatment is further complicated by the fact that patients in pain are often under great stress and may feel fear and anxiety about the treatment (see Chapter 16); therefore a condition may appear more severe than it actually is and thus prompt a more invasive procedure than is needed.

Cases where the pulp is not exposed and where the painful condition is about hypersensitivity or only short-lasting pain to external stimuli are especially amenable to a conservative, or wait and see, kind of treatment. A

recent restorative procedure or recent periodontal therapy are examples of these cases; the symptoms are often of a temporary nature and will disappear over a few weeks without active treatment. If symptoms are pronounced or have persisted for some time, removal of the restoration and replacement with a new or temporary restoration may take care of the problem. However, root exposure subsequent to periodontal therapy or tooth wear is not managed as easily and requires some form of therapeutic agent that can block the permeability of the involved dentinal tubules so that pain transmission via the hydrodynamic mechanism is not possible (see Chapter 3).

The alpha and omega of emergency pain treatment is to listen very carefully to the story given by the patient before any intraoral examination and treatment. By spending sufficient time on listening and asking relevant questions many mistreatments may be avoided (see Chapter 14).

In cases where the condition of the pulp is deemed to be of an irreversible nature, the first step in the emergency treatment is to expose the pulp. If there is a carious lesion, all carious dentin should be excavated first. From then on several options are available, although time pressure often decides the choice of treatment. Several studies have indicated that pulpectomy with complete debridement of the root canals is the emergency treatment with the highest probability of pain relief (60, 82). Sufficient time is often not available to relieve pain in the acute patient by this procedure. An alternative faster treatment with a high rate of success is pulpotomy, where the coronal pulp is removed (33, 60) (Clinical procedure 4.3). The fastest and simplest treatment, but the least predictable, is to cover the pulpal exposure with a cotton pellet and a temporary filling. Where pulp is exposed after caries removal in an asymptomatic tooth, the latter procedure is normally sufficient until the patient can be scheduled for pulpectomy.

Clinical procedure 4.3   Emergency pulpotomy

(1) Prepare access opening to the pulp and remove the coronal pulp with a bur in an air-rotor.
(2) Irrigate with copious amounts of 0.1% chlorhexidine or 0.5% NaOCl.
(3) Control hemorrhage by pressure with sterile cotton pellets. In the case of profuse bleeding, soak pellets in 3% hydrogen peroxide or an aqueous mixture of $Ca(OH)_2$.
(4) Apply a small sterile cotton pellet to the pulpal wound at the canal orifices.
(5) Restore access cavity with a temporary filling.
(6) Perform pulpectomy as soon as possible.

Special considerations

It was previously held that a sedative or antibacterial dressing, such as eugenol, camphorated phenol or steroids, was a necessary adjunct to obtain pain relief. Comparative studies have shown that there is no additional effect from using agents of this nature over what is gained by the placement of a sterile dry cotton pellet (33, 86). The cotton pellet also may be omitted because its function is merely to ease the location of the canal orifices at the next sitting upon removal of the temporary filling. If a pellet is placed it must be small to permit a 4–5 mm thick layer of temporary filling material (e.g. zinc oxide–eugenol cement) to prevent bacterial leakage and infection of the pulp between sessions.

Although pulpectomy has shown the highest success rate of pain relief, pulpotomy has given total or partial pain relief in about 95% of cases in clinical follow-ups (42, 60). In situations where pain relief is not accomplished by pulpotomy, pulpectomy should be performed and the patient should be made aware that some postoperative tenderness or a slight dull pain in the affected region is to be expected for a couple of days after the emergency procedure. If severe pain continues, the patient should be advised to call and ask for a new appointment.

Pulp exposure by trauma or caries in a non-painful tooth

In the case of pulp exposure of an asymptomatic pulp by trauma or caries, direct pulp capping or partial pulpotomy may be considered. Either treatment should be given as soon as possible following injury and then a permanent filling to preclude bacterial contamination should be carried out. If proper conditions for capping or pulpotomy do not exist, then pulpectomy is the treatment of choice and may be scheduled for a later appointment. In this case pulpal exposure should be managed by a temporary dressing as described above.

Mid-treatment or post-treatment emergency

A painful condition may remain after emergency pulpectomy or arise following pulpectomy of an initially non-painful tooth. The latter condition is termed endodontic flare-up. The cause is likely to be of bacterial origin combined with an inadequate technical procedure. Contamination due to not applying a rubber dam, an unsatisfactory temporary restoration, displacement of carious dentin and bacterial plaque into the canal are key factors (1, 42, 69, 86). In combination with inappropriate intracanal medication, incomplete instrumentation, non-instrumented canals and apical over-

---

> **Core concept 4.6**
>
> Adherence to basic endodontic principles – including aseptic treatment, complete removal of accessible pulpal tissue and filling of canal to proper length – favors pain relief and precludes endodontic flare-ups.

instrumentation, it is easy to comprehend that conditions for bacterial multiplication are created in the root canal system. It should be emphasized that complications of this nature should be rare and only occur at a low rate in a properly managed clinical practice (42, 82) (Core concept 4.6). Cracked tooth substance and traumatic occlusion are other factors to consider when examining patients for causes of an endodontic flare-up.

In painful conditions after pulpectomy, the first step is to assess the need to carry out a re-entry procedure. This is particularly relevant if the tooth is already permanently filled. The condition is often self-healing and may be controlled simply by over-the-counter pain medication and a reduction of the functional cusps. If re-entry is deemed necessary, the endodontic procedure should follow the same strict routine as described above, which includes proper rubber dam application and disinfection. If necessary, the access opening should be adjusted to gain optimal entry to the root canal system. It is advantageous to enter without anesthesia for the control of any missed canals or incomplete removal of pulpal tissue. Of course, the control should be carried out with great care under gentle probing of potential canal orifices and root canals. Special notice should be given to the high frequency of maxillary molars with two mesial canals; the one that is most often missed is the mesiolingual canal. In lower molars the distal root may also harbor two canals. Copious irrigation and reinstrumentation of the canals should then follow, if necessary under local anesthesia. On carrying out the procedure, ensure proper working length and temporize the canal with a dressing of calcium hydroxide. In order to secure a bacteria-tight temporary filling of sufficient strength, a mix of a zinc oxide–eugenol cement or similar compound should be applied over the calcium hydroxide dressing, followed by a surface seal of hard-setting cement.

An endodontic flare-up may also be associated with an overfilled root canal. Normally, a small extrusion of root filling material does not cause more than slight tenderness, if at all, over a couple of days and subsides over the following days. If a severe pain condition has developed along with apical tenderness and some swelling, there is often a bacterial cause where, along with the root filling material, microorganisms have been pushed into the periodontal tissues. Gross overfills may by themselves cause severe tissue responses due to a strong toxic effect.

A rare but severe complication is associated with root filling material being forced into the mandibular canal. This is especially true if a paraform-releasing paste has been used (see Chapter 12). In such instances the patient may be numb for a few days, which later may lead to a severe pain condition due to neuritis. Such a painful condition may last for weeks or months.

Case study 1

Sequelae following the use of toxic endodontic medicaments

A patient appeared in the dental clinic with pain and swelling related to the first right mandibular molar, a reduced capability of opening the mouth and paresthesia of the right lower lip. Root canal treatment had been initiated by another dentist some time previously and paraform used as a deposit between sittings. The intra-oral examination revealed exposed cortical bone between the molar and the second premolar (a). Removal of a temporary filling in the molar released a strong smell of camphorated paramonochlorphenol from a cotton pellet and revealed devitalized pulp tissue and a mesial perforation of the pulp chamber.

The pulp chamber and the root canals were irrigated with copious amounts of sterile saline and the canals were further cleaned and shaped, followed by an intra-canal deposit of a calcium hydroxide suspension. Antibiotics were prescribed.

Surgical removal of the necrotic tissue the following day revealed a mesial perforation of the molar (b).

The swelling was resolved and the paresthesia was reduced after 1 week.

One month later a bone sequestrum was removed and a deep periodontal pocket was probed mesially and in the furcation area (c, d), after which it was decided to extract the molar: (e) shows the mesial aspect of the extracted tooth, with perforation and apical remnants of the periodontal membrane. An implant was inserted later.

The case emphasizes the problematic use of highly toxic endodontic medicaments, which under adverse circumstances may leach to the surrounding periodontal tissues, resulting in serious destruction. (Courtesy of Dr K. Bröndum.)

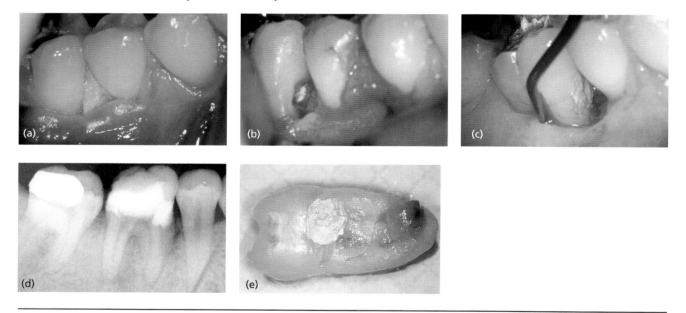

Case study 2

Pulpitis may be accompanied by severe painful symptoms. While the cause is often a deep carious lesion, painful pulpitis may also follow pulp capping or restoration placed close to the pulp. Especially in a dentition that is fully and properly restored the offending tooth may be difficult to identify. The following case demonstrates the dilemma the clinician may be faced with in cases like this.

The emergency patient, a 40-year-old woman, had suffered from excruciating pain over several days. The pain, which is typical in cases of painful pulpitis, varied from none to intense. Also suggestive of pulpitis was that the pain was poorly localized and was felt to variably originate from the lower as well as from the upper jaw on the left hand side. Occasionally the symptoms radiated peripherally to involve the temporal region and the temporomandibular joint. There was, according to the patient, no clear association with intake of hot and cold drinks or food and provocation tests were inconclusive. Paracetamol gave relief, albeit only for a few hours.

The patient, who had been a regular attendant to the clinic, was well restored and had no obvious carious lesion (a and b). Teeth 27 and 35 had received their resin-composite fillings 3 years and 2 years prior to the visit, respectively, while 26 had been restored just a few months earlier. Periodontal conditions were fair without any remarkable pocket probing depths around these teeth although there was some exposure of root dentin that gave highly sensitive responses to cold testing. Sensitivity to percussion or apical palpation was negative. The root filled lower molar had no signs of apical periodontitis although the mesial root was filled somewhat short.

The patient had dental anxiety and refused local anesthetic with epinephrine. Yet, selective anesthesia, normally useful in cases like this, at least to confirm or exclude the location of the pain to one or the other jaw, was attempted. A prerequisite for this measure to be effective is that pain condition is more or less permanent, which was not quite the case. Nevertheless, a mandibular block attaining lower left lip numbness had no effect suggesting location to one of the teeth in the upper, left jaw. A block near the fairly recently restored 26 gave no definitive clue pointing to 27, which in a bitewing radiograph (c) displayed a restoration very close to pulp. Because of the inconclusive anesthetic test, it was elected to postpone emergency treatment for the risk of entering the wrong tooth. Three days later the patient was seen again after having been on analgesics. Tooth 27 was now severely percussion sensitive. Upon accessing the pulp, the causative tooth was confirmed by the finding of a partially necrotic pulp in this tooth.

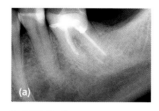
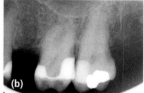
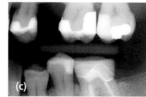

References

1. Abbott PV. Factors associated with continuing pain in endodontics. *Aust. Dent. J.* 1994; 39: 157–61.
2. Accorinte MLR, Loguercio AD, Reis A, Muench A, Araújo VC. Response of human pulp capped with bonding agent after bleeding control with hemostatic agents. *Oper. Dent.* 2005; 30-2: 147–55.
3. Accorinte MLR, Reis A, Loguerico AD, Araújo VC, Muench A. Influence of rubber dam isolation on human pulp responses after capping with calcium hydroxide and an adhesive system. *Quintessence Int.* 2006; 37: 205–12.
4. Accorinte MLR, Holland R, Reis A, Bortoluzzi MC, Murata SS, Dezan E. Jr., *et al.* Evaluation of mineral trioxide aggregate and calcium hydroxide cement as pulp-capping agents in human teeth. *J. Endod.* 2008; 34: 1–6.
5. Barthel CR, Rosenkranz B, Leuenberg A, Roulet J-F. Pulp capping of carious exposures: treatment outcome after 5 and 10 years: a retrospective study. *J. Endod.* 2000; 26: 528–8.
6. Baume LJ. Diagnosis of diseases of the pulp. *Oral Surg.* 1980; 29: 102–16.
7. Baume LJ, Holz J. Long term clinical assessment of direct pulp capping. *Int. Dent. J.* 1981; 31: 251–60.
8. Bergenholtz G. Evidence for bacterial causation of adverse pulpal responses in resin-based dental restorations. *Crit. Rev. Oral Biol. Med.* 2000; 11: 467–80.
9. Bergenholtz G. Advances since the paper by Zander and Glass (1949) on the pursuit of healing methods for pulpal exposures: historical perspectives. *Oral Surg. Oral Med. Oral Pathol. Oral Radiol. Endod.* 2005; 100: 5102–8.

10. Bergenholtz G, Spångberg L. Controversies in endodontics. *Crit. Rev. Oral Med. Biol.* 2004; 15: 99–114.

11. Caliskan MK. Pulpotomy of carious vital teeth with periapical involvement. *Int. Endod. J.* 1995; 28: 172–6.

12. Cox CF, Bergenholtz G, Fitzgerald M, Heys DR, Heys RJ, Avery JK. Capping of the dental pulp mechanically exposed to the oral microflora – a 5 week observation of wound healing in the monkey. *J. Oral Pathol.* 1982; 11: 327–39.

13. Cox CF, Bergenholtz G, Heys DR, Syed SA, Fitzgerald M, Heys RJ. Pulp capping of dental pulp mechanically exposed to oral microflora: a 1–2 year observation of wound healing in the monkey. *J. Oral Pathol.* 1985; 14: 156–68.

14. Cox CF, Keall Cl, Keall HJ, Ostro E, Bergenholtz G. Biocompatibility of surface-sealed dental materials against exposed pulps. *J. Prosthet. Dent.* 1987; 57: 1–8.

15. Cox CF, Hafez AA, Akimoto N, Otsuki M, Suzuki S, Tarim B. Biocompatibility of primer, adhesive and resin composite systems on non-exposed and exposed pulps of non-human primates. *Am. J. Dent.* 1998; 11: S56–63.

16. Cvek M. A clinical report on partial pulpotomy and capping with calcium hydroxide in permanent incisors with complicated crown fracture. *J. Endod.* 1978; 4: 232–7.

17. Cvek M, Cleaton-Jones PE, Austin JC, Andreasen JO. Pulp reactions to exposure after experimental crown fractures on grinding in adult monkeys. *J. Endod.* 1982; 9: 391–7.

18. Cvek M, Granath L, Cleaton-Jones P, Austin J. Hard tissue barrier formation in pulpotomized monkey teeth capped with cyanoacrylate or calcium hydroxide for 10 and 60 minutes. *J. Dent. Res.* 1987; 66: 1166–74.

19. Cvek M. Prognosis of luxated non-vital maxillary incisors treated with calcium hydroxide and filled with gutta-percha. A retrospective clinical study. *Endod. Dent. Traumatol.* 1992; 8: 45–55.

20. De Munck J, Van Landuyt K, Peumans M, Poitevin A, Lambrechts P, Braem M, Van Meerbeek B. A critical review of the durability of adhesion to tooth tissue: methods and results. *J. Dent Res.* 2005; 84: 118–32.

21. de Souza Costa CA, Lopes do Nascimento AB, Teixeira HM, Fontana UF. Response of human pulps capped with a self-etching adhesive system. *Dent. Mater.* 2001; 17: 230–40.

22. Dummer PM, McGinn JH, Rees DG. The position of topography of the apical canal constriction and apical foramen. *Int. Endod. J.* 1984; 17: 192–8.

23. Farsi N, Alamoudi N, Balto K, Mushayt AA. Clinical assessment of mineral trioxide aggregate (MTA) as direct pulp capping in young permanent teeth. *J. Clin. Pediatr. Dent.* 2006; 31: 72–6.

24. Fitzgerald M. Cellular mechanics of dentinal bridge repair using ³H-thymidine. *J. Dent. Res.* 1979; 58: 2198–206.

25. Fitzgerald M, Chiego D, Heys DR. Autoradiographic analysis of odontoblast replacement following pulp exposure in primate teeth. *Arch. Oral Biol.* 1990; 35: 707–15.

26. Fuks AB, Gavra S, Chosack A. Long-term follow up of traumatized incisors treated by partial pulpotomy. *Pediatr. Dent.* 1993; 15: 334–6.

27. Gesi A, Hakeberg M, Warfwinge J, Bergenholtz G. Incidence of osteolytic lesions and clinical symptoms after pulpectomy – a clinical evaluation of one- versus two-session treatment. *Oral Surg. Oral Med. Oral Pathol. Oral Radiol. Endod.* 2006; 101: 379–88.

28. Goldberg M, Smith AJ. Cells and extracellular matrices of dentin and pulp: a biological basis for repair and tissue engineering. *Crit. Rev. Oral Biol. Med.* 2004; 15: 13–27.

29. Gwinnet AJ, Tay FR. Early and intermediate time response of the dental pulp to an acid etch technique *in vivo*. *Am. J. Dent.* 1998; 11: S35–44.

30. Hargreaves KM, Giesler T, Henry M, Wang Y. Regeneration potential of the young permanent tooth: what does the future hold? *Pediatr. Dent.* 2008; 30: 253–60.

31. Hashimoto M, Ohno H, Kaga M, Endo K, Sano H, Oguchi H. *In vivo* degradation of resin–dentin bonds in humans over 1 to 3 years. *J. Dent. Res.* 2000; 79: 1385–91.

32. Hasselgren G, Olsson B, Cvek M. Effects of calcium hydroxide and sodium hypochlorite on the dissolution of necrotic porcine muscle tissue. *J. Endod.* 1988; 14: 125–7.

33. Hasselgren G, Reit C. Emergency pulpotomy: pain relieving effect with and without the use of sedative dressings. *J. Endod.* 1989; 15: 254–6.

Seventy-three patients seeking emergency treatment because of acute pulpal pain were subjected to pulpotomies. After removal of the coronal portion of the pulp a cotton pellet moistened with camphorated phenol, eugenol, cresatin or isotonic saline, or simply a dry pellet, was placed on the remaining pulp tissue by random selection. Alternatively, zinc oxide–eugenol cement was placed directly on the pulpal tissue, which also was used for sealing the access cavities in the 73 teeth. Three of the patients returned for further treatment with pulpectomies after the anesthetic effect had disappeared. The residual 70 patients had no pain 1 day after the emergency treatment, irrespective of whether a medicament was used or not. The common use of sedative dressings seems thus to have no pain-relieving effect. The important part of the emergency treatment is removal of the irritants and the most inflamed part of the pulp tissue, followed by a bacteria-tight temporary filling.

34. Hayashi Y, Imai M, Yanagiguchi K, Viloria IL, Ikeda IL, Ikeda T. Hydroxyapatite applied as direct pulp capping medicine substitutes for osteodentin. *J. Endod.* 1999; 25: 225–9.

35. Heide S, Kerekes K. Delayed partial pulpotomy in permanent incisors of monkeys. *Int. Endod. J.* 1986; 19: 78–89.

36. Heide S, Mjör IA. Pulp reactions to experimental exposures in young permanent monkey teeth. *Int. Endod. J.* 1983; 16: 11–19.

37. Hunter FA. Saving pulps. A queer process. *Items of Interest* 1883; 352.

38. Hørsted P, El Attar K, Langeland K. Capping of monkey pulps with Dycal and a Ca-eugenol cement. *Oral Surg.* 1981; 52: 531–53.

39. Hørsted P, Nygaard-Östby B. Tissue formation in the root canal after total pulpectomy and partial root filling. *Oral Surg.* 1978; 46: 275–82.

40. Hørsted P, Søndergaard B, Thylstrup A, El Attar K, Fejerskov O. A retrospective study of direct pulp capping with calcium hydroxide compounds. *Endod. Dent. Traumatol.* 1985; 1: 29–34.

41. Hørsted-Bindslev P, Vilkinis V, Sidlauskas A. Direct capping of human pulps with a dentin bonding system or with calcium hydroxide cement. *Oral Surg. Oral Med. Oral Pathol. Oral Radiol. Endod.* 2003; 96: 591–600.

42. Imura N, Zuolo ML. Factors associated with endodontic flare-ups: a prospective study. *Int. Endod. J.* 1995; 28: 261–5.

43. Iwamoto CE, Adachi E, Pameijer CH, Barnes D, Romberg EE, Jefferies S. Clinical and histological evaluation of with ProRoot MTA in direct pulp capping. *Am. J. Dent.* 2006; 19: 85–90.

44. Jaber L, Mascrès C, Donohue WB. Electron microscope characteristics of dentin repair after hydroxyapatite direct pulp capping in rats. *J. Oral Pathol. Med.* 1991; 20: 502–8.

45. Kardos TB, Hunter AR, Hanlin SM, Kirk EEJ. Odontoblast differentiation: a response to environmental calcium? *Endod. Dent. Traumatol.* 1998; 14: 105–11.

46. Kerekes K, Tronstad L. Long-term results of endodontic treatment performed with a standardized technique. *J. Endod.* 1979; 5: 83–90.

47. Ketterl W. Kriterien für den Erfolg der Vitalexstirpation. *Dtsch. Zahnärztl. Z.* 1965; 20: 407–16.

48. Kitasako Y, Inokoshi S, Tagami J. Effects of direct resin pulp capping techniques on short-term response of mechanically exposed pulps. *J. Dent.* 1999; 27: 257–63.

49. Malamed S. *Handbook of Local Anesthesia*, 5th edn. St. Louis: Mosby, 2004.

50. Mejàre I, Cvek M. Partial pulpotomy in young permanent teeth with deep carious lesions. *Endod. Dent. Traumatol.* 1993; 9: 238–42.

51. Michaelson PL, Holland GR. Is pulpitis painful? *Int. Endod. J.* 2002; 35: 829–32.

    Two-thousand endodontically treated maxillary incisors were checked with regard to history of pain prior to treatment. It was observed that many diseased pulps (40%) progressed to necrosis without producing a painful condition. Elderly individuals experienced painless pulpitis more often than younger patients.

52. Modaresi J, Dianat O, Soluti A. Effect of pulp inflammation on nerve impulse quality with or without anesthesia. *J. Endod.* 2008; 34: 438–41.

53. Murray PE, Garcia-Godoy F, Hargreaves KM. Regenerative endodontics: a review of current status and a call for action. *J. Endod.* 2007; 33: 377–90.

54. Myer SL. The efficacy of an intraosseous injection. System of delivering local anesthetic. *J. Am. Dent. Assoc.* 1995; 126: 81–6.

55. Nair PNR, Duncan HF, Pitt Ford TR, Luder HU. Histological, ultrastructural and quantitative investigations on the response of healthy human pulps to experimental capping with mineral trioxide aggregate: a randomized controlled trial. *Int. Endod. J.* 2008; 41: 128–50.

56. Nyborg H. Capping of the pulp. The processes involved and their outcome. A report of the follow-ups of a clinical series. *Odontol. Tidskr.* 1958; 66: 296–364.

57. Nyborg H, Tullin B. Healing processes after vital extirpation. An experimental study of 17 teeth. *Odontol. Tidskr.* 1965; 73: 430–46.

58. Nygaard-Östby B. *Introduction to Endodontics.* Oslo: Universitetsforlaget, 1971.

59. Nygaard-Östby B, Hjortdal O. Tissue formation in the root canal following pulp removal. *Scand. J. Dent. Res.* 1971; 79: 333–49.

60. Oguntebi BR, DeSchepper EJ, Taylor TS, White CL, Pink FE. Postoperative pain incidence related to the type of emergency treatment of symptomatic pulpitis. *Oral Surg.* 1992; 73: 479–83.

61. Oguntebi BR, Heaven T, Clark AE, Pink FE. Quantitative assessment of dentin bridge formation following pulp-capping miniature swine. *J. Endod.* 1995; 21: 79–82.

62. Pereira JC, Stanley HR. Pulp capping: influence of the exposure site on pulp healing – histologic and radiographic study in dogs' pulp. *J. Endod.* 1981; 7: 213–23.

63. Pereira JC, Seagale AD, Costa CAS. Human pulpal response to direct pulp capping with an adhesive system. *Am. J. Dent.* 2000; 13: 139–47.

64. Pitt Ford TR, Torabinejad M, Abedi HR, Bakland LK, Kariyawasam SP. Using mineral trioxide aggregate as a pulp-capping material. *J. Am. Dent. Assoc.* 1996; 127; 1491–8.

65. Potocnik I, Bajrovic F. Failure of inferior alveolar nerve block in endodontics. *Endod. Dent. Traumatol.* 1999; 15: 247–51.

66. Qudeimat KM, Barrieshi-Nusair KM, Owais AI. Calcium hydroxide vs. mineral trioxide aggregates for partial pulpotomy of permanent molars with deep caries. *Eur. Arch. Paediatr. Dent.* 2007; 8: 2.

67. Ricucci D. Apical limit of root canal instrumentation and obturation, part 1. Literature review. *Int. Endod. J.* 1998; 31: 384–93.

68. Ricucci D, Langeland K. Apical limit of root canal instrumentation and obturation, part 2. A histological study. *Int. Endod. J.* 1998; 31: 394–409.

    Report presents histological observations of the apical and periapical tissue from 41 root filled human teeth. Inflammatory tissue reactions were seen many years after completion of root fillings in cases with extrusion of root filling material into the periapical tissue, whereas the most favorable histological conditions were observed when obturation remained at or short of the apical constriction.

69. Rosenberg PA, Babick PJ, Schertzer L, Leung A. The effect of occlusal reduction on pain after endodontic instrumentation. *J. Endod.* 1998; 24: 492–6.

70. Rutherford B, Fitzgerald M. A new biological approach to vital pulp therapy. *Crit. Rev. Oral Biol. Med.* 1995; 6: 218–29.

71. Safavi K, Hørsted P, Pascon EA, Langeland K. Biological evaluation of the apical dentin chip plug. *J. Endod.* 1985; 11: 18–24.

72. Schröder U. Effects of calcium hydroxide-containing pulp capping agents on pulp cell migration, proliferation, and differentiation. *J. Dent. Res.* 1985; 64: 541–8.

73. Schuurs AHB, Gruythuysen RJM, Wesselink PR. Pulp capping with adhesive resin-based composite versus calcium hydroxide: a review. *Endod. Dent. Traumatol.* 2000; 16: 240–50.

74. Sedgley CM, Messer HH. Are endodontically treated teeth more brittle? *J. Endod.* 1992; 18: 332–5.

75. Seltzer S, Bender IB, Ziontz M. The dynamics of pulp inflammation: correlations between diagnostic data and actual histologic findings in the pulp. *Oral Surg.* 1963; 16: 846–71.

76. Spångberg L, Engström B. Studies on root canal medicaments II. Cytotoxic effect of medicaments used in root filling. *Acta Odontol. Scand.* 1967; 25: 183–6.

77. Stanley HR, Lundy T. Dycal therapy for pulp exposures. *Oral Surg.* 1972; 34: 818–27.

78. Stein P, Brueckner J, Milliner M. Sensory Innervation of mandibular teeth by the nerve to the mylohyoid: implications in local anesthesia. *Clin. Anat.* 2007; 20: 591–5.

79. Sübay RK, Asci S. Human pulpal response to hydroxyapatite and a calcium hydroxide material as direct capping agents. *Oral Surg.* 1993; 76: 485–92.

80. Tronstad L. Reaction of the exposed pulp to Dycal treatment. *Oral Surg.* 1974; 38: 945–53.

81. Tronstad L. Tissue reactions following apical plugging of the root canal with dentin chips in monkey teeth subjected to pulpectomy. *Oral Surg.* 1978; 45: 297–304.

82. Trope M. Flare-up rate of single-visit endodontics. *Int. Endodont. J.* 1991; 24: 24–7.

83. Tziafas D, Smith AJ, Lesot H. Designing new treatment strategies in vital pulp therapy. *J. Dent.* 2000; 28: 77–92.

84. Tziafas D, Pantelidou O, Alvanou A, Belibasakis G, Papadimitriou S. The dentinogenic activity of mineral trioxide (MTA) in short-term capping experiments. *Int. Endod. J.* 2002; 35: 245–54.

85. Wallace JA, Michanowicz AE, Mundell RD, Wilson EG. A pilot study of the clinical problem of regionally anesthetizing the pulp of an acutely inflamed mandibular molar. *Oral Surg.* 1985; 59: 517–21.

86. Walton R, Fouad A. Endodontic interappointment flare-ups: a prospective study of incidence and related factors. *J. Endod.* 1992; 18: 172–7.

87. Yoshiba K, Yoshiba N, Nakamura H, Iwaku M, Ozawa H. Immunolocalization of fibronectin during reparative dentinogenesis in human teeth after pulp capping with calcium hydroxide. *J. Dent. Res.* 1996; 75: 1590–7.

88. Zilberman U, Mass E, Sarnat H. Partial pulpotomy in carious permanent molars. *Am. J. Dent.* 1989; 2: 147–50.

Chapter 5
Endodontics in primary teeth

Ingegerd Mejàre

Introduction

The need for endodontic treatment in primary teeth is usually related to caries in molars, with the main objective being to maintain space in order to prevent crowding of the permanent teeth. Normally, the most important time period is before the first permanent molars have reached occlusion. The special features of the primary molar, such as the complicated root anatomy and close relation to the permanent tooth germ and its restricted period of function, make the treatment principles somewhat different from those of permanent teeth. These principles will be reviewed in this chapter.

The normal pulp

The histological appearance of the normal pulp in a primary tooth is no different from that of the permanent tooth. Physiological aging occurs in both, although the time span during which this occurs is shorter in primary teeth. A common misunderstanding is that the primary tooth is not as sensible to pain as the permanent tooth and that operative treatment therefore would not require local anesthesia to the same extent. Even though it has been observed that the quantity of nerve fibers is smaller in the pulp of primary teeth (62), there is no proof that the primary tooth would not be equally sensible to pain. The only exception would be just before exfoliation, when the number of nerves within the pulp decreases.

Pulpal inflammation in the primary tooth

Even though there has been some controversy in the literature as to the capacity of the pulp of primary teeth to respond to caries by forming reparative dentin, several histological studies have demonstrated a frequent occurrence of reparative dentin in primary molars with deep caries (33, 60, 63, 72). Magnusson and Sundell (42) found a significantly lower frequency of pulp exposure with a stepwise excavation procedure compared with direct complete excavation of deep caries in primary molars, suggesting that the pulp has good potential to produce reparative dentin.

The morphology of the primary molar implies that the clinical symptoms of pulp tissue reactions to damage may differ from those of permanent teeth (Core concept 5.1). Thus, owing to the relatively small distance from the coronal pulp floor to the bifurcation and the frequent presence of accessory canals through the pulpal floor, pulpal inflammation by caries in primary molars more often results in pathological changes in the interradicular area. Fistula and abscesses due to pulp infection also are seen more often in primary teeth, probably because of the relatively thin buccal cortical bone in young children.

Internal root resorption is the most common sequel to inflammation after pulpotomy, the origin of which is not understood. It may be due to the different way in which the pulp tissue in primary teeth reacts to irritating agents. Thus, it has been shown that the physiological process of shedding occurs in areas lacking predentin, which has been shown to increase the risk of internal resorption (50, 78). By using calcium hydroxide as a dressing material after pulpotomy, the presence of a remaining blood clot between the dressing and the wound surface has been suggested to enhance the internal root resorption process (73).

Diagnosis

Pulpotomy, that is removal of the coronal portion of the pulp tissue, has been and probably still is the most commonly used treatment for primary teeth with carious exposure. As a consequence, focus has been on the ability to assess the extent of preoperative pulpal inflammation. Two diagnostic terms are often used in the literature: *partial pulpitis*, designated for teeth without preoperative clinical and/or radiographic symptoms of pulpal inflammation; and *total pulpitis*, designated for teeth with preoperative symptoms of pulpal inflammation extending into the root pulp (10, 11, 72).

Although essential for the outcome of the treatment, there is at present no means of clinically determining the

Core concept 5.1   Special features of the pulp and root morphology of primary molars in comparison with permanent molars

- The molar has practically no root socle.
- The coronal pulp chamber is comparatively large and wide and the distance to the surface of the tooth is small, in both the occlusal and approximal directions.
- The pulp horns are relatively large, in both the occlusal and approximal directions, making the tooth vulnerable to mechanical and carious exposure.
- The distance from the pulpal floor to the bifurcation is short and the area between the pulp floor and the bifurcation often contains accessory canals. Because of this and a possible less well-mineralized dentin in this area, an interradicular widened periodontal membrane with loss of lamina dura or bone loss is a common radiographic sign of extensive inflammatory changes or necrosis of the pulp tissue.
- The roots are often flared and bent and then converge in the apical part and are in close relation to the permanent tooth. In the coronal part the root canals are reasonably wide and accessible, whereas in the apical part they often show intricate morphology with narrow, ribbon-shaped and curved canals. Instrumentation may therefore be difficult, particularly in upper molars.

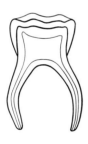 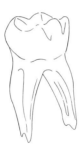

precise histological status of the pulp. Teeth judged to be without signs of total pulpitis might have profound pulpal inflammation. The proportion of correctly diagnosed pulps in histological terms judged from preoperative clinical findings has been investigated, with results varying from 56 to 81%. Most investigators have reported a poor correlation between clinical and histological findings (11, 12, 37, 60, 63), whereas others have found a relatively high agreement of about 80% (38, 72). Several of these studies suffer from a relatively small number of teeth and it is often not stated how the teeth were selected. Overall, it seems that the probability of arriving at a histologically correct pulp diagnosis based on clinical symptoms is rather poor.

In the clinic, it may be sufficient to know whether the pulp is treatable with vital pulp therapy or not, and it has been suggested that if teeth are divided into two treatment categories only, i.e. 'treatable' (= partial pulpitis; vital pulp treatment) or 'not treatable' (= total pulpitis or

necrosis; extraction), the agreement between clinical and histological findings will improve (11, 38). However, these studies also suffer from a small number of selected patients and in one (11) the difference between the two groups was not statistically significant. In the other (38), the basis for grouping the teeth focused on the character of the bleeding of the exposed pulp combined with the character of pain, a variable that is difficult to make unequivocal and reliable.

Along with the introduction of treatment options such as partial pulpotomy, indirect pulp capping and stepwise excavation as alternatives to pulpotomy, the diagnostic terms reversible and irreversible pulpal inflammation have been suggested. However, these terms are not supported by any more reliable or accurate markers than those for partial and total pulpitis.

It follows that there are no clinical means to determine accurately the extent and severity of pulpal inflammation. There are, however, various clinical symptoms that can be used to enhance the probability of arriving at a proper pulp diagnosis (Core concept 5.2). It has to be realized though, that teeth with deep carious lesions without any of these symptoms and accordingly classified as partial pulpitis may be classified correctly in histological terms in no more than 60–70% and at best in 80% of cases.

Importantly, it is less difficult to predict total pulpitis from clinical symptoms than it is to predict a healthy pulp or a pulp with partial pulpitis (11, 12, 37, 60), and the obvious presence of any of the listed symptoms (apart from pain from percussion and/or pressure, which is often difficult to interpret) indicates total pulpitis. Particular notice should be given to radiographic pathological changes such as widened and diffusely outlined lamina dura and the presence of spontaneous pain, particularly at night, both of which strongly suggest total pulpitis. Severe symptoms, such as swelling, fistula or an abscess, suggest pulp necrosis.

Core concept 5.2   Clinical signs of total pulpitis

- Radiographic pathological changes, such as widened periodontal membrane with loss of lamina dura, interradicular or periapical resorptive periodontitis (owing to superimposed structures, radiographic changes may be difficult to discover in maxillary molars)
- Abnormal tooth mobility
- Spontaneous or persistent pain, particularly at night
- Radiographic signs of calcifications in the pulp chamber
- Dark red and/or thick–viscous bleeding of the exposed pulp
- Pulp exposed after removal of demineralized dentin – large pulp exposure
- Profuse bleeding of the exposed pulp
- Pain from percussion and/or pressure (often difficult to interpret, particularly in younger children)

Healing

A proper preoperative pulp diagnosis is decisive for successful endodontic treatment in primary teeth. Presupposing that the cause is removed, the extent to which inflammation can be present in the pulp while the pulp recovers and undergoes repair and healing is not known. In other words, the stage at which the inflammatory process is irreversible is uncertain but essential, because endodontic treatment in primary teeth focuses mainly on vital pulp therapy.

Results from recent clinical studies on direct or stepwise excavation of deep carious lesions in young permanent teeth and partial pulpotomy of cariously exposed pulps in both primary and young permanent teeth suggest that the pulp has good potential to recover once the irritants are removed (35, 39, 47, 74, 93). Thus, for example, a 100% clinical and radiographic success rate was observed after stepwise excavation in young permanent molars with deep carious lesions after observation periods of at least 2 years. Important prerequisites for successful treatment were the absence of clinical and/or radiographic pathological symptoms.

The operative technique must be pointed out as an important factor for successful endodontic treatment. It has been shown that presumably infected dentin fragments unintentionally left behind in the pulp tissue cause widespread inflammatory reactions (36). Therefore, meticulous cleansing of the exposed pulp is crucial, particularly when using capping techniques (35).

Repair and healing after pulpotomy where the amputation site is situated at the orifices of the root canals, depend on whether or not preoperative inflammatory reactions also involve the root pulp, on the operative technique and on the characteristics of the wound dressing used. Furthermore, infection due to bacterial leakage is a prime threat to both repair and healing (5), and the importance of a bacteria-tight seal cannot be overemphasized.

Wound dressings – characteristics, modes of action and reported clinical success rates

The ideal dressing material for either unexposed or exposed vital pulps should be bactericidal and enhance the repair and healing of the pulp. The dressing also should be biocompatible and not interfere with the physiological process of root resorption. The cost of the material should also be reasonable. Unfortunately, the ideal dressing has still to be discovered. Meanwhile, various dressing materials are used. A detailed list of clinical success rates observed for different treatment procedures with different dressing materials is presented in Table 5.1.

The most commonly used wound dressings are: calcium hydroxide, formocresol (FC), glutaraldehyde, corticosteroids (Ledermix®), zinc oxide–eugenol cement and ferric sulfate. Although still not used much in clinical practice, mineral trioxide aggregate (MTA) is also described since promising clinical results have been obtained with this material.

Calcium hydroxide

Calcium hydroxide is used as a dressing material on both unexposed and exposed pulps. It is a strong alkaline compound with a pH of about 12 that causes a superficial necrosis of about 1.5–2 mm in the area underneath its placement on an exposed pulp. After the initial irritation of the underlying tissue, the pulp produces new collagen and thereafter a bone-like hard tissue. Avoidance of an extrapulpal blood clot is essential when using calcium hydroxide as a wound dressing, because its presence may interfere with pulp healing (73). Therefore, it is important to use a gentle technique, including cutting with high-speed equipment and diamond burs followed by irrigation with water or saline in order to achieve hemostasis.

The formation of a hard-tissue barrier, although seldom complete, protects the pulp mechanically and gives partial protection from bacterial infection (Fig. 5.1). It should be noted though that the presence of such a barrier, often considered a criterion of successful treatment, is no guarantee of a healthy residual pulp (57, 71).

Unsuccessful outcomes of pulpotomies using calcium hydroxide as a wound dressing have been attributed to a blood clot left behind between the dressing and wound surface (73). An *in vitro* laboratory study showed that blood and serum substantially lowered the pH of calcium hydroxide and thereby reduced its bactericidal effect (45). The presence of bacteria combined with a blood clot may therefore be an important cause of failure. Because

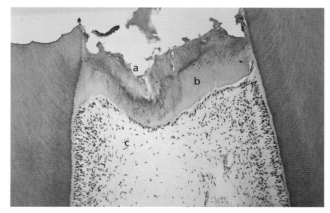

Fig. 5.1 Hard-tissue barrier in a primary molar formed after pulpotomy using calcium hydroxide as a wound dressing (H & E, ×40). a = wound surface; b = hard-tissue barrier; c = normal pulp tissue. (Courtesy of M. Cvek.)

Table 5.1 Reported clinical/radiographic success rates of various vital pulp treatment procedures of primary molars with deep carious lesions along with type of dressing material, number of teeth included in the study and follow-up times.

First author (Reference)	Type of study	Treatment procedure	Dressing material	Number of teeth	Follow-up time	Success rate (%)
Al-Zayer (2)	Retrospective	Indirect pulp capping*	Calcium hydroxide	187	1 yr	96
Falster (14)	RCT	Indirect pulp capping*	Adhesive resin vs Dycal®	48	2 yrs	96 vs 83 (ns)**
Marchi (43)	RCT	Indirect pulp capping*	Dycal vs Vitremer®	27	4 yrs	89 vs 93 (ns)
Farooq (15)	Retrospective	Indirect pulp capping* vs pulpotomy	Vitrebond® FC diluted to 1/5	133	2–7 yrs	93 vs 74
Davies (7)	Cohort	Direct pulp capping	Calcium hydroxide	71	2–3 yrs	60
Pritz (59)	Cohort	Direct pulp capping	Calcium hydroxide	20	2 yrs	57
Tuna (86)	RCT	Direct pulp capping	MTA vs calcium hydroxide	44	2 yrs	100 vs 100[a]
Jeppesen (35)	Cohort	Partial pulpotomy	Calcium hydroxide	78	4 yrs	78
Schröder (72)	Cohort	Partial pulpotomy	Calcium hydroxide	93	1 yr	83
Gruythuysen (24)	Cohort	Pulpotomy	Calcium hydroxide	196	2 yrs	80
Schröder (71)	Cohort	Pulpotomy	Calcium hydroxide	33	2 yrs	59
Via (89)	Retrospective	Pulpotomy	Calcium hydroxide	103	2 yrs	31
Hicks (27)	Cohort	Pulpotomy	FC[a], Buckley's formula	164	3.5 yrs	89
Mejàre (46)	Cohort	Pulpotomy	FC, Buckley's formula	74	2.5 yrs	55[b]
Rölling (69)	Cohort	Pulpotomy	FC, Buckley's formula	98	3 yrs	70
Fuks (18)	Cohort	Pulpotomy	FC, diluted to 1/5	77	2 yrs	94
Morawa (51)	Cohort	Pulpotomy	FC, diluted to 1/5	125	6–60 mo	98
Huth (30)	RCT	Pulpotomy	Laser vs ferric sulfate vs FC vs calcium hydroxide	200	2 yrs	78 vs 86 vs 85 vs 53
Waterhouse (91)	RCT	Pulpotomy	FC vs calcium hydroxide	79	6–38 mo	84 vs 77 (ns)
Smith (77)	Cohort	Pulpotomy	Ferric sulfate	242	4–57 mo	74[c]
Fuks (20)	Cohort	Pulpotomy	Ferric sulfate	55	6–34 mo	93
Fei (17)	Cohort	Pulpotomy	Ferric sulfate	29	1 yr	97
Ibricevic (32)	Comparative	Pulpotomy	Ferric sulfate vs FC, Buckley's formula	164	3.5–4 yrs	92 vs 95 (ns)
Shumayrikh (76)	Cohort	Pulpotomy	Glutaraldehyde, 2%	61	1 yr	74
Tsai (85)	Cohort	Pulpotomy	Glutaraldehyde, 2 or 5%	150	3 yrs	79
Fuks (19)	Cohort	Pulpotomy	Glutaraldehyde, 2%	53	2 yrs	82
Garcia-Godoy (22)	Cohort	Pulpotomy	Glutaraldehyde, 2%	49	1.5–3.5 yrs	96
Gerdes (23)	Retrospective	Pulpotomy	Ledermix®[d]	101	3 yrs	76[e]
Hansen (26)	Cohort	Pulpotomy	Ledermix®	14	1–42 mo	79
Magnusson (41)	Cohort	Pulpotomy	Zinc oxide–eugenol	40	6–39 mo	55
Hansen (26)	Cohort	Pulpotomy	Zinc oxide–eugenol	14	1–42 mo	57
Maroto (44)	Cohort	Pulpotomy	MTA	69	6–42 mo	99
Eidelman (10)	RCT	Pulpotomy	MTA vs FC	32	6–30 mo	100 vs 83 (ns)
Agamy (1)	CCT	Pulpotomy	MTA vs FC	60	1 yr	90 vs 90
Holan (28)	RCT	Pulpotomy	MTA vs FC	62	38 mo	97 vs 83 (ns)
Farsi (16)	RCT	Pulpotomy	MTA vs FC	120	2 yrs	99 vs 87 (radiographic)
Moretti (52)	RCT	Pulpotomy	MTA vs FC vs calcium hydroxide	43	2 yrs	100 vs 100 vs 36
Casas (6)	RCT	Pulpectomy vs pulpotomy	Ferric sulfate	29	3 yrs	92 vs 62

* Without re-entry.

** ns = no statistically significant difference.

[a] Size of pulp exposure <1 mm.

[b] 61% of the molars had obvious preoperative clinical signs of total pulpitis.

[c] The success rate after 2–3 years was 81% ($n = 57$) and after >3 years it was 74% ($n = 31$).

[d] Contains a synthetic corticosteroid and Ledermycin®.

[e] Successful was defined as functioning, i.e. teeth with radiographic evidence of internal root resorption were included in successful cases (15%).

FC = formocresol; MTA = mineral trioxide aggregate; RCT = randomized clinical trial.

the blood clot probably serves as a buffer, it also prevents calcium hydroxide from exerting its superficial necrotizing effect on the pulp tissue. Another reason for failure could be an incorrect preoperative pulp diagnosis. Thus, it has been suggested that calcium hydroxide has no other effect besides promoting the formation of a hard-tissue barrier and therefore cannot be used successfully on an inflamed pulp tissue (73). The latter suggestion is, however, not consistent with recent reports on relatively high rates of successful treatments using partial pulpotomy in cariously exposed pulps (47, 74).

After pulpotomy with calcium hydroxide as a wound dressing, reported success rates vary between 31 and 80% (24, 52, 71, 89). Using the same diagnostic criteria, the overall success rates were higher when calcium hydroxide was used as a dressing material after partial pulpotomy (78–83%) (35, 74) (Table 5.1). As judged from these studies, it seems that the partial pulpotomy technique is more favorable than direct pulp capping. Randomized clinical studies comparing the two techniques have yet to confirm this assumption.

Formocresol

Formocresol (FC) is used as a dressing material after pulpotomy. The original compound, Buckley's FC, contains concentrated formalin (19% formaldehyde), cresol (35%) and glycerol (7%) in an aqueous solution, the main active component being formaldehyde. Nowadays, Buckley's formula is often diluted to one-fifth of its original strength. Depending on the concentration and time of exposure to formaldehyde, part of the root pulp tissue is devitalized. Importantly, it has been shown that even after prolonged application of the full concentration of FC the entire pulp was not devitalized (48, 66).

The most common histological appearance when using FC as a wound dressing is devitalized pulp tissue in the upper part of the root canal, inflammatory changes with internal root resorption and apposition of hard tissue in the middle section, with the most apical part usually showing normal pulp tissue (66) (Fig. 5.2). Thus, the use of FC does not result in repair and healing in histological terms, and a hard-tissue barrier underneath the dressing is not formed. This makes the tooth vulnerable to contamination from bacterial leakage and emphasizes the importance of a bacteria-tight seal when restoring the tooth.

As shown in Table 5.1, in most studies on pulpotomy the clinical success rates using Buckley's formula are higher than those obtained with calcium hydroxide as a dressing material (18, 27, 46, 51, 69). Also, when diluted 1:5, the clinical success rates of FC are considerably higher than those of calcium hydroxide (18, 51). Fuks and Bimstein (18), reporting a clinical success rate of 94% after 2 years of observation, recommended the use of the diluted formula of FC instead of Buckley's FC.

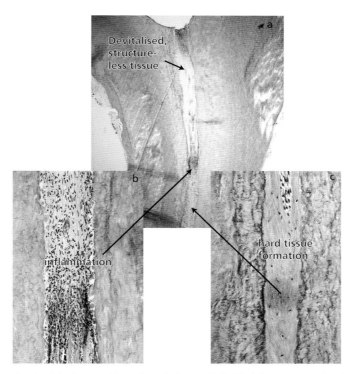

Fig. 5.2 Palatal root of upper second molar. Pulp tissue reactions after pulpotomy with Buckley's formocresol as dressing, 2.5 years postoperatively: (a) overview (H & E, ×25); (b, c) middle part of the root (H & E, ×60).

The most probable reason for the relatively high clinical success rate with FC as a dressing material is that, as long as the devitalized tissue does not become infected, the tooth usually stays asymptomatic. Furthermore, because of the more extensive devitalization of the pulp compared with calcium hydroxide, the use of FC is not as sensitive to a correct preoperative diagnosis of the inflammatory status of the root pulp as when calcium hydroxide is used. The clinical success rate when using Buckley's FC on molars with obvious clinical signs of total pulpitis amounted to 82% after 1.5 years of observation but dropped to 50% after 3 years (46).

Glutaraldehyde

Glutaraldehyde (GA) – a dialdehyde – has gained increasing attention as a possible substitute for FC as a wound dressing, the suggestion being less pulp devitalization but similar clinical results. Glutaraldehyde has not been produced commercially yet, the main reason being its instability, even when refrigerated.

Like FC, GA can cause allergic skin reactions, and hand dermatitis has been reported in dental assistants after using the disinfecting agent Cidex® (56). There are no unequivocal indications of mutagenic properties of GA. The full concentration or a 1:5 dilution of FC was 2–3 times more cytotoxic to human fibroblasts than 2.5% GA (34). In another study, however, little difference in the relative toxicities was observed between formaldehyde and GA when the data were calculated in terms of molar concentrations rather than dilution (81). Interestingly, GA appeared more toxic to rat nasal epithelium than FC (80). Owing to cross-linking, GA is less penetrative than formaldehyde and consequently causes less immediate damage to pulp tissue. However, in a study on monkeys GA did not result in repair and healing in histological terms (82) and it cannot be ruled out that, under a narrow zone of fixation, partial cell damage and/or a slow death of cells deeper within this zone may lead to chronic cell injury (81).

Studies reporting on the clinical success rate of GA as a wound dressing are listed in Table 5.1. Using 2 or 5% GA, the reported success rates vary from 74 to 96%, the periods of observation being between 1 and 3.5 years (19, 22, 76, 85).

It has been suggested that buffered GA solution is more effective than unbuffered solution. The concentration and time of exposure to the tissue show a strong interaction (81), implying that GA needs a relatively long contact time with the pulp tissue to achieve optimal fixation. Whether this problem can be circumvented in the clinic by raising the concentration is debatable. Thus, the optimal strength of GA is, as yet, uncertain and there are also varying opinions about whether it should be included in the permanent dressing of zinc oxide–eugenol

cement or not. Considering the suggested similar cytotoxicity of GA and FC, it is doubtful whether GA has any advantage over FC as a wound dressing material.

Corticosteroids

The concept behind using corticosteroids as a wound dressing is to suppress and, ideally, reverse any inflammatory reactions in the pulp tissue. Ledermix® – the only commercially available dressing material for this purpose – is a synthetic glucocorticoid with some Ledermycin® (demethylchlortetracycline) added to it, mixed with calcium hydroxide, zinc oxide and eugenol.

There is a great deal of controversy associated with the efficacy of corticosteroids and their capacity, when used locally, to reverse pulpal inflammation. Hansen (25) showed that the active component of Ledermix was decomposed after 18 days. It has been argued also that any anti-inflammatory effect is restricted to the contact area between the dressing and the pulp tissue (3). Furthermore, the dressing does not induce the formation of a hard-tissue barrier, a characteristic considered to be important in protecting the pulp of primary molars from bacterial leakage and subsequent infection. These factors may explain why Ledermix has not gained widespread acceptance as a dressing material.

Hansen et al. (26) compared zinc oxide–eugenol with Ledermix as a wound dressing after pulpotomy in cariously exposed pulps and found less severe internal root resorptions and inflammatory reactions in teeth where Ledermix was used. Although a lenient material without any observed side-effects, only a few studies report on the success rate with a corticosteroid as the wound dressing. In a small study of 30 molars and varying observation times, Hansen et al. (26) reported a success rate of 79%. In a 3-year study with 101 molars, Gerdes et al. (23) reported a success rate of 76% (defined as functioning teeth and including 12 teeth with internal root resorptions and four teeth with radiographic and clinical symptoms). From these studies it might be expected that corticosteroids are superior to calcium hydroxide as a dressing material (see Table 5.1). However, because of the lack of randomized prospective clinical studies using different wound dressing materials, it is not possible to propose the best material.

Zinc oxide–eugenol cement

Zinc oxide–eugenol cement is probably not so often used today as a dressing material alone after pulpotomy; it results in a high percentage of internal resorptions and reported clinical success rates are low (55–57%) (26, 41).

Ferric sulfate

Ferric sulfate ($Fe_2(SO_4)_3$) in a 15.5% solution has been used as a coagulative and hemostatic agent in crown and bridgework. Blood proteins agglutinate when they are exposed to the ferric and sulfate ions but the exact mechanisms of action are still debated.

When used as a wound dressing after pulpotomy, a metal–protein blood clot forms at the site of pulp exposure. Ferric sulfate has been investigated as a possible alternative to FC (17, 19, 77). The reported clinical success rates are similar to those of diluted FC and vary from 78 to 97%. In the retrospective study by Smith *et al.* (77) the clinical success rate was 74% after 3 years of observation ($n = 242$); Fei *et al.* (17) reported a 97% success rate after 3–12 months ($n = 29$); and Fuks *et al.* (19) found a success rate of 93% after observation times varying from 6 to 34 months ($n = 55$). Three systematic reviews comparing formocresol and ferric sulfate medicaments conclude that they are likely to have similar clinical/radiographic results (21, 40, 58).

Mineral trioxide aggregate (MTA)

MTA is a powder composed of tricalcium silicate, bismuth oxide, dicalcium silicate, tricalcium aluminate, tetracalcium aluminoferrite and dicalcium sulfate dihydrate. It sets via hydration to become a collodial gel with a pH of 12.5, similar to that of calcium hydroxide. The setting time is 3–4 hours, and its compressive strength is comparable to that of IRM® (Intermediate Restorative Material, Dentsply, York, PA, USA) (75, 83, 84). MTA in a set state is biocompatible, has good sealing properties and promotes hard-tissue formation (28).

Overall, high success rates (>95%) have been achieved with MTA as dressing material for treating cariously exposed pulps in primary teeth (1, 10, 16, 28, 44, 52, 86). The studies are summarized in Table 5.1. One study compares MTA with calcium hydroxide for direct pulp capping (86). Both materials gave 100% success rate after 2 years. This is contradictory to the other two studies on direct pulp capping where relatively low success rates were obtained. According to the authors, the main reason for the high success rates is that a tight seal was secured by using resin-bonded zinc oxide–eugenol. Other reasons could be that only small exposures (<1 mm) were accepted, and that only occlusal lesions were included. Furthermore, it cannot be ruled out that some pulp exposures were of traumatic origin.

In five studies evaluating MTA as an alternative to formocresol (FC) in pulpotomized primary molars, the success rate of MTA was equal or superior to FC. As a consequence, the authors suggest that MTA is a proper alternative to FC as a pulp dressing material. Moretti *et al.* (52) compared MTA with FC or calcium hydroxide as dressing material and found MTA and FC superior to calcium hydroxide.

To summarize, MTA seems to be the dressing material of choice for treating cariously exposed pulps in primary teeth. Longer follow-up periods are, however, needed before any definite conclusions can be made as to the suitability of MTA as dressing material in pulpotomized primary molars. At present, the major drawbacks with MTA seem to be its cost and perceived problem with storage. Commercially available MTA is expensive and once the package is opened, the material should be sealed in an airtight and waterproof container.

Objectives of pulp treatment

Strictly, the objectives of pulp treatment are repair and healing of the residual pulp tissue in histological terms and a well-functioning tooth until normal exfoliation. At present, calcium hydroxide is the only dressing that, theoretically, has the potential to fulfill these criteria.

Because of the relatively low clinical success rate reported for calcium hydroxide after pulpotomy and because of the restricted lifespan of the primary tooth, less strict criteria for the success of pulp treatment are accepted in many countries. This means that, besides no general harm, no damage should be inflicted to the permanent tooth and the primary tooth should be symptom free until normal exfoliation. Formocresol is considered by many to meet these criteria and, owing to the comparatively high clinical success rate, is still a commonly used dressing material, although healing in histological terms does not occur (Advanced concept 5.1).

Operative treatment procedures

Indications and clinical success

Based on clinical and radiographic symptoms and other possible considerations for deciding the best therapy, the following operative treatment options are available (see Core concept 5.3):

- indirect pulp capping:
  - stepwise excavation
  - without re-entry and further excavation;
- direct pulp capping;
- partial pulpotomy;
- pulpotomy;
- pulpectomy and root canal treatment;
- extraction.

Indirect pulp capping – stepwise excavation

The purpose of stepwise excavation is to prevent pulp exposure by intermittent removal of carious dentin. By comparing the number of pulp exposures from stepwise excavation with those from direct complete excavation, it has been demonstrated both in primary and permanent

Advanced concept 5.1   Concerns about the use of formocresol as a wound dressing in primary teeth

The use of formocresol (FC) as a wound dressing after pulpotomy in primary molars has been critically reviewed (61, 90). Besides its cyto-toxicity, the main concerns are possible carcinogenicity, mutagenicity and the fact that formaldehyde is a potent allergen.

Formaldehyde (CH_2O), the main active agent of FC, is a small, highly reactive molecule that rapidly converts to water and carbon dioxide. It is cytotoxic and causes devitalization when applied to pulp tissue, the extent of which is dose and time dependent (48). Damage to the permanent successor, due to possible diffusion of FC through the pulpal floor, has not been observed, however (18, 67).

Animal studies have shown that formaldehyde has mutagenic and carcinogenic effects. Carcinoma in humans due to formaldehyde exposure is, however, extremely rare (79) and the carcinogenic potential from a single application of FC to the pulp tissue of a primary tooth is negligible. It is to be noted that most of us inhale formalde-hyde daily, mainly from cars, wooden products, textiles, perfumes and other cosmetics and burning wood.

Any increase in positive reactions to patch tests in children who have had a previous FC pulpotomy could not be found (68), but aller-gic reactions to formaldehyde after root canal treatment have been observed in adults (9, 13). There are no known studies on a possible immune response from applying an antigen (allergen) directly to exposed pulp tissue. Although potential antigen-presenting cells mediating the immune response are present in pulp tissue, it seems very unlikely that a single dose of FC applied directly on pulp tissue would sensitize a person. Immunoglobulin E-mediated sensitivity to formaldehyde also seems to be rare (9). In contrast, contact allergy from the handling of the medicament is of major concern for dental personnel.

For the above-mentioned reasons and the lack of healing proper-ties, FC is far from ideal as a wound dressing and efforts to find an efficient substitute for formaldehyde-containing wound-dressing materials in pediatric dentistry are important.

Core concept 5.3   Deep carious lesions

Pulp treatment procedures and their indications	Indicated pulp status

Indirect pulp capping – stepwise excavation

Indications: deep carious lesions, where the bulk of necrotized dentin has not yet reached the pulp; no clinical and/or radiographic signs of pathology, such as persistent pain, widened periodontal membrane or interradicular or periapical periodontitis.

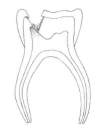

Indirect pulp capping – without re-entry and further excavation

Indication: as for stepwise excavation (no clinical and/or radiographic signs of pathology). The technique differs in that the innermost layer of carious dentin is deliberately and permanently left behind.

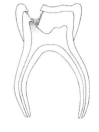

Direct pulp capping

Indication: accidental or pinpoint carious pulp exposure of a symptom-free tooth.

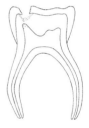

Partial pulpotomy

Indications: traumatic exposure or pulp exposure due to caries; no clinical or radiographic signs of pathology.

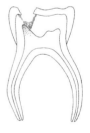

Pulpotomy

Indication: clinical and/or radiographic symptoms indicating coronal pulpal inflammation.

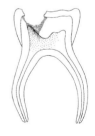

Pulpectomy/root canal treatment

Indications: inflammation extending into the root pulp, pulp necrosis and where special concern makes the tooth valuable.

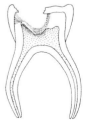

molars that pulp exposures can often be prevented by stepwise excavation (39, 42) (Key literature 5.1). In a systematic review on minimal versus complete caries removal in permanent and primary teeth it was conclud-ed that partial caries removal is preferable to complete caries removal in deep lesions in order to reduce the risk of carious exposure (64).

It is assumed that by placing calcium hydroxide tem-porarily on the remaining innermost layer of carious dentin, the pulp tissue is stimulated to produce repara-tive dentin, allowing complete excavation without pulp exposure to be carried out at a subsequent treatment occasion. It is also possible that, by alleviating the bacte-rial load, pulpal healing and repair are facilitated. Other mechanisms, such as remineralization of the remaining dentin, may be involved but whether and to what extent they contribute to the lower frequency of pulp exposures following stepwise excavation is not known.

Key literature 5.1

In the study by Leksell et al. (39), the prevalence of pulp exposure after stepwise versus direct complete excavation of permanent posterior teeth with deep carious lesions was assessed in 127 teeth from 116 patients aged 6–16 years (mean = 10.2 years). Included were teeth with radiographs revealing carious lesions to such a depth that pulp exposure could be expected if direct complete excavation was performed, but teeth with clinical symptoms other than transient pain shortly before treatment were not accepted. The teeth were randomly selected for either treatment procedure.

Stepwise excavation implied removal of the bulk of carious tissue and application of calcium hydroxide, followed by sealing of the cavity with zinc oxide–eugenol cement. After a period of 8–24 weeks, the rest of the carious dentin was removed and the cavity sealed with calcium hydroxide, zinc oxide–eugenol and a restorative material. Direct complete excavation entailed removal of all carious dentin followed by sealing, as mentioned above. In the case of pulp exposure, a pulp treatment was performed.

The pulp was exposed in 40% of the teeth treated by direct complete excavation. The corresponding figure for those treated by stepwise excavation was 17.5%. The difference was statistically significant. The teeth with no pulp exposure after direct or stepwise excavation showed normal clinical and radiographic conditions at the last check-up (mean = 43 months).

In conclusion, stepwise excavation can prevent pulp exposure in teeth with deep carious lesions and the results indicate that this treatment procedure is successful provided that no preoperative symptoms of irreversible pulpal inflammation are present.

Based on animal studies, Bergenholtz (4) suggested that the healing capacity of the pulp could be substantial once the irritating agents are removed. This assumption was confirmed by the favorable results of the >90% clinical success rate when stepwise excavation was used to treat deep carious lesions in young permanent posterior teeth (39). Although there are no clinical studies confirming the value of stepwise excavation in primary teeth, there is no reason to believe that this procedure should not also be favorable in primary molars. Stepwise excavation is therefore recommended for deep carious lesions in primary molars, presupposing that there are no or only minor preoperative subjective symptoms and no radiographic signs of pathology (i.e. no signs of irreversible pulpal inflammation).

Indirect pulp capping without re-entry and further excavation

Indirect pulp capping is similar to stepwise excavation but differs in the sense that the innermost layer of carious dentin is deliberately and permanently left behind. Four studies using this technique show high clinical success rates (Table 5.1) suggesting that indirect pulp capping is as appropriate as stepwise excavation. Two of them are randomized clinical trials (RCTs) but the

samples are small. Furthermore, there are no RCTs that have compared the two techniques and therefore, there is insufficient evidence to know whether it is necessary to re-enter and excavate further or not. It seems logical to assume that a restoration that gives a tight seal becomes particularly important if indirect pulp capping without re-entry is used.

Direct pulp capping

Direct pulp capping means that a minimal pulp exposure is just cleaned and covered with a wound dressing. Except for one study comparing MTA with calcium hydroxide (86) (see under Wound dressings, MTA), reported clinical success rates after direct pulp capping in primary teeth are low (7, 59) and the procedure should therefore be restricted to accidental or pinpoint carious exposures. In an RCT on hard-tissue formation after direct pulp capping in healthy young permanent teeth, a calcium hydroxide cement was compared clinically and histologically with a dentin bonding material as wound dressing material (31). The calcium hydroxide cement was superior in that complete hard-tissue formation occurred more frequently and fewer inflammatory changes were observed. In principle, de Souza Costa et al. obtained the same results (8). It is therefore recommended to use calcium hydroxide cement as dressing material for direct pulp capping.

Partial pulpotomy

Partial pulpotomy implies removal of only the most superficial part of the pulp tissue adjacent to the exposure, and is indicated for a traumatic pulp exposure or a pulp exposure from a deep carious lesion. Important prerequisites for a favorable result are the same as for stepwise excavation, i.e. no or only minor preoperative subjective symptoms, no radiographic signs of pathology and normal bleeding of the exposed pulp tissue. Two studies report on the clinical success rate in primary molars, varying from 78 to 83% after 1–4 years of observation (35, 74).

Pulpotomy

The indications for pulpotomy (implying removal of the entire coronal pulp) are the same as for partial pulpotomy, i.e. teeth with carious exposures with no or only minor preoperative subjective symptoms, no radiographic signs of pathology and normal bleeding of the exposed pulp tissue. Pulpotomy has been the most commonly used vital pulp therapy and numerous reports have been presented on the success rates. Depending on the status of the pulp, the operative technique, wound dressing and observation time, success rates vary between 31 and 98% (Table 5.1).

Although randomized prospective studies comparing partial pulpotomy and pulpotomy are lacking, the relatively high success rates reported for partial pulpotomy suggest that pulpotomy may be restricted to borderline cases, i.e. when clinical and/or radiographic findings are not easily interpreted and possibly indicate irreversible inflammation in the coronal pulp tissue.

Pulpectomy and root canal treatment

Usually, a primary tooth with clinical and/or radiographic symptoms indicating total pulpitis or pulp necrosis should be extracted. However, if the tooth is considered of special importance (e.g. when the permanent successor is missing) or if the child and the parents appreciate this type of service, pulpectomy or root canal treatment can be performed. The size and shape of the root canals are often considered hindrances but root canal instrumentation might be performed if the canals are considered accessible. In order not to damage the underlying permanent tooth, broaches and files must be handled with extreme care and a resorbable medicament such as calcium hydroxide should be placed in the canals.

Extraction

Generally, clinical and/or radiographic signs of total pulpitis or pulp necrosis suggest extraction of the tooth. This is particularly important in a child with a history of severe acute or chronic illness, because the child should not be subjected to the possibility of further infection resulting from pulp therapy.

How to do it – procedures and important points

Several studies have shown that the type of restoration impacts success rate (15, 24, 29). Irrespective of treatment procedure, a restoration that gives a tight seal is crucial and a stainless steel crown is probably the most effective for preventing bacterial leakage.

Stepwise excavation

Procedure: After local anesthesia, all peripheral caries, the bulk of the necrotic and part of the demineralized dentin are removed. A layer of calcium hydroxide is placed on the remaining carious dentin and covered with zinc oxide–eugenol cement. After 6–8 weeks the rest of the carious dentin is removed and the bottom of the cavity is again covered with a calcium hydroxide layer. A layer of slow-setting zinc oxide–eugenol cement or fast-setting calcium hydroxide-containing cement is placed and the cavity is permanently restored (see Case study 1). Alternatively, another intermediate excavation can be performed.

Partial pulpotomy

Procedure: Local anesthesia and a rubber dam are applied. All caries is removed and 1–1.5 mm of the exposed pulp tissue is removed with a spherical diamond bur and high-speed equipment (with water). It is not critical to use sterile saline but a coolant with ample flow is important. Remove all carious dentin adjacent to the pulp exposure before cutting the pulp tissue. Jeppesen (35) emphasized the importance of careful cleansing of possibly injected dentin chips from the area of amputation before applying the wound dressing. Bleeding is stopped by irrigation with sterile saline or water. Dry gently with sterile cotton pellets. A layer of calcium hydroxide is applied and gently pressed in contact with the wound surface. A layer of slow-setting zinc oxide–eugenol cement or fast-setting calcium hydroxide-containing cement is placed and the cavity restored.

Pulpotomy using calcium hydroxide

Procedure: Local anesthesia and a rubber dam are applied. Access is gained to the pulp chamber. The coronal pulp is removed with a spherical diamond bur and high-speed equipment. The wound surface is irrigated with saline or water. Applying cotton pellets using slight pressure stops bleeding. After hemostasis, the wound surfaces at the orifices of the root canals are covered by a layer of gently pressed calcium hydroxide. A layer of slow-setting zinc oxide–eugenol cement covered with fast-setting cement is placed and the cavity is restored.

Pulpotomy using ferric sulfate (FS)

Procedure: Local anesthesia and a rubber dam are applied. The coronal pulp is removed with a spherical bur and high-speed equipment. A small amount of FS (Astringdent™ Ultradent Products, Salt Lake City, UT, provided as a 15.5% aqueous solution with a plastic syringe and a cotton pellet needle) is applied by gently wiping the cotton tip of the needle against the wound surfaces at the orifices of the root canals for 10–15 s. In order to remove any blood clot formation, the FS is then thoroughly flushed from the pulp chamber with distilled water. After drying with sterile cotton pellets, a layer of slow-setting zinc oxide–eugenol cement is placed on the wound surfaces and covered with fast-setting cement and the cavity is restored.

Pulpotomy using formocresol (FC)

Procedure: Local anesthesia and a rubber dam are applied. The coronal pulp is removed with a spherical bur and high-speed equipment. The wound surfaces at the orifices of the root canals are irrigated with saline or water. Bleeding is stopped by applying cotton pellets using slight pressure. After hemostasis, a cotton pellet soaked in FC is applied to each wound surface and left in place for 3–5 min. Full-strength FC (19% formaldehyde) is recommended if signs of total pulpitis are present, otherwise a one-fifth dilution is sufficient. The pellets are removed and a paste of one drop of FC mixed with zinc oxide–eugenol is placed on the wound surface. Avoid placing the pellets on the pulpal floor. A layer of slow-setting zinc oxide–eugenol cement covered with fast-setting cement is placed and the cavity is restored (see Case study 2).

Pulpotomy using glutaraldehyde

Procedure: Local anesthesia and a rubber dam are applied. The operative procedure is in principle the same as for FC. Pellets soaked in a 2% buffered freshly prepared glutaraldehyde solution are placed on the wound surfaces and left in place for 3–5 min. The pellets are removed and slow-setting zinc oxide–eugenol cement covered with a fast-setting cement is placed and the cavity restored.

Follow-up principles

Clinical and radiographic follow-ups should be done 6 months postoperatively and then at yearly intervals; in general, primary teeth subjected to endodontic treatment should be observed until exfoliation.

Long-term follow-ups are essential (35, 70). In most studies, success or failure has been judged from clinical and radiographic examinations only. However, in a study by Jeppesen (35) on partial pulpotomy, 43/76 clinically successful cases were judged histologically after 4 years of observation and were considered to be successful in 88%. With due respect to the restricted proportion of teeth that could be examined histologically, this is an important observation. It suggests that the majority of cases judged to be successful clinically and radiographically is also successful histologically, even though a potential for new failures may still be present even after a follow-up time of 4 years.

Treatment failure

The clinical means for revealing an unsuccessful treatment include clinical inspection and radiographic examination. The earliest signs of failure are most often radiographically detected internal root resorption and/or interradicular bone loss, with subjective symptoms, such as pain, being unusual. Particularly in small children, electronic pulp testing is often unreliable and instead careful inspection of the tooth and the surrounding oral mucosa should be made. Pathological tooth mobility,

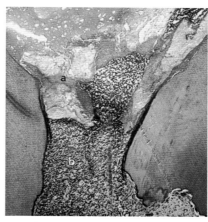

Fig. 5.3 Unsuccessful pulpotomy using calcium hydroxide as dressing material: (a) remnants of hard-tissue barrier; (b) heavy infiltration with inflammatory cells; (c) internal root resorption (H & E, ×40). (Courtesy of Ulla Schröder.)

swelling or fistulae constitute late and definite signs of an unsuccessful treatment.

As mentioned earlier, the formation of a hard-tissue barrier when using calcium hydroxide as a wound dressing is no proof of healing (57), but failure to produce hard tissue at the amputation site always means marked pathological changes histologically (35) (Fig. 5.3).

Radiographic signs of failure

Internal root resorption: This is the most common complication after pulpotomy in primary teeth, particularly after pulpotomy with zinc oxide–eugenol or calcium hydroxide as wound dressings. When zinc oxide–eugenol was used (41) internal root resorption was observed in 18/40 (45%) teeth within a follow-up time of 3 years, whereas it was found in 11/33 (33%) after 2 years with calcium hydroxide as wound dressing (71). The prevalence was considerably lower when the partial pulpotomy technique was used – 4/93 (4%) (74) – although the follow-up time in that study was only 1 year. Jeppesen (35), also using the partial pulpotomy technique, did not report any failures due to internal root resorption after almost 4 years of observation. With calcium hydroxide as a wound dressing, most internal root dentin resorptions were observed within the first year after pulpotomy (71).

Internal root dentin resorption occurs also after pulpotomy using FC, glutaraldehyde or Ledermix as wound dressings (Fig. 5.4). In a study by Mejàre (46), 16/74 (22%) molars with FC as dressing showed internal root resorptions after 2.5 years of observation, whereas the prevalence after 2 years of observation was only 1/70 (1%) when the diluted formula of FC was used (18). With glutaraldehyde as a dressing, 6/50 (12%) showed internal root resorption after 2 years of observation (19). The use

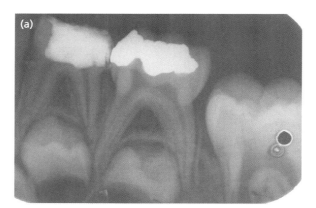

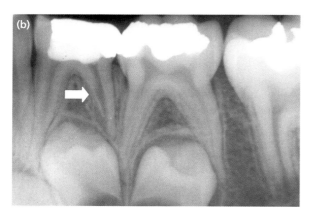

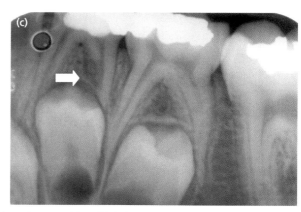

Fig. 5.4 Lower left first molar with radiographic evidence of internal root resorption after pulpotomy with Buckley's formocresol as dressing material: (a) at the time of treatment; (b) 18 months postoperatively; (c) 3 years postoperatively.

of Ledermix resulted in internal root resorptions in 18/101 (18%) after 3 years of observation (23).

As mentioned earlier, the reason for the emergence of internal root resorption after pulpotomy is not clear. Concerning calcium hydroxide, it has been suggested to be the result of either preoperative pulpal inflammation in the root pulp or an extrapulpal blood clot left behind between the dressing and the remaining pulp tissue. Regarding FC or glutaraldehyde, the reason is probably the irritating effects of the medicaments.

Interradicular periodontitis: This was a common cause of failure after FC pulpotomies using Buckley's formula (46, 69) and was found in 29/74 (39%) teeth in a study by Mejàre (46) (Fig. 5.5). It should be noted, though, that in this study more than half of the teeth had obvious clinical signs of total pulpitis at the time of treatment, indicating a poor pulp condition and thus probably reducing the prerequisites for successful treatment. When using the one-fifth dilution of FC or glutaraldehyde, interradicular periodontitis has been less commonly observed: 3–4% (18, 19).

Periapical periodontitis: This was the most common reason for failure after partial pulpotomy and occurred in 10/93

(11%) teeth 1 year postoperatively in one study (74) but only in 2/78 (3%) teeth during a follow-up time of almost 4 years in another study (35). After 3 years of observation with Ledermix as a dressing, periapical periodontitis was observed in 9/101 molars (23).

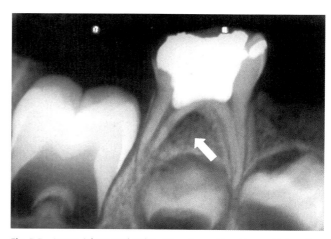

Fig. 5.5 Lower right second molar with radiographic evidence of interradicular osteitis 2.5 years after pulpotomy with Buckley's formocresol as dressing material.

Pulp obliteration: This has been observed mostly after pulpotomies using FC or glutaraldehyde as a wound dressing (Fig. 5.6). Radiographic evidence of pulp obliteration was seen in 62–80% of molars pulpotomized using Buckley's formula of FC (27, 46, 69, 92). When the diluted formula was used (18), pulp obliteration was observed in 20/70 (29%) after 2 years of follow-up. With glutaraldehyde, pulp obliteration occurred in 20/50 (40%) after 2 years of observation (19), whereas Tsai *et al.* (85) reported a lower prevalence of 26/150 (17%) after 3 years of observation.

The reason for pulp obliteration is probably a response to the irritating effects of these agents, particularly the vascular damage inflicted upon the remaining vital pulp. It was shown that the formaldehyde component of FC is rapidly transported through the vascular system, causing severe thrombosis and hemorrhage at varying and seemingly unpredictable distances from the wound surface (49). As a consequence, remote parts of the original pulp tissue are damaged and may react by producing hard tissue. Similar reactions probably occur with glutaraldehyde as a wound dressing. It should be noted that this common reaction following FC and glutaraldehyde pulpotomies implies that vital tissue remains in the root canals. In most clinical studies this complication is not judged as a failure.

Premature exfoliation: This complication is not considered as a failure but deserves to be mentioned. Exfoliation of a molar after FC or glutaraldehyde pulpotomy may occur faster than for the symmetrically opposite tooth. It has been suggested that glutaraldehyde is superior to FC in this respect, because it resulted in a lower percentage of premature exfoliation: 15 versus 47% with Buckley's FC and 39% with the diluted formula (19). Although not properly evaluated, the clinical significance of a possible premature exfoliation of, at most, 6 months is probably of minor importance.

Indications and contraindications for pulp treatment in primary teeth

The most important reason for keeping a primary tooth until exfoliation is to preserve the space to prevent crowding in the permanent dentition. Concerning the molars, normally the most important time period is before the first permanent molars have reached occlusion. Other important reasons are to maintain masticatory functions, to prevent tongue habits and to preserve esthetics. Furthermore, it might be important to keep the primary teeth for psychological reasons and the age and/or mental condition of the child may require special handling and consideration. When the permanent tooth is missing, it may be important to keep the primary tooth for an extended period of time.

The following conditions generally contradict pulp treatment and the tooth should be extracted:

- presence of clinical and/or radiographic symptoms indicating severe inflammatory reactions in the pulp, pulp necrosis, swelling, fistula or abscess;
- medically compromised children, particularly those with a lowered resistance to infection, e.g. children with severe cardiac conditions;
- an unrestorable tooth or less than two-thirds of the root is present, i.e. the remaining function time of the tooth is short.

Future directions

The degree and extent to which an existing pulpal inflammation can be treated successfully using vital pulp therapy has still not been determined and there is no precise definition of what "irreversible" pulpal inflammation means. In order words, the capacity of the inflamed pulp to recover is largely unknown. Because

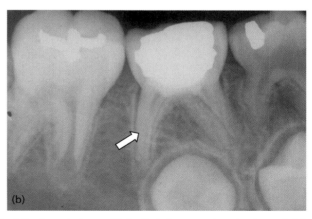

Fig. 5.6 Radiographic evidence of pulp obliteration in a lower right second molar following pulpotomy with Buckley's formocresol as dressing material: (a) preoperatively; (b) 2 years postoperatively.

Advanced concept 5.2   Comments on studies included in Table 5.1 concerning validity and knowledge gaps

Table 5.1 gives an overall picture of clinical/radiographic success rates subsequent to different procedures for treatment of primary molars with deep dentinal lesions with or without carious pulp exposures. Reported studies are heterogeneous; data differ in diagnostic criteria for pulp treatment, in follow-up periods and criteria for successful treatment, making direct comparisons problematic. Furthermore, the effect of clustering of teeth within individuals has not been taken into consideration and allocation concealment is not reported in the majority of the studies, both of which may overestimate treatment effects.

In a randomized clinical trial (RCT) four different techniques/dressing materials after pulpotomy were tested by Huth *et al.* (30). The authors concluded that calcium hydroxide resulted in a lower success rate compared with Er:YAG laser, ferric sulfate and formocresol. Another RCT with shorter follow-up time found no statistically significant difference between FC and calcium hydroxide (91). One reason for the contrasting results could be that the latter study was underpowered (too small number of subjects) and/or that follow-up time was too short.

It is noteworthy that the two indirect pulp capping procedures, stepwise excavation versus no re-entry, have not been compared in RCTs. A retrospective study compared the effect of indirect pulp capping (without re-entry) with diluted formocresol pulpotomy and found a higher success rate for indirect pulp capping (15). The finding is intriguing and ought to be further evaluated in RCTs.

Overall, no conclusions can be made as to the optimum treatment or techniques for primary molars with pulp involvement owing to the scarcity of relevant scientific research (21, 54).

Advanced concept 5.3   New biological approaches to vital pulp therapy

New approaches to treatment strategies in vital pulp therapy focus on cellular and molecular activities during tissue repair. The key elements of dentinal regeneration are pulp stem cells, bioactive molecules, so-called growth factors and the scaffold of extracellular matrix (55). A good understanding of the molecular and cellular processes involved in dental tissue repair is critical since it provides an important basis for development of new biological approaches to vital pulp therapy. However, the mechanisms behind odontoblast differentiation and dental tissue repair are still not fully understood. An example is the role of growth factors that regulate cell activities. How these molecules trigger odontoblast activities has received particular attention and current advances involve the stimulation of pulp stem cells to regenerate the damaged dentin–pulp complex. Murray *et al.* (53) and Tziafas (87, 88) give excellent overviews of current approaches to and challenges of regenerative endodontic techniques.

Transdentinal treatment
The stepwise excavation procedure, where calcium hydroxide is often used to induce the formation of reparative dentin, is an example of transdentinal treatment. A layer of reparative dentin deep within the remaining dentin would provide extra protection from external irritants. The reduced permeability of this reparative dentin provides an additional protection of the pulp from thermal and mechanical challenges. A controlled amount of reparative dentin immediately following extensive dentin loss without pulp exposure would therefore be a desirable clinical goal. The new transdentinal approach implies the use of biological agents to control pulp response through an existing layer of dentin. Although no materials are presently available to satisfy these criteria, there are indications that a network of extracellular matrix molecules and growth factors is potentially capable of working in this direction (88).

---

endodontic treatment in primary teeth focuses on vital pulp therapy, this is an essential future research field. In this respect, well-designed and well-conducted randomized clinical studies are of vital importance. Comparison between the two indirect pulp capping techniques (with and without re-entry) and comparison between the partial pulpotomy technique and the pulpotomy technique are examples of important research fields. Another important task is to find better assays for the clinician to decide the status of the pulp from clinical symptoms.

The fundamental biological processes leading to reparative dentinogenesis are not fully understood, nor are the mechanisms behind tissue regeneration and healing. This is essential in order to understand new efforts in biological approaches to vital pulp therapy (65) (Advanced concept 5.3).

Acknowledgment

The author would like to thank Nils Pyk for providing some of the illustrations for this chapter.

Case study 1

Stepwise excavation in a 5-year-old

History

A healthy 5-year-old boy presented with a deep carious lesion in the upper right second molar. There was no complaint of toothache other than sporadic pain in connection with meals and there were no visible pathological periapical changes.

Treatment

In order to avoid mesial drifting of the first permanent molar, it was important to keep the second primary molar at least until the first permanent molar had reached occlusion. Because there were no clinical or radiographic symptoms indicating irreversible pulpal inflammation, the diagnosis was partial pulpitis and stepwise excavation was the therapy of choice.

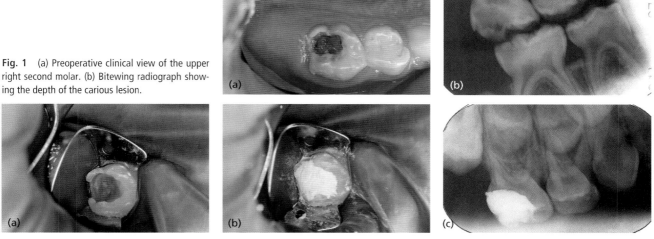

Fig. 1 (a) Preoperative clinical view of the upper right second molar. (b) Bitewing radiograph showing the depth of the carious lesion.

Fig. 2 (a) Clinical view after excavation of the bulk of demineralized dentin. (b) Calcium hydroxide was applied and the cavity was filled with a slow-setting zinc oxide–eugenol cement. (c) The radiograph shows no signs of periapical pathological changes.

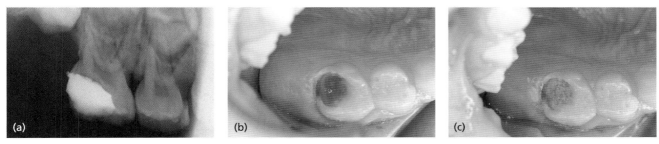

Fig. 3 At the second visit 8 weeks later, the tooth is without symptoms: (a) the radiograph shows no pathological changes; (b) the clinical view after re-entry and removal of the temporary filling; (c) the clinical view after removal of the remaining carious dentin. A new layer of calcium hydroxide was applied to the deeper parts of the lesion, a layer of fast-setting calcium hydroxide was placed and the tooth was restored with glass ionomer cement.

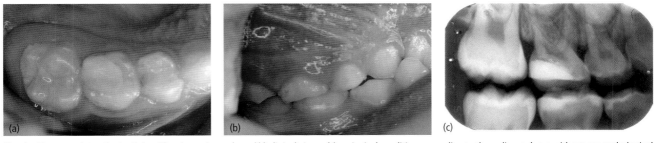

Fig. 4 Two years later, the tooth is without symptoms: (a and b) clinical views; (c) periapical conditions according to the radiograph are without any pathological changes. Note that the first permanent molar has erupted and reached normal occlusion, in which the second primary molar has played an important role as a space maintainer.

Case study 2

Pulpotomy using formocresol in a 5-year-old

History

A healthy 5-year-old boy presented with a deep carious lesion in the lower right second primary molar. There was no history of pain other than occasionally after sweet food intake. There were no signs of swelling of the gingiva or fistula and the tooth mobility was normal. The radiograph revealed a deep carious lesion and the interradicular area showed a widened periodontal membrane and a diffusely outlined lamina dura. At caries excavation, soft, demineralized dentin reached the pulp chamber and the bleeding at pulp exposure was profuse and dark.

Treatment

In order to avoid mesial drifting of the first permanent molar it was important to keep the second primary molar at least until the first permanent molar had reached occlusion. In this case there were obvious signs of total pulpitis, such as demineralized dentin reaching the pulp tissue, dark profuse bleeding at exposure and periradicular pathological signs, as judged radiographically. With the pulp diagnosis being total pulpitis, the prognosis using calcium hydroxide as a wound dressing after pulpotomy would be poor. An alternative to extraction is to use formocresol as the wound dressing. In this case pulpotomy was carried out and full-strength formocresol was chosen as the wound dressing.

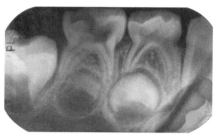

Fig. 1 Preoperative radiograph revealing a deep carious lesion in the lower right second primary molar. Note the position of the lower first permanent molar with its angled direction of eruption.

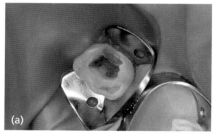

Fig. 2 (a) Formocresol has been applied to the root canal orifices for 5 min and the bleeding has stopped. (b) The formocresol-containing wound dressing has been applied to the root canal orifices. Note that the pulpal floor is not covered with the dressing.

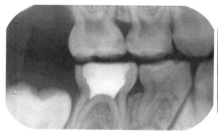

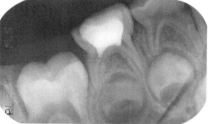

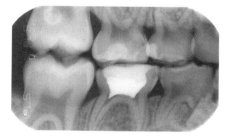

Fig. 3 Radiographs taken 6 months postoperatively. The right image of the interradicular area towards the mesial root still shows a diffusely outlined lamina dura, although the picture is not easily interpreted. Otherwise the tooth is symptomless.

Fig. 4 Radiograph taken 2 years postoperatively. There are no obvious signs of periradicular pathology, the tooth is clinically symptomless and the first permanent molar has erupted and reached occlusion.

References

1. Agamy HA, Bakry NS, Mounir MM, Avery DR. Comparison of mineral trioxide aggregate and formocresol as pulp-capping agents in pulpotomized primary teeth. *Pediatr. Dent.* 2004; 26: 302–9.
2. Al-Zayer MA, Straffon LH, Feigal RJ, Welch KB. Indirect pulp treatment of primary posterior teeth: a retrospective study. *Pediatr. Dent.* 2003; 25: 29–36.
3. Baume LJ. The use of corticosteroids in endodontic therapy. *Int. Dent. J.* 1968; 18: 471–2.
4. Bergenholtz G. Inflammatory response of the dental pulp to bacterial irritation. *J. Endod.* 1981; 7: 100–4.
5. Bergenholtz G, Cox C, Loesche W, Sved S. Bacterial leakage around dental restorations: its effect on the dental pulp. *J. Oral. Pathol.* 1982; 11: 439–50.
6. Casas MJ, Kenny DJ, Johnston DH, Judd PL. Long-term outcomes of primary molar ferric sulfate pulpotomy and root canal therapy. *Pediatr. Dent.* 2004; 26: 44–8.
7. Davies G. Pulp therapy in primary teeth. *Aust. Dent. J.* 1962; 7: 111–20.

8. de Souza Costa CA, Lopes do Nascimento AB, Teixeira HM, Fontana UF. Response of human pulps capped with a self-etching adhesive system. *Dent. Mater.* 2001; 17: 230–40.

    Study comparing pattern of healing after capping experimental pulp exposures in healthy human teeth where either calcium hydroxide or a resin composite was used as wound medicament. While calcium hydroxide gave complete dentinal repair the response to the bonding agent was characterized by a lingering inflammatory response.

9. Ebner H, Kraft D. Formaldehyde-induced anaphylaxis after dental treatment? *Contact Dermatitis* 1991; 24: 307–9.

10. Eidelman E, Holan G, Fuks AB. Mineral trioxide aggregate vs. formocresol in pulpotomized primary molars: a preliminary report. *Pediatr. Dent.* 2001; 23: 15–18.

11. Eidelman E, Touma B, Ulmansky M. Pulp pathology in deciduous teeth. Clinical and histological correlations. *Israel J. Med. Sci.* 1968; 4: 1244–8.

12. Eidelman E, Ulmansky M, Michaeli Y. Histopathology of the pulp in primary incisors with deep dentinal caries. *Pediatr. Dent.* 1992; 14: 372–5.

13. el Sayed F, Seite-Bellezza D, Sans B, Bayle-Lebey P, Marguery MC, Bazex J. Contact urticaria from formaldehyde in a root-canal dental paste. *Contact Dermatitis* 1995; 33: 353.

14. Falster CA, Araujo FB, Straffon LH, Nor JE. Indirect pulp treatment: *in vivo* outcomes of an adhesive resin system vs calcium hydroxide for protection of the dentin–pulp complex. *Pediatr. Dent.* 2002; 24: 241–8.

15. Farooq NS, Coll JA, Kuwabara A, Shelton P. Success rates of formocresol pulpotomy and indirect pulp therapy in the treatment of deep dentinal caries in primary teeth. *Pediatr. Dent.* 2000; 22: 278–86.

16. Farsi N, Alamoudi N, Balto K, Mushayt A. Success of mineral trioxide aggregate in pulpotomized primary molars. *J. Clin. Pediatr. Dent.* 2005; 29: 307–11.

17. Fei A, Udin R, Johnson R. A clinical study of ferric sulfate as a pulpotomy agent in primary teeth. *Pediatr. Dent.* 1997; 19: 327–32.

18. Fuks AB, Bimstein E. Clinical evaluation of diluted formocresol pulpotomies in primary teeth of school children. *Pediatr. Dent.* 1981; 3: 321–4.

19. Fuks AB, Bimstein E, Guelmann M, Klein H. Assessment of a 2 percent buffered glutaraldehyde solution in pulpotomized primary teeth of schoolchildren. *ASDC J. Dent. Child.* 1990; 57: 371–5.

20. Fuks AB, Holan G, Davis JM, Eidelman E. Ferric sulfate versus dilute formocresol in pulpotomized primary molars: long-term follow up. *Pediatr. Dent.* 1997; 19: 327–30.

21. Fuks AB, Papagiannoulis L. Pulpotomy in primary teeth: review of the literature according to standardized assessment criteria. *Eur. Arch. Paediatr. Dent.* 2006; 7: 64–71.

22. Garcia-Godoy F. A 42 month clinical evaluation of glutaraldehyde pulpotomies in primary teeth. *J. Pedod.* 1986; 10: 148–55.

23. Gerdes I, Ravn J, Lambjerg.Hansen H. Vital pulpotomy in primary molars with Ledermix cement used as amputation material (In Danish, English summary). *Tandlaegebladet* 1977; 81: 421–6.

24. Gruythuysen RJ, Weerheijm KL. Calcium hydroxide pulpotomy with a light-cured cavity-sealing material after two years. *ASDC J. Dent. Child.* 1997; 64: 251–3.

25. Hansen H. Corticoids in endodontia. A clinical–histological study of 109 cases. *Tandlaegebladet* 1969; 73: 539–56.

26. Hansen HP, Ravn JJ, Ulrich D. Vital pulpotomy in primary molars. A clinical and histologic investigation of the effect of zinc oxide–eugenol cement and Ledermix. *Scand. J. Dent. Res.* 1971; 79: 13–25.

27. Hicks MJ, Barr ES, Flaitz CM. Formocresol pulpotomies in primary molars: a radiographic study in a pediatric dentistry practice. *J. Pedod.* 1986; 10: 331–9.

28. Holan G, Eidelman E, Fuks AB. Long-term evaluation of pulpotomy in primary molars using mineral trioxide aggregate or formocresol. *Pediatr. Dent.* 2005; 27: 129–36.

29. Holan G, Fuks AB, Ketlz N. Success rate of formocresol pulpotomy in primary molars restored with stainless steel crown vs amalgam. *Pediatr. Dent.* 2002; 24: 212–16.

30. Huth KC, Paschos E, Hajek-Al-Khatar N, Hollweck R, Crispin A, Hickel R, *et al.* Effectiveness of 4 pulpotomy techniques – randomized controlled trial. *J. Dent. Res.* 2005; 84: 1144–8.

31. Hørsted-Bindslev P, Vilkinis V, Sidlauskas A. Direct capping of human pulps with a dentin bonding system or with calcium hydroxide cement. *Oral Surg. Oral Med. Oral Pathol. Oral Radiol. Endod.* 2003; 96: 591–600.

32. Ibricevic H, Al-Jame Q. Ferric sulphate and formocresol in pulpotomy of primary molars: long term follow-up study. *Eur. J. Paediatr. Dent.* 2003; 4: 28–32.

33. Ireland R. Secondary dentin formation of deciduous teeth. *Am. Dent. J* 1941; 28: 1626–32.

34. Jeng HW, Feigal RJ, Messer HH. Comparison of the cytotoxicity of formocresol, formaldehyde, cresol, and glutaraldehyde using human pulp fibroblast cultures. *Pediatr. Dent.* 1987; 9: 295–300.

35. Jeppesen K. Direct pulp capping on primary teeth – a long-term investigation. *J. Int. Assoc. Dent. Child.* 1971; 12: 10–19.

36. Kalnins V, Frisbie H. Effect of dentine fragments on the healing of the exposed pulp. *Arch. Oral. Biol.* 1960; 2: 96–103.

37. Kisling E. Histologiske undersögelser af mælketændernes pulpae som grundlag for en klinisk diagnose (In Danish). *Dens Sapiens* 1957; 17: 52–61.

38. Koch G, Nyborg H. Correlation between clinical and histological indications for pulpotomy for deciduous teeth. *J. Int. Assoc. Dent. Child.* 1970; 1: 3–10.

39. Leksell E, Ridell K, Cvek M, Mejàre I. Pulp exposure after stepwise versus direct complete excavation of deep carious lesions in young posterior permanent teeth. *Endod. Dent. Traumatol.* 1996; 12: 192–6.

40. Loh A, O'Hoy P, Tran X, Charles R, Hughes A, Kubo K, *et al.* Evidence-based assessment: evaluation of the formocresol versus ferric sulfate primary molar pulpotomy. *Pediatr. Dent.* 2004; 26: 401–9.

41. Magnusson B. Therapeutic pulpotomy in primary molars – clinical and histological follow-up. II. Zinc oxide–eugenol as wound dressing. *Odontol. Revy* 1971; 22: 45–54.

42. Magnusson BO, Sundell SO. Stepwise excavation of deep carious lesions in primary molars. *J. Int. Assoc. Dent. Child.* 1977; 8: 36–40.

Study reporting fewer pulp exposures in deciduous teeth with deep carious lesions by stepwise excavation and re-entry after 4–6 weeks than following direct complete excavation.

43. Marchi JJ, de Araujo FB, Froner AM, Straffon LH, Nor JE. Indirect pulp capping in the primary dentition: a 4 year follow-up study. *J. Clin. Pediatr. Dent.* 2006; 31: 68–71.

44. Maroto M, Barberia E, Vera V, Garcia-Godoy F. Mineral trioxide aggregate as pulp dressing agent in pulpotomy treatment of primary molars: 42-month clinical study. *Am. J. Dent.* 2007; 20: 283–6.

45. Mejàre B. Bactericidal effect of calcium hydroxide on enterococci in blood and serum. *J. Dent. Res.* 1986; 65: Abstr. 12.

46. Mejàre I. Pulpotomy of primary molars with coronal or total pulpitis using formocresol technique. *Scand. J. Dent. Res.* 1979; 87: 208–16.

47. Mejàre I, Cvek M. Partial pulpotomy in young permanent teeth with deep carious lesions. *Endod. Dent. Traumatol.* 1993; 9: 238–42.

48. Mejàre I, Hasselgren G, Hammarström LE. Effect of formaldehyde-containing drugs on human dental pulp evaluated by enzyme histochemical technique. *Scand. J. Dent. Res.* 1976; 84: 29–36.

49. Mejàre I, Larsson A. Short-term reactions of human dental pulp to formocresol and its components – a clinical–experimental study. *Scand. J. Dent. Res.* 1979; 87: 331–45.

50. Mjör I. Dentine and pulp. In: *Reaction Patterns in Human Teeth* (Mjör IA, ed.). Boca Raton, FL: CRC Press, 1983; 101.

51. Morawa AP, Straffon LH, Han SS, Corpron RE. Clinical evaluation of pulpotomies using dilute formocresol. *ASDC J. Dent. Child.* 1975; 42: 360–3.

52. Moretti AB, Sakai VT, Oliveira TM, Fornetti AP, Santos CF, Machado MA, *et al.* The effectiveness of mineral trioxide aggregate, calcium hydroxide and formocresol for pulpotomies in primary teeth. *Int. Endod. J.* 2008; 41: 547–55.

53. Murray PE, Garcia-Godoy F, Hargreaves KM. Regenerative endodontics: a review of current status and a call for action. *J. Endod.* 2007; 33: 377–90.

54. Nadin G, Goel BR, Yeung CA, Glenny AM. Pulp treatment for extensive decay in primary teeth. *Cochrane Database Syst. Rev.* 2003: CD003220.

55. Nakashima M, Akamine A. The application of tissue engineering to regeneration of pulp and dentin in endodontics. *J. Endod.* 2005; 31: 711–18.

56. Nethercott JR, Holness DL, Page E. Occupational contact dermatitis due to glutaraldehyde in health care workers. *Contact Dermatitis* 1988; 18: 193–6.

57. Nyborg H. Capping of the pulp. The processes involved and their outcome. A report of the follow-ups of clinical series. *Odontol. Tidskrift* 1958; 66: 296–364.

58. Peng L, Ye L, Guo X, Tan H, Zhou X, Wang C, *et al.* Evaluation of formocresol versus ferric sulphate primary molar pulpotomy: a systematic review and meta-analysis. *Int. Endod. J.* 2007; 40: 751–7.

59. Pritz W. Erfahrungen mit Calxyl zur pulpenüberkappung. *Zahnärztl. Welt* 1957; 58: 120–4.

60. Prophet A, Miller J. The effect of caries on the deciduous pulp. *Br. Dent. J.* 1955; 99: 105.

61. Ranly DM. Formocresol toxicity. Current knowledge. *Acta Odontol. Pediatr.* 1984; 5: 93–8.

62. Rapp R AK, Strachan DS. Possible role of acetylcholinesterase in neural conduction within the dental pulp. In: *Biology of the Dental Pulp Organ: A Symposium* (Finn SB, ed.). Alabama: University of Alabama Press, 1968; 309–31.

63. Rayner J, Southam J. Pulp changes in deciduous teeth associated with deep carious lesions. *J. Dent.* 1979; 7: 39–42.

64. Ricketts DN, Kidd EA, Innes N, Clarkson J. Complete or ultraconservative removal of decayed tissue in unfilled teeth. *Cochrane Database Syst. Rev.* 2006; 3: CD003808.

65. Rutherford B, Fitzgerald M. A new biological approach to vital pulp therapy. *Crit. Rev. Oral Biol. Med.* 1995; 6: 218–29.

66. Rölling I, Hasselgren G, Tronstad L. Morphologic and enzyme histochemical observations on the pulp of human primary molars 3 to 5 years after formocresol treatment. *Oral Surg. Oral Med. Oral Pathol.* 1976; 42: 518–28.

67. Rölling I, Poulsen S. Formocresol pulpotomy of primary teeth and occurrence of enamel defects on the permanent successors. *Acta Odontol. Scand.* 1978; 36: 243–7.

68. Rölling I, Thulin H. Allergy tests against formaldehyde, cresol, and eugenol in children with formocresol pulpotomized primary teeth. *Scand. J. Dent. Res.* 1976; 84: 345–7.

69. Rölling I, Thylstrup A. A 3-year clinical follow-up study of pulpotomized primary molars treated with the formocresol technique. *Scand. J. Dent. Res.* 1975; 83: 47–53.

70. Sawusch RH. Direct and indirect pulp capping with two new products. *J. Am. Dent. Assoc.* 1982; 104: 459–62.

71. Schröder U. A 2-year follow-up of primary molars, pulpotomized with a gentle technique and capped with calcium hydroxide. *Scand. J. Dent. Res.* 1978; 86: 273–8.

72. Schröder U. Agreement between clinical and histologic findings in chronic pulpitis in primary teeth. *Scand. J. Dent. Res.* 1977; 85: 583–7.

73. Schröder U. Effect of an extra-pulpal blood clot on healing following experimental pulpotomy and capping with calcium hydroxide. *Odontol. Revy* 1973; 24: 257–69.

74. Schröder U, Szpringer-Nodzak M, Janicha J, Wacinska M, Budny J, Mlosek K. A one-year follow-up of partial pulpotomy and calcium hydroxide capping in primary molars. *Endod. Dent. Traumatol.* 1987; 3: 304–6.

75. Schwartz R, Mauger M, Clemet D, Walker W III. Assessment of a novel alternative to conventional formocresol–zinc oxide eugenol pulpotomy for the treatment of pulpally involved human primary teeth: diode laser–mineral trioxide aggregate pulpotomy. *J. Am. Dent. Assoc.* 1999; 130: 967–75.

76. Shumayrikh NM, Adenubi JO. Clinical evaluation of glutaraldehyde with calcium hydroxide and glutaraldehyde with zinc oxide eugenol in pulpotomy of primary molars. *Endod. Dent. Traumatol.* 1999; 15: 259–64.

77. Smith NL, Seale NS, Nunn ME. Ferric sulfate pulpotomy in primary molars: a retrospective study. *Pediatr. Dent.* 2000; 22: 192–9.

78. Soskolne W, Bimstein E. A histomorphological study of the shedding process of human deciduous teeth at various chronological stages. *Arch. Oral Biol.* 1977; 22: 331–5.

79. Squire RA, Cameron LL. An analysis of potential carcinogenic risk from formaldehyde. *Regul. Toxicol. Pharmacol.* 1984; 4: 107–29.

80. St Clair MB, Gross EA, Morgan KT. Pathology and cell proliferation induced by intra-nasal instillation of aldehydes in

the rat: comparison of glutaraldehyde and formaldehyde. *Toxicol. Pathol.* 1990; 18: 353–61.

81. Sun HW, Feigal RJ, Messer HH. Cytotoxicity of glutaraldehyde and formaldehyde in relation to time of exposure and concentration. *Pediatr. Dent.* 1990; 12: 303–7.

82. Tagger E, Tagger M. Pulpal and periapical reactions to glutaraldehyde and paraformaldehyde pulpotomy dressing in monkeys. *J. Endod.* 1984; 10: 364–71.

83. Torajinebad M, Chivian N. Clinical applications of mineral trioxide aggregate. *J. Endod.* 1999; 25: 197–205.

84. Torajinebad M, Hong C, McDonald F, Pitt Ford T. Physical and chemcial properties of a new root-end filling material. *J. Endod.* 1995; 21: 349–53.

85. Tsai TP, Su HL, Tseng LH. Glutaraldehyde preparations and pulpotomy in primary molars. *Oral Surg. Oral Med. Oral Pathol.* 1993; 76: 346–50.

86. Tuna D, Olmez A. Clinical long-term evaluation of MTA as a direct pulp capping material in primary teeth. *Int. Endod. J.* 2008; 41: 273–8.

87. Tziafas D. Designing new treatment strategies in vital pulp therapy. *J. Dent.* 2000; 28: 77–92.

88. Tziafas D. The future role of a molecular approach to pulp–dentinal regeneration. *Caries Res.* 2004; 38: 314–20.

89. Via F. Evaluation of deciduous molars treated by pulpotomy and calcium hydroxide. *J. Am. Dent. Assoc.* 1955; 50: 34–43.

90. Waterhouse PJ. Formocresol and alternative primary molar pulpotomy medicaments: a review. *Endod. Dent. Traumatol.* 1995; 11: 157–62.

91. Waterhouse PJ, Nunn JH, Whitworth JM. An investigation of the relative efficacy of Buckley's Formocresol and calcium hydroxide in primary molar vital pulp therapy. *Br. Dent. J.* 2000; 188: 32–6.

92. Willard RM. Radiographic changes following formocresol pulpotomy in primary molars. *ASDC J. Dent. Child.* 1976; 43: 414–15.

93. Zilberman U, Mass E, Sarnat H. Partial pulpotomy in carious permanent molars. *Am. J. Dent.* 1989; 2: 147–50.

Part 2
The Necrotic Pulp

Chapter 6
The microbiology of the necrotic pulp

Gunnel Svensäter, Luis Chávez de Paz and Else Theilade

Introduction

Breakdown of the dental pulp by any cause (Chapter 2) results in loss of defense mechanisms that can counter microorganisms in the oral cavity from entering the root canal system of teeth. In direct exposure by, for example, caries or fracture, microorganisms readily occupy the available pulpal space. In apparently intact teeth micro-organisms may also find ways of accessing root canals, where the vital functions of the pulp have been lost (Fig. 6.1): the attractant is the necrotic tissue, which will serve as a primary nutrient for microbial growth and multiplication. The root canal space is also a sanctuary where colonizing microorganisms can build up microbial communities in the form of biofilms without much inter-ference from the defense system of the host. Infection of root canals, described in detail in this chapter in terms of microbial biofilms, ecological determinants and patho-genic potential, will initiate and maintain inflammatory lesions in the periodontium. While this may occur at any portal of exit from the root canal system, these lesions are often established near the root tip and therefore go under the term *apical periodontitis* (see Chapter 7).

Evidence for the essential role of microorganisms in apical periodontitis

Historical background

Microorganisms colonizing the necrotic pulp of teeth have long been recognized as the cause of acute and chronic manifestations of apical periodontitis (Chapter 7). The first observation of microorganisms in root canals was by Antony van Leeuwenhoek (Key literature 6.1), whose home-made microscope also enabled him to make the first drawing of dental plaque in 1683. However, it was 200 years before root canal microorganisms came under biological investigation. Willoughby D. Miller (1853–1907), the father of oral microbiology, described the clinical effects of 'gangrenous tooth pulps' as centers of infections varying from hardly perceptible apical inflammation to severe local and general symptoms, sometimes even with fatal outcome (Key literature 6.1). He cultured and characterized bacteria from necrotic pulps and studied their pathogenic potential in animal experiments (40).

Pulp exposure due to   *Dentinal tubules exposed due to*

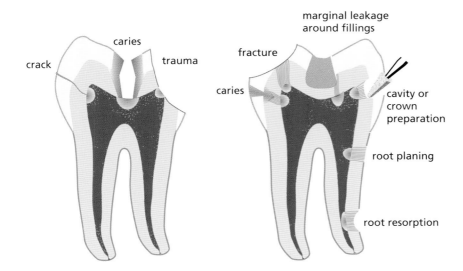

Fig. 6.1 Drawing illustrating the pathways of entry for microorganisms into the root canal. Obvious ways of entry are pulp exposures due to caries or trauma. Potential pathways are cracks in enamel and dentin due to trauma, and dentinal tubules exposed by caries, fracture, cavity or crown preparation, marginal leakage around filling, root resorption or root planing.

Key literature 6.1   Citations from classics

"… I took this stuff out of the hollows in the roots, and mixed it with clean rain water, and set it before the magnifying-glass so as to see if there were as many living creatures in it as I had aforetime discovered; and I must confess that the whole stuff seemed to me to be alive …"

Antonie van Leeuwenhoek, 1683,
cited from (9)

"The vulgar and even certain authors have believed and still believe that toothache and caries are caused by dental worms and these worms gnaw away little by little the tissue of the bony fibers or nervous filaments."

Pierre Fauchard, 1723,
cited from (9)

"In the mouth we find certain conditions which are presented by no other part of the human body, in that a direct way is furnished for parasites through the medium of the root canals and diseased tooth-pulps into the deeper parts …

Infections through gangrenous tooth-pulps are to be ranked among the most frequent pyogenic infections of the human body; they by no means always have the harmless character commonly ascribed to them …

Apical infections exhibit all transitions from a hardly perceptible reaction to the most dangerous phlegmonous inflammations, accompanied by general symptoms, such as high fever, chills, etc. which, as many instances show, may lead to meningitis, as well to pyæmic and septicæmic processes, with fatal termination …

Small particles of such pulps brought under the skin of mice, occasioned in the majority of cases inflammation and swelling … At the end of the second or third day a small abscess was generally found … In 36.8 per cent the infections were accompanied by severe symptoms, in 7 per cent the disease resulted fatally …"

Willoughby D. Miller, 1890 (40)

With the publication in 1911 of William Hunter's book *Oral Sepsis as a Cause of Disease* (cited in Ref. 9), the theory of focal infection emerged: the concept that infected teeth cause infections in other parts of the body and also cause many systemic diseases. Hunter accused dentists of producing masses of oral sepsis with their procedures for fillings, crowns and bridges, which often caused pulpitis, pulp necrosis and apical periodontitis. He proposed that a more suitable name for 'conservative dentistry' was 'septic dentistry'. His publication (26) led to the view that all teeth suspected of infection should be extracted. This concept gained widespread acceptance for years and resulted in mass extractions of teeth. It probably caused a delay in the development of modern endodontics, but eventually led to biologically sound treatment methods, including the elimination of root canal infections.

Observations in animal experiments and human studies

The view that microorganims in root canals play a key role in the pathogenesis of apical periodontitis has not always been universally shared. A primary reason has been failure to produce cultures from root canals in humans to confirm a clear-cut association of apical periodontitis with presence of bacteria in sampled teeth. Some early authors therefore suggested that decomposition of necrotic pulp tissue or stagnant tissue fluid in the pulpal space might cause apical periodontitis alone, in the absence of root canal infection. However, animal experiments proved this theory wrong and demonstrated that empty tubes or sterile dead tissue implanted subcutaneously caused only transient inflammation that did not prevent healing, whereas necrotic tissue infected with bacteria caused intense inflammation and often abscess formation (35).

A key piece of evidence for the crucial role of microorganisms in the pathogenesis of apical inflammatory lesions was provided by the classical study by Kakehashi, Stanley and Fitzgerald in 1965 (28). These investigators used germ-free and conventional rats to demonstrate that only in the presence of bacteria could pulp necrosis and apical periodontitis be induced in teeth where pulps were exposed to the oral environment. In germ-free animals, on the other hand, the exposed pulps healed with hard-tissue repair at the exposure site in spite of gross food impaction. In agreement with this study, aseptically devitalized pulps that were sealed and kept sterile for 6–7 months in experimental monkeys did not result in inflammatory responses of the apical tissues. In contrast, pulps lacerated by instrumentation and contaminated with oral bacteria caused clinical, radiographic and histological signs of apical periodontitis (42).

Cultural studies in humans, when taking account of the fastidious and often obligate anaerobic nature of the root canal microbiota, were also eventually able to show a connection of apical periodontitis with the presence of bacteria in root canals. In these studies (6, 43, 63) non-vital tooth pulps with closed necrosis after trauma were accessed and sampled for bacterial culture under strict aseptic conditions. Indeed a strong association was confirmed in that absence of bacterial growth correlated with cases without radiographic signs of apical inflammation, while most cases with an obvious lesion gave bacterial growth.

Routes of microbial entry to the pulpal space

The root canals of teeth are normally sterile and the presence of microorganisms is dependent on their invasion.

As long as the pulp is vital and has a functioning infection defense, bacterial entry will usually be opposed, especially in cases where there is no direct exposure of the pulpal tissue to the oral cavity (see Chapter 2). On the other hand, when a deep carious lesion reaches the pulp the massive bacterial exposure will eventually cause the inflammatory defense barrier to recede, thereby giving access for the bacteria at the caries front to invade and colonize the pulpal space. A similar route of entry will occur in teeth with pulp exposure due to trauma, fracture and cracks as well as following unprotected iatrogenic exposure in restorative procedures. Direct pathways to the root canal space may be present in teeth with periodontal disease. From subgingival plaque, bacteria can enter through accessory lateral and furcal canals and, in ultimate periodontal breakdown, through the apical foramen.

A direct pathway from the external environment is not necessarily a prerequisite for microbial colonization of the pulpal space, however. In cases of a damaged pulp, oral microorganisms may enter along the dentinal tubules following their exposure by trauma, root resorption, root caries, gaps in the cementum in the cervical area and by cavity and crown preparation or under restorations with marginal gaps. Even in seemingly intact teeth following breakdown of the pulp, as in trauma cases (Chapter 15), microorganisms may cross the hard-tissue barrier (6, 63). In fact, a route of entry is possible through minor cracks in enamel and dentin that occurred in conjunction with the injury (34). Anachoresis has also been suspected of leading to infection in these cases. This term means that bacteria have been disseminated to the site of inflammation out of the blood stream. It is well known that bacteremia is common in humans (Chapter 8). Yet, bacteria normally are eliminated from the blood stream and the fact that species from other body sites are rarely recovered in traumatized teeth has cast the significance of anachoresis as a route of entry to necrotic pulps in doubt. Figure 6.1 summarizes the most common pathways for microorganisms in the oral cavity to enter the root canal in cases of pulp necrosis.

Modes of colonization

Microorganisms colonizing a body site such as the root canal space may either be free-floating as single cells (planktonic form) or attached to each other or on to the root canal walls or both. Organisms dwelling in a planktonic state require a liquid phase. In root canals the fluid is primarily inflammatory exudate that is released at the host defense–bacterial front interface. Saliva may also be the vehicle where there is direct communication of the root canal system with the oral environment.

When bacterial cells become densely packed and embedded in an extracellular matrix of polymers of host and microbial origin, the term *microbial biofilm* is used. Bacteria residing in such microbial communities have gained a great deal of interest in recent years because infections, including those of root canals, often involve microbial biofilms. While planktonic microorganisms can be easily eliminated, there is a major challenge for root canal therapy to combat bacteria firmly attached to the root canal walls. This is especially so when microorganisms are in all areas of the canal space as well as in the dentinal tubules (Fig. 6.2) (53).

Microbial biofilms are ubiquitous in nature in all situations where natural liquid and microorganisms come in contact with surfaces (16). Dental plaque is one of the most studied biofilms and most members of the oral microflora contribute to the extensive biofilm formation on tooth surfaces. What is known about this particular biofilm also has implications for biofilms in the root canal environment (Fig. 6.6).

Independent of milieu, the development of biofilms seems to follow essentially the same sequence of events, starting with the adsorption of macromolecules to which microorganisms attach. Coadhesion of other microorganisms subsequently occurs and their attachment may be strengthened through polymer production and unfolding of cell surface structures. The multiplication and metabolism of adhering microorganisms ultimately result in the development of a structurally organized microbial community that is in a state of balance with the local environment (7, 37). Many natural biofilms have a highly diverse microflora with the individual species also organized functionally. When mature biofilms are viewed using non-invasive and non-destructive techniques (e.g. confocal laser scanning microscopy, CLSM), significant structural features observed include microcolonies of bacteria embedded in an extracellular matrix with channels or pores traversing the depth of the biofilm (4, 15).

Biofilms in root canals

The most direct evidence for biofilms in root canals comes from light microscopy, transmission electron microscopy and scanning electron microscopy studies *in situ* of extracted teeth with apical periodontitis (33, 47). Biofilms, most often composed of several morphotypes, grow in multilayers or as aggregates on the dentin walls of the root canal (Figs 6.3 and 6.4) or as dense aggregates in the necrotic tissue (Fig. 6.5). The amorphous material filling the interbacterial spaces in biofilms has been interpreted as being an extracellular matrix of bacterial origin. In many cases, the spatial organization described for root canal biofilms resembles that reported for dental biofilms (32). Hence, palisade structures of filaments and chains

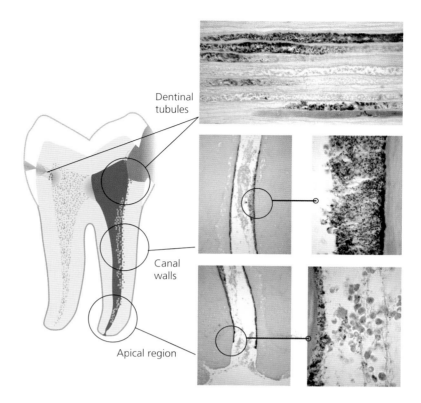

Fig. 6.2 Microbial biofilms in dentinal tubules and on dentinal walls of the root canal. (Histological specimen courtesy of Dr D. Ricucci.)

Dentinal tubules

Canal walls

Apical region

of cocci perpendicular to the canal wall (46), or corn-cob-like structures of cocci attached to filaments (44) have been described.

Because of difficulty in accessing naturally occurring root canal biofilms with CLSM, information on their detailed architecture is limited. However, an open architecture is likely to exist enabling molecules, such as nutrients and microbial products, to move readily in and out of the biofilms.

Extraradicular colonization

The necrotic tissue of a non-vital pulp is the major location of microorganisms causing apical periodontitis, but the lesion *per se* may also harbor microorganisms. They may be attached to the root tip, or occur either as free-floating single cells or in clusters.

Indeed, multispecies biofilms have been described on the outer root surface of teeth adjacent to the apical foramen (30, 33). Such aggregations have been composed of various microbial forms, even including yeasts (46, 65) (Fig. 6.7). These colonizers are of particular significance from a treatment aspect in that an orthograde approach for endodontic treatment will not be able to eliminate the infection. However, it is not clear how common such extraradicular microbial aggregations are. They have been demonstrated mainly in cases with acute symptoms with and without sinus tracts (fistulae), or in cases not responding to endodontic treatment.

Microorganisms continuously detach from the surface of biofilms for colonization of other sites. In endodontic infections, released organisms may exit the apical foramen and may, at least temporarily, be present in the periapical tissue lesion *per se*, either in a free-floating state or inside phagocytes or both. This is normally the case in apical abscesses, which may harbor a variety of microbial forms.

Although microorganisms, including rods, spirochetes and cocci, have also been identified in asymptomatic periapical lesions of root filled teeth (59), well-organized tissue lesions, so-called apical granulomas (Chapter 7), are not normally found to be infected. An exception to this rule is the occasional finding of typical actinomyces-containing colonies (48). Radicular cysts may also harbor clusters of microorganisms (49).

Ecological determinants for microbial growth in root canals

As is the case for dental plaque (for review, see Ref. 38), adherence and coadherence are key ecological determinants for the survival and persistence of oral bacteria in the root canal environment. Low oxygen tension and the level of nutrients available from the host are other important ecological factors determining the success or failure of microorganisms entering the root canal to survive and grow (Core concept 6.1). The root canal biofilms contain

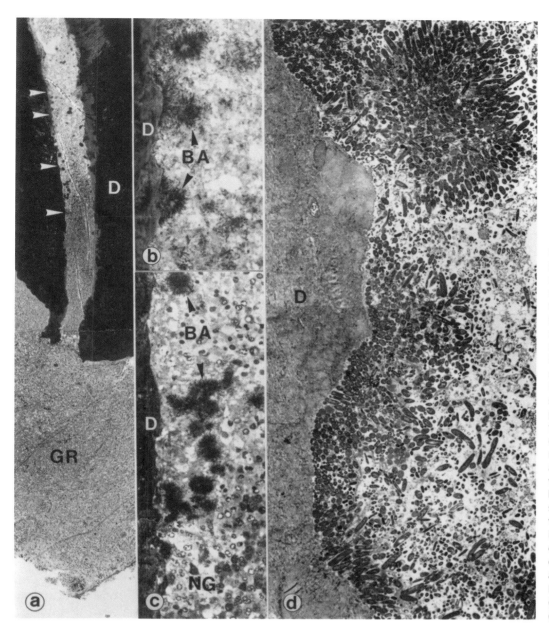

Fig. 6.3 Microbial biofilm in the apical part of a human tooth with apical periodontitis (GR). The areas between the upper two and the lower two arrowheads in (a) are magnified in (b) and (c), respectively. Note the dense bacterial aggregates (BA) sticking (in b) to the dentinal (D) wall and also remaining suspended among neutrophilic granulocytes (NG) in the fluid phase of the root canal content (in c). The neutrophilic granulocytes appear to form a defensive wall, against the advancing bacterial front. A transmission electron microscopic view (d) of the pulpodentinal interphase shows bacterial condensation on the surface of the dentinal wall, forming a thick layered plaque. Magnification: (a) ×46; (b) ×600; (c) ×370; (d) ×2350. (From Nair (49).)

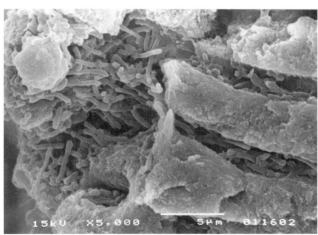

Fig. 6.4 A community consisting of cocci and rods in an ecological niche on the root canal wall. The aggregated bacteria also show some penetration into the dentinal tubules. Scanning electron microscopy, magnification ×5000. (From Sen *et al.* (53).)

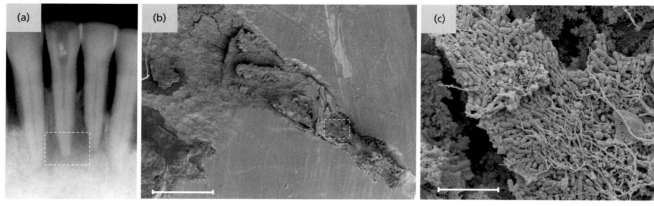

Fig. 6.5   Microbial biofilm in the apical region of a root canal. (a) Radiograph showing a lower incisor with apical periodontitis. (b) Scanning electron microscopic view of the apical region of the root canal. Scale bar: 500 μm. The delimited area is zoomed in in (c) where bacterial biofilm formation within the necrotized tissues is apparent. Scale bar: 5 μm. (Courtesy of Dr D. Jaramillo and Dr C. Schaudinn.)

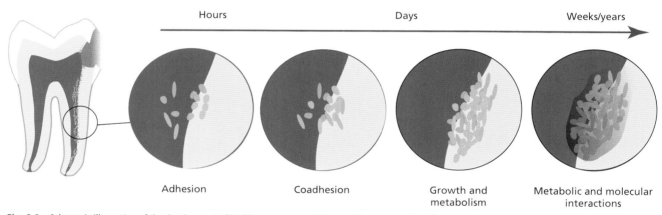

Fig. 6.6   Schematic illustration of the development of biofilms on root canal tissues. Adherence and coadherence of microorganisms are followed by division and growth which are dependent on nutrients from the environment. The final composition reflects the outcome of metabolic and molecular interactions between members of the microbial community of the biofilm. (Adapted from the model designed by Dr G. Bowden.)

> ### Core concept 6.1   Ecological determinants of the endodontic microflora
>
> - Adhesion to root canal tissues
> - Coaggregation of populations
> - Low oxygen concentration and redox potential
> - Nutrition
>   - necrotic tissue
>   - tissue fluid
>   - tissue exudate
>   - microbial food chains
> - Microbial interactions
>   - synergistic
>   - antagonistic
> - Endodontic treatment
>   - mechanical debridement
>   - antimicrobial agents

multiple species in close physical contact, and this increases the probability of both synergistic and antagonistic interactions between microbial cells. With time, a multispecies microbial community is established and microbial interactions eventually give stability to the community. This mode of colonization gives rise to a chemical heterogeneity in the biofilm environment, which encourages phenotypic diversity. It also enhances the ability of the microorganisms to resist environmentally derived stressful conditions (see Advanced concept 6.1). Once a stable biofilm is established, disruption of the habitat, such as application of mechanical forces and antiseptics, must occur before the microbial community is significantly affected.

Nutrition

Microorganisms entering the necrotic tissue in root canals encounter suitable conditions for growth. The

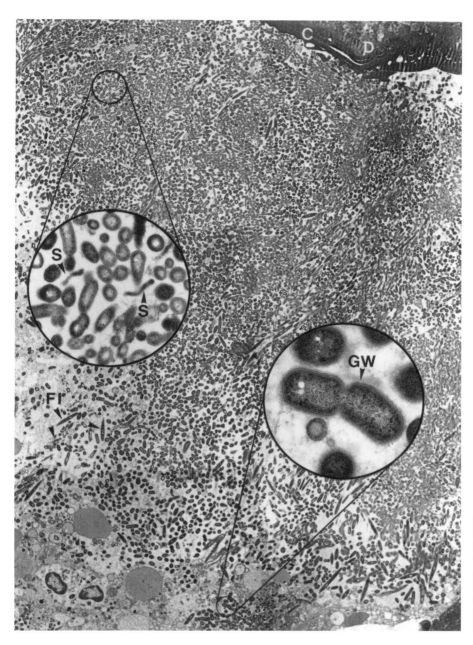

Fig. 6.7 Microbial biofilm at the periapex of a human tooth with acute apical periodontitis. Note the mixed bacterial flora consisting of numerous dividing cocci, rods (lower inset), filaments (Fl) and spirochetes (S, upper inset). Rods often reveal a Gram-negative cell wall (GW, lower inset). C = cementum; D = dentin. Magnification: ×2680; upper inset: ×19 200; lower inset: ×36 400. (From Nair (49).)

necrotic tissue, tissue fluid and inflammatory exudates from the apical tissue supply the basic requirements for carbon, nitrogen, salts and energy as well as the special requirements for amino acids, nucleotides, vitamins and hemin (62). Nutrients can be derived directly from these sources but also from degradation of macromolecules such as proteins and glycoproteins, a process that requires the concerted action of enzymes released from different species in the microbial community. The resulting carbohydrates, small peptides and amino acids then serve as nutrients and an energy source for many inhabitants of the biofilm. The biofilm organisms may also benefit from intermicrobial food chains where metabolic end-products (e.g. NH_3, CO_2 and organic acids) of one species serve as nutrients for others. Owing to the small amount of carbohydrate available directly or liberated from degradation of glycoproteins, growth of microorganisms requiring carbohydrate for energy is limited, whereas proteolytic and amino-acid degrading microorganisms are favored. This is reflected in the high proportion of proteolytic bacteria present in the endodontic microbiota. The nutrient conditions in the root canal appear, in many ways, to be similar to those experienced by subgingival dental biofilms (for a review, see Ref. 58).

In clinical situations where the necrotic tissues in root canals have been removed and the apical inflammatory process controlled, nutrients will be scarce. In nature, many microorganisms can survive such hostile environ-

Advanced concept 6.1   Microbial biofilms are marked by their heterogeneity

The environmental heterogeneity of biofilms is followed by a phenotypical heterogeneity among microorganisms in the community. Bacteria alter their pattern of gene and protein expressions as a response to the local environmental heterogeneity within the biofilm, one consequence of which might be an enhanced virulence or a greater resistance to antimicrobial agents. Recently, it has been recognized that oral bacteria use both inter- and intraspecies signaling molecules for cellular communication. Once released, these molecules (peptides for Gram-positive bacteria and autoinducer-2 for Gram-positive and Gram-negative bacteria) diffuse in the local environment and influence properties of neighboring cells, such as their resistance to environmental stress and antimicrobials.

Core concept 6.2   Microbial interactions in a polymicrobial community

Synergism
- Coaggregation
- Maintenance of anaerobic environment
- Enzyme complementation for concerted degradation of macromolecules
- Food chains
- Joint defense

Antagonism
- Competition for space and nutrients
- Inhibitory metabolic products
- Bacteriocins

ments by inducing a starvation response. While information on the starvation response in root canal bacteria is limited, microorganisms are likely to regulate their metabolic balance away from multiplication, towards the acquisition of energy for survival (21). It is quite possible that the adoption of a non-growing state could be an important mechanism for survival in nutrient-deprived environments of the root canal (12).

Redox potential

Generally, the oxygen tension and redox potential in root canals are low, which select for obligately anaerobic microorganisms, with only a few facultative anaerobes and the rare occurrence of obligate aerobes. As for dental biofilms, any oxygen entering the root canal, e.g. with saliva, will be consumed by the facultative anaerobes, which tolerate oxygen due to their enzymes that catalyze removal of toxic oxygen products. It should be emphasized that the failure of oxygen to penetrate biofilms is not a result of physical exclusion, since the extracellular matrix of biofilms allows diffusion of oxygen (19). Oxygen will not reach the inner parts, however, because it is actively consumed by facultative anaerobes in the biofilm. Thus, in dense microbial biofilms, low oxygen levels and a low redox potential suitable for obligate anaerobes will prevail.

Microbial interactions in biofilms

Root canal biofilms contain multiple oral species that are able to interact. Evidence is accumulating that members of the microbial community in biofilms are actively involved in a wide range of metabolic, molecular and physical interactions that may well be essential for the attachment, growth and survival of species at a site, enabling microorganisms to persist in harsh environments (Core concept 6.2). One good example of how the

participating microorganisms utilize a community lifestyle is the consumption of oxygen by facultatively anaerobic species. Combined with the accumulation of reduced metabolic end-products this creates an environment suitable for obligate anaerobes (8). Another example of interactions that benefit participating microorganisms are those necessary to metabolize complex host glycoproteins and proteins. These molecules are normally recalcitrant to catabolism by individual microorganisms but can easily be broken down by the concerted action of the microbes in microbial communities.

In addition to the conventional metabolic interactions, more subtle interactions such as cell–cell signaling might occur among microorganisms in root canal biofilms. Many species of oral bacteria have evolved signaling systems that probably help them to adapt and survive host-imposed fluctuations in their local environment (17). Some of these communication systems may also function between different oral species and can lead to coordinated gene and protein expression within the microbial community. Such signaling strategies might also play a role in the establishment and regulation of the microbial community in an infected root canal and are currently being viewed as potential targets for new therapeutic methods (for a review, see Ref. 52).

Examples have already been given about how the bacterial organisms at the surface of the biofilm provide protection to those in the inner or deeper portion of the biofilm. All the members of the community may also benefit from the ability of some species to inactivate host defense by degrading antibodies and inhibiting phagocytosis. Nevertheless antagonistic relationships will occur. For example, some metabolic end-products (e.g. H_2O_2, fatty acids and sulfur compounds) may accumulate in concentrations that are inhibitory or toxic for other species. In addition, antimicrobial peptides, so-called bacteriocins, generated by some species target others that are sensitive, so that their growth is suppressed.

Antimicrobial resistance

Central to the theme of biofilm control is the use of surfactants, antimicrobial agents and preservatives. Antimicrobial agents have often been developed and optimized for their activity against fast-growing, single species. Numerous studies have now demonstrated that biofilm growth protects bacteria from killing by biocides, disinfectants and antibiotics, a feature that is highly relevant to root canal infections. There are reports showing that microorganisms grown in biofilms could be two- to 1000-fold more resistant than the corresponding planktonic forms (22). With respect to oral bacteria, the inhibitory concentrations for chlorhexidine and amine fluoride are 300 and 75 times greater, respectively, when *Streptococcus sobrinus* is grown as a biofilm compared with free-floating bacteria (54). Biofilms of oral bacteria have also been found to be more resistant to amoxicillin, doxycycline and metronidazole (29).

The protective mechanisms underlying biofilm antimicrobial resistance are not well known, although several mechanisms have been proposed (22). The structure and dense organization of the biofilm community within the polymeric matrix may restrict the penetration of the agent into the biofilm, leaving microorganisms in the depths of the biofilm unaffected. In the process the agent might also be inactivated. In addition, in an established biofilm bacteria grow only slowly under nutrient-deprived conditions. As a consequence they are much less susceptible than fast-dividing bacteria. Biofilm bacteria may also display a distinct phenotype that accounts for the enhanced resistance. For example, biofilm bacteria might not express the drug target or may use different metabolic pathways than planktonic bacteria.

Of special interest for root canal infections are the experimental *in vitro* studies showing that cultures of *Enterococcus faecalis*, added to calcium hydroxide-medicated and non-medicated root canals, are able to form biofilm structures on the canal walls (20) and that biofilm formation seems to allow the microorganism to resist treatment. As well as possible variations in the concentration of hydroxyl ions to which root canal bacteria are exposed, they are also known to vary in their intrinsic ability to withstand alkaline pH changes (10, 11).

Methods for studying the root canal microflora

The microflora of necrotic pulps has been studied for more than 100 years, mainly by direct microscopy and cultivation. Much knowledge has been gained through research into the composition, ecology and pathogenic potential of the microflora. In clinical practice, root canal cultures may be used to determine the microbiological

---

Core concept 6.3   Problems in root canal cultures

Sampling
- Location is not accessible
- Contamination

Transport
- Death of microorganisms
- Overgrowth of microorganisms

Cultivation
- Media are not adequate
- Anaerobiosis is not adequate
- Microorganisms are not cultivatable

Identification
- Time-consuming laboratory procedures
- Expensive
- Taxonomy not yet defined

Culture-independent, molecular genetic techniques can solve some of the problems.

---

status and to assess the efficacy of the treatment measures given prior to completion of the treatment by root filling. Owing to the location of the microorganisms and the high species diversity of the microflora, there are, however, several methodological problems with this technique (Core concept 6.3).

For many years, the methods for sampling, transport, cultivation and identification were rather inadequate for the many fastidious, often anaerobic microorganisms present. Therefore, false-negative cultures (no growth in spite of microorganisms living in the root canal) were common. False-positive cultures (growth of contaminating microorganisms not present in the root canal) were also a common event. Of course, optimal techniques to minimize such false results and to secure the growth of all members of the mixed microflora are essential (43). Methods for microbial identification with and without culturing are developing rapidly, and the names and taxonomic position of many bacteria change with the newly acquired knowledge. The common steps followed for detection and identification of root canal microorganisms are shown in Fig. 6.8.

Sampling

Asepsis is necessary during sampling to avoid contamination from teeth, oral mucosa, saliva, fingers and instruments. Caries must be excavated, fillings, crowns, plaque and calculus removed, a rubber dam applied and the tooth and rubber dam disinfected. Sterile burs and instruments are used to gain access to the root canals, and samples are taken with sterile paper points. The canal may contain inflammatory exudate that can be

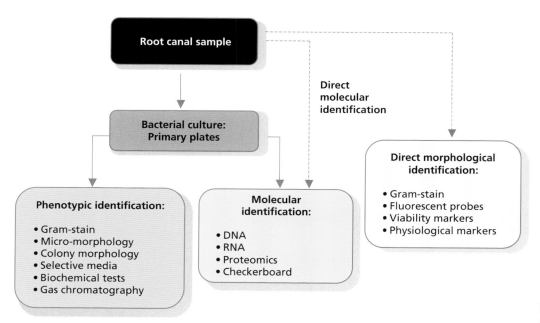

Fig. 6.8 Protocol for visualization and identification of endodontic microorganisms.

used in the sampling process. If absent, it is necessary to introduce a small amount of sterile fluid. By slight instrumentation with a file of a size fitting the canal space, necrotic tissue and material from the root canal wall are dispersed in the fluid, which is then absorbed with a sufficient number of paper points to soak up all the fluid. The paper points should be transferred immediately to a tube of reduced transport medium designed to keep the organisms alive, but not growing, during transport to the laboratory.

Cultivation

In the laboratory, the microorganisms must first be evenly dispersed in the fluid, e.g. by vigorous mixing with glass beads before cultivation. Dilutions of the dispersed sample are spread on agar media, which are then incubated long enough (10–14 days) to allow even slow growers to form colonies. In a broth culture, the fastest growing bacteria will overgrow the others and members of a mixed microflora will be missed (62). Non-selective agar media containing hemolyzed blood (Fig. 6.9) fulfill many special nutrient requirements and are best suited to culture the many bacterial types as well as yeasts (43). Selective media may be included, e.g. Sabouraud agar for yeasts, mitis salivarius agar for streptococci, or Rogosa SL agar selective for lactobacilli. Special media are required for the growth of mycoplasms and spirochetes, but only some of the latter can be cultivated even when special techniques are used (43).

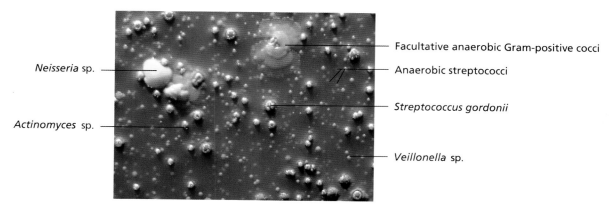

Fig. 6.9 Growth of root canal microorganisms on blood agar. A paper point sample from root canal with necrotic pulp was inoculated to blood agar and microorganisms were allowed to grow under anaerobic conditions. After 10 days of growth, several colony types are seen. Later identification of microorganisms revealed a mixed infection with various types of microorganisms involved.

As microorganisms colonizing root canals are facultative and obligate anaerobes, anaerobic techniques for handling and incubation of cultures are essential for accurate results. This requirement can be fulfilled by incubation in anaerobic jars or even better in an anaerobic box, which allows work with samples and cultures as well as incubation in an oxygen-free atmosphere. In order to facilitate the identification of facultative anaerobic and capnophilic (thrives in conjunction with carbon dioxide) bacteria, a set of agar plates is incubated in air supplemented with carbon dioxide. Generally, one or two colonies of each type are subcultured for identification. Because different bacteria may have similar colony morphologies, for some purposes it is better to isolate a large number of colonies.

Direct microscopy

Direct observation with phase-contrast or dark-field microscopy, scanning electron microscopy or microscopy of Gram-stained smears, enables observation of all morphological types present – even those not recovered in cultures (18). The presence of specific bacteria may be assessed in smears stained with the indirect immuno-fluorescent technique (3). Fluorescence microscopy in conjunction with live/dead stains can be used to visualize morphologically different types (Fig. 6.10), although the reliability of such stains for viable versus non-viable is far from optimal (31). A wide range of fluorescent probes is commercially available; when combined with fluorescence microscopy these allow assessment of the physiological state of individual microorganisms in a sample. These physiological probes are designed to target different cellular functions such as metabolic activity, cell-membrane integrity, membrane potential, enzyme activities and nucleic acid synthesis (for review, see Ref. 27). They are valuable tools, e.g. when evaluating the antimicrobial effect of bactericidal compounds on complex microbial communites, such as those existing in root canals.

One promising approach that allows visualization and also permits examination of microorganisms in complex matrices is the use of fluorescence in situ hybridization (FISH) techniques. The preferred mode of observation is by CLSM with fluorescent oligonucleotide probes targeting the ribosomal RNA (rRNA) of bacteria (2). Using this approach, microorganisms are fixed to stabilize the morphology and make the cell membrane permeable to allow the labeled probes to diffuse to their intracellular rRNA targets (45). Failure to detect target cells by FISH is most often caused by lack of cell permeability, low cellular ribosome content or inaccessibility of the probe binding site based on the higher-order structure of the ribosome (1). FISH techniques have been successfully employed to detect and also, to a certain extent, identify specific bacteria species in sections of apical lesions (59).

Methods for identification

Precise identification, at the species level, of endodontic isolates is time consuming and costly and sometimes not possible because many members of the oral microflora are not yet sufficiently characterized. Some are even impossible to culture. Detailed identification of microorganisms is, however, essential for research, e.g. concerning the etiology of different periapical disease states and the role of certain bacteria or microbial combinations in disease progression and treatment outcome.

Bacterial isolates from culture can be grouped simply on the basis of certain characteristics, such as colony morphology and pigmentation, cell morphology, the presence or absence of motility, Gram-staining reaction and facultative or obligate anaerobe. Genus or species identification requires several biochemical tests for enzyme activities and end-products, possibly with commercial test kits. Unknown isolates must be compared with

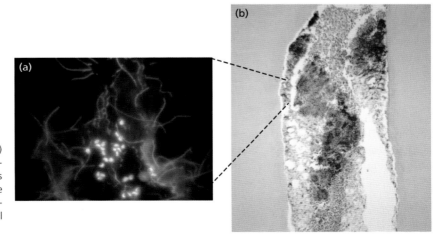

Fig. 6.10 Visualization of bacteria in root canals. (a) Viability stain (BacLight LIVE/DEAD) of a microbial biofilm containing numerous filamentous microorganisms and coccoid forms. Fluorescent green represents viable whereas orange represents membrane-damaged bacteria. (b) This biofilm was obtained from a root canal with a necrotic pulp. (From Chávez de Paz (14).)

reference strains of defined species. Similarities between strains can be examined with advanced methods such as DNA–DNA homology analysis or protein profiles of cell extracts by polyacrylamide gel electrophoresis. With the "checkerboard" DNA–DNA hybridization method, DNA extracted from endodontic samples has been reacted with DNA probes from up to 40 bacterial species, with results indicating the presence of many of these species (67). Such methods designed to detect specific bacteria are only reliable if appropriate specific DNA probes are available. So far, they seem less suitable for endodontic microbiology, where the presence of any of a large number of oral as well as non-oral species is of interest.

Molecular genetic techniques hold great promise for the examination of endodontic samples (67). Elimination of the need for culturing means that the (probably numerous) unculturable bacteria can be included. The method currently dominating the field is based on sequence analysis of the 16S subunit rRNA gene, which can be applied to identification on different levels (bacteria in general, bacterial order- or family-specific, species-specific and subspecies). In this approach, nucleic acids are directly extracted from samples without any prior cultivation; amplification is then performed using universal primers targeting conserved segments of the 16S rRNA gene, and identification is based on similarity with sequences deposited in public ribosomal gene data bases (50). Even if the sequence is unknown from previous work, it can be placed in relation to known organisms and other sequences in nature. Methods have focused on 16S rRNA genes because the molecule is universally distributed, has some extremely conserved segments as well as variable regions, and yields an RNA product that has many copies per cell and can be used directly as a hybridization target. With this approach, 16S rRNA gene sequencing has been used to identify both known and currently unknown microbial species in samples of infected root canals (56).

Composition of the endodontic microflora

The recent application of molecular methods to the identification of oral bacteria has resulted in the detection and identification of a large number of novel taxa; previously uncultivated or cultivated but not identified. An estimated 700 oral bacterial species have been identified by nucleotide sequence analysis of the 16S rRNA subunit and less than 50% of these species cannot, as yet, be cultured in the laboratory (66). The polymicrobial nature of root canal infections has been confirmed by 16S rRNA gene sequencing (55) and future studies using culture-independent approaches will ensure characterization of the full diversity and improvements in the taxonomy of the endodontic microflora.

Oral microorganisms in the necrotic pulp

The microorganisms in root canal samples from deciduous as well as permanent teeth are predominantly the same bacteria as those found in dental plaque, periodontal pockets and carious lesions (36, 51). The majority of isolates in initial cultures are obligate anaerobic bacteria. These constituted 91% of the isolates from closed necrosis (63), 90% of isolates from necrotic pulps of deciduous teeth (51) and 68% from the apical part of necrotic pulps in carious teeth (5). A large proportion of the anaerobes are asaccharolytic, peptide- and amino acid-degrading bacteria (51, 62).

The many genera and species currently identified in root canal samples comprise obligate anaerobic and facultative anaerobic oral bacteria (5, 6, 43). The genera most commonly isolated from root canals are summarized in Core concept 6.4. Among the streptococci, *S. anginosus*, *S. intermedius*, *S. constellatus*, *S. mitis*, *S. oralis*, *S. gordonii*, *S. sanguinis* and *S. parasanguinis* are common, and in carious teeth also *S. mutans*. It was suggested (39) that *S. sanguinis* and *S. salivarius* often occur in root canal cultures due to contamination with saliva or invasion through leaking temporary fillings. Lactobacilli are mainly found in teeth with caries. *Actinomyces israelii* (as well as other *Actinomyces* species) may be present, and sometimes actinomycotic apical lesions develop (48).

Black-pigmented bacteria of the genera *Porphyromonas* and *Prevotella* have attracted much attention as potential pathogens in endodontic as well as in periodontal microbiology (24). These anaerobic, Gram-negative rods are common isolates from necrotic pulps before treatment, especially the *Prevotella* species *Pr. nigrescens*, *Pr. intermedia*, *Pr. tannerae*, *Pr. melaninogenica*, *Pr. denticola* and *Pr. buccae*, as well as the *Porphyromonas* species *P. endodontalis* and *P. gingivalis*. Other oral bacteria commonly found are species of *Peptostreptococcus*, *Eubacterium*, *Veillonella*, *Fusobacterium*, *Selenomonas*, *Campylobacter*, *Neisseria*, *Capnocytophaga*, *Eikenella* and *Treponema*, the latter generally demonstrated by direct microscopy. Some species such as *Treponema denticola* and *Bacteroides forsythus*, which are difficult to culture, have been demonstrated with DNA techniques applied directly to root canal samples (57).

Yeasts of the genus *Candida* and sometimes other fungi are common members of the resident oral microflora (36). Yeasts have also been observed by electron microscopy in root canals that had been exposed to the oral cavity (33, 53), and in biopsy specimens from root filled teeth with therapy-resistant apical lesions (47). In many older cultural studies, yeasts alone or together with bacteria are reported in up to 17% of cases (for a review, see Ref. 68). In a study of 967 samples cultured from unfilled root canals with therapy-resistant infection (68), yeasts were found in 7%, sometimes in pure culture but

Core concept 6.4   The microbiota of the root canal

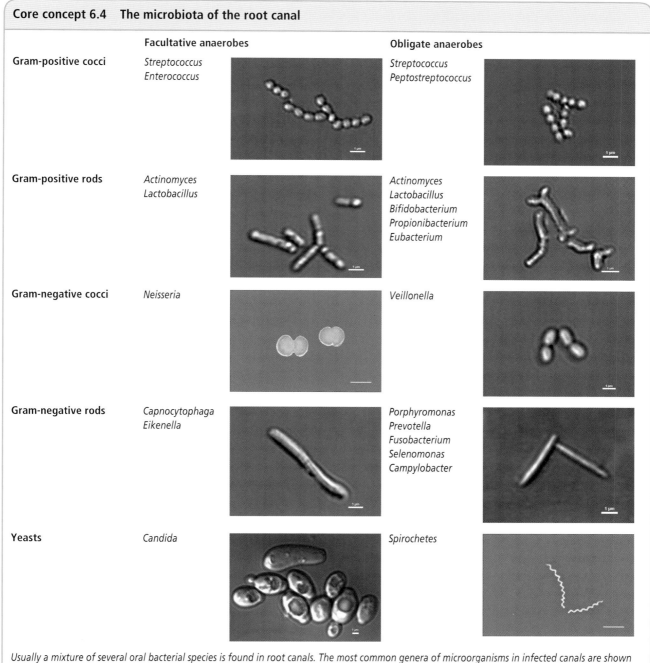

	Facultative anaerobes	Obligate anaerobes
Gram-positive cocci	*Streptococcus* *Enterococcus*	*Streptococcus* *Peptostreptococcus*
Gram-positive rods	*Actinomyces* *Lactobacillus*	*Actinomyces* *Lactobacillus* *Bifidobacterium* *Propionibacterium* *Eubacterium*
Gram-negative cocci	*Neisseria*	*Veillonella*
Gram-negative rods	*Capnocytophaga* *Eikenella*	*Porphyromonas* *Prevotella* *Fusobacterium* *Selenomonas* *Campylobacter*
Yeasts	*Candida*	Spirochetes

Usually a mixture of several oral bacterial species is found in root canals. The most common genera of microorganisms in infected canals are shown above.

more often together with bacteria. A surprisingly high prevalence (40%) of yeasts (in most cases together with bacteria) was demonstrated in pus from dentoalveolar abscesses from deciduous teeth in children with nursing bottle caries, a condition known to favor the growth of yeasts in the mouth (64). In case endodontic treatment fails to eliminate the infection, a wide range of microorganisms may be recovered (see Key literature 6.2).

Bacteria of extraoral origin in the necrotic pulp

Facultatively anaerobic, enteric bacteria are frequently found in root canals, sometimes in initial samples but especially in samples taken later during treatment in the case of poor response or during retreatment of failed root fillings (13, 41, 61). By far the most common species in this group is *Enterococcus faecalis* (formerly *Streptococcus*

Key literature 6.2 Bacteria persisting after root canal treatment

Gram-positive cocci
- *Staphylococcus* (19)
- *Enterococcus* (46)
- *Peptostreptococcus* (15)
- *Streptococcus* (100)

Gram-positive rods
- *Actinomyces* (20)
- *Bifidobacterium* (22)
- *Clostridium* (4)
- *Eubacterium* (11)
- *Lactobacillus* (97)
- *Propionibacterium* (20)

Gram-negative cocci
- *Veillonella* (10)

Gram-negative rods
- *Enterobacteria* (11)
- *Fusobacterium* (11)
- *Porphyromonas* (1)
- *Prevotella* (16)

Yeasts
- *Candida* (2)

Gram-positive cocci
- *Enterococcus* (18)
- *Streptococcus* (24)

Gram-positive rods
- *Actinomyces* (7)
- *Bifidobacterium* (3)
- *Clostridium* (1)
- *Eubacterium* (2)
- *Lactobacillus* (23)
- *Propionibacterium* (7)

Gram-negative rods
- *Enterobacteria* (1)

Gram-positive cocci
- *Enterococcus* (2)
- *Streptococcus* (1)

Gram-positive rods
- *Actinomyces* (1)
- *Lactobacillus* (4)
- *Propionibacterium* (3)

Sample 1   Sample 2   Sample 3

The most commonly found microorganisms in root canals during root canal treatment. The number within brackets represents the isolation frequency of the microorganism.

In a series of studies, a total of 276 teeth with apical periodontitis undergoing root canal treatment were microbiologically analyzed (13). In samples taken after initiation of treatment (**Sample 1**), microorganisms were detected in 183 teeth of which Gram-positive cocci and rods accounted for 87% of the total number of isolates. In a subsequent sample after 2 weeks (**Sample 2**), microorganisms were found in 78 teeth and the most frequently isolated microorganisms belonged to the genera *Enterococcus*, *Lactobacillus* and *Streptococcus*. In a third sample in another 2 weeks (**Sample 3**), 11 teeth presented growth, with *Lactobacillus* spp., *Propionibacterium* spp. and *Enterococcus* spp. being the most prevalent.

---

faecalis), which is the only isolate from many of these cases. Other enteric bacteria isolated comprise species of *Enterobacter*, *Acinetobacter*, *Proteus*, *Klebsiella* and *Pseudomonas*. It is not clear whether these bacteria are present initially and become predominant during treatment, or enter the canals later owing to failures in aseptic technique and temporary seals. *Staphylococcus* species are also among the bacteria occasionally present in root canal cultures, in some cases probably as a contaminant from the skin.

Virulence factors

The oral microorganisms are opportunistic (potential) pathogens and can cause disease if they colonize a location where host defense mechanisms are unable to eliminate them (Core concept 6.5). Any microflora which succeed in colonizing the root canal seem to produce

quite severe disease. Yet, there is no single or unique pathogen. Therefore endodontic treatment should be directed at combating the entire microbiota (see Chapter 9). The presence of different complex mixtures of microorganisms in root canals is typical. The sum of several virulence factors produced by the consortia of microorganisms present will determine the degree of pathogenicity (Advanced concept 6.3). Information on virulence factors is limited to examples in certain oral species that have attracted attention, mainly as potential pathogens in periodontal disease (36). Some of these are also common in endodontic samples and similar pathogenic mechanisms are likely to be active in apical periodontitis lesions (62).

A distinct feature of apical periodontitis is that host defense mechanisms are unable to remove microorganisms located outside their reach in the necrotic pulp and on the walls of the root canal. In addition, some

Core concept 6.5   Polymicrobial opportunistic infection

- Apical periodontitis is a polymicrobial, opportunistic infection caused by resident oral microorganisms becoming pathogenic when they colonize the necrotic pulp, root canal walls, dentin and cementum.
- There is no single or unique pathogen.
- Several potential virulence factors expressed by various species in root canal environments may contribute to the collective pathogenicity of the endodontic microflora.

Advanced concept 6.2   Some microbial virulence factors implicated in apical periodontitis

Colonization of root canal
- Surface components for adhesion and coaggregation
- Enzymes to get nutrients
- Microbial food chains

Evasion of host defenses
- Location
- Immunoglobulin-degrading proteases
- Complement-degrading proteases
- Capsules
- Inhibition of phagocytes

Direct tissue damage
- Proteases and other enzymes
- Cytotoxic metabolic products
- Lipopolysaccharide endotoxins

Indirect tissue damage due to inflammatory response to the microorganisms
- Cytokines
- Proteases and other enzymes from host cells

microorganisms can impair host defense, with enzymes degrading plasma proteins such as immunoglobulins, complement factors, proteinase inhibitors and proteins involved in the clotting, fibrinolytic and kinin systems (62). Such enzymes have been demonstrated in *Porphyromonas* and *Prevotella* species and may offer protection to the whole microbial community, not only to the producers. Phagocytosis is of paramount importance in host defense. Although leukotoxin-producing (phagocyte-killing) bacteria are rare in the endodontic microflora, several of the bacteria commonly found can evade phagocytosis or resist intracellular killing in various ways. One such mechanism is the above-mentioned degradation of plasma proteins essential for opsonization, and another is the presence of a capsule around some bacteria (36).

Direct damage to the apical connective tissue and bone may be caused by extracellular bacterial enzymes such as proteases, collagenase, hyaluronidase and chondroitin sulfatase. These enzymes are produced by several species isolated from root canals, notably *Prevotella*, *Porphyromonas*, *Peptostreptococcus*, *Eubacterium* and *Treponema* species (25). The endodontic microflora also produce cytotoxic metabolites, which may damage the tissues and cause inflammation. Examples are: ammonia, amines, indole, hydrogen sulfide, methyl mercaptan, butyrate, propionate, succinate and others (36, 62). Another group of cytotoxic substances are the lipopolysaccharide endotoxins of Gram-negative bacteria. These agents act as antigenic and toxic compounds, which cause inflammation and induce bone resorption.

Many virulence factors of the endodontic microflora can induce inflammation, and this will lead indirectly to host tissue damaging itself (Advanced concept 6.2). Although the inflammatory process serves a protective function, aimed at elimination of the microorganisms and their products, it also causes degradation of peri-apical connective tissue fibers and extracellular matrix, and osteoclasts are activated leading to bone resorption. In addition, dormant epithelial rests may be stimulated to proliferate (49). These intricate processes are described in Chapter 7.

Association of signs and symptoms with specific bacteria

Although most apical inflammatory processes run silently without giving subjective symptoms, acute manifestations will occur (see Chapter 7). It is logical to assume that some microorganisms and certain mixtures are more virulent than others and therefore more likely to cause acute symptoms. However, no firm correlations have yet been established owing to the often small number of cases studied (25, 60, 63). Nevertheless the risk seems increased where large quantities of microorganisms prevail in canals with mixtures of several, mainly anaerobic species. In some studies *Porphyromonas*, *Prevotella*, *Peptostreptococcus*, *Fusobacterium* and *Eubacterium* species were associated with an increased incidence of symptoms (24, 63).

The *Porphyromonas* and *Prevotella* species forming black colonies on blood agar have attracted special attention in endodontic as well as periodontal microbiology. The important role of these black-pigmented bacteria in mixed anaerobic infections has been known for more than 35 years and for some of them was confirmed in a study of experimental infections induced in guinea pigs by subcutaneous injections of combinations of root canal bacteria (60). Persistent abscesses and transmissible infections could only be produced with mixtures comprising *Po. endodontalis* or *Pr. intermedia/nigrescens*. (These studies were conducted before "*Bacteroides intermedius*" was divided into *Pr. intermedia* and *Pr. nigrescens*.)

Studies of black-pigmented bacteria in cases of apical inflammation with and without acute symptoms (24) suggest that the presence of *Po. endodontalis, Po. gingivalis* or *Pr. intermedia/nigrescens* in the mixed microflora increases the risk of clinical symptoms and abscess formation. In one of these studies of 62 cases of apical periodontitis (35 acute and 27 clinically asymptomatic cases), 37 strains of black-pigmented bacteria were isolated from 31 (50%) of the teeth, always in a mixed anaerobic microflora (24). These bacteria were cultured from both symptomatic and asymptomatic teeth, and there were also several symptomatic cases from which they were not isolated. However, the proteolytic species *Po. gingivalis* and *Po. endodontalis* were present only in acute infections, whereas *Pr. intermedia/nigrescens* was found in both symptomatic and asymptomatic cases and *Pr. denticola* occurred mostly in asymptomatic root canals. If the canal contains black-pigmented bacteria, the method of canal instrumentation is an especially important determinant in the development of post-treatment abscess, because these bacteria are likely to cause acute symptoms if pushed outside the apical foramen.

One study (23) suggests that statistically significant associations exist between individual endodontic symptoms and particular combinations of specific bacteria. Thus, pain was associated with mixtures of anaerobes comprising *Peptostreptococcus* and *Prevotella* species. Swelling was particularly associated with isolation of *Eubacterium, Peptostreptococcus* or *Prevotella* species, and even more strongly with a combination of *Peptostreptococcus* and *Prevotella* species. Exudate in the canal was significantly associated with combinations of *Prevotella/Eubacterium* species and *Peptostreptococcus/Eubacterium* species.

In some cases root canal bacteria seem resistant to treatment, as indicated by persisting exudation, lingering symptoms and sinus tracts. Cultures from such cases after several treatment sessions often show presence of streptococci, enterobacteria and yeasts. While these organisms may have been present from the very beginning and be relatively resistant to treatment, their presence may often be due to contamination of canals left open to the oral cavity or inadequately sealed, or to other failures in aseptic technique (68). In studies of root filled teeth retreated due to persisting apical lesions, the microflora cultured differed markedly from that of untreated teeth. It consisted mostly of one or two species of mainly Gram-positive bacteria, and the most common isolate was *Enterococcus faecalis* (41, 60).

Concluding remarks

Bacteria in the root canal environment should be seen as a multicellular, microbial community, which concomitantly behaves, responds and adapts for survival.

Root canals – whether they contain necrotic tissue, have been emptied by debridement or are filled with cement and gutta-percha – provide an environment with limited oxygen and fluctuating nutrient availability, in which many different oral microorganisms may survive and grow. The degree to which microorganisms tolerate these environmental conditions determines their success in establishing themselves as the cause of apical periodontitis. The presence of multiple species in root canal biofilms gives a greater overall potential for survival, growth and tolerance of environmental challenges, such as antimicrobial agents, than any single microbial species would possess. The pathogenic potential of microorganisms can be modulated through the close proximity within a biofilm which increases the probability of interactions between bacteria through signal molecules and in response to environmental factors. Thus, a more complete understanding of the role of microorganisms in apical periodontitis relies on an appreciation, not only of the composition of the root canal biofilms, but also of the interactions between species and impact of the microenvironment upon their virulence. Such knowledge is critical to more readily explaining the resistance of root canal microorganisms to antimicrobial agents and sudden acute presentations of apical periodontitis as well as opening up new opportunities for the control and treatment of these mixed-species biofilm infections.

References

1. Amann R, Fuchs BM. Single-cell identification in microbial communities by improved fluorescence *in situ* hybridization techniques. *Nat. Rev. Microbiol.* 2008; 6: 339–45.
2. Amann RI. Ludwig W, Schleifer KH. Phylogenetic identification and *in situ* detection of individual microbial cells without cultivation. *Microbiol. Rev.* 1995; 59: 143–69.
3. Assed S, Ito IY, Leonardo MR, Silva LA, Lopatin DE. Anaerobic microorganisms in root canals of human teeth with chronic apical periodontitis detected by indirect immunofluorescence. *Endot. Dent. Traumatol.* 1996; 12: 66–9.
4. Auschill TM, Arweiler NB, Netuschil L, Brecx M, Reich E, Sculean A. Spatial distribution of vital and dead microorganisms in dental biofilms. *Arch. Oral Biol.* 2001; 46: 471–6.
5. Baumgartner JC, Falkler WA. Bacteria in the apical 5mm of infected root canals. *J. Endodont.* 1991; 17: 380–3.
6. Bergenholtz G. Micro-organisms from necrotic pulp of traumatized teeth. *Odontol. Revy* 1974; 25: 347–58.
7. Bowden GH, Hamilton IR. Survival of oral bacteria. *Crit. Rev. Oral Biol. Med.* 1998; 9: 54–85.
8. Bradshaw DJ, Marsh PD, Allison C, Schilling KM. Effect of oxygen, inoculum composition and flow rate on development of mixed culture oral biofilms. *Microbiology* 1996; 142: 623–29.
9. Burnett GW, Scherp HW. *Oral Microbiology and Infectious Disease*, 3rd edn. Baltimore: Williams & Wilkins, 1968; 27–31, 467, 485.

10. Byström A, Claesson R, Sundqvist G. The antibacterial effect of camphorated paramonochlorophenol, camphorated phenol and calcium hydroxide in the treatment of infected root canals. *Endod. Dent. Traumatol.* 1985; 1: 170–5.

11. Chávez de Paz LE, Bergenholtz G, Dahlén G, Svensäter G. Response to alkaline stress by root canal bacteria in biofilms. *Int. Endodont. J.* 2007; 40: 344–55.

12. Chávez de Paz LE, Hamilton, IR, Svensäter G. Oral bacteria in biofilms exhibit slow reactivation from nutrient deprivation. *Microbiology* 2008; 154: 927–38.

13. Chávez de Paz LE. *On bacteria persisting root canal treatment.* Doctoral Thesis, University of Gothenburg, 2005.

14. Chávez de Paz LE. Redefining the persistent infection in root canals: possible role of biofilm communities. *J. Endod.* 2007; 33: 652–62.

15. Costerton JW, Lewandowski Z, Caldwell DE, Korber DR, Lappin-Scott HM. Microbial biofilms. *Annu. Rev. Microbiol.* 1995; 49: 711–45.

16. Costerton JW, Stewart PS, Greenberg EP. Bacterial biofilms: a common cause of persistent infections. *Science* 1999; 284: 1318–22.

17. Cvitkovitch DG, Li YH, Ellen RP. Quorum sensing and biofilm formation in streptococcal infections. *J. Clin. Invest.* 2003; 112: 1626–32.

18. Dahle UR, Tronstad L, Olsen I. Observation of an unusually large spirochete in endodontic infection. *Oral Microbiol. Immunol.* 1993; 8: 251–3.

19. De Beer D, Stoodley P, Roe F, Lewandowski Z. Effects of biofilm structures on oxygen distribution and mass transport. *Biotechnol. Bioeng.* 1994; 43: 1131–8.

20. Distel JW, Hatton JF, Gillespie MJ. Biofilm formation in medicated root canals. *J. Endod.* 2002; 28: 689–93.

21. Giard JC, Hartke A, Flahaut S, Boutibonnes P, Auffray Y. Glucose starvation response in *Enterococcus faecalis* JH2-2: survival and protein analysis. *Res. Microbiol.* 1997; 148: 27–35.

22. Gilbert P, Das J, Foley I. Biofilm susceptibility to antimicrobials. *Adv. Dent. Res.* 1997; 11: 160–7.

23. Gomes BPFA, Lilley JD, Drucker DB. Associations of endodontic symptoms and signs with particular combinations of specific bacteria. *Int. Endod. J.* 1996; 29: 69–75.

24. Haapasalo M, Ranta H, Ranta K, Shah H. Black-pigmented *Bacteroides* spp. in human apical periodontitis. *Infect. Immun.* 1986; 53: 149–53.

25. Hashioka K, Suzuki K, Yoshida T, Nakane A, Horiba N, Nakamura H. Relationship between clinical symptoms and enzyme-producing bacteria isolated from infected root canals. *J. Endod.* 1994; 20: 75–7.

26. Hunter W. The role of sepsis and of antisepsis in medicine. *Dent. Cosmos* 1918; 60: 585–602.

27. Joux F, Lebaron P. Use of fluorescent probes to assess physiological functions of bacteria at single-cell level. *Microbes Infect.* 2000; 2: 1523–35.

28. Kakehashi S, Stanley HR, Fitzgerald RJ. The effects of surgical exposures of dental pulps in germ-free and conventional laboratory rats. *Oral Surg.* 1965; 20: 340–9.
    Key reference in the endodontic literature confirming the crucial role of bacteria in pulpal and periapical disease processes.

29. Larsen T. Susceptibility of *Porphyromonas gingivalis* in biofilms to amoxicillin, doxycycline and metronidazole. *Oral Microbiol. Immunol.* 2002; 17: 267–71.

30. Leonardo MR, Rossi MA, Silva LA, Ito IY, Bonifacio KC. EM evaluation of bacterial biofilm and microorganisms on the apical external root surface of human teeth. *J. Endod.* 2002; 28: 815–18.

31. Leuko S, Legat A, Fendrihan S, Stan-Lotter H. Evaluation of the LIVE/DEAD BacLight kit for detection of extremophilic archaea and visualization of microorganisms in environmental hypersaline samples. *Appl. Environ. Microbiol.* 2004; 70: 6884–6.

32. Listgarten MA, Lai CH. Comparative microbiological characteristics of failing implants and periodontally diseased teeth. *J. Periodontol.* 1999; 70: 431–7.

33. Lomcali G, Sen BH, Cankaya H. Scanning electron microscopic observations of apical root surfaces of teeth with apical periodontitis. *Endod. Dent. Traumatol.* 1996; 12: 70–6.

34. Love RM. Invasion of dentinal tubules by root canal bacteria. *Endod. Topics* 2004; 9: 52–65.

35. Makkes PC, Thoden van Velzen SK, Wesselink PR. Reactions of the living organism to dead and fixed dead tissue. *J. Endod.* 1978; 4: 17–21.

36. Marsh P, Martin M. *Oral Microbiology*, 5th edn. Oxford: Wright, 2009; 74–95, 128–32.

37. Marsh PD. Are dental diseases examples of ecological catastrophes? *Microbiology* 2003; 149: 279–94.

38. Marsh PD. Dental plaque: biological significance of a biofilm and community life-style. *J. Clin. Periodontol.* 2005; 32: 7–15.

39. Mejàre B. The incidence and significance of *Streptococcus sanguis*, *Streptococcus mutans* and *Streptococcus salivarius* in root canal cultures from human teeth. *Odontol. Revy* 1974; 25: 359–78.

40. Miller WD. *The Micro-organisms of the Human Mouth* (unaltered reprint of the original work published in 1890 in Philadelphia). Basel: S. Karger, 1973; 96–9, 285–95.

41. Molander A, Reit C, Dahlén G, Kvist T. Microbiological status of root filled teeth with apical periodontitis. *Int. Endod. J.* 1998; 31: 1–7.

42. Möller ÅJR, Fabricius L, Dahlén G, Öhman AE, Heyden G. Influence on periapical tissues of indigenous oral bacteria and necrotic pulp tissue in monkeys. *Scand. J. Dent. Res.* 1981; 89: 475–84.
    In this experimental study in monkeys, pulps were aseptically necrotized. In 26 teeth they were kept sterile by sealing and 52 were infected with the oral microflora. After 6–7 months, the teeth and periapical tissues were examined. The non-infected root canals were all sterile and there was no apical inflammation in these teeth. The teeth with infected necrotic tissue showed inflammation clinically (12/52 teeth) and radiographically (47/52 teeth). All infected teeth histologically examined displayed pronounced inflammation in the apical tissue.

43. Möller ÅJR. *Microbiological Examination of Root Canals and Periapical Tissues of Human Teeth. Methodological Studies.* Doctoral Thesis. Göteborg: Akademiförlaget, 1966.

44. Molven O, Olsen I, Kerekes K. Scanning electron microscopy of bacteria in the apical part of root canals in permanent teeth with periapical lesions. *Endod. Dent. Traumatol.* 1991; 7: 226–9.

45. Moter A, Gobel UB. Fluorescence *in situ* hybridization (FISH) for direct visualization of microorganisms. *J. Microbiol. Methods* 2000; 41: 85–112.

46. Nair P. Light and electron microscopic studies on root canal flora and periapical lesions. *J. Endod.* 1987; 13: 29–39.

In this report bacterial condensations in biofilm-like structures were described for the first time to occur in infected root canals. The observations were based on a series of cases comprising 31 teeth severely damaged by caries examined by light microscopy and transmission electron microscopy. Bacterial organisms were rarely found in the apical inflammatory tissue attached to the teeth.

47. Nair PN, Sjogren U, Krey G, Kahnberg KE, Sundqvist G. Intraradicular bacteria and fungi in root-filled, asymptomatic human teeth with therapy-resistant periapical lesions: a long-term light and electron microscopic follow-up study. *J Endod.* 1990; 16: 580–8.

48. Nair PNR, Schroeder HE. Periapical actinomycosis. *J. Endod.* 1984; 10: 567–70.

49. Nair PNR. Apical periodontitis: a dynamic encounter between root canal infection and host response. *Periodontol. 2000* 1997; 13: 121–48.

50. Paster BJ, Bosches SK, Galvin JL, Ericson RE, Lau CN, Levanos VA, *et al.* Bacterial diversity in human subgingival plaque. *J. Bacteriol.* 2001; 183: 3770–83.

51. Sato T, Hoshino E, Uematsu H, Noda T. Predominantly obligate anaerobes in necrotic pulps of human deciduous teeth. *Microb. Ecol. Health Dis.* 1993; 6: 269–75.

52. Scheie AA, Petersen FC. The biofilm concept: consequences for future prophylaxis or oral diseases? *Crit. Rev. Oral Biol. Med.* 2004; 15: 4–12.

53. Sen BH, Piskin B, Demirci T. Observation of bacteria and fungi in infected root canals and dentinal tubules by SEM. *Endod. Dent. Traumatol.* 1995; 11: 6–9.

54. Shani S, Friedman M, Steinberg D. The anticariogenic effect of amine fluorides on *Streptococcus sobrinus* and glucosyltransferase in biofilms. *Caries Res.* 2000; 34: 260–7.

55. Siqueira JF Jr, Rocas IN, Paiva SS, Magalhaes KM, Guimaraes-Pinto T. Cultivable bacteria in infected root canals as identified by 16S rRNA gene sequencing. *Oral Microbiol. Immunol.* 2007; 22: 266–71.

56. Siqueira JF Jr, Rocas IN. Exploiting molecular methods to explore endodontic infections: Part 1 – current molecular technologies for microbiological diagnosis. *J. Endod.* 2005; 31: 411–23.

57. Siqueira JF, Rocas IN, Souto R, de Uzeda M, Colombo AP. Checkerboard DNA–DNA hybridization analysis of endodontic infections. *Oral Surg.* 2000; 89: 744–8.

58. Socransky SS, Haffajee. Dental biofilms: difficult therapeutic targets. *Periodontol. 2000* 2002; 28: 12–55.

59. Sunde PT, Olsen I, Gobel UB, Theegarten D, Winter S, Debelian GJ, *et al.* Fluorescence *in situ* hybridization (FISH) for direct visualization of bacteria in periapical lesions of asymptomatic root-filled teeth. *Microbiology* 2003; 149: 1095–102.

60. Sundqvist G, Eckerbom MI, Larsson ÅP, Sjögren UT. Capacity of anaerobic bacteria from necrotic dental pulps to induce purulent infections. *Infect. Immun.* 1979; 25: 685–93.

61. Sundqvist G, Figdor D, Persson S, Sjögren S. Microbiological analysis of teeth with failed endodontic treatment and outcome of conservative re-treatment. *Oral Surg.* 1998; 85: 86–93.

62. Sundqvist G. Taxonomy, ecology, and pathogenicity of the root canal flora. *Oral Surg.* 1994; 78: 522–30.

63. Sundqvist G. *Bacteriological Studies of Necrotic Dental Pulps.* Umeå, Sweden: Umeå University Odontological Dissertations, 1976; no. 7.

Teeth with intact crowns injured by trauma were selected for microbiological analysis under strict asepsis. Anaerobic conditions were maintained for sampling, transport and cultivation. No bacteria could be isolated from any of the samples from 13 teeth free from radiographic signs of apical periodontitis. From 18 of 19 teeth with apical lesions 1–12 strains of bacteria were recovered by culture, the majority being anaerobes. Teeth with acute symptoms had a complex anaerobic flora comprising Bacteroides melaninogenicus.

64. Terheyden H, Knospe HJ, Dunsche A, Meunier D. Keimspektrum odontogener Abszesse im Milchgebiss. *Dtsch. Zahnärztl. Z.* 1997; 52: 124–5.

65. Tronstad L, Barnett F, Cervone F. Periapical bacterial plaque in teeth refractory to endodontic treatment. *Endod. Dent. Traumatol.* 1990; 6: 73–7.

66. Wade W. Unculturable bacteria in oral biofilms. In: *Dental Plaque Revisited* (Newman HN, Wilson M, eds). Cardiff: BioLine, 1999; 313–22.

67. Wade WG, Spratt DA, Dymock D, Weightman AJ. Molecular detection of novel anaerobic species in dentoalveolar abscesses. *Clin. Infect. Dis.* 1997; 25: 235–6.

68. Waltimo TMT, Sirén EK, Torkko HLK, Olsen I, Haapasalo MPP. Fungi in therapy-resistant apical periodontitis. *Int. Endod. J.* 1997; 30: 96–101.

Among 967 microbiological samples taken by general practitioners from persistent endodontics infections 692 gave growth and yeasts were isolated from 477 (7%). The yeasts were found in pure culture in six (13%) and together with bacteria in 41 (87%) of these samples. The accompanying bacteria were mostly streptococci and other Gram-positive facultative anaerobes.

Chapter 7
Apical periodontitis

Zvi Metzger, Itzhak Abramovitz and Gunnar Bergenholtz

Introduction

Apical periodontitis is an inflammatory lesion in the periodontal tissues that is caused mostly by bacterial elements derived from the infected root canal system of teeth (Core concept 7.1). In non-treated teeth apical periodontitis represents a defensive response to a primary infection in a necrotic pulp. Apical periodontitis may also develop due to a secondary infection subsequent to endodontic treatment procedures. Post-treatment apical periodontitis is most commonly due to either unsuccessful control of primary root canal infection by endodontic treatment measures, or infection or reinfection of the root canal system due to inadequate obturation and/or inadequate coronal seal that allowed bacterial leakage to take place. Inadvertent extrusion of certain medicaments and root filling materials into the periapical tissue compartment may also cause tissue toxic effects as well as precipitate foreign body reactions (Chapter 12). In this chapter the focus will be on apical periodontitis associated with non-endodontically treated teeth affected by root canal infection. It will be described in terms of biological function, pathogenesis and clinical as well as histological presentation.

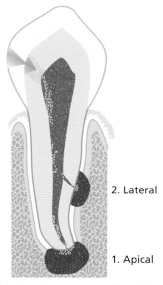

Fig. 7.1 Potential sites for emergence of endodontic lesions in the periodontium.

The nature of apical periodontitis

Apical periodontitis serves an important protective function, aimed at confining bacteria discharged from the root canal space and preventing them from spreading into adjacent bone marrow spaces and other remote sites. The process is unique in the sense that it cannot eradicate the source of infection. The reason is that once a pulp has become necrotic, defense mechanisms cannot operate far into the root canal owing to the lack of vascular support. Although these mechanisms can act at the apical margins of the necrotic tissue, they are unable to penetrate it in a fully developed tooth. Consequently, without proper endodontic treatment apical periodontitis may prevail chronically.

Bone resorption is a most conspicuous feature of apical periodontitis and is an unavoidable side-effect of the defensive process. Some may view it as a "price" paid by the host to provide the necessary, effective, immune response to the root canal infection. Bone loss that appears in radiographs serves as the main clinical indicator for

---

Core concept 7.1   Apical periodontitis

As indicated by the term "apical periodontitis", the lesion typically develops near the tips of roots, where the root canal communicates with the periodontium via the apical foramen. Inflammatory periodontal lesions of endodontic origin may also emerge at other anatomical or iatrogenic openings, which may be present in the lateral aspects of roots or in furcations of multirooted teeth (Fig. 7.1). In these instances the causative agents are released along lateral or accessory canals. This led to the more comprehensive term *periradicular* lesion. Since most portals of exit are in the apical portion of roots, and for the sake of convenience, the term *periapical* or *apical* lesion is used in this text to designate all inflammatory lesions of endodontic origin in the periodontium.

the presence of apical periodontitis (Fig. 7.2c), as many of these lesions are silent and prevail without overt clinical symptoms. Such lesions will be referred to in this text as *asymptomatic apical periodontitis*. Asymptomatic apical periodontitis is mostly biofilm derived (39). Yet, acute forms do occur and may develop during the expanding phase of the initial lesion. Lesions of *symptomatic apical periodontitis* may also emerge as a result of a disturbed equilibrium between the host defense and the bacterial infection in an already established lesion. Symptomatic apical periodontitis results mostly from the action of planktonic bacteria (11, 39). Hence, single lesions of apical periodontitis can be symptomatic or asymptomatic at different stages of their development and progression. By far, most cases of apical periodontitis are asymptomatic.

Pain, tenderness to biting pressure, percussion or palpation as well as swellings are typical clinical expressions of symptomatic apical periodontitis (Fig. 7.2a, b). The symptoms may vary from mild to severe. More dramatic clinical symptoms of apical periodontitis may appear and dominate when the local immune defense has failed to detain the infection resulting in an apical abscess. Although very rare, acute apical periodontitis may develop into a very serious and even life-threatening condition. Phlegmonous spread of the infection into the connective tissue around the upper respiratory tract, orbit, neck or even to the brain is alarming. Infectious elements released in conjunction with symptomatic apical periodontits may also be distributed via the blood stream and cause heart valve and myocardial infections (see Chapter 8). Even though apical periodontitis may be associated with such severe clinical manifestations, it needs to be stressed that its basic function is to contain root canal bacteria and not allow their dissimenation to distant sites (Core concept 7.2). Identification of apical periodontitis is directly related to the resolution of our examination tools; many apical periodontitis lesions that

> **Core concept 7.2   Nature of the periapical lesion**
>
> Apical periodontitis develops following pulp tissue breakdown and the emergence of root canal infection. It represents an important host defense response aiming to confine root canal bacteria and prevent them from spreading into adjacent bone marrow spaces and other remote sites. Single lesions of apical periodontitis may or may not present with clinical symptoms including pain, tenderness and swelling. Periapical bone resorption, although representing tissue destruction, occurs as part of the defensive process. When bacteria are eliminated by root canal treatment the active inflammatory lesion gradually subsides and bone regeneration usually takes place.

are not seen on conventional radiographs are identified on CBCT (cone beam computed tomography) and many more may be identified only upon histological examination.

On a microscopic level, different structural frameworks of apical periodontitis can be identified. These forms include *apical granuloma*, *apical abscess* and *apical cyst*. These lesions will be described here in terms of their general histological features while their clinical presentation will be detailed later in the chapter. Clinically and radiographically these histopathological entities cannot be distinguished from each other or recognized, with the exception of abscesses with a sinus tract.

Apical granuloma is the most common form of apical periodontitis and consists of an inflammatory lesion dominated by lymphocytes, macrophages and plasma cells (see also Key literature 7.1 and Advanced concept 7.1) (Fig. 7.3). Numerous fibroblasts and connective tissue fibers are usually present with abundant capillaries. At its periphery an encapsulation attempt may often be found but great structural heterogeneity is the norm for apical periodontitis (31, 34).

Epithelial cell proliferation is a common finding in longstanding apical granulomas and may occur in up to 50% of the lesions (31, 33, 34, 45). The epithelium is

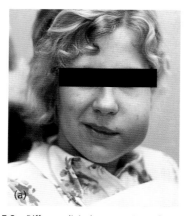
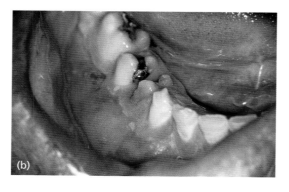
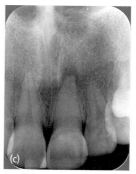

Fig. 7.2   Different clinical presentations of apical periodontitis due to an infected necrotic pulp: (a) extraoral swelling in the left cheek region; (b) intraoral vesitibular swelling associated with the severely broken down first premolar; (c) apically positioned radiolucent area (upper left incisor).

Key literature 7.1   Antigen presentation in apical periodontitis

Major histocompatibility complex class II (MHC II) molecule-expressing macrophages and dendritic cells were found by Kaneko *et al.* in experimentally induced periapical lesions in rats (19). The presence of HLA-DR+ cells, which are the human equivalent of the MHC II positive cells, was studied in human granulomas, in a dispersed-cell cytometric flow immunochemistry study (23). Activated macrophages (HLA-DR+, CD14+) and mature dendritic cells (HLA-DR+, CD83+) were found in great numbers. Thus, antigen presentation is possible and likely to occur within the apical granuloma.

Advanced concept 7.1   Dendritic cell function

Mature dendritic cells regulate the specific immune responses occurring during the initial phases of apical periodontitis. The activation phase includes cloning in regional lymph nodes of antigen specific lymphocytes (T-cells), which soon appear at the lesion site and later become a dominant cell type in the lesion. During the early active phase helper T-cells (CD4+) predominate over cytotoxic T-cells (CD8+), whereas in the more established chronic phase the situation becomes reversed (42, 43). This feature suggests that helper T-cells are active during the expansion of the inflammatory process. Thus, they are likely to be involved with the bone-resorptive process by activating macrophages to produce bone-resorptive mediators.

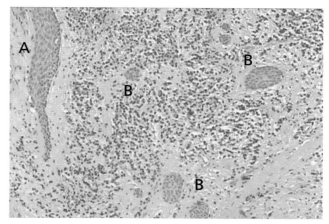

Fig. 7.4   Epithelial strands in a periapical granuloma. Epithelial cell masses, originating from the epithelial rests of Mallasez, proliferate in periapical granulomas and form strands. Some are cut longitudinally (A) and some perpendicular to the long axis of the strand (B).

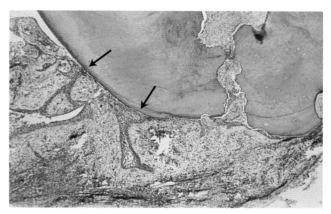

Fig. 7.5   Epithelial strands in a periapical granuloma that seem to attach to the root tip (arrows).

believed to originate from the epithelial cell rests of Mallasez. Under the influence of cytokines and growth factors released in the inflammatory process, the normally resting cells divide and migrate. They may form more or less continuous strands that seem to take a random course (Fig. 7.4). They may also become attached to the root surface (Fig. 7.5).

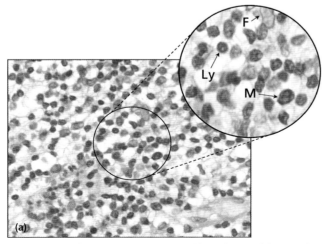
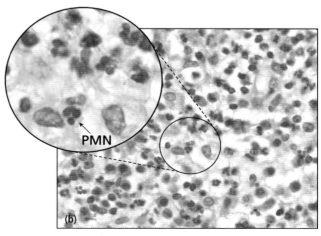

Fig. 7.3   Cells of the periapical granulomas: (a) lymphocytes (Ly), macrophages (M) and connective tissue fibroblasts (F) are the three main cells in the periapical granuloma. (b) Other cells like PMNs are also found but they are newcomers, not residents of the granuloma: each of them was recently recruited and will die in a few days.

Polymorphonuclear leukocytes (PMNs) are found in varying numbers. Often they appear close to the bacterial front. They may reach local dominance within a given area of the lesion and even form an abscess cavity. Thus, abscess formation can be a transient or persistent event within an existing apical granuloma.

Apical abscess denotes the presence of pus within the lesion. Abscess formation may reflect a shift in cellular dynamics within a pre-existing apical granuloma or be a direct outcome of an acute primary infection. The influx of PMNs is now dramatically increased. Upon the intense phagocytic activity of these cells and upon their death, tissue-destructive elements (e.g. hydrolytic enzymes and reactive oxygen species) are released to the extent that macrophages are no longer able to keep up with clearing and repairing the cell and tissue damage induced. Connective tissue constituents such as collagen and hyaluronic acid are degraded and the tissue in the center of the lesion is liquefied. In the periphery, granulomatous tissue may persist.

Consequently, a continuum exists between apical abscesses and apical granulomas. While in some cases apical granulomas may contain only small numbers of infiltrating PMNs, other cases present with a massive influx of PMNs, leading to tissue liquefaction and pus formation.

An *apical cyst* is an epithelium-lined cavity that contains fluid or semi-solid material and is commonly surrounded by dense connective tissue variably infiltrated by mononuclear leukocytes and PMNs (Figs 7.6 and 7.7). The cyst cavity is most commonly lined with stratified squamous epithelium of varying thickness that originates from the epithelial rest cells of Malassez. Rarely, the lining may be ciliary epithelium originating from the adjacent maxillary sinus. The epithelial lining may be continuous, but may also be disrupted or even completely missing in certain areas of the cavity. It should be noted that apical cysts may also become abscessed.

In contrast to periapical granulomas, some apical cysts appear never to arrive at a steady state. They may slowly expand over time and eventually, if left untreated, may consume a considerable portion of the surrounding bone (Fig. 7.8).

Apical cysts are divided into *pocket cysts* (*bay cyst*) and *true cysts* (29, 33, 34) (Fig. 7.9). A pocket cyst is an apical inflammatory cyst that contains a sac-like, epithelium-lined cavity that is open to and continuous with the root canal space. True apical cysts, on the other hand, are located within the periapical granuloma with no apparent connection between their cavity and that of the root canal space.

The mechanism by which cysts are formed, grow and expand is not well understood, but is most likely to involve inflammatory mediators that are present in the

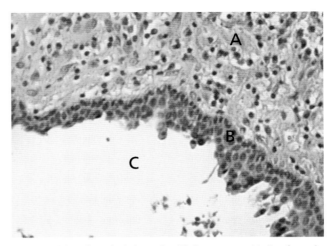

Fig. 7.6 Lining of a periapical cyst. Stratified squamous epithelium forms the lining of a periapical cyst which formed within a granuloma. A = granuloma; B = epithelial lining; C = cyst cavity.

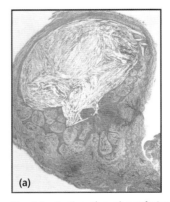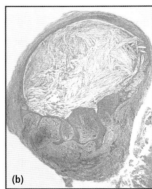

Fig. 7.7 Sections through a soft-tissue lesion encompassing an apical cyst. In this case, the cyst lumen was filled with cholesterol crystals. (From Ricucci and Bergenholtz (38). Reproduced with permission from Wiley-Blackwell.)

tissue lesion (13) (for cyst formation theories see also Advanced concept 7.2).

Given the presumed mechanisms of pathogenesis (Advanced concept 7.2), epithelial growth in some apical cysts ceases when the stimulating factors are eliminated, for example after proper endodontic treatment. Subsequently the epithelium lining may become thin and even disappear and thus provide conditions for healing.

In some cases both the cyst capsule and the cyst cavity may contain cholesterol, which forms oblong needle-like crystals (Fig. 7.7). In tissue sections the crystals are not seen but appear as typical tissue clefts resulting from the dissolution of the cholesterol during histological tissue processing. The crystals are formed in the connective tissue of the cyst capsule and are gradually moved towards and into the cyst cavity. They attract multinuclear giant cells of the foreign body type and, thus, elicit a foreign body response in the connective tissue (28). The

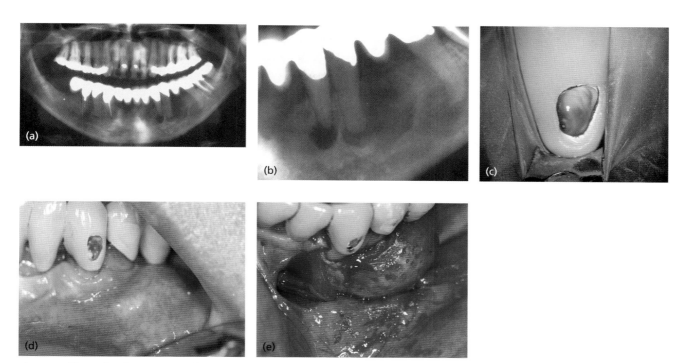

Fig. 7.8   Different clinical presentations of apical cysts. Radiographs in (a) and (b) demonstrate two radiolucent areas; one small associated with tooth 33 and one large with extension in a distal–coronal direction on tooth 34. Although the size and shape of a radiolucent lesion are not definitive criteria for cyst formation, there are other features suggestive of apical cyst. On opening tooth 33 for endodontic treatment, clear exudates drew off from the root canal (c). It was not possible to stop the exudation and this prevented completion of endodonic therapy. At the buccal and distal aspects of tooth 34 there was a distinct prominence that was hard and not tender to palpation (d). On raising a flap for enucleation of both processes, the expansive process is more clearly visible (e). Thin bone tissue limited the fluid-filled process at the surface. Histological examination of a tissue specimen confirmed the diagnosis.

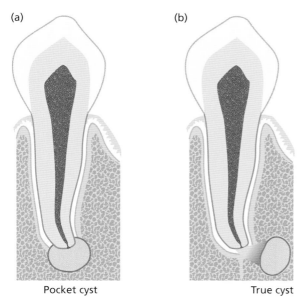

Fig. 7.9   Radicular cysts may appear in two configurations: a pocket cyst (a) where there is direct communication between the cyst cavity and the root canal space; and a true cyst (b) where no such pathway exists.

Advanced concept 7.2   Cyst formation mechanisms

The mechanism of cyst formation in periapical inflammatory lesions has been the subject of much debate (34, 45, 52). Two main theories were proposed. The "nutritional deficiency theory" assumes that epithelial proliferation results in an epithelial mass that is too large for nutrients to reach its core, resulting in necrosis and liquefaction of the cells in the center. PMNs are attracted by the necrotic material, which, together with tissue exudate, result in microcavities that eventually coalesce to form the cystic cavity (34). The "abscess theory" assumes that tissue liquefaction occurs first, at the central part of an abscess. The peripheral aspect of the cavity is later lined by proliferating epithelium, owing to the inherent nature of epithelial cells to cover exposed connective tissue surfaces.

The exact mechanism for the subsequent slow increase in the size of radicular cysts has not received an explanation. Some believe that increased osmotic pressure in the cyst's cavity is a key element (41). Increased osmosis leading to passage of fluid from the surrounding tissue into the cyst lumen is likely to occur owing to breakdown of epithelial and inflammatory cells. Furthermore, cyst expansion is also related to the release of bone-resorbing factors from mononuclear leukocytes present in the cyst wall, including interleukins, mast cell tryptase and prostaglandins (10, 13, 24, 53).

crystals are thought to derive from disintegrating red blood cells in stagnant vessels of the lesion. Inflammatory cells and circulating plasma lipids are other proposed sources (2).

Interactions with the infecting microbiota

Microbial infection is an absolute prerequisite for the emergence of apical periodontitis in a non-treated tooth (6, 46). Necrotic tissue alone in the pulpal space is unable to sustain inflammatory lesions in the periapical tissue environment. For example, following an ischemic injury by trauma, total pulp necrosis may develop without bacterial involvement (see Chapter 15); apical periodontitis will not be established unless the pulpal space is infected (6, 46). This may occur sooner or later as necrotic tissue, like anywhere in the body, serves as a growth medium ready for microbial colonization.

The course and the severity of the tissue response to root canal infection depend on the microbial load

(number of organisms and their pathogenic potential, see Chapter 6), the state of the defense potential of the host and time. Acute and severe forms may develop at initial stages when microorganisms have rapidly increased in numbers and overwhelmed the local immune defense. This scenario is related mostly to bacteria in their planktonic state, which allows fast growth of organisms. Certain pathogens seem prone to cause acute processes. Organisms belonging to the anaerobic segment of the microbiota, including genera of *Porphyromonas*, *Prevotella*, *Fusobacterium* and *Peptostreptococcus*, are more often associated with symptomatic and painful lesions of apical periodontitis than are other types of organisms (12, 46, 49).

Bacterial elimination

Bacterial elimination in periapical lesions is carried out by PMNs. All other constituents and processes in apical periodontitis may be viewed as *serving this ultimate goal* (Fig. 7.10). Local recruitment of PMNs from the capillaries,

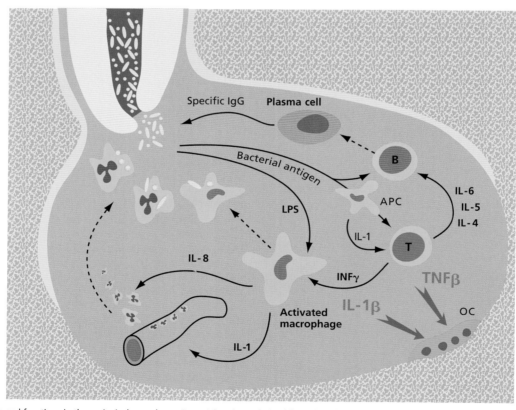

Fig. 7.10 Cells and functions in the periapical granuloma. Bacterial antigens derived from the infected root canal are taken by antigen presenting cells (APC), processed and presented to the T-lymphocytes (T). A dual signal of antigen presentation with IL-1 activates the T-lymphocytes. Cytokines produced by these activated cells include (a) IL-4, IL-5 and IL-6, which induce proliferation and maturation of a specific clone of B-lymphocytes (B) that were exposed to this specific antigen, to result in plasma cells producing IgG specific to this antigen; (b) INFγ which serves to activate macrophages which in turn will produce the IL-1 essential for local recruitment of circulating PMNs and IL-8 which activates these PMNs. Bacterial endotoxin (LPS), derived from Gram-negative bacteria, synergistically participates in the activation of macrophages. All the above is aimed to allow effective specific phagocytosis by the PMNs of any bacterium emerging from the apical foramen. Bone resorption is a side-effect of the above defensive process, mediated by TNFβ, produced by the activated T-lymphocytes and IL-1β, produced by the activated macrophages. Both activate osteoclastic bone resorption (OC).

by ICAM-1-mediated *margination*, depends on inter-leukin-1 (IL-1) and tumor necrosis factor alpha (TNFα) derived from activated macrophages. Specific immuno-globulins are essential for effective phagocytosis. Their local production requires antigen presentation followed by activation of specific T-lymphocytes to produce a set of cytokines that will allow proliferation of antigen-specific B-lymphocytes and their maturation into specific IgG-producing plasma cells, and interferon gamma (INFγ) activates macrophages to produce the IL-1 and TNFα required for the above tasks, as well as IL-8 which further activates the PMNs. All this elaborate network of cells and events serves one cause: bacterial elimination by PMNs (Fig. 7.10). See also Advanced concept 7.3.

The bacterial front line

Bacteria causing apical periodontitis will normally remain confined to the root canal space and rarely be able to survive and establish themselves in the apical lesion *per se*. In the process of pulpal breakdown, for example after carious exposure, bacteria will gradually gain terrain and move their front towards the apex, depending on how effective the host response is in limit-ing further bacterial colonization in the pulp tissue. In due course, however, the host tissue–bacterial front will be established in the vicinity of or at the exit of the apical foramen. In fact observations by Nair (28), following histological examination of teeth with severe caries, indicated that the exact position of the bacterial front is unpredictable. He found that the level could often be well inside the apical foramen, where PMNs were engaged in phagocytic activities and obviously prevented further dispersion of bacterial elements detached from the root canal biofilm. Yet, PMNs have a hard task deal-ing with those organisms that are already attached in a

biofilm structure. This means that there is a constant battle between the attempts of organisms to spread and the host defense to curb dissemination of detached bacteria.

Although bacteria are most often only transient visi-tors which are readily killed, they may nevertheless find their way into the lesion tissue and establish themselves in the lesion more or less permanently (Fig. 7.11). The term *extraradicular infection* has been introduced in this context. Two types of such infections can be discerned:

1. *Bacteria in chronic abscesses, with a persistent sinus tract.* Viable bacteria can usually be isolated from the exudate in these cases. The source may be bacteria that emerged from the root canal space which the PMNs failed to kill. This may be attributed to various phagocytosis-evading mechanisms held by these bacteria. Such bacterial presence will cease in most cases after adequate endodontic treatment (see below).
2. *Bacterial cluster formation in the lesion tissue per se.* Some strains of *Actinomyces israeli* and *Propionibacterium propionicum* have an inherent ability to grow in clumps and thereby prevail in the soft-tissue lesion of apical periodontitis (39). Such aggregations may become too large for phagocytosis. Because the bacte-rial cells are out of reach for phagocytosis a chronic infection may ensue that cannot be managed by con-ventional endodontic treatment.

Evidence has also accumulated to indicate that other bacteria may aggregate and survive outside the root canal space (Advanced concept 7.4).

Another form of bacterial aggregate may sometimes be found on the external root tip surface with a biofilm structure (36, 37, 54) (Fig. 7.12). The frequency at which such bacterial biofilms occur is not well established, but they have been described in several case reports.

Advanced concept 7.3 Complement functions in apical periodontitis

The complement system has a crucial role in recruitment of PMNs to the lesion site. Complement activation may occur either through bacterial antigens reacting with specific IgG or IgM (the classical pathway) or directly by bacterial cell wall constituents such as LPS (the properidine pathway). It results in formation of C3a and C5a that cause mast cell degranulation thus releasing vasoactive amines that cause local vasodilation and increased vascular permeability. C5a serves also as a chemotactic factor, which directs the migration of PMNs. The opsonin C3b is another essential complement activation product, which binds to the surface of bacteria to allow effective phagocytosis by PMNs via their C3b receptor. Thus, complement activation is essential for bacterial elimination by the PMNs. It also has a major role in causing edema, a key mechanism in endodontic flare-ups.

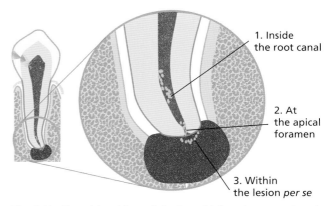

Fig. 7.11 Potential positions of the bacterial front in a necrotic pulp: (1) inside the root canal at a small distance from the apical foramen; (2) at the apical foramen; (3) within the lesion *per se*.

Advanced concept 7.4   Evading phagocytosis by bacterial coaggregation

Certain bacteria, such as *Actinomyces israeli* and *Propniobacterium proprionicum*, may survive and grow in the periapical tissue as aggregates that can escape phagocytosis by PMNs. Other bacteria may gain a similar benefit from coaggregation between cells of different species, mediated by cell surface adhesins. *Fusobacterium nucleatum* and certain strains of *Porphyromonas gingivalis* coaggregate through surface adhesins on the former (*F. nucleatum*) that recognize galactose residues on the latter (*P. gingivalis*) (26, 57). The same adhesin also allows adhesion of *F. nucleatum* to host cells that express galactose residues (57). This may in turn mediate attachment of bacterial coaggregates to host cells in the periapical lesion, thus facilitating colonization and extraradicular persistence of bacteria.

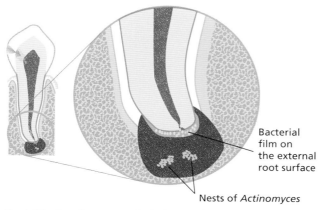

Bacterial film on the external root surface

Nests of *Actinomyces*

Fig. 7.12 Bacteria may occur in the lesion either as a film on the external root surface or as nests, as in this example.

Bacterial clusters within the tissue as well as bacterial biofilms on the external root structure may persist after conventional endodontic treatment even though the root canal infection has been eliminated. Both types of infection, thus, represent a true *extraradicular infection*.

The formation of the lesion

Bone resorption is the hallmark of apical periodontitis. It has been, traditionally, presented as a deliberate removal of the bone from the source of infection to form a "buffer zone" but should rather be viewed as a negative, unavoidable, side-effect of the battle between the immune response and the infection in the root canal.

The process of bone resorption is carried out by osteoclasts. The recruitment and activation of these cells are mediated by a variety of potential mediator molecules. Among these the cytokines IL-1β and TNFβ are the two most important and are produced by activated macrophages (IL-1β) and T-lymphocytes (TNFβ) (see Key literature 7.2, 7.3 and Advanced concept 7.5). These cells are activated in the periapical tissue in order to enable an

Key literature 7.2   Bone resorption in apical periodontitis

Many molecules that may cause bone resorption in organ culture *in vitro* were also found in periapical lesions. It was *postulated* that they were involved in the process of bone resorption, allowing development and maintenance of the lesions. It was not until the critical study by Wang and Stashenko (56) that the agents *actually responsible* for bone resorption in human periapical lesions were identified from the large number of those that *could potentially* be involved in the process. Extracts from surgically removed human periapical lesions were processed by gel chromatography and fractions with bone resorbing activity were subjected to the neutralizing effect of antibodies specific to the various inflammatory cytokines. It was concluded that the two agents responsible for most of the bone resorbing activity found in these extracts were IL-1β and TNFβ (56). The first is mainly produced by activated macrophages; the second by activated T-lymphocytes.

Key literature 7.3   Are T-cells essential for formation of periapical lesions?

For a long time activated T-lymphocytes were considered the key cells responsible for the formation of periapical inflammatory lesions. Studies by Tani-Ishii *et al.* (50) and Wallstrom *et al.* (55) were concomitantly carried out with the aim of confirming this point. In both studies athymic animals, which lack T-lymphocytes, were used. Contrary to previous assumptions, both studies observed that experimental periapical lesions developed *at the same rate* in both groups of animals, i.e. in those lacking T-lymphocytes as well as in normal animals. This finding served as a turning point for the understanding of the central role of activated macrophages in the process (25, 27). In the athymic animals macrophages were probably activated directly by bacterial endotoxin (LPS) with *no vital role* for the T-lymphocyte-derived interferon-γ (INFγ); until then INFγ was considered to be essential to the formation of the lesion (42).

Advanced concept 7.5   Helper T-cell functions in apical periodontitis

T helper (CD4+) lymphocytes may be divided according to their cytokine expression pattern and classified as either T helper-1 (Th1) cells that produce and secrete IL-2 and interferon-γ (INFγ) or Th2 cells that produce and secrete IL-4, IL-5, IL-6, IL-10 and IL-13. Th1 type cytokines augment cytotoxic T-cell functions and stimulate proinflammatory cytokine production in other cells, such as macrophages, while Th2-type cytokines participate in B-cell stimulation, to mount a humoral immune response, and in downregulation of inflammatory reactions (14, 35).

effective protective immune response (see Core concept 7.2 and Advanced concept 7.6). Cyclooxygenase products, such as PGE₂, also contribute to the process of periapical bone resorption (43, 56).

Advanced concept 7.6   Regulation of local bone resorption.

IL-1β, produced by activated macrophages, and TNFβ, produced by activated T-lymphocytes, are responsible for the local bone resorption in apical periodontitis. Nevertheless, osteoclasts do not have receptors for these cytokines and require other cells to trigger them. IL-1β and TNFβ engage receptors on osteoblasts and bone stromal cells, thus triggering these cells to express the surface ligand *osteoprotegerin ligand* (OPGL, RANK ligand) (21, 44, 51) (Fig. 7.13). OPGL-receptors (*receptor activator of nuclear factor κB*, RANK) are found on preosteoclasts and on osteoclasts. Engagement of the receptors on nearby preosteoclasts activates these cells to become multinucleated osteoclasts. Similar engagement of the receptors on existing osteoclasts activates them to express an active ruffled border and resorb bone. Both OPGL (RANK ligand) and its receptor on the preosteoclasts and osteoclasts (RANK) are *cell-bound molecules*. Thus, proximity of the cells expressing OPGL and those carrying its receptor is essential for this process to take place (51). This activation process is downregulated by a soluble mediator, osteoprotegerin (OPG), which competitively inhibits osteoclast activation by binding to the OPGL, thus blocking it and preventing the engagement of the receptors on the osteoclasts and preosteoclasts (51). This process explains how osteoclasts, which do not have IL-1β- or TNFβ-receptors, are *locally* activated by these cytokines.

In the early phases of apical periodontitis, osteoclasts are abundant and outperform bone-forming osteoblasts. Consequently the net result is loss of bone tissue within a limited area near the exit of main apical foramina and/or accessory canals. For the lesion to be visible radiographically, a certain amount of bone must be removed. Therefore early developing lesions are not detectable in radiographs.

Along with the process of bone resorption some apical parts of the root may be lost as well. However, root resorption will be much less pronounced, and is often visible only in microscopic sections and seldom in radiographs. Yet, root tips may sometimes be shortened and the apical end of the root canal widened to the extent that the original configuration of the apical foramen anatomy is altered (Fig. 7.14) (38).

The equilibrium between bacteria and the host

Apical granuloma and apical abscesses represent two distinct types of equilibrium established between the bacterial attack and the host defense. A major difference between these two conditions is in the extent of PMN influx to the area.

In the apical granuloma bacteria that occasionally emerge through the apical foramen are readily phagocytosed and eliminated (Core concept 7.2). PMNs recruited to the lesion site play a central role here and form the first line of defense. Following leaving the vasculature they are relatively short-lived and, once engaged in phagocytosis and bacterial killing, PMNs will spontaneously die within a short period of time. The disintegrated PMNs and the remaining dead bacteria will be taken up by an abundance of macrophages. Histological sections of such lesions will show mainly the long-lived cells such as macrophages and lymphocytes. PMNs will be seen only in small numbers within established periapical granulomas, either at the apical foramen or on their way from adjacent blood vessels to where bacteria are found.

As already stated, an apical granuloma may occasionally develop either into an acute apical abscess or into a chronic abscess that maintains a suppurating sinus tract. This event is most likely induced by a shift in the bacteria–host equilibrium. The shift may be quantitative, qualitative, or both. If the amount of bacteria introduced into the lesion suddenly increases, the amount of

Stimulation of osteoblasts/stromal cells

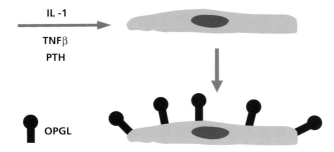

Osteoclast activation

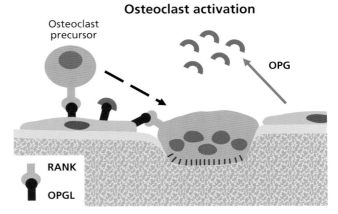

Fig. 7.13 Osteoclast activation by RANK. When exposed to bone-resorbing cytokines, osteoblasts and stromal cells express RANK on their surfaces. Engagement of OPGL (RANK ligand) on the surface of osteoclasts with RANK activates them to express ruffled border and resorb bone. Mononuclear preosteoclasts are similarly activated to develop into mature multinucleated osteoclasts. The process is downregulated by a soluble mediator OPG which competitively inhibits the above activation.

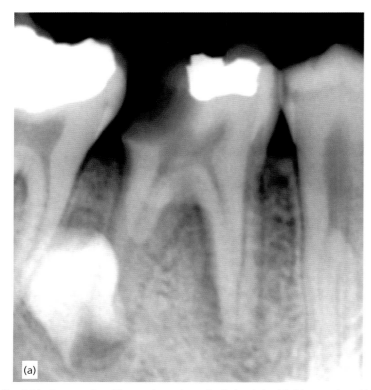
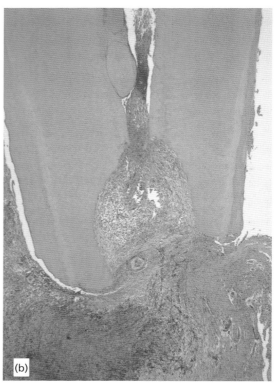

Fig. 7.14 Lower molar with extensive caries and apical periodontitis (a) presenting with a large area of root resorption inside the most apical portion of the mesial root (b). (From Ricucci and Bergenholtz (38). Reproduced with permission from Wiley-Blackwell.)

complement-derived chemotactic factors will increase, followed by an increased number of PMNs reaching the area per given time period as well as increased vascular permeability and fluid extravasation. As this response can be associated with pain and swelling it is known as an endodontic flare-up (see further bellow). In cases when the increased amount of bacteria is transient, host defense will gradually clean the area and the lesion will return to one that contains mainly mononuclear leukocytes, i.e. macrophages and lymphocytes.

The shift in the bacteria–host equilibrium may also be of a qualitative nature. Some bacterial organisms have developed mechanisms that allow them to circumvent killing by PMNs. Some strains of *Porphyromonas gingivalis*, isolated from suppurative apical periodontitis, for example, have developed an antiphagocytic capsule allowing each individual bacterial cell to evade phagocytosis (48).

Other *P. gingivalis* strains contain a specific enzyme that cleaves IgG at the hinge region, thus removing the Fc portion of the immunoglobulin and leaving the bacterial cell coated with host-derived Fab fragments (18). Other strains have a survival strategy based on the capacity to cleave the complement C3 molecules in the area, thus offsetting essential components of the host response. This in turn may allow them, as well as other bacterial by-standers, to colonize the site (47). Another strategy is the ability to cleave cell-bound C3b molecules

faster than they attach to the bacterial cell walls (8). Consequently, all this will cause a frustrated host response, which will continue to pour PMNs into the area with no ability to eradicate the infectious elements. The PMN influx will be large and continuous, well beyond the cleaning capacity of the macrophages. Continuous formation of liquefied tissue (pus) will result in a chronic abscess with a suppurating sinus tract.

Clump formation by *Actinomyces israeli* and *Propionibacterium propionicum*, as discussed above, represents another strategy of evading phagocytosis. A similar strategy has been adopted by bacterial strain combinations that *coaggregate* to form mixed bacterial clumps (26, 57) or grow as a biofilm on the outer surface of the apical area of the root (36, 37, 54). Bacteria in all these structures are protected from the phagocytes, thus resulting in a chronic abscess.

The endodontic flare-up

A flare-up represents a shift from or disruption of an established balance between bacteria and the host and is induced when bacteria are suddenly dispersed into the lesion. Exacerbation is another term used, which implies worsening of a clinical condition from a silent, asymptomatic process to one presenting with overt clinical symptoms, i.e. pain, tenderness and swelling.

An endodontic flare-up may have a variety of causes. It may occur spontaneously without any obvious cause and is likely to be explained by an ecological change within the root canal microbiota favoring growth and dispersion of especially aggressive endodontic pathogens. Exacerbation may also be iatrogenic in nature (iatrogenic = a condition caused by the practitioner). Such a condition is not uncommon in conjunction with endodontic treatment of infected root canals whereupon canal content may be inadvertently moved into the lesion site. The risk is particularly high following piercing and passing through the apical foramen with an endodontic instrument or when a piston-like movement of a larger endodontic instrument pushes some of the root canal content into the lesion. While the mechanical trauma is inconsequential *per se*, the immediate immune reaction to the bacterial antigens may result in a flare-up.

An exacerbation may also be explained by an increased flow of nutrients into the root canal space following mechanical opening and widening of the apical foramen. Release of blood or inflammatory exudates into the root canal may thus break the harsh nutritional conditions that normally existed in the infected root canal and favor enhanced growth of those proteolytic bacteria that may have escaped killing by the endodontic treatment procedure.

The symptoms associated with an endodontic flare-up are a function of edema formation in the periapical area, resulting from local activation of the complement system. As bacterial antigens are introduced in the periapical tissue, specific immunoglobulins present against these bacteria will immediately engage the antigen and form immune complexes that activate the complement system. C3a and C5a formation will cause mast cell degranulation which will induce local vasodilation and increased vascular permeability resulting in edema (see also Key literature 7.4). Since the tissue is encased in a solid structure, the only direction a swelling can take is pushing the tooth occlusally, as far as the periodontal ligament will allow. The effect is a tooth which is extremely sensitive to occlusal load and percussion. Viable bacteria carried into the periapical tissue may also start multiplying in the lesion *per se*, to an extent that an acute apical abscess and/or facial cellulitis may be initiated (see below).

Clinical manifestations and diagnostic terminology

Diagnostic terminology discussed here includes *normal periapical conditions, asymptomatic apical periodontitis* (syn.; chronic apical/periradicular periodontitis), *symptomatic apical periodontitis* (syn.: acute apical/periradicular periodontitis), *acute apical abscess* (syn.: acute periradicular

Key literature 7.4   Specificity of immunoglobulins to root canal bacteria

The presence of immunoglobulins in apical periodontitis may be random and does not necessarily mean that they are specific for the bacteria present in the necrotic pulp. Baumgartner and Falkler (3) and Kettering *et al.* (20) have tested immunoglobulins from human apical granulomas for reactivity against a large number of oral bacteria, using a modified enzyme-linked immunosorbent assay (ELISA). They demonstrated that the immunoglobulins found in apical periodontitis are specific for the bacteria commonly residing in the apical part of necrotic root canals. Baumgartner and Falkler extended these findings further and demonstrated that local production of IgG takes place in human periapical tissues (4,5).

abscess), *chronic apical abscess* (syn.: chronic periradicular abscess, suppurative apical/periradicular periodontitis), *cellulitis, condensing osteitis* (syn.: focal sclerosing osteomyelitis, periradicular osteosclerosis, sclerosing osteitis, sclerotic bone). It needs be recognized that these entities reflect clinical conditions and may not directly define the histopathological character of the lesion. Indeed there is a rather *limited* potential, under clinical conditions, to tell a granuloma from a cyst or even from an abscess. This applies in particular to asymptomatic lesions including abscesses with no evident sinus tract (see also Chapter 14).

Normal periapical conditions

Recognition of "normality" is essential to estimate changes that may occur with disease, as well as their gradual disappearance with healing (1). It is therefore necessary to recognize what is a normal healthy condition. A healthy tooth is comfortable to the patient, it is not tender to percussion or occlusal pressure neither is it sensitive to palpation of the mucosa overlying the periapical region. There should furthermore be no sinus tract, or swelling or complaint of painful symptoms. Pocket-probing should not be deep: while indicating periodontal disease, pocketing may also imply a sinus tract from a chronic periapical abscess draining along the periodontal ligament space. Normal periapical conditions are also recognized in periapical radiographs by unbroken lamina dura and a distinct periodontal ligament space of normal width, comparable to adjacent and contralateral teeth.

Asymptomatic apical periodontitis

Asymptomatic apical periodontitis is a longstanding periapical inflammatory process with radiographically visible periapical bone resorption but with no clinical signs and symptoms. The designation of this diagnostic term should only be done in association with a tooth with a non-vital pulp (untreated or treated). It needs be recognized that progressive pulpitis, e.g. in response to a carious exposure, can also manifest itself radiographically by loss of lamina dura, and a small periapical radiolucent area. Such a periapical tissue response may emerge before major breakdown of the pulp tissue.

The development of asymptomatic apical periodontitis may go unnoticed by the patient and is often discovered only by routine radiographic examination. It may also be surmised from a carefully taken disease history in cases when patient has experienced a prior painful event.

The radiological appearance may take a wide range of forms. This has tempted clinicians to search for a correlation between size and morphology of the lesion with its histological nature, but there are no diagnostic means currently available to distinguish a granuloma from a cyst.

Symptomatic apical periodontitis

Symptomatic apical periodontitis may develop as a direct consequence of the breakdown and infection of the pulp within a previously healthy periapical region. It then reflects a response to an initial exposure of the periapical periodontium to bacteria or their products emerging from the infected root canal.

Symptomatic apical periodontitis may also appear in a tooth with previous asymptomatic apical periodontitis. This may either reflect a natural shift in the balance previously established between the bacteria and the host or occur in response to endodontic treatment (endodontic flare-up).

The typical symptoms include pain of an aching nature that may become severe or even unbearable to the patient and which brings the patient to the dentist. The tooth will usually be tender to percussion, with the mucosa and bone overlying the apical area sensitive to palpation. The tooth may occlude prematurely, owing to occlusal displacement caused by the edema in the periapical area.

Acute apical abscess

An acute apical abscess is characterized by rapid onset, spontaneous pain, tenderness of the tooth to pressure, pus formation and eventual swelling of associated tissues. At the initial stages of its formation, the process may be extremely painful, as pressure builds up in the restricted periapical bony crypt or periodontal space. The overlying cortical plate may eventually perforate and pus will accumulate under the periosteum producing a most severe painful condition. Only with the perforation of the periosteum will the pus be able to drain and allow pain to subside. At this stage, a tender local swelling will appear. In some cases, natural drainage will be established within a few days by perforation of the covering tissue. In other cases, the swelling will remain for some time before it gradually subsides.

Drainage of an apical abscess will take the "path of least resistance" which is usually defined by the thickness of overlying bone (Fig. 7.15). Following penetration of the bone and periosteum, drainage will often be visible in the oral cavity but it may also occur into perioral tissues or into the maxillary sinus.

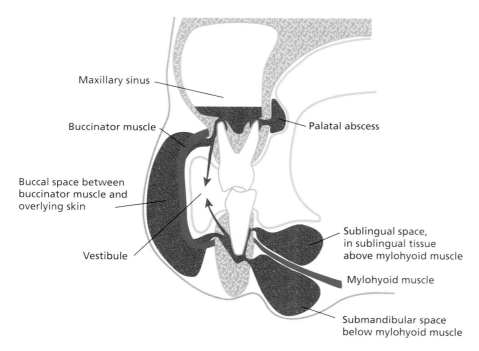

Maxillary sinus

Buccinator muscle

Buccal space between buccinator muscle and overlying skin

Vestibule

Palatal abscess

Sublingual space, in sublingual tissue above mylohyoid muscle

Mylohyoid muscle

Submandibular space below mylohyoid muscle

Fig. 7.15 Common pathways of an apical abscess. The route depends on the location of the roots in relation to the surrounding anatomical structures: (1) sublingual space, in the sublingual tissue above the mylohyoid muscle; (2) submandibular space below the mylohyoid muscle; (3) palatal abscess; (4) buccal space between buccinator muscle and overlying skin; (5) maxillary sinus; (6) vestibule.

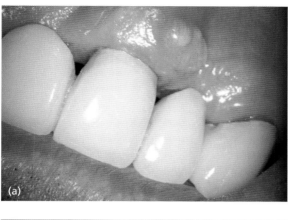
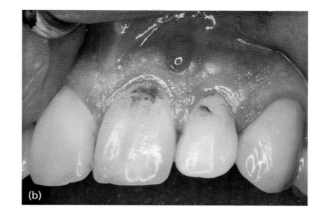
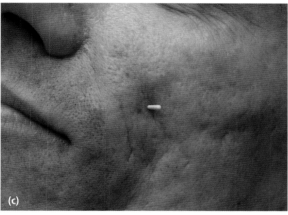
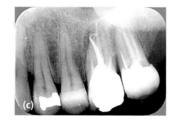

Fig. 7.16 Clinical photographs demonstrating different presentation of fistulous tracts. (a, b) Typical intraoral fistulations. (c) Extraoral fistulation to which a gutta-percha cone has been inserted in order to trace its origin. (d) Radiograph showing gutta-percha cone pointing to the tip of the mesiobuccal root of the first molar, where there is a radiolucent zone.

Chronic apical abscess

A sinus tract is the typical feature of the chronic apical abscess. The inflammatory process has perforated one of the cortical plates and a draining sinus tract is established which allows continuous discharge of pus forming in the periapical lesion through an opening in the oral mucosa. In rare cases, a sinus tract may drain extraorally through the skin (Fig. 7.16). Typically, a stoma of a parulis can be detected that, from time to time, will discard pus. A sinus tract may establish exit with drainage into the gingival sulcus, in a periodontal pocket (Fig. 7.17) or in a furcation area and must be differentiated from periodontal disease and from a pocket associated with a vertical root fracture. A sinus tract may also lead into the maxillary sinus and cause unilateral chronic sinusitis.

A chronic apical abscess is most commonly, but not always, associated with an apical radiolucency. It is asymptomatic or only slightly symptomatic and the patient may often be unaware of its presence. This may last as long as the sinus tract is not obstructed. Even when such an obstruction occurs, it is most likely that any swelling will be of limited duration and will be limited to the local area of the sinus tract, as both the bone and the periosteum are already perforated.

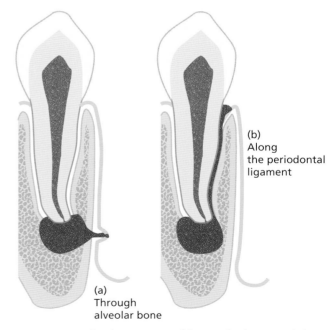

(b)
Along
the periodontal
ligament

(a)
Through
alveolar bone

Fig. 7.17 Examples of various routes of draining of a chronic apical abscess to the oral environment: (a) through the alveolar bone; (b) along the periodontal ligament.

Cellulitis

Cellulitis is a symptomatic edematous inflammation associated with diffuse spreading of invasive microorganisms through connective tissue and fascial planes. Its main clinical feature is diffuse swelling of facial or cervical tissues. Cellulitis is usually a sequela of an apical abscess that penetrated the bone, allowing the spread of pus along paths of least resistance, between facial structures. This usually implies the fascial planes between the muscles of the face or neck. Spreading of an infection may or may not be associated with systemic symptoms such as fever and malaise. Since cellulitis is usually a sequela of an uncontrolled apical abscess, other clinical features typical of an apical abscess are also expected. Spreading of an infection into adjacent and more remote connective tissue compartments may, rarely, result in serious or even life-threatening complications. Cases of Ludwig's angina (17), orbital cellulitis (7), cavernous sinus thrombosis (9) and even death from a brain abscess (16, 22) originating from a spreading dental infection have been reported.

Condensing osteitis

Condensing osteitis is a diffuse radiopaque lesion believed to represent a localized bone reaction to a low-grade inflammatory stimulus, usually seen at an apex of a tooth (or its extraction site) in which there has been a longstanding pulp disease. It is characterized by over-production of bone in the periapical area, mostly around the apices of mandibular molars and premolars that had longstanding chronic pulpitis. The pulp of the involved tooth may be vital and chronically inflamed or may have become necrotic with time, leaving the radiopaque sequella. Normally the condition does not prompt treatment *per se*, unless the pulp undergoes further breakdown leading to necrosis. The radiopacity may or may not disappear after endodontic treatment or tooth extraction (15) (see also Chapter 14).

References

1. Abbott PV. Classification, diagnosis and clinical manifestation of apical periodontitis. *Endod. Topics* 2004; 8: 36–54.
2. Arwill T, Heyden G. Histochemical studies on cholesterol formation in odontogenic cysts and granulomas. *Scand. J. Dent. Res.* 1973; 81: 406–10.
3. Baumgartner JC, Falkler WA Jr. Reactivity of IgG from explant cultures of periapical lesions with implicated microorganisms. *J. Endod.* 1991; 17: 207–12.
4. Baumgartner JC, Falkler WA Jr. Biosynthesis of IgG in periapical lesion explant cultures. *J. Endod.* 1991; 17: 143–6.
5. Baumgartner JC, Falkler WA Jr. Detection of immunoglobulins from explant cultures of periapical lesions. *J. Endod.* 1991; 17: 105–10.
6. Bergenholtz G. Microorganisms from necrotic pulp in traumatized teeth. *Odontol. Revy.* 1974; 25: 347–58.
7. Bullock JD, Fleishman JA. The spread of odontogenic infections to the orbit: diagnosis and management. *J. Oral Maxill. Surg.* 1985; 43: 749–55.
8. Cutler CW, Arnold RR, Schenkein HA. Inhibition of C3 and IgG proteolysis enhances phagocytosis of *Porphyromonas gingivalis*. *J. Immunol.* 1993; 151: 7016–29.
9. Fielding AF, Cross S, Matise JL, Mohnac AM. Cavernous sinus thrombosis: report of case. *J. Am. Dent. Assoc.* 1983; 106: 342–5.
10. Formigli L, Orlandini SZ, Tonelli P, Giannelli M, Martini M, Brandi ML, *et al.* Osteolytic processes in human radicular cysts: morphological and biochemical results. *J. Oral Pathol. Med.* 1995; 24: 216–20.
11. Furukawa S, Kuchma SL, O'Toole GA. Keeping their options open: acute versus persistent infections. *J. Bacteriol.* 2006; 188: 1211–17.
12. Gomes BPFA, Drucker DB, Lilly JD. Association of specific bacteria with some endodontic signs and symptoms. *Int. Endod. J.* 1994; 27: 291–8.
13. Harris M, Jenkins MV, Bennett A, Wills MR. Prostaglandin production and bone resorption by dental cysts. *Nature* 1973; 245: 213–15.
14. Harris DP, Goodrich S, Mohrs K, Mohrs M, Lund FE. Cutting edge: the development of IL-4-producing B cells (B effector 2 cells) is controlled by IL-4, IL-4 receptor alpha, and Th2 cells. *J. Immunol.* 2005; 175: 7103–7.
15. Hedin M, Polhagen L. Follow-up study of periradicular bone condensation. *Scand. J. Dent. Res.* 1971; 79: 436–40.
16. Henig EF, Derschowitz T, Shalit M, Toledo E, Tikva P, Aviv T. Brain abcess following dental infection. *Oral Surg. Oral Med. Oral Pathol. Oral Radiol. Endod.* 1978; 45: 955–8.
17. Hought RT, Fitzgerald BE, Latta JE, Zallen RD. Ludwig's angina: report of two cases and review of the literature from 1945 to January 1979. *J. Oral Surg.* 1980; 38: 849–55.
18. Jansen HJ, van-der Hoeven JS, van-den Kkiboom CWA, Goertz JH, Camp PJ, Bakkeren JA. Degradation of immunoglobulin G by periodontal bacteria. *Oral Microbiol. Immunol.* 1994; 9: 345–51.
19. Kaneko T, Okiji T, Kan L, Takagi M, Suda H. Ultrastructural analysis of MHC class II molecule-expressing cells in experimentally induced periapical lesions in the rat. *J. Endod.* 2001; 27: 337–42.
20. Kettering JD, Torabinejad M, Jones SL. Specificity of antibodies present in human periapical lesions. *J. Endod.* 1991; 17: 213–16.
21. Lacey DL, Timms E, Tan HL, Kelley MJ, Dunstan CR, Burgess T. Osteoprotegerin ligand is a cytokine that regulates osteoclast differentiation and activation. *Cell* 1998; 93: 165–76.
22. Li X, Tronstad L, Olsen I. Brain abscess caused by oral infection. *Endod. Dent. Traumatol.* 1999; 15: 95–101.
    Review paper analyzing potential pathways by which root canal infection can initiate brain abscess.
23. Lukic A, Vasilijic S, Majstorovic I, Vucevic D, Mojsilovic S, Gazivoda D, *et al.* Characterization of antigen-presenting cells in human apical periodontitis lesions by flow cytometry and immunocytochemistry. *Int. Endod. J.* 2006; 39: 626–36.

24. Meghji S, Harvey W, Harris M. Interleukin 1-like activity in cystic lesions of the jaw. *Br. J. Oral Maxillofac. Surg.* 1989; 27: 1–11.

25. Metzger Z. Macrophages in periapical lesions. *Endod. Dent. Traumatol.* 2000; 16: 1–8.

26. Metzger Z, Featherstone L, Ambrose W, Trope M, Arnold RR. Kinetics of coaggregation of *Porphyromonas gingivalis* HG405 with *Fusobacterium nucleatum* PK1594. A study with a novel V-max automated kinetic coaggregation assay. *Oral Microbiol. Immunol.* 2001; 16: 163–9.

27. Metzger Z, Abramovitz I. Periapical lesions of endodontic origin. In: *Ingle's Endodontics*, 6th edn (Ingle JI, Bakland LK, Baumgartner JC, eds). Hamilton, Ontario: BC Decker, 2008; 494–519.

28. Nair PNR. Light and electron microscopic studies of root canal flora and periapical lesions. *J. Endod.* 1987; 13: 29–39.
    Classic paper describing patterns of bacterial colonization in teeth with infected pulp necrosis and the microscopic features of the associated periapical inflammatory lesions.

29. Nair PNR, Sjögren U, Schumacher E, Sundqvist G. Radicular cyst affecting a root-filled human tooth: a long-term post-treatment follow-up. *Int. Endod. J.* 1993; 26: 225–33.

30. Nair PNR, Pajarola G, Schroeder HE. Types and incidence of human periapical lesions obtained with extracted teeth. *Oral Surg. Oral Med. Oral Pathol. Oral Radiol. Endod.* 1996; 81: 93–102.

31. Nair PNR. Apical periodontitis: a dynamic encounter between root canal infection and host response. *Periodontol. 2000* 1997; 13: 121–48.

32. Nair PNR, Henry S, Cano V, Vera J. Microbial status of apical root canal system of human mandibular first molars with primary apical periodontitis after "one visit" endodontic treatment. *Oral Surg. Oral Med. Oral Pathol. Oral Radiol. Endod.* 2005; 99: 231–52.

33. Nair PNR. On the causes of persistent apical periodontitis: a review. *Int. Endod. J.* 2006; 39: 249–81.

34. Nair PNR. Pathobiology of primary apical periodontitis. In: *Pathways of the Pulp*, 9th edn (Cohen S, Hargreaves KM, eds). Philadelphia: Elsevier, 2006; 541–79.

35. Naldini A, Morena E, Filippi I, Pucci A, Bucci M, Cirino G, Carraro F. Thrombin inhibits IFN-gamma production in human peripheral blood mononuclear cells by promoting a Th2 profile. *J. Interfer. Cytok. Res.* 2006; 26: 793–9.

36. Noguchi N, Noiri Y, Narimatsu M, Ebisu S. Identification and localization of extraradicular biofilm-forming bacteria associated with refractory endodontic pathogens. *Appl. Environ. Microbiol.* 2005; 71: 8738–43.

37. Noiri Y, Ehara A, Kawahara T, Takemura N, Ebisu S. Participation of bacterial biofilms in refractory and chronic apical periodontitis. *J. Endod.* 2002; 28: 679–83.

38. Ricucci D, Bergenholtz G. Histologic features of apical periodontitis in human biopsies. *Endod. Topics* 2004; 8: 68–87.

39. Siqueria JF. Periapical actinomycosis and infection with *Propionobacterium propionicum*. *Endod. Topics* 2003; 6: 78–95.

40. Siquerira JF, Rocas IN. Bacterial pathogenesis and mediators in apical periodontitis. *Braz. Dent. J.* 2007; 18: 267–80.

41. Skaug N. Soluble proteins in fluid from non-keratinizing jaw cysts in man. *Int. J. Oral Surg.* 1977; 6: 107–21.

42. Stashenko P, Yu SM. T helper and T suppressor cell reversal during the development of induced rat periapical lesions. *J. Dent. Res.* 1989; 68: 830–4.

43. Stashenko P, Teles R, D'Souza R. Periapical inflammatory responses and their modulation. *Crit. Rev. Oral Biol. Med.* 1998; 9: 498–521.
    The nature of the periapical inflammatory response to root canal infection and the immunopathological mechanisms involved by which it is controlled are the focus of this review article.

44. Suda T, Takahashi N, Udagawa N, Jimi E, Gillespie MT, Martin TJ. Modulation of osteoclast differentiation and function by the new members of the tumor necrosis factor receptor and ligand families. *Endocr. Rev.* 1999; 20: 345–57.

45. Summers L. The incidence of epithelium in periapical granulomas and the mechanism of cavitation in apical dental cysts in man. *Arch. Oral Biol.* 1974; 19: 1177–80.

46. Sundqvist G. *Bacteriological studies of necrotic dental pulps.* Thesis, Umeå University, 1976.

47. Sundqvist G, Carlsson J, Herrmann B, Tärnvik A. Degradation of human immunoglobulins G and M and complement factors C3 and C5 by black-pigmented *Bacteroides*. *J. Med. Microbiol.* 1985; 19: 85–94.

48. Sundqvist G, Figdor D, Hänström L, Sörlin S, Sandström G. Phagocytosis and virulence of different strains of *Porphyromonas gingivalis*. *Scand. J. Dent. Res.* 1991; 99: 117–29.

49. Sundqvist G. Associations between microbial species in dental root canal infections. *Oral Microbiol. Immunol.* 1992; 7: 257–62.

50. Tani-Ishii N, Kuchiba K, Osada T, Watanabe Y, Umemoto T. Effect of T-cell deficiency on the formation of periapical lesions in mice: histological comparison between periapical lesion formation in BALB/c and BALB/c nu/nu mice. *J. Endod.* 1995; 21: 195–9.

51. Teitelbaum SL. Bone resorption by osteoclasts. *Science* 2000; 289: 1504–8.

52. Ten Cate AR. The epithelial cell rests of Malassez and the genesis of the dental cyst. *Oral Surg. Oral Med. Oral Pathol. Oral Radiol. Endod.* 1972; 34: 956–64.

53. Teronen O, Hietanen J, Lindqvist C, Salo T, Sorsa T, Eklund KK, *et al.* Mast cell-derived tryptase in odontogenic cysts. *J. Oral Pathol. Med.* 1996; 25: 376–81.

54. Tronstad L, Barnett F, Gervone F. Periapical bacterial plaque in teeth refractory to endodontic treatment. *Endod. Dental Traumatol.* 1990; 6: 73–7.

55. Wallstrom JB, Torabinejad M, Kettering J, McMillan P. Role of T cells in the pathogenesis of periapical lesions. A preliminary report. *Oral Surg. Oral Med. Oral Pathol. Oral Radiol. Endod.* 1993; 76: 213–18.

56. Wang CY, Stashenko P. Characterization of bone-resorbing activity in human periapical lesions. *J. Endod.* 1993; 19: 107–11.

57. Weiss EI, Shaniztki B, Dotan M, Ganeshkumar N, Kolenbrander PE, Metzger Z. Attachment of *Fusobacterium nucleatum* PK1594 to mammalian cells and its coaggregation with periopathogenic bacteria are mediated by the same galactose-binding adhesin. *Oral Microbiol. Immunol.* 2000; 15: 371–7.

Chapter 8
Systemic complications of endodontic infections

Nils Skaug and Vidar Bakken

Introduction

Infectious processes associated with the root canal system of teeth may give rise to various complications that not only result in local manifestations but may also produce lesions in other body sites. As outlined in Fig. 8.1, there are three means by which a root canal infection may cause metastatic infections:

1. Through an acute periapical abscess whereby pus, microorganisms and their products are spread.
2. By an endodontic treatment procedure where microorganisms are disseminated to other body compartments along the circulatory system.
3. By the release of bacterial products and proinflammatory mediators from a chronic periapical inflammatory lesion.

The clinical significance of these mechanisms for the spread of infection and the measures to be undertaken to prevent systemic complications in otherwise healthy patients or patients compromised by a systemic disease are discussed in this chapter.

Acute periapical infections as the origin of metastatic infections

Acute manifestations of endodontic lesions involve the formation of abscesses in the periapical tissues (Chapter 7). Although these lesions are often confined to the oral region, they may extend to both nearby and distant body compartments along anatomical pathways (fascial planes and spaces). Hence, a periapical abscess may spread and reach the maxillary sinuses, the brain, the cavernous sinus, the eye or the mediastinum. Needless to say, some of these conditions are truly life threatening. In addition to the direct spread of pus and bacterial components, brain and lung abscesses may be caused by septic emboli. Furthermore, oral bacteria involved in endodontic infections may be aspirated into the lung and cause serious infections. Acute osteomyelitis is yet another condition that can arise from an endodontic infection. Before the antibiotic era, all these non-oral infections caused by disseminating oral bacteria were often fatal. In contrast to the status in developing countries, complications of this nature are now rare in the

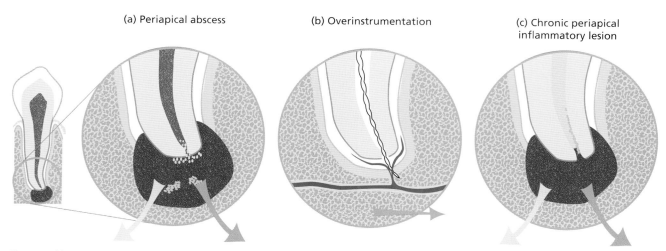

(a) Periapical abscess   (b) Overinstrumentation   (c) Chronic periapical inflammatory lesion

Fig. 8.1 (a) A periapical abscess at a root tip, (b) a root canal overinstrumentation and (c) an established periapical inflammatory lesion.

industrialized world. Yet, when they do occur, they still represent a threatening situation that demands proper dental and medical attention.

Spread of oral microorganisms by the circulation

Invasion of the circulation by bacteria and their dissemination by the blood stream throughout the body is called bacteremia. Bacteremias may occur as a result of surgical and other invasive procedures. They are generally asymptomatic and transient (duration <15–30 min) because the number of bacterial cells in the blood is usually low (<10 colony-forming units per ml). The host's mononuclear phagocytes and the humoral immune response, furthermore, readily eliminate the organisms. Therefore, in healthy individuals transient bacteremias are usually of no clinical significance and are asymptomatic. However, in individuals who lack normal protection against infections (compromised hosts) the bacteria may start to multiply in the blood resulting in sepsis, a serious infection that is accompanied by systemic manifestations of inflammation. In compromised hosts (e.g. patients with cancer, unregulated diabetes or immunodeficiency), sepsis may proceed to a generalized fatal infection.

Oral microorganisms may gain access to the blood after loss of oral mucosal integrity from trauma or manipulation. In connection with endodontic treatment procedures, for example, the placement of a rubber dam clamp often causes transient bacteremia. Bacteremias may also follow instrumentation of root canals (see below). Bacteremia can occur spontaneously as well as in conjunction with various types of professional dental treatments and other oral manipulations, including oral health procedures and mastication (Table 8.1).

It is important to note that bacteremia occurs frequently from routine daily oral activities. In fact, bacteremias are 1000–8000 times more likely to be caused by daily oral manipulations than by dental treatment procedures (42). The incidence and magnitude of bacteremias of oral origin have been found to be directly proportional to the degree of oral inflammation and infection (9, 41) and occur more frequently in persons with high dental plaque scores and gingivitis than in individuals maintaining adequate oral hygiene (48). Calculations have been done to estimate how different types of dental treatment and oral manipulations may lead to risk of exposure to transient bacteremia. Roberts (47) estimated that tooth brushing twice daily for 1 year had a 154 000 times greater risk of exposure to bacteremia than that resulting from a single tooth extraction. He also compared a single tooth extraction and the cumulative exposure during 1 year to bacteremia from routine, daily activities and estimated the latter to be as high as 5.6 million times greater. One study in which the gingival health and

Table 8.1 Frequency of treatment-induced and self-induced transient bacteremias.

Dental procedure	Frequency of bacteremias	Reference
Intraligamental anesthetic injections in children	16–97	46
Tooth extractions	10–94	29
Periodontal surgery	36–88	19
Gingival scaling	8–80	19
	25–61	2
Endodontics	31–54	16
	0–5	4
Ultrasonic scaling	53	44
Periodontal probing	43	14
Prophylaxis	0–40	19
Matrix band with wedge placement	32	45
Subgingival irrigation	30	31
Rubber dam clamp placement	29	45
Polishing teeth	24	45
Suture removal	11–16	8
Routine daily oral activities		
Dental flossing	0–58	19
Chewing	17–51	19
Water irrigation device	7–50	19
Oral rinsing	50	20
Toothpicks	20–40	9
Tooth brushing	0–26	19

plaque scores were the same in both test groups, found that the Sonicare electronic toothbrush induced significantly more (78%) bacteremias than did conventional toothbrushes (10).

Bacteremia and endodontic treatment

The actual number of microorganisms introduced into the blood stream depends upon the size of the apical foramen, the degree of infection of the root canal and the method of root canal treatment (2). A variety of oral bacteria, and species that are found in infective endocarditis, have been isolated from infected root canals and periapical lesions (27), yet there are relatively few reports in the literature describing how often bacteremia occurs following endodontic therapy and few provide bacteriological findings (Table 8.2).

Studies performed during the 1960s were not able to demonstrate positive blood cultures even if the root canal system had been instrumented vigorously in the presence of saliva. However, when canals were instrumented beyond the root apex, there was a 25–30% incidence of bacteremia (8). Baumgartner et al. (4) used an aseptic technique to culture the blood of 20 patients and registered bacteremia in only one case when a root canal

Table 8.2 Studies showing bacteria isolated from blood samples obtained in conjunction with non-surgical or surgical endodontic therapy.

Author (Ref.)	No. of teeth/ patients studied	Procedure	Frequency of positive blood samples	Number of isolates (n)
Rahn et al. (43)	56/56	Peripheral blood samples were obtained aseptically prior to apicoectomy and 3, 6 and 9 min postoperatively. Blood samples were cultivated aerobically and anaerobically	6/56 (10%)	*Streptococcus viridans* (n = 1) *Corynebacterium* sp. (n = 1) *Micrococcus* sp. (n = 1) *Staphylococcus* (n = 1) (coagulase-negative) *Lactobacillus fermentum* (n = 1) *Peptostreptococcus* sp. (n = 1)
Heimdahl et al. (26)	4/20	Blood samples were obtained aseptically in Vacutainer® tubes before, during and after intracanal endodontic instrumentation. After lysis-filtration, the blood samples were incubated anaerobically for 10 days	4/20 (20%)	*Micrococcus* spp. (n = 1) *Streptococcus* spp. (n = 1) *Corynebacterium hofmanii* (n = 1) *Neisseria* spp. (n = 1) Viridans group streptococci (n = 4) Anaerobic streptococci (n = 1)
Debelian et al. (15)	26/26	Blood samples were obtained aseptically during and after the endodontic procedure. See further Heimdahl et al. (26)	11/26 (42%)	*Prevotella intermedia* (n = 3) *Fusobacterium nucleatum* (n = 1) *Propionibacterium acnes* (n = 3) *Streptococcus intermedius* (n = 1) *Streptococcus sanguis* (n = 1) *Actinobacillus israelii* (n = 1) *Saccharomyces cerevisiae* (n = 1) (fungus)

had been overinstrumented. Debelian *et al.* (15), on the other hand, found a comparatively high frequency of bacteremias subsequent to endodontic therapy (42%), particularly in cases where the endodontic instrumentation had been deliberately carried out beyond the apical foramen (7/13 versus 4/13 for non-overinstrumented cases). In this latter study anaerobes were frequently isolated from the positive blood cultures, as opposed to previous studies where facultative organisms had predominated. These authors later verified that, for each patient in which a positive blood culture had been found, there was phenotypic and genotypic homology between the bacteria isolated from the root canal and the blood, suggesting that the blood bacteria originated from the treated root canals (16). Interestingly, in one patient the fungus *Saccharomyces cerevisiae* was recovered from both the root canal and the blood sample (Advanced concept 8.1).

Infective endocarditis

Bacteremia is considered a risk factor for the development of endocarditis. Bacterial endocarditis is a bacterial infection of the heart valves and the epithelial lining (endocardium) of the heart. The term infective endocarditis has recently been proposed to emphasize the fact that microbes other than bacteria also may cause endocarditis (25). According to new terminology, infective endocarditis is named after the infective microorganism, e.g. streptococcal endocarditis, staphylococcal endocarditis or fungal endocarditis (Table 8.3). Although currently

termed infective endocarditis, bacterial endocarditis is still used by many authors in the dental and medical literature.

Infective endocarditis results from a complex interaction among the endocardium, local hydrodynamic effects, circulating microorganisms and local and systemic host defense factors. In many countries it is a relatively uncommon life-threatening disease (approximately 50 cases are officially registered in Norway and 300 in Denmark per year). Infective endocarditis usually occurs in individuals with underlying congenital or acquired structural cardiac defects who develop bacteremia with bacteria prone to causing endocarditis. Symptoms of endocarditis generally start within 2 weeks of the incited bacteremia, although the time to diagnosis may be shorter or longer (51). An incubation period longer than 2 weeks between the invasive procedure and the onset of symptoms significantly lessens the likelihood of the procedure being the proximate cause (30).

The symptoms are non-specific and include fever, malaise, anorexia, cardiac murmurs, splenomegaly, anemia and weight loss. Before the antibiotic era the mortality of bacterial endocarditis was 100%, and it still is if not treated adequately. Currently, the death rate is less than 10% for viridans (alpha-hemolytic) streptococcal endocarditis (21, 55) and 30% for staphylococcal endocarditis (21).

The organism(s) in the circulation causing the disease adheres to and forms vegetations in a focal area of the heart valves. A prerequisite is often a prior injury where fibrin and platelets have been released, which can cap-

> **Advanced concept 8.1   Accuracy of testing blood samples for bacterial presence**
>
> When drawing blood by venipuncture for culturing circulating oral bacteria, there is always a risk of contaminating the blood sample with skin commensals. The presence in blood cultures of typical skin bacteria, such as coagulase-negative staphylococci, corynebacteria or propionibacteria, indicates contamination from the skin. Recently it was shown that skin disinfection with alcoholic chlorhexidine is more efficacious than skin preparation with aqueous providone–iodine in reducing contamination of blood cultures (37). However, bacteria known to be skin commensals also may be present in the oral microbiota, therefore it has been hard to tell whether such bacteria, when present in blood cultures, originate from the skin or the oral cavity. Recently developed molecular identification techniques may overcome this problem (16). A previous study (46) on bacteremias following local anesthetic injections in children showed blood culture with bacterial growth in 8% of the children prior to the injections. Both coagulase-negative staphylococci (a dominant member of the constant skin flora) and the oral bacterium *Streptococcus sanguinis* were isolated from these preinjection blood cultures. Brown et al. (12) eliminated patients from their bacteremia study who demonstrated blood cultures positive for coagulase-negative staphylococci, corynebacteria and propionibacteria because they were thought to be indicative of skin contamination. In the study by Debelian et al. (16), homology was found between *Propionibacterium acnes* isolated in both the blood samples and the root canal samples, suggesting that in these cases the organism was not a skin contaminant.
>
> The volume of blood used for culturing, the concentration of bacteria in the blood, the type of blood culturing system and the identification procedure employed determine the frequency of positive blood cultures with respect to type and number of species. With improved blood culture procedures and improvements in the isolation of anaerobic and fastidious microorganisms from blood, recovery of microorganisms from transient bacteremias has markedly increased during recent years. Therefore, not only higher frequencies of bacteremia but also more species and a higher number of microorganisms are expected when the results of more recent studies are compared with those of studies performed decades ago.

Table 8.3   Relative frequency of oral viridans streptococci associated with infective endocarditis at the New York Hospital from 1944 to 1983 (51).

Species	Frequency (%)
Streptococcus mitis	33–41
Streptococcus sanguis	31–47
Streptococcus anginosus	5–8
Streptococcus mutans	3–10
Streptococcus salivarius	1–2
Nutritionally variant	6–7
Unspeciated	1–3

ture circulating microbes. Multiplication within the vegetations leads to discharges of the infecting organism(s) back to the circulation, producing a constant bacteremia that gives multiple positive blood cultures. The clinical symptoms, including embolization to organs, are a direct result of this mechanism.

A wide variety of bacteria has been isolated from blood of patients with infective endocarditis. Viridans streptococci are the most common (50–63%) followed by staphylococci (25–26%) (21, 54). Various other microorganisms account for less than 10% (34). Among the oral viridans streptococci associated with infective endocarditis, *Streptococcus mitis* and *Streptococcus sanguinis* dominate and account for more than two-thirds of the registered cases.

The reason why viridans streptococci are more likely than other types of streptococci to cause endocarditis relates to their release of extracellular polysaccharides, which provides them with an exceptional adhesion mechanism. Other adhesins like lipoteichoic acid, fibrinogen-binding protein, fibronectin-binding protein and platelet-interactive molecules are putative virulence factors of bacteria associated with endocarditis (21). It was suggested recently that the majority of infected root canals contain bacteria that may have the potential to cause bacterial infective endocarditis (3).

Staphylococcus aureus is another important pathogen that may originate from the oral cavity, although there is no convincing evidence that oral staphylococci can cause infective endocarditis (59). However, this organism is capable of infecting even structurally normal heart valves and is the most commonly isolated organism in infective endocarditis of intravenous drug abusers (54).

It should be recognized that oral microorganisms presumed to cause infective endocarditis in a given case are not normally specific to the oral cavity only. Furthermore, the incubation period (the time between a procedure resulting in bacteremia and the onset of symptoms) is often well outside the accepted time frame, which should be within 10–14 days, depending on the causative organism (30). This means that it is often hard to establish the origin of a given heart infection.

Cardiac conditions and dental treatment procedures as risk factors for infective endocarditis

The American Heart Association (AHA) has made recommendations for the prevention of infective endocarditis for more than half a century. Nine documents were published from 1955 to 1997 (13, 58). During these years the guidelines became more and more complicated and increasingly difficult for both practitioners and patients to follow. Risk assessment of patients for infective endocarditis was based on types of heart diseases and oral intervention. The AHA now recommends that only patients at greatest risk of negative outcomes from infective endocarditis should take short-term preventive antibiotics before routine dental procedures. According to the AHA, patients who should continue to take preventive antibiotics include those with artificial heart valves, a history of infective endocarditis, certain congenital heart conditions (including a patch to repair the heart defect within the past 6 months) and a cardiac transplant that develops heart valve problems. Thus an extremely small number of cases of infected endocarditis might be prevented by antibiotic prophylaxis even if it were 100% effective (58).

Certain cardiac conditions are thought to predispose individuals for infective endocarditis more often than others. Most at risk are those patients with a prior history of infective endocarditis and those with a prosthetic heart valve. In line with this knowledge, the AHA (58) has defined high-risk and moderate-risk categories for infective endocarditis (Core concept 8.1). This body has also defined dental and oral treatment procedures that are likely to cause hazardous bacteremia in these two infective endocarditis categories (Core concept 8.2). Hence, a variety of invasive dental procedures is felt to pose a risk for infective endocarditis, although the associations have never been firmly documented. Endodontic surgery, including incision and drainage of abscesses and instrumentation beyond the tooth apex, belong to the dental procedures that, according to the AHA, should be regarded as risk factors to individuals with cardiac conditions.

Core concept 8.1   Cardiac conditions associated with the highest risk of adverse outcome from endocarditis for which prophylaxis with dental procedures is reasonable (58)

- Prosthetic cardiac valve or prosthetic material used for cardiac valve repair
- Previous infective endocarditis
- Congenital heart disease (CHD):*
  - Unrepaired cyanotic CHD, including palliative shunts and conduits
  - Completely repaired congenital heart defect with prosthetic material or device, whether placed by surgery or by catheter intervention, during the first 6 months after the procedure†
  - Repaired CHD with residual defects at the site or adjacent to the site of a prosthetic patch or prosthetic device (which inhibit endothelialization)
- Cardiac transplantation recipients who develop cardiac valvulopathy

* Except for the conditions listed above, antibiotic prophylaxis is no longer recommended for any other form of CHD.

† Prophylaxis is recommended because endothelialization of prosthetic materials occurs up to 6 months after the procedure.

Core concept 8.2   Dental procedures for which endocarditis prophylaxis is reasonable for patients in Core concept 8.1 (58)

All dental procedures that involve manipulation of gingival tissue or the periapical region of teeth or perforation of the oral mucosa.*

* The following procedures and events do not need extra prophylaxis: routine anesthetic injections through non-infected tissue, taking dental radiographs, placement of removable prosthodontic or orthodontic appliances, adjustment of orthodontic appliances, placement of orthodontic brackets, shedding of primary teeth and bleeding from trauma to the lips or oral mucosa.

About 40% of all infective endocarditis cases occur in patients without previously identified risk factors. It has been estimated that 20% of cases can be related to dental treatment procedures or infections (21) but the vast majority are due to oral organisms and are not related to dental procedures (41).

Even if the oral focal infection theory (see below) no longer enjoys widespread acceptance, it has retained its position when it comes to the etiology of infective endocarditis. This is in spite of the lack of firm evidence for a cause–effect relationship. Therefore, to determine the cause of a given case of endocarditis, physicians often ask patients if they have received dental treatment in recent months. If the answer is yes, the dental treatment is usually blamed for the condition (55). There are few well-controlled studies of dental risk factors for infective endocarditis (28, 52). One of these studies found no increased risk associated with dental procedures in the preceding 90 days (28), although borderline increased risks were noted for endodontic treatment and dental scaling. In another large, population-based, case–control study (52) none of the dental procedures that were observed, except possibly tooth extraction, was found to be a risk factor. This was true even in cases where there were underlying cardiac valvular abnormalities (prosthetic valves, previous history of endocarditis). The study did confirm, however, the importance of these heart abnormalities as risk factors for infective endocarditis.

The recent AHA guidelines state:

"In patients with dental disease, the focus on the frequency of bacteremia associated with a specific dental procedure and the AHA guidelines for prevention of IE have resulted in an overemphasis on antibiotic prophylaxis and an underemphasis on maintenance of good oral hygiene and access to routine dental care, which are likely more important in reducing lifetime risk of IE than the administration of antibiotic prophylaxis for a dental procedure. However, no observational or controlled studies support this contention." (58)

Good oral hygiene is the most important factor in reducing the risk of endocarditis in susceptible individuals, and access to high-quality dental care is also emphasized by the Working Party of the British Society for Antimicrobial Chemotherapy (BSAC) (22).

Therefore, even if dental procedures have not been confirmed as risk factors for infective endocarditis, cases are often infected with microorganisms common to the oral microbiota (52) and transient bacteremias due to dental treatment procedures cannot be excluded as causative factors. Consequently, dentists must always be aware of the potential risk of dental infections and dental procedures, and follow established guidelines for prevention.

Preventive measures

Current recommendations on antibiotic prevention of bacteremia sequelae

The AHA has issued widely accepted recommendations stating that antibiotics should be given to prevent endocarditis when a patient is undergoing dental risk treatment and when qualifying for the moderate- or high-risk category (Core concept 8.1). New guidelines have recently been published by the Working Party of the BSAC, recommending that dental prophylaxis should be restricted to patients who have a history of previous endocarditis, patients with cardiac valve replacement surgery, or those with surgically constructed pulmonary shunts or conduits (22).

Dental risk treatment is defined as a treatment procedure that is known to produce bacteremia, which includes endodontic surgery and root canal instrumentation (Core concept 8.2). Certain procedures that are not recommended for antibiotic prophylaxis may nevertheless cause significant bleeding in patients with poor oral hygiene. In such cases prophylaxis is also appropriate. Consequently, the dentist is always responsible for the final decision as to whether antibiotic prophylaxis should be instituted. See Core concept 8.3 for guidelines on antibiotic prophylaxis and risk assessment of patients.

Prophylaxis is most effective when given preoperatively in doses that are sufficient to ensure adequate antibiotic concentrations in the blood during and 10 hours after the procedure. To minimize the risk of anaphylactic reactions and antibiotic resistance, the AHA recommends oral regimens as the standard route. A single dose of 2 g (AHA) (58) or 3 g (BSAC) (22) amoxicillin in adults should be given orally 1 hour before the dental treatment. In the case of penicillin allergy, 600 mg of clindamycin is recommended preferentially as an alternative. Amoxicillin, when given at the recommended doses, is preferred to other penicillins because it ensures adequate antibiotic concentrations in the serum for

---

Core concept 8.3   Risk assessments and antibiotic prophylaxis

Patients
- Oral bacteremias are transient, occur frequently and represent a negligible risk for infective endocarditis or metastatic infections in healthy individuals.
- Bacteremias following certain dental treatment procedures can provoke infective endocarditis in moderate- and high-risk individuals. Antibiotic prophylaxis should therefore be instituted.
- Immunocompromised patients (individuals with reduced granulocyte count, leukemic patients, bone marrow transplant patients with leukemia) are at high risk of bacteremia-induced infections. Antibiotic prophylaxis is needed and should be determined in consultation with the patient's physician because universal guidelines are not available.
- Recipients of organ transplants and cancer patients, although they have increased susceptibility to infections, do not normally require routine antibiotic prophylaxis in conjunction with dental treatment.

Dental procedures
- The vast majority of infective endocarditis cases are not associated with dental treatment procedures.
- Dental procedures that involve manipulation of gingival tissue or the periapical region (root canal instrumentation beyond the apical foramen and endodontic surgery) are associated with transient bacteremias and require antibiotic prophylaxis in patients at highest risk of infective endocarditis (see Core concept 8.1).

Preventive measures
- Any use of antibiotic prophylaxis must take into consideration the adverse effects of antibiotic toxicity and allergy, selection of resistant microorganisms, superinfections and effects on the microbial ecology.
- Under any circumstance, the dentist is ultimately responsible for the final decision as to whether antibiotic prophylaxis should be instituted and the selection of drug.

Failure to give proper antibiotic prophylaxis may generate malpractice claims.

---

10 hours postoperatively. For patients who are unable to take or absorb oral medication, 2 g of ampicillin may be administered intramuscularly or intravenously just before the procedure. Ampicillin-allergic patients may be treated with parenterally administered clindamycin (600 mg in adults) (58).

If the patient has forgotten to take the prescribed antibiotic prior to the treatment, the medication can still be effective if given in conjunction with the procedure, but not later than 2 hours after it was started. The rationale is that the antimicrobial effect primarily is due to inhibition of bacterial growth on the damaged heart valves and not, as thought before, to the colonization *per se* or to the killing of microorganisms in the blood stream (24).

It is well documented that antibiotic prophylaxis, according to the recommended regimens, may select for microorganisms that are resistant to the drug. Resistance is likely not to persist for more than 9–14 days after termination of prophylactic treatment, therefore dental treatments requiring an antibiotic umbrella should be scheduled with at least 14-day intervals. If a shorter interval is needed, an alternative antibiotic should be selected (Table 8.4). If a situation were to emerge where antibiotic prophylaxis is required twice within a short time interval (12–24 hours), it is unlikely that a significant selection of resistant microorganisms would have occurred. In such instances the use of the same prophylactic regimen is acceptable.

Antibiotic prophylaxis in compromised hosts

The antibiotic prophylaxis regimens of the AHA and BSAC seem to be appropriate for the prevention of bacteremia in cancer chemotherapy patients but might be inappropriate in patients with suppressed granulocyte count, leukemic patients or bone marrow transplant patients. In the latter category of patients more effective agents against Gram-negative organisms are required (41). This is because the oral flora of such immunocompromised patients can be different from that of normal individuals and includes Gram-negative bacteria (e.g. *Klebsiella pneumoniae*, *Enterobacter cloacae*, *Escherichia coli*) that are highly resistant to the beta-lactam antibiotics, aminoglycosides, vancomycin and fluoroquinolones. The most obvious risk for bone marrow transplant patients with leukemia is, however, septic shock caused by viridans streptococci (41). Hence, the latter authors recommend that dental patients with low granulocyte counts should be treated only on an emergency (non-elective) basis. Because of significant interindividual differences in the oral microflora of immunocompromised patients and the lack of controlled clinical studies, antibiotic prophylaxis in these patients should be based on microbiological evaluation and in collaboration with the patient's physician.

Patients in need of organ (e.g. heart, kidney, liver) transplantation should have a pretransplant dental evaluation. All required endodontic treatment should be completed in due time prior to the transplantation because of the increased risk of infection that these patients will be exposed to due to immunosuppression. Antibiotic prophylaxis in such patients still has an empirical base and no guidelines have been issued so far. Root canal instrumentation beyond the tooth apex should always be avoided and any antibiotic prophylaxis prior to periapical surgery should be determined in consultation with the patient's physician.

An expert panel of dentists, orthopedic surgeons and infectious disease specialists concluded that antibiotic prophylaxis is not routinely indicated for most dental patients with total joint replacements, nor is it recommended for dental patients with pins, plates and screws (1). Antibiotic prophylaxis for the prevention of systemic infections is not recommended in hemodialysis patients, heart transplant patients or splenectomized patients, or to prevent brain abscess (41).

Surgical intervention in an infected area is sometimes necessary. In addition to the risk for bacteremia, local spread of microorganisms will always occur and may present a risk for metastatic infection. Yet, surgical antibiotic prophylaxis is only justified in immunocompromised patients and should begin 2 hours before and be terminated when the surgery is finished and no later than 24–48 hours after the surgery (for references, see Ref. 41).

Table 8.4 The American Heart Association's recommendations of 2007 on antibiotic regimen for a dental procedure (58).

Situation	Agent	Regimen: single dose 30–60 min before procedure
Oral	Amoxicillin	Adults: 2.0 g; children: 50 mg/kg
Unable to take oral medications	Ampicillin	Adults: 2.0 g intramuscularly (IM) or intravenously (IV); children: 50 mg/kg IM or IV
Allergic to penicillins or ampicillin – oral	Clindamycin	Adults: 600 mg; children: 20 mg/kg
	or	
	Cephalexin[a]	Adults: 2.0 g; children: 50 mg/kg
	or	
	Azithromycin or clarithromycin	Adults: 500 mg; children: 15 mg/kg
Allergic to penicillins or ampicillin and unable to take oral medication	Clindamycin	Adults: 600 mg IM or IV; children: 20 mg/kg IM or IV
	or	
	Cefazolin[a]	Adults: 1.0 g IM or IV; children: 50 mg/kg IM or IV

[a] Cephalosporins should not be used in individuals with immediate-type hypersensitivity reactions to penicillins or ampicillins (e.g. urticaria, angioedema or anaphylaxis).

It needs to be recognized that in order to achieve a satisfactory risk–benefit ratio any use of antibiotic prophylaxis must take into consideration the adverse effects of antibiotic toxicity and allergy, the selection of resistant microorganisms, superinfections and effects on the microbial ecology (41).

Are the current antibiotic prophylaxis recommendations appropriate?

The most important rationale for antibiotic prophylaxis has been to prevent infective endocarditis because this disease carries high morbidity and mortality. Studies in experimental animals have indeed demonstrated that antibiotics can prevent infective endocarditis (17) and that penicillin is the drug of choice in the case of viridans streptococcal bacteremia. Yet, the effectiveness of antibiotics to prevent infective endocarditis in humans has not been proven and probably never will be because it is a rare disease and controlled studies cannot be conducted for ethical reasons (17). In the Strom et al. (52) study, a minority (<10%) of the cases had received antibiotic prophylaxis but the risk for infective endocarditis remained the same regardless of whether prophylactic antibiotics had been taken or not.

The lack of firm evidence that dental treatment is a frequent cause of infective endocarditis, the report of well-documented cases where antibiotic prophylaxis has failed to prevent infective endocarditis (30), the low compliance with the current guidelines for antibiotic prophylaxis, the unfavorable cost–benefit and risk–benefit relationships and the risk for selection of antibiotic resistance have initiated qualified questions as to the appropriateness of the current guidelines for prophylaxis against infective endocarditis before dental treatment. It has been proposed that antibiotic prophylaxis should be given only to patients with prosthethic heart valves or previous history of endocarditis and only in conjunction with procedures resulting in high-level bacteremias (extractions and gingival surgery, including implant surgery) (18). Because infective endocarditis of oral origin is more likely to be due to poor oral health and hygiene than dental treatment per se, patients with cardiac abnormalities should be encouraged to maintain a high level of oral health (30).

The significance of the contribution of acute oral infections to prosthetic joint infections has been discussed for years. The current view is that it is likely that bacteremias associated with such infections can, and do, cause implant infection. Therefore, elimination of the source of infection (e.g. endodontic therapy or tooth extraction) is required in these patients (1). There is still significant debate as to which dental procedures require antibiotic prophylaxis and what antibiotic regimen should be prescribed (11).

Chronic periapical infections as the origin of metastatic infections

Systemic effects of chronic dental infections

From "oral sepsis" to "focal infection"

"Gold fillings, gold caps, gold bridges, gold crowns, fixed dentures, built in, on, and around diseased teeth, form a veritable mausoleum of gold over a mass of sepsis to which there is no parallel in the whole realm of medicine or surgery.

"It is therefore not a matter of teeth and dentistry, it is an all important matter of sepsis and antisepsis."

Sir William Hunter, 1861–1937

The belief that infected teeth are the cause of certain systemic diseases (e.g. arthritis) emerged at the beginning of the 19th century, but the notion may be tracked back to ancient times and Hippocrates (40). On the basis of his studies of the oral microbiota, the American dentist W.D. Miller drew attention to the possible interrelationship between oral infections and systemic diseases (35, 36). At the turn of the 20th century the English physician W. Hunter introduced the term oral sepsis. It implied that in addition to dissemination of bacteria from the oral cavity, particularly from long-term low-grade oral infections, oral bacteria act specifically and selectively on different target organs by liberating toxins, thereby producing adverse systemic effects (42). According to Hunter's theory, the mouth was the most important septic focus and oral sepsis the most common source of sepsis. He alleged that conservative dentistry was synonymous with septic dentistry.

In 1912 the American physician F. Billings replaced the term oral sepsis with focal infection (40, 42). Focal infection occurs when microorganisms disseminate from a localized area of infection (focus of infection) and establish themselves elsewhere in the body as a secondary infection. When an oral infection is the source of focal infection, the term oral focal infection is used. Dental focal infection implies that an infected tooth is the focus. When the focal infection theory was most popular, periapical infections were thought to play a major role. During recent years, asymptomatic lesions of apical periodontitis have been examined for microorganisms using conventional cultivation, electron microscopy, DNA–DNA hybridization, polymerase chain reaction (PCR), fluorescence in situ hybridization (FISH) in combination with epifluorescence and confocal laser scanning microscopy (CLSM). FISH demonstrated coaggregating bacteria in mixed consortia located in different tissue layers of the 50% of the examined granulomas while the remaining ones seemed bacteria free (53). Several authors have therefore suggested that granulomas are protective reactions aiming at preventing the spread of periapical bacteria. Bacteremia from asymptomatic apical periodontitis has never been reported.

Figure 8.2 shows how dental infection was once thought to be responsible for dental sepsis and various connected systemic conditions. Common to these conditions, at that time, was that no cause other than oral focal infection could be found. Therefore, even the extraction of healthy teeth became justified to prevent systemic infections and diseases. As a consequence, endodontic therapy nearly disappeared in the USA for many years (7). Fellow colleagues even maintained that dentists who performed root canal therapy should be considered criminals and be sentenced to 6 months of hard labour (42). Later, the true etiology of many of the infectious conditions that were associated with oral foci was disclosed. It became obvious that over the years many healthy teeth had been removed for no good reason. The dental focal infection theory therefore gradually lost its influence. However, owing to the continued release of new case reports with claims that patients had been cured from arthritis or other chronic diseases after extraction of their infected or root filled teeth, and in spite of lack of scientific evidence, the dental focal infection theory never died (40, 42).

Potential mechanisms by which a chronic inflammatory periapical lesion may cause adverse systemic effects

The dental focal infection theory acquired a new dimension when immunopathological mechanisms were added to disseminated bacteria and microbial toxins as causative factors of systemic diseases (Fig. 8.3). Recent data suggest that chronic subclinical infections (e.g.

chronic periodontal infections), as indicated by raised values within the normal range of C-reactive protein (34) and other acute-phase proteins (57), may induce systemic inflammation leading to such conditions as atherosclerosis, cardiovascular disease, cerebrovascular disease or preterm low birth-weight delivery. These observations have led to a paradigm shift in our understanding of the pathobiology of these complex associations. It is now realized that oral bacteria and their products, particularly lipopolysaccharides and proinflammatory cytokines, induced locally in response to oral infections, enter the blood stream and may subsequently activate systemic responses in certain susceptible individuals. It is not yet known whether these relationships are causal or consequential.

Deliberations in recent years

Spurred by epidemiological findings in large patient populations, a renewed interest has emerged in recent years on the role of chronic oral infections in certain systemic diseases such as coronary heart disease. Data from Finland, for example, have demonstrated a significant association in male patients to dental infections (32, 33, 49) and primarily to periodontal disease (23). Evidence from the literature also suggests that there is an association between severe periodontal infections and spontaneous preterm birth (56). It is now believed that systemic inflammations have common biological triggering mechanisms (IL-1β, IL-6, TNFα, PGE2) and that they occur more frequently in individuals with hyperinflammatory monocyte/macrophage phenotype than in individuals with normal monocyte phenotype. The monocytes of the former phenotype secrete three- to ten-fold more of these mediators in response to lipopolysaccharides than those of the normal monocyte phenotype (5, 6).

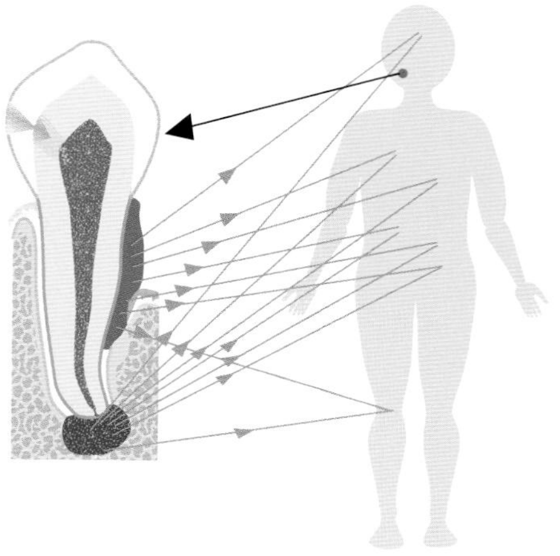

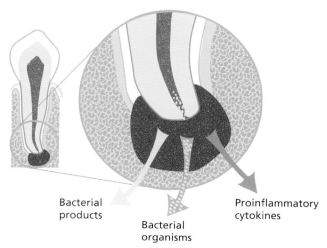

Fig. 8.2 According to the dental focal infection theory, several systemic diseases affecting the brain, eyes, lung, heart, liver, joints and the skin are caused by dental sepsis, involving dissemination of bacteria and bacterial products from chronic periapical and marginal periodontitis.

Bacterial products

Bacterial organisms

Proinflammatory cytokines

Fig. 8.3 Potential mechanisms of focal infection.

Case study

A 57-year-old male with a chief complaint of intense intermittent pain in his lower right quadrant presented at the School of Dentistry, University of Bergen, Norway. The pain had started spontaneously about 3 weeks earlier and it occurred when he drank or ate something hot. In the beginning, cold water in the mouth relieved the pain. However, after some days cold water no longer had any effect on the pain intensity. As the pain-free intervals became shorter, the pain intensity increased and he awoke occasionally at night in pain. The pain had been controlled by analgesics. The clinical examination revealed that the lower right quadrant was asymptomatic to palpation and that 36 and 37 were slightly sensible to percussion. Both the molars had gold crowns and did not respond to thermal or electrical vitality testing. Periapical radiographs of 36 and 37 revealed neither periapical pathoses nor periodontal ligament space widening.

One week later in the morning the patient was seen in severe pain by an endodontist in Bergen. The pain intensity had increased during recent days and there had been almost no pain-free intervals. Also, the pain could no longer be relieved by analgesics. The patient who had had very little sleep during the previous 2 nights now insisted on being relieved of his pain. The clinical examination showed that there was a tender moderate swelling along the buccal aspect of the alveolar ridge of 36 and 37 and that these teeth were more sensitive to percussion than before. Periapical radiographs were taken. Still no definitive widening of periodontal ligaments could be verified. The patient's medical history was unremarkable, but for the following information. First, the patient had a history of reaction to oral penicillin with signs and symptoms indicating an immediate-type hypersensitivity reaction. The patient had never taken any other antibiotics. Second, he had a prosthetic heart valve. The endodontist decided to treat the patient later the same day, but only after he had taken antibiotic prophylaxis. The patient received a prescription for clindamycin, was asked to buy the drug and to take 600 mg (two 300 mg capsules of Dalacin) 1 hour prior to the appointment for the endodontic treatment. The patient did so and the pulp chamber of 36 could be explored without anesthesia. The root canals were totally debrided and then obturated using laterally condensed gutta-percha points and sealer.

Two days later the patient returned to the endodontist with a buccal abscess in the 35–37 region. The endodontist immediately called a nearby oral surgeon who agreed to see the patient 30 min later. The oral surgeon's treatment plan included an antibiotic prophylaxis and incision of the abscess. This time 500 mg of a macrolide antibiotic (one 500 mg tablet of Azitromax) was given 1 hour prior to incision of the abscess. The patient recovered rapidly and after some days all clinical symptoms were gone. He was referred to a dermatologist to be examined for allergy to penicillin. This examination revealed no such allergy.

Comments

1. When antibiotic prophylaxis is needed, it is highly recommended to adhere to the current guidelines on antibiotic prophylaxis of the American Heart Association (AHA) or the British Society for Antimicrobial Therapy and not to another antibiotic regimen.

2. According to the current AHA guidelines (2007), only endodontic procedures involving instrumentation beyond the apical foramen require prophylaxis. Based on the clinical findings in the present case, the endodontist felt that microbes had already spread periapically of 36 and because more bacteria might be transported to the same area during the root canal instrumentation, antibiotic prophylaxis was chosen. Therefore, 36 was root filled even with some acute clinical symptoms.

3. Because the patient's medical history indicated allergy to penicillin and this could neither be professionally confirmed nor invalidated at that time, the endodontist correctly chose an alternative antibiotic (clindamycin) other than cephalosporins. The latter antibiotics should not be used in individuals with immediate-type hypersensitivity reactions to penicillins.

4. For the second antibiotic prophylaxis the oral surgeon changed from clindamycin to a macrolide antibiotic (Azitromax). This was done to reduce the probability of selecting resistant microorganisms in the oral cavity because such resistance is likely not to persist 9–14 days after the antibiotic is terminated. In this case a shorter interval was necessary. If a longer interval had been possible, clindamycin would have been appropriate.

Demonstration of DNA from *Aggregatibacter actinomycetemcomitans*, *Porphyromonas gingivalis* and *Prevotella intermedia* in atheromas strongly indicates a role for these oral bacteria in atherosclerosis (5). Although they are known as periodontal pathogens, they are also involved in endodontic infections. Activated macrophages in periapical infections produce the proinflammatory cytokines (IL-1β and TNFα) (39). It is currently not known whether there is a relationship between the phenotypes of monocytes/macrophages, chronic periapical infection and systemic inflammation (38). The latest studies concerning possible relationships between periodontal disease and cardiovascular disease have shown a significant, albeit modest, positive association, even after adjusting for confounders (50).

References

1. Advisory Statement. Antibiotic prophylaxis for dental patients with total joint replacements. *J. Am. Dent. Assoc.* 1997; 128: 1004–8.
2. Baltch AL, Schaffer C, Mark RDH, Hammer MS, Suthpen NT, Smith RP, *et al.* Bacteremia following dental cleaning in patients with and without penicillin prophylaxis. *Am. Heart J.* 1982; 104: 1335–9.
3. Bate AL, Ma JK-C, Pitt Ford TR. Detection of bacterial virulence genes associated with infective endocarditis in infected root canals. *Int. Endod. J.* 2000; 33: 194–203.
4. Baumgartner CJ, Heggers P, Harrison JW. The incidence of bacteremias related to endodontic procedures. I. Nonsurgical endodontics. *J. Endod.* 1976; 2: 135–40.
5. Beck JD, Offenbacher S. Oral health and systemic disease: periodontitis and cardiovascular disease. *J. Dent. Educ.* 1998; 62: 859–70.
6. Beck JD, Slade G, Offenbacher S. Oral disease, cardiovascular disease and systemic inflammation. *Periodontol. 2000* 2000; 23: 110–20.
7. Bellizzi R, Cruse WP. A historic review of endodontics, 1689–1963. Part 3. *J. Endod.* 1980; 6: 576–80.
8. Bender IB, Seltzer S, Tashman S, Meloff G. Dental procedures in patients with rheumatic heart disease. *Oral Surg.* 1963; 16: 466–73.
9. Bender IB, Naidorf IJ, Garvey GJ. Bacterial endocarditis: a consideration for physicians and dentists. *J. Am. Dent. Assoc.* 1984; 109: 415–20.
10. Bhanji S, Williams B, Sheller B, Elwood T, Mancl L. Transient bacteremia induced by toothbrushing: a comparison of the Sonicare toothbrush with a conventional toothbrush. *Pediatr. Dent.* 2002; 24: 295–9.
11. Brincat M, Savarrio L, Saunders M. Endodontics and infective endocarditis – is antimicrobial chemoprophylaxis required? *Int. Endod. J.* 2006; 39: 671–82.
12. Brown AR, Christopher J, Schultz P, Theisen FC, Schultz RE. Bacteremia and intraoral suture removal: can an antimicrobial rinse help? *J. Am. Dent. Assoc.* 1998; 129: 1455–61.
13. Dajani AS, Taubert KA, Wilson W, Bolger AS, Bayer A, Ferrieri P, *et al*. Prevention of bacterial endocarditis: recommendations by the American Heart Association. *J. Am. Dent. Assoc.* 1998; 128: 1142–51.
14. Daly C, Mitchell D, Grossberg D, Highfield J, Stewart D. Bacteremia caused by periodontal probing. *Aust. Dent. J.* 1997; 42: 77–80.
15. Debelian GJ, Olsen I, Tronstad L. Bacteremia in conjunction with endodontic therapy. *Endod. Dent. Traumatol.* 1995; 11: 142–9.
16. Debelian GJ, Olsen I, Tronstad L. Anaerobic bacteremia and fungemia in patients undergoing endodontic therapy: an overview. *Ann. Periodontol.* 1998; 3: 281–7.
17. Durack DT. Prevention of infective endocarditis. *N. Engl. J. Med.* 1995; 332: 38–44.
18. Durack DT. Antibiotics for prevention of endocarditis during dentistry: time to scale back? *Ann. Intern. Med.* 1998; 129: 829–31.
19. Epstein JP. Infective endocarditis: dental implications and new guidelines for antibiotic prophylaxis. *J. Can. Dent. Assoc.* 1998; 64: 281–92.
20. Felix C, Rosen S, App G. Detection of bacteremia after use of oral irrigation device in subjects with periodontitis. *J. Periodontol.* 1971; 42: 785–7.
21. Franklin C. Infective endocarditis: a review of the etiology, epidemiology and pathogenesis. In: *Clinical Oral Science* (Harris M, Edgar M, Meghji S, eds). Bristol: Wright, 1998; 213–21.
22. Gould FK, Elliot TSJ, Foweraker J, Fulford M, Perry JD, Roberts GJ, *et al.* Guidelines for the prevention of endocarditis: report of the Working Party of the British Society for Antimicrobial Chemotherapy. *J. Antimicrob. Chemother.* 2006; 57: 1035–42.
23. Grau AJ, Buggle F, Ziegler C, Schwarz W, Meuser J, Tasman A-J, *et al.* Association between acute cerebrovascular ischemia and chronic and recurrent infection. *Stroke* 1997; 28: 1724–9.
24. Hall G, Heimdahl A, Nord CE. Bacteremia after oral surgery and antibiotic prophylaxis for endocarditis. *Clin. Infect. Dis.* 1999; 29: 1–8.
25. Harris SA. Definitions and demographic characteristics. In: *Infective Endocarditis* (Kaye D, ed.). New York: Raven Press, 1992; 1–18.
26. Heimdahl A, Hall G, Hedberg M, Sandberg H, Söder P-Ö, Tunér K, *et al.* Detection and quantitation by lysis-filtration of bacteremia after different oral surgical procedures. *J. Clin. Microbiol.* 1990; 28: 2205–9.
27. Kettering JD, Torabinejad M. Microbiology and immunology. In: *Pathways of the Pulp*, 7th edn (Cohen S, Burns RC, eds). St. Louis, MO: Mosby, 1998; 463–75.
28. Lacassin F, Hoen B, Leport C, Selton-Suty C, Delahaye F, Goulet V, *et al.* Procedures accociated with infective endocarditis in adults. A case control study. *Eur. Heart J.* 1995; 16: 1869–974.
29. Lockhart PB. An analysis of bacteremias during dental extractions. *Arch. Intern. Med.* 1996; 156: 513–20.
30. Lockhart PB. The risk for endocarditis in dental practice. *Periodontol. 2000* 2000; 23: 127–35.
31. Lofthus JE, Waki MY, Jolkovsky DL, Otomo-Corgel J, Newman N, Flemming T. Bacteremia following subgingival irrigation and scaling and root planing. *J. Periodontol.* 1991; 62: 602–7.

32. Mattila K, Nieminen MS, Voltonen VV, Rasi VP, Käsaniemi YA, Syrjälä SL, et al. Association between dental health and acute myocardial infection. *Br. Med. J.* 1989; 298: 779–81.

   Designed a cumulative score system based upon the number of carious lesions, the extent of periodontal pocketing, the presence and magnitude of periapical lesions and the presence or absence of pericoronitis for correlation to coronary heart disease.

33. Mattila KJ, Vantonen VV, Nieminen M, Huttunen JK. Dental infection and the risk of new coronary events: prospective study of patients with documented coronary artery disease. *Clin. Infect. Dis.* 1995; 20: 588–92.

34. Mendall M, Patel P, Ballam L, Strachan D, Northfield T. C reactive protein and its relation to cardiovascular risk factors: a population based cross sectional study. *Br. Med. J.* 1996; 312: 1061–5.

35. Miller WD. The human mouth as a focus of infection. *Dent. Cosmos* 1891; 33: 689–95.

36. Miller WD. *The Micro-organisms in the Human Mouth. The Local and General Diseases Which are Caused by Them.* Philadelphia, PA: S.S. White, 1890; 274–341.

37. Mimoz O, Karim A, Mercat A, Cosseron M, Falissard B, Parker F, et al. Chlorhexidine compared with providone-iodine as skin preparation before blood culture. A randomized, controlled trial. *Ann. Intern. Med.* 1999; 131: 834–7.

38. Murray CA, Saunders WP. Root canal treatment and general health: a review of the literature. *Int. Endod. J.* 2000; 33: 1–18.

39. Nair PNR. Apical periodontitis: a dynamic encounter between root canal infection and host response. *Periodontol. 2000* 1997; 13: 121–48.

40. O'Reilly PG, Claffey NM. A history of oral sepsis as a cause of disease. *Periodontol. 2000* 2000; 23: 13–18.

41. Pallasch TJ, Slots J. Antibiotic prophylaxis and the medically compromised patient. *Periodontol. 2000* 1996; 10: 107–38.

   Describing the principles of antibiotic prophylaxis, reviewing bacteremia, discussing various aspects of infective endocarditis, including dentist and physician compliance, and indicating proper use of antibiotic prophylaxis in patients with severely impaired resistance to infections.

42. Pallasch TJ. The focal infection theory: appraisal and re-appraisal. *Calif. Dent. Assoc. J.* 2000; 28: 194–200.

43. Rahn R, Shah PM, Scäfer V, Frenkel G, Seibold K. Bakteriämie nach chirurgish endodontischen Eingriffen. *ZWR* 1987; 96: 903–7.

44. Reinhardt R, Bolton R, Hlava G. Effect of non sterile versus sterile water irrigation with ultrasonic scaling and postoperative bacteremias. *J. Periodontol.* 1982; 53: 96–9.

45. Roberts GJ, Holzel HS, Sury MR, Simmons NA, Gardner P, Longhurst P. Dental bacteremia in children. *Pediatr. Cardiol.* 1997; 18: 24–7.

46. Roberts, GJ, Simmons NB, Longhurst P, Hewitt PB. Bacteremia following local anesthetic injections in children. *Br. Dent. J.* 1998; 185: 295–8.

47. Roberts GJ. Dentists are innocent! "Everyday" bacteremia is the real culprit: a review and assessment of the evidence that dental surgical procedures are a principal cause of bacterial endocarditis in children. *Pediatr. Cardiol.* 1999; 20: 317–25.

48. Sconyers JR, Crawford JJ, Moriarty JD. Relationship of bacteremia to toothbrushing in patients with periodontitis. *J. Am. Dent. Assoc.* 1973; 87: 616–22.

49. Seymour RA, Steele JG. Is there a link between periodontal disease and coronary heart disease? *Br. Dent. J.* 1998; 184: 33–8.

50. Seymour GJ, Ford PJ, Cullinan MP, Leishman S, Yamazaki K. Relationship between periodontal infections and systemic disease. *Clin. Microbiol. Infect.* 2007; 13 (Suppl. 4): 3–10.

51. Starkebaum M, Durack D, Beeson P. The "incubation period" of bacterial endocarditis. *Yale J. Biol. Med.* 1977; 50: 49–58.

52. Strom BL, Abrutyn E, Berlin JA, Kinman JL, Seldman RS, Stolley PD, et al. Dental and cardiac risk factors for infective endocarditis. A population-based, case–control study. *Ann. Intern. Med.* 1998; 129: 761–9.

   This population-based, case–control study concludes that dental treatment seems not to be a risk factor for infective endocarditis, even in patients with valvular abnormalities. Consequently, the policies for antibiotic prophylaxis in such patients should be reconsidered.

53. Sunde PT, Olsen I, Göbel UB, Theegarten D, Winter S, Debelian GJ, et al. Fluorescence *in situ* hybridization (FISH) for direct visualization of bacteria in periapical lesions of asymptomatic root-filled teeth. *Microbiology* 2003; 149: 1095–102.

54. Tunkel AR, Mandell GL. Infecting micro-organisms. In: *Infective Endocarditis* (Kaye D, ed.). New York: Raven Press, 1992; 85–97.

55. Wahl MJ. Myths of dental-induced endocarditis. *Comp. Cont. Educ. Dent.* 1994; 15: 1100–19.

56. Williams CECS, Davenport ES, Sterne JAC, Sivapathasundaram V, Fearne JM, Curtis MA. Mechanisms of risk in preterm low-birthweight infants. *Periodontol. 2000* 2000; 23: 142–50.

57. Williams RC, Offenbacher S. Periodontal medicine: the emergence of a new branch of periodontology. *Periodontol. 2000* 2000; 23: 9–12.

58. Wilson W, Taubert KA, Gewitz M, Lockhart PB, Baddour LM, Levison M, et al. American Heart Association Rheumatic Fever, Endocarditis and Kawasaki Disease Committee, Council on Cardiovascular Disease in the Young; Council on Clinical Cardiology; Council on Cardiovascular Surgery and Anesthesia; Quality of Care and Outcomes Research Interdisciplinary Working Group; American Dental Association. Prevention of infective endocarditis: guidelines from the American Heart Association: a guideline from the American Heart Association Rheumatic Fever, Endocarditis and Kawasaki Disease Committee, Council on Cardiovascular Disease in the Young, and the Council on Clinical Cardiology, Council on Cardiovascular Surgery and Anesthesia, and the Quality of Care and Outcomes Research Interdisciplinary Working Group. *Circulation* 2007; 116: 1736–54.

59. Younessi OJ, Walker DM, Ellis P, Dwyer DE. Fatal *Staphylococcus aureus* infective endocarditis. The dental implications. *Oral Surg. Oral Med. Oral Pathol. Oral Radiol. Endod.* 1998; 85: 168–72.

Chapter 9
Treatment of the necrotic pulp

Paul Wesselink and Gunnar Bergenholtz

Introduction

This chapter details the procedures utilized to carry out conservative root canal therapy (RCT) of teeth with necrotic pulps. The treatment principles described apply to teeth where the root canal system may or may not be infected. Treatment of non-infected cases is a prophylactic measure to prevent colonization and multiplication of microbes in the more or less empty root canal space and the subsequent development of symptomatic or non-symptomatic presentations of apical periodontitis (Chapter 7). In most instances, however, RCT is curative and initiated to eliminate a root canal infection, thereby remedying periapical inflammatory tissue lesions (Fig. 9.1). Treatment in such cases is also essential to impede the spread of root canal bacteria and their prod-

ucts to distant organs (Chapter 8). Although extraction of the tooth in question solves the infection problem, it is a radical procedure not usually acceptable to patients. RCT offers a realistic alternative, provided the tooth is restorable. Hence, if properly conducted, RCT of teeth with infected pulp necrosis enjoys a high rate of success and can be expected to result in complete resolution of clinical and radiographic signs of apical periodontitis in almost nine out of ten cases (29, 56).

Objectives and general treatment strategies

The overall objective of RCT is to exclude the root canal system as a source of microorganisms. Therefore a

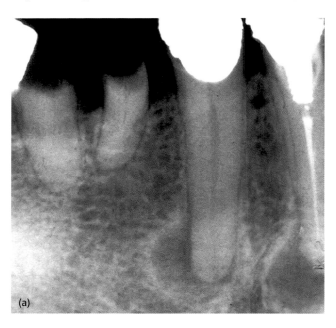
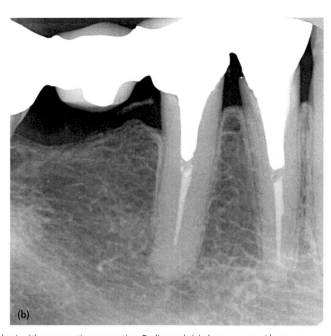

Fig. 9.1 The reason for carrying out root canal therapy of teeth with necrotic pulps is either preventive or curative. Radiograph (a) shows a second lower premolar with a well-delineated apical radiolucency in a 57-year-old woman, indicating infected pulp necrosis and apical periodontitis. The neighboring root filled first premolar also has an apical lesion suggesting an unsuccessful prior root canal treatment. Radiograph (b) is a follow-up radiograph taken 24 years after completion of endodontic treatment of both teeth that were included as abutments in a bridgework. There is now no evidence of apical bone lesions. The case demonstrates the potentials of carefully conducted RCT for a long-term successful outcome.

primary task includes efforts to eradicate bacteria resident in the root canal system (Fig. 9.2). A second charge is to provide measures to ensure that root canal infection will not recur. The procedure includes several phases, of which mechanical instrumentation to clean and shape root canals (Chapter 11), irrigation and disinfection are critical elements. To prevent reinfection, a filling is subsequently placed in the instrumented root canal(s) (Fig. 9.1b).

If successfully conducted, teeth with clinical symptoms of apical periodontitis (tenderness, pain, swelling, fistulae) become non-symptomatic. Successful treatment also demands that any radiographic evidence of apical periodontitis that existed prior to treatment should resolve and result in complete reorganization of the periapical tissue (Figs 9.1b and 9.3).

Historical perspective

Over the years, different approaches to combat endodontic infections have been in vogue. At the beginning of the 20th century, following the discovery of the role bacteria play in disease processes in general and apical periodontitis in particular, emphasis was placed on the use of strong antiseptics. Such agents were phenol derivatives and their mixtures, e.g. methylacresylacetate and camphorated monochlorophenol, and formaldehyde and its derivatives, e.g. formocresol and paraformaldehyde (12). Antiseptic agents were administered either to the orifice or to the interior of root canals in paste or liquid form. By evaporation of the medicament, bacterial organisms could be killed without a cleaning procedure or filling of the root canal system. In other modes of

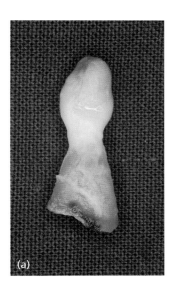
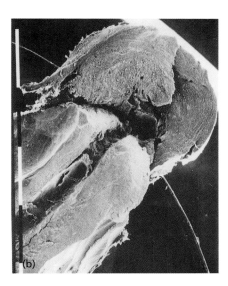
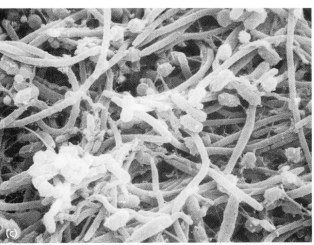
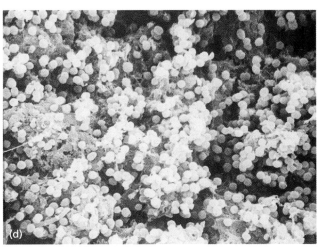

Fig. 9.2 (a) An extracted tooth with attached inflammatory soft-tissue lesion. On cracking the tooth open (b) and observing the interior (c, d) in the scanning electron microscope, various forms of bacterial morphotypes may be identified on the root canal walls, including filaments, spirochetes, rods and cocci. (Figures (b)–(d) are from Molven et al. (37) and published with permission of Munksgaard.) (Courtesy of Dr O. Molven.)

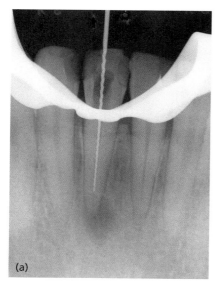

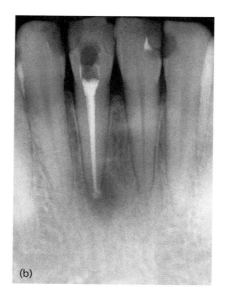

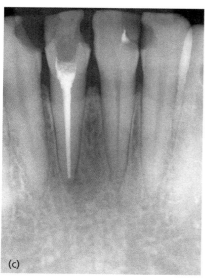

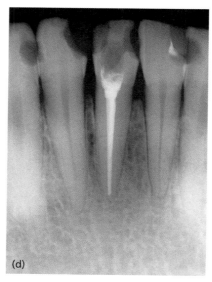

Fig. 9.3 A series of radiographs demonstrating the successful outcome of root canal therapy in a lower incisor. (a) A root canal instrument is placed in the canal, which is used to clean the canal and determine the length of instrumentation in relation to the radiographic apex. In this case working length had to be extended. Note the apical radiolucency, indicating apical periodontitis. (b) The instrumented canal has received a slightly overextended root filling. (c) A radiograph taken 2 years later. (d) Radiograph taken 6 years later, showing complete resolution of the previous lesion. The tooth now rests on a healthy periodontium and there are no symptoms (tenderness, pain, swellings) suggesting ongoing root canal infection.

treatment strong antiseptics were combined with mechanical instrumentation, followed by filling the instrumented canal(s) with a paste containing a strong antiseptic agent. It was felt that incorporation of antiseptics in the root filling material would allow a continuous release of the antiseptic agent which would prevent survival and regrowth of any organisms that had not been killed by the instrumentation procedure. Indeed, such treatment approaches gained great popularity and are practiced even today. However, the use of strong antiseptics in endodontics raises several serious concerns:

- Although they are effective against microbes, strong antiseptics cause substantial cell and tissue damage, particularly if extruded to the periapical tissue environment (59) (see also Chapter 12).
- These disinfectants, also in diluted form, have the disadvantage of sensibilization and hypersensitivity responses (Chapter 12). Some chemicals even carry carcinogenic and mutagenic risks (32).
- In liquid form, chemicals are rapidly inactivated by inflammatory exudate and therefore provide antibacterial effects only of a short duration, becoming inactive within hours or a few days (22, 34).
- Since antiseptics included in root filling materials will eventually lose their antibacterial activity infection can reappear if canals were improperly filled or poorly sealed coronally, or both.

In recent decades the strategy for treatment of necrotic and infected pulps has changed in the move to more biocompatible methods. Thorough biomechanical instrumentation, combined with extensive irrigation with light antiseptics and with the use of minimally toxic and allergenic disinfectants, is now emphasized and will be detailed here.

Scheme for a routine procedure in root canal therapy

To achieve an optimal result by RCT, several critical steps can be identified:

1. Assessing, prior to treatment, the technical difficulties that may be encountered during the procedure in terms of being able to access and negotiate the root canal anatomy (see Chapter 11).
2. Opening the tooth to be treated in order to localize all canals, so-called access opening preparation.
3. Providing an aseptic field of operation including the use of rubber dams.
4. Carrying out mechanical instrumentation of the canal interior.
5. Irrigating the canal system to remove debris and provide chemical disinfection.
6. Placing an antimicrobial dressing until the next appointment.
7. Closing the root canal system between appointments.
8. Assessing the result of the initial treatment.
9. Carrying out root canal filling.
10. Recalling the patient in 6–12 months to assess long-term outcome.

Access opening

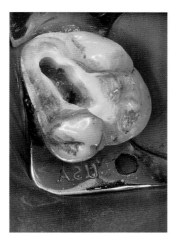

Once a decision for treatment has been taken and the difficulties assessed as to the presence of canal obstacles, length of canals and extent of curvatures, the root canal system needs be accessed. The most important quality of the access opening preparation is to uncover all the canal orifices present, so that an unobstructed mechanical preparation of each root canal can be carried out (see further Chapter 11). It is often advantageous to enter the tooth interior prior to the placement of a rubber dam to reduce the risk of going in the wrong direction and causing a perforation to the periodontal ligament space. Aligning the direction of the bur to the long axis of the tooth facilitates the procedure. This is particularly significant in the teeth of elderly patients, where the pulp chamber is often reduced by mineralization and is then difficult to find. It applies also to teeth with artificial crowns.

Aseptic technique

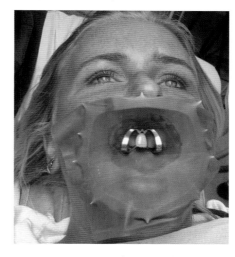

Even though teeth with necrotic pulps are most often infected, RCT requires an aseptic technique of operation. Asepsis is maintained first of all to exclude contamination with organisms that have greater resistance to treatment than members of the root canal microbiota. Common contaminants, which are difficult to manage, belong to the facultative Gram-positive segment, most notably enterococci; other enteric bacteria and yeasts may be introduced into the canal system owing to failure to maintain proper asepsis. Other sources of contaminating organisms are along leaky temporary restorations applied between treatment sessions and by leaving canals open to the oral cavity for drainage (54, 65). Elimination of microorganisms from root canals naturally requires prevention of oral contaminants. As stated in Chapter 4, procedures in this context include removal of plaque and calculus, defective fillings and crowns and carious dentin prior to the initiation of treatment. For the subsequent RCT, proper rubber dam application is indispensable and sterile burs and instruments must be used.

Mechanical instrumentation

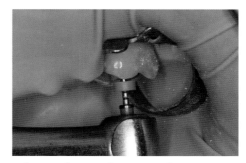

Cleaning the canal interior with hand and rotary instruments is a most important technique to remove the bulk of the infecting bacterial mass and its nutritional supply. The instrumentation, if possible, should be carried out throughout the entire extension of each root canal and ideally end at its exit or slightly short of the apical foramen. The procedure aims to:

• Physically remove as much as possible of the bacterial mass, including those bacteria attached to the root

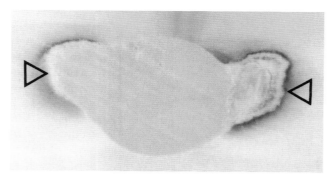

Fig. 9.4 Cross-sectional cut through a root canal partly filled with gutta-percha. Note the unfilled lateral extensions (arrow heads), which may provide space for bacterial growth and leakage of bacterial elements to the periapical tissue environment.

canal walls in a biofilm structure and those free-floating in the canal.

- Remove sources of substrate for bacterial regrowth and multiplication, including necrotic tissue and tissue-breakdown products.
- Remove the inner portion of the root canal walls, where dentin is most heavily infected.
- Provide access for irrigation solutions to all parts of the root canal system for cleaning and chemical disinfection.
- Create a clean and properly shaped canal that facilitates the insertion of a well-sealing root filling.

The task is not an easy one. Not only are microorganisms located in the main canal(s) (Fig. 9.2) but they will also enter any space and ramification available to them, including dentinal tubules (45), isthmuses and lateral canals. This makes the cleaning and disinfection procedure precarious as well as demanding. In this context it needs to be recognized that crevices and lateral areas of oval-shaped canals (Fig. 9.4) are especially difficult to reach. If untouched by the instruments, both substrate and bacterial organisms may remain in such locations and, if they are allowed a pathway to the apical environment, a failure may ensue. In fact, studies examining the extent to which root canals are rendered clean after instrumentation often find remnants of necrotic tissue and debris on the canal walls, especially in oval-shaped canals (69) and in isthmuses of mesial roots of mandibular molars (39). Bacteria lodged in dentinal tubules also may remain unaffected.

Narrow, partially blocked canals and canals in severely curved roots further challenge the instrumentation procedure (Fig. 9.5a, b). Instrumentation is also a demanding task where canals are extremely wide, e.g. in young immature teeth (Fig. 9.5c). One reason for this is that the armamentarium normally is not designed for treatment of teeth with incomplete root development. Another is that instrumentation in such cases has to be limited owing to the already thin root structure to limit risk for

subsequent root fracture. Therefore, combating infection in such root canals has to rely more on chemical disinfection and proper root filling than the mechanical instrumentation *per se* (see also Chapter 11).

The instrumentation procedure is a highly important step in RCT. By enlarging and preparing canals and giving them shape for access to irrigants, chemical disinfectants and filling, the bulk of the infecting microbiota is physically removed (3–6). Therefore the time spent in cleaning and shaping root canals according to the principles described in Chapter 11 is well worthwhile.

To enhance the cleaning capacity over and beyond what the mechanical preparation with hand and rotary instruments can do, it has been shown that ultrasonic activation of the irrigating solution has a positive effect. It is important that the ultrasonic instrument moves freely within the canal without active preparation, so-called passive ultrasonic irrigation (64). This measure is therefore applied after the mechanical instrumentation. The use of a small ultrasonic file, preferably with a smooth surface in order to prevent damage to the canal wall or ledge formation, is advocated (Fig. 9.6).

Considerations in routine cases

The instrumentation technique in routine cases, i.e. when the canal anatomy is within a fairly normal range in terms of width, length and curvature (Figs 9.1 and 9.3), is no different to that carried out in conjunction with pulpectomy (Chapter 4). Yet, there are certain precautions that need be undertaken to avoid three complications:

- Blocking the canal patency.
- Causing an endodontic flare-up.
- Overextending the apical foramen.

Blocking the canal patency can occur by fracturing an instrument, by causing a ledge or pushing dentin debris into the apical portion of the canal. These complications are particularly common in narrow and curved canals and are often the result of improper technique. Obviously, effective removal of the infecting microbiota is hampered by such errors. Therefore it is important that the instrumentation procedure follows a well-proven scheme of steps (see Chapter 11).

To reduce the risk of causing an *endodontic flare-up* (Chapter 7) and *overextension of the apical foramen*, proper determination of the length of instrumentation (working length) is especially important in RCT (Core concept 9.1). This measure is undertaken primarily to ensure that the entire length of each canal is treated, if possible. If instrumentation is carried out too short, substantial amounts of bacteria may be left behind and continue to sustain apical periodontitis. Indeed, this is a major cause of failure in RCT (56).

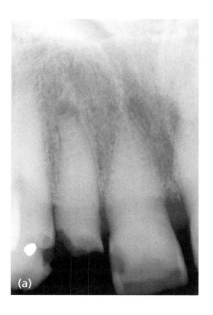
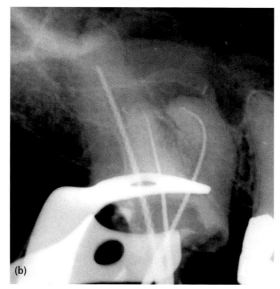
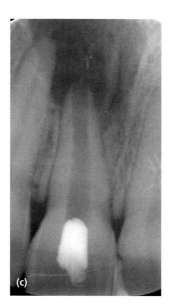
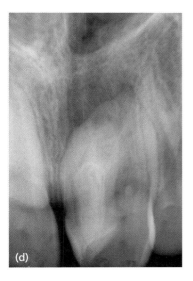
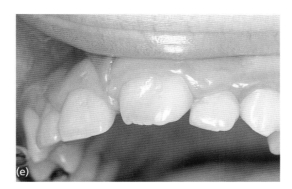
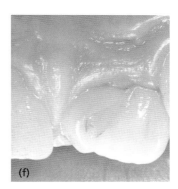
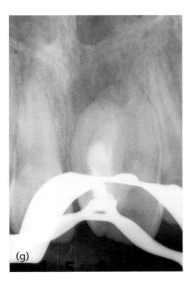
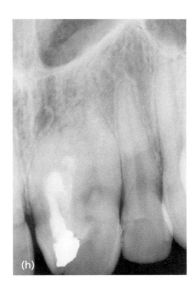

Fig. 9.5 Examples of cases displaying various degrees of difficulty: (a) a partially blocked canal in 12 due to previous mineralization processes in the pulp; (b) a tooth with severely curved root canal anatomy in the mesial root; (c) a tooth with incomplete root development; (d) a supernumerary tooth with a dense invaginatus fused to the permanent incisor; (e) buccal aspect; (f) lingual aspect. Following instrumentation and filling of the invagination only (g), the periapical lesion resolved (h). The tooth responded to an electronic pulp tester and cold, indicating that the other root portion had a vital pulp.

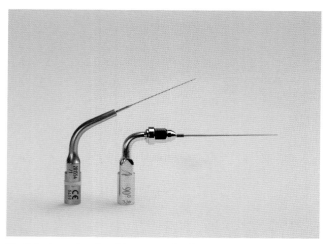

Fig. 9.6 Examples of small instruments for ultrasonic activation of root canal irrigant.

Core concept 9.1

Working length is a term used for the length a given root canal should be mechanically instrumented. Two methods are currently in use to determine this length:

(1) Radiographic assessment with a file inserted into the canal to the vicinity of the apex (Fig. 9.3a).
(2) Electronic apex locator.

For detailed descriptions on the use of these methods see Chapter 11.

Core concept 9.2

Overextension of the apical foramen in conjunction with RCT is a serious complication because:

- Bacterial organisms and infected debris may be extruded into the periapical tissue and cause a flare-up of a non-painful lesion, aggravate a painful lesion and/or perpetuate apical periodontitis on a long-term basis.
- It may result in enhanced nutritional supply of any remaining organisms and boost their growth to cause endodontic flare-ups and/or long-term failure.
- It enhances the risk of overfilling.
- The potential to carry out a permanent root filling, which seals the apical portion bacteria-tight, is often impaired.

Careful working length determination is also important to prevent a set of complications that may ensue if instrumentation is carried out beyond the apical foramen (Core concept 9.2). One complication relates to the risk of extruding bacteria and infected dentin debris into the periapical tissue. If especially virulent, such organisms

may aggravate a periapical inflammatory condition and cause the development of painful symptoms, including an apical abscess (endodontic flare-up). Extruded infected debris may also perpetuate apical periodontitis, despite complete elimination of bacterial organisms from the canal system itself (70).

Over-instrumentation also extends the apical foramen and promotes entry of inflammatory exudate into the canal. Owing to its content of serum proteins, the growth of proteolytic organisms is then likely to be boosted. This latter mechanism may also lead to an endodontic flare-up.

Another grave complication of overpreparation is so-called apical zipping (Chapter 11). This is when the canal orifice has been not only enlarged but also transported in a lateral direction. Similar to an incompletely developed root, such canals are extremely difficult to fill properly. Besides the risk of overfilling, the root canal filling is often unable to provide an apical seal (68). In fact, unfilled spaces (pockets) often remain along the apical portion of the root filling, where bacteria may continue to grow and maintain apical periodontitis (40).

Controlling pain during instrumentation

Usually treatment of a necrotic pulp does not require anesthesia. However, even in the presence of a radiolucency, functional sensory nerve fibers may remain in the apical portion of the canal (33). Once canal instruments touch these fibers, a pain response is initiated. Thus, for painless completion of treatment, anesthesia may be required. Some patients may allow the necessary instrumentation without anesthesia, but this should not be conducted unless complete agreement with the patient has been sought. Pain is usually gone after instrumentation with one or two file sizes.

There is some benefit in carrying out the treatment without anesthesia for length control. Hence, a pain response during instrumentation of a necrotic pulp may indicate that the foramen has been inadvertently pierced and that the working length should be reassessed. This should be carried out in spite of what appears to be a correctly recorded working length. Distinction between nerve fiber remnants and overpreparation is not always obvious and to ensure proper length of instrumentation one may:

1. Take a control radiograph under a 20° distal or mesial angle with a file in place to obtain a good image of the buccal or lingual aspect of the root (such a radiograph shows more clearly than an orthogonal picture if the tip of the file extends into the periodontium).
2. Carry out additional measurements with an apex locator.

3. Insert paper points to the presumed working length and observe whether moisture (bleeding or exudation) is picked up.

In other words, because of the sometimes deviant exit of the apical foramen into the periodontium, it is advantageous to carry out RCT in the absence of anesthesia because this draws attention to the risk of overinstrumenting the canal. Yet, the comfort of the patient should always be given the highest priority.

Irrigation and chemical disinfection

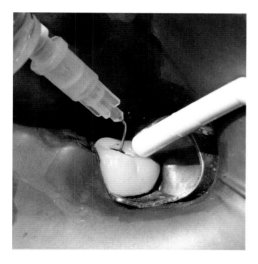

Mechanical instrumentation of root canals needs to be supported by frequent irrigation. There are several important purposes of such a measure:

- To clean out debris and dentinal shavings and to keep canals moist so that instruments run smoothly.
- To exert antibacterial effects.
- To augment the efficacy of the instrumentation procedure by dissolving necrotic tissue remnants, especially in areas mechanical instrumentation cannot reach, including crevices, isthmuses and accessory canals.
- To dissolve the smear layer.

Another desirable property of the agent to be used is that it should cause minimal tissue damage and thus be minimally toxic in case it is extruded into the periapical tissue environment.

Various irrigating solutions are available, but none can be said to satisfy all these requirements. Furthermore, it should be recognized that efficacy of agents as far as their disinfecting ability is limited by interactions with dentin, dentin debris and organic compounds present in the root canals of necrotic pulps, *viz.* serum proteins and microbial biomasses. This means that endodontic disin-

fectants may not be as potent as indicated by trials carried out *in vitro* (25). Commonly used irrigants are sodium hypochlorite (NaOCl) and ethylenediaminetetraacetic acid (EDTA). The specific properties of these agents will be described here in some detail.

Sodium hypochlorite

The most commonly employed solution for endodontic irrigation is NaOCl, which unites three important qualities essential to RCT:

- It dissolves organic material.
- It is a potent disinfectant.
- It is minimally irritating to tissue in low concentrations.

The tissue-dissolving capacity of NaOCl is well established (2, 38). Both vital and necrotic tissue are affected and dissolved in excess of NaOCl. The speed of tissue dissolution is dependent on the extent of contact between active solution and tissue. Thus, stirring or the use of ultrasound will speed up the tissue-dissolving process considerably (38).

The effect of NaOCl is quickly inactivated in the presence of oxidizable material, such as dentin debris and organic material, because it dissociates into Na^+ and Cl^- ions (24, 38). Therefore, during RCT, the solution has to be replenished consistently. Although NaOCl breaks down collagen, it hardly affects the canal walls (23, 52). The addition of surfactant, which should promote its flow into areas inaccessible for mechanical instrumentation, or hydrogen peroxide has not been confirmed to provide significant therapeutic effects.

Sodium hypochlorite is a strong and fast-acting disinfectant with a low tissue-irritating potential at low concentrations (0.5–1%) (48). Yet, it is a potent tissue irritant in higher concentrations (2.5–5%) (26, 28, 31, 48). High concentrations should therefore be either avoided or used with great care so that no solution is dropped into the eyes of the patient or extruded beyond the apical foramen, which may cause severe tissue irritation (Clinical procedure 9.1). The risk–benefit ratio of the use of high concentrations of NaOCl can be questioned further on the basis of the limited gain in antibacterial effect found in clinical trials (6, 71).

Ethylenediaminetetraacetic acid

EDTA is a calcium binder (chelator) that aids in removal of the smear layer. The smear layer is mainly composed of dentin particles embedded in an amorphous mass of organic material that forms on the inner root canal walls during the instrumentation procedure. Sodium hypo-

<table>
<tr><td>

Clinical procedure 9.1   Prevention and treatment of complications due to extrusion of irrigating solutions beyond the apical foramen

To prevent extrusion
- Use a small-diameter needle (0.4 mm), apply a rubber stop on the needle for length control, and insert no further than 2 mm short of the working length.
- Ensure that the needle is never locked into the canal.
- Do not use excessive pressure to force the fluid out of the syringe.

Sequelae to extrusion
- Immediate pain response, which may or may not be followed by edema.
- Within a few hours extensive swelling may occur in lip and eyelid.
- After some days there may be an extraoral hematoma and some local soft-tissue necrosis.

Treatment of severe sequelae
- Administer strong analgesics. Local anesthetic may be administered but no vasoconstriction should be used in order to prevent the development of further tissue necrosis.
- Cold compresses during the first 6 hours may give some relief.

</td></tr>
</table>

chlorite is unable to dissolve this debris, which often contains bacterial organisms. Some contend that it is advantageous to leave the smear layer intact because it acts as a physical barrier for bacteria lodged in dentinal tubules and thereby locks them in. On the other hand, the smear layer counteracts disinfectants and blocks the penetration of medicaments into the dentinal tubules. It also interferes with adhesion and penetration of root filling material. For effective removal of the smear layer after preparation and irrigation with NaOCl one may leave EDTA in the canal for approximately 1 min. Alternatively, citric acid may be used for smear layer removal.

Other irrigants and methods for canal disinfection

A variety of other irrigants have also found application in RCT including detergents, chemotherapeutics and combinations thereof. Only brief comments are given here as supporting clinical evidence for these agents is limited.

Chlorhexidine. This agent is of interest because of its extensive use as an effective antimicrobial in other medical and dental contexts. It is biocompatible and adheres to hydroxyapatite (25). Because of its affinity to dentin, chlorhexidine has been suggested as a final rinse, as, once bound to the surface, it has prolonged activity, a

phenomenon called substantivity. Good clinical evidence confirming the advantage of the use of chlorhexidine as a final rinse is, however, lacking (71). As a sole iririgant in RCT it has the disadvantage of not being tissue-dissolving (47).

Antibiotics. The local use of antibiotics in RCT has been regarded as inappropriate owing to the limited clinical efficacy attained in clinical trials and the potential for sensitization and induction of bacterial resistance. Recently, a mixture of doxycycline, a semi-synthetic tetracycline, citric acid and a detergent (Tween 80) termed MTAD was introduced and has gained some popularity as a final rinse after NaOCl irrigation by virtue of promising *in vitro* results (50).

Photodynamic therapy. Photodynamic therapy is also under exploration (20). This method does not make use of active chemicals but uses light of a specific wavelength to generate oxygen-based free radicals in a non-toxic compound by photoactivation. This so-called photosensitizer is then administered to the instrumented root canals, where it may penetrate areas untouched by the instrumentation procedure and aid in killing residual bacteria following light activation.

Interappointment dressing

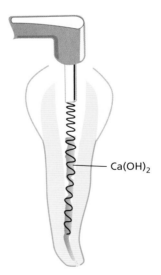

Ca(OH)$_2$

Mechanical instrumentation and irrigation with an antimicrobial solution (*biomechanical preparation*) has been found to render root canals free of cultivable organisms in approximately 50–80% of treated cases (3–6, 44, 51, 55). In teeth where bacteria were still recovered the number was nonetheless greatly reduced, showing that biomechanical preparation and irrigation, if carefully conducted, is quite an effective means of bacterial removal in RCT. Nevertheless, if there are space and potential for nutritional supply after the procedure, regrowth to original numbers may occur. Therefore, further measures need be taken to control the root canal infection.

Essentially, there are two approaches to render the low number of remaining bacteria harmless:

1. To further enhance bacterial elimination before the permanent root filling by applying a long-acting disinfectant in the instrumented canal(s) between two treatment sessions; a so-called *interappointment dressing*.
2. To entomb the remaining bacteria in the permanently filled root canal space. Root filling is then carried out after completion of the biomechanical preparation in the same visit. It is expected that the antibacterial activity of the root canal sealer, in its unset stage, kills the organisms and/or they become deprived of nutritional supply and space for regrowth if pathways from and to the periapical tissue are effectively blocked. This procedure is often referred to as *one-appointment endodontics*.

In straightforward, non-symptomatic teeth, where treatment can be carried out without complications and within a reasonable time span, a case can be made for completion of RCT in one session (62). A one-visit treatment saves time and further offers the advantage that the peculiarities of the canal anatomy (e.g. curvatures, irregularities) are current to the operator and canals are therefore likely to be easier to fill than at a second appointment a week, or weeks or months later. Furthermore, any residual organisms in fins and crevices of the canal or in dentinal tubules, or both, may be enclosed by the root filling, thus offsetting their pathogenic potential. Against this approach can be argued that root fillings do not invariably seal root canals hermetically and any residual organisms may find both space and nutritional supply for regrowth, which may result in an endodontic failure. Indeed, Sjögren *et al.* (57), in a clinical follow-up, observed that the outcome of RCT of teeth with apical periodontitis was significantly less successful if cultivatable bacterial organisms were recovered at the time of filling rather than if not. Similar findings have been reported from an experimental study in monkeys (16). Although several studies support the view that, after biomechanical preparation and before the permanent filling, root canals should be medicated with an antibacterial dressing until a second treatment session (3–6, 61), conflicting data exist as to the merit of such a measure (36, 44, 67). Nonetheless, RCT should never be rushed at the expense of proper instrumentation and chemical disinfection in order to finish it in one session. Furthermore, awaiting the disappearance of clinical signs of ongoing infection is another strong argument for postponing permanent root filling to a later appointment (Core concept 9.3).

Core concept 9.3   Reasons for withholding root filling until a later appointment after completion of biomechanical instrumentation

(1) To observe the direct effect of the treatment on the prevailing clinical symptoms, including pain, swellings and fistulae, and on lesions where the prognosis is regarded doubtful (if not resolving, renewed treatment can be carried out without having to remove the permanent root filling).
(2) To control apical suppuration, exudation or bleeding.
(3) To ensure that sufficient time is available for completion of the biomechanical preparation.

Selecting an intracanal dressing

Over the years a multitude of antimicrobial agents has been used for intracanal dressing in RCT, including pastes, various forms of tinctures and aqueous solutions (12, 17). Iodine–potassium iodide (IKI, 5% and 10%) is an example of an aqueous solution with appealing properties. It is a potent disinfectant (41) because iodine evaporates to reach far into the dentinal tubules, crevices and fins of root canals (41, 49). Furthermore, its cytotoxic potential is low (59). However, in root canals the antimicrobial activity is of short duration and IKI is therefore unsuitable for use over extended periods of time. In fact, this applies to any liquid medicament because such agents are rapidly inactivated in root canals, particularly when there is seepage of exudate from an apical inflammatory process. As a consequence, there is potential for regrowth of bacteria in the interim phase (5, 6). If liquid medicaments are to be used they should ideally be applied only for a short period (5–10 min) followed by a temporary or permanent root filling in an attempt to kill organisms in spaces inaccessible to instrumentation (30). The clinical efficacy of such a measure is, however, equivocal (36).

As an interappointment dressing, a substance should be selected that is not easily replaced by tissue fluid and that can remain physically intact over weeks or months. As such a water-slurry of calcium hydroxide ($Ca(OH)_2$) combines several attractive features (17, 53). It is a strongly alkaline substance (pH 12.5) that dissociates into calcium and hydroxyl ions in aqueous solution; the latter provide antimicrobial effects (5) (Advanced concept 9.1) and tissue-dissolving capacity (27). With its fairly low solubility and mere physical presence, it may be used as an intracanal dressing over long periods of time (Fig. 9.7). Its most essential function is then to obstruct bacterial regrowth, which may occur by:

• filling the instrumented root canal space and thereby serve as a space-holder;

- blocking nutritional supply of inflammatory exudates derived from the apical lesion;
- serving as a deterrent for bacterial entry of the instrumented canal by the release of bactericidal hydroxyl ions.

It should be noted that because of its low solubility the antibacterial capacity of $Ca(OH)_2$ is limited to the near vicinity of the microorganisms. Therefore it cannot be expected to effectively kill organisms in non-instrumented parts of the root canal or bacteria lodged in dentinal tubules (41, 53) (see also Advanced concept 9.1). Yet, $Ca(OH)_2$ serves as an ideal intracanal dressing for follow-up of treatment effects and thus offers convenient scheduling of the patients. Thereby, ample time can be reserved for observation of tissue healing in progress, e.g. for large lesions, symptomatic lesions or when prognosis for a successful outcome in any other respect appears questionable (Fig. 9.7).

In RCT, $Ca(OH)_2$ also serves an important function in controlling seepage of inflammatory exudates into root canals. This type of leakage is a particular problem in conjunction with symptomatic periapical lesions, where suppuration hampers effective disinfection and adhesion of root filling material to the canal walls. In such instances permanent root filling is contraindicated. Healing of the acute phase of the lesion is promoted by blocking the canal space for bacterial multiplication and the associated release of inflammatogenic substances to the periapical tissue. Normally this will occur within 1 week and RCT can subsequently be continued. In other instances, for example in cases of large cyst-like lesions, repeated change of calcium hydroxide paste may be necessary before a treatment effect can be attained (7).

Advanced concept 9.1   The antibacterial effect of calcium hydroxide in RCT

Calcium hydroxide is mainly used in saturated aqueous suspensions but also has been combined with many other vehicles (for overview see Ref. 17). An aqueous suspension generates high pH, which provides great cytotoxic potential and kills bacteria and host cells by cell membrane protein denaturation and DNA damage (53). In spite of its tissue-damaging potential, $Ca(OH)_2$ has gained wide acceptance as an effective antimicrobial agent in endodontic therapies. An important rationale is that the substance is reasonably tissue compatible owing to its slow water solubility and diffusibility. Because of these properties, cytotoxicity is limited to the tissue area which it contacts, where limited necrosis is normally induced. Its lethal effects on bacterial cells also relate to its caustic action by the release of hydroxyl ions. Yet, owing to its poor solubility and diffusibility, $Ca(OH)_2$ is a rather inefficient antimicrobial for microorganisms lodged in pulpal remnants, crevices of the canal and dentinal tubules (41, 49). It has been shown also that hydroxyapatite inhibits its antibacterial capacity (24) and that $Ca(OH)_2$ is effective against only a limited spectrum of the root canal microbiota. For example, both enterococci and yeasts sustain a high alkaline environment and are able to survive in root canals medicated with $Ca(OH)_2$ (54, 65). These are likely reasons why controversy has emerged over its usefulness as an antimicrobial agent in RCT. Although several clinical trials have observed that root canals are rendered free of cultivable bacteria following its application for a week or more (6, 51), others have found that microorganisms can still be recovered from a substantial number of treated root canals (30, 42, 44). Differences in findings may relate to the type of teeth included in the studies and the associated effectiveness of the biomechanical preparation, sampling technique and the extent to which $Ca(OH)_2$ was eliminated from the root canals prior to the sampling procedure.

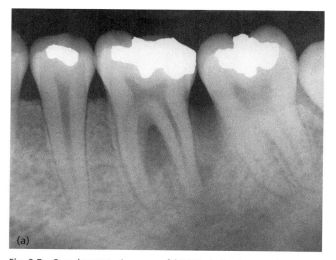 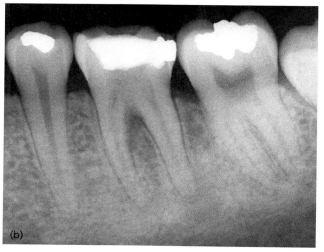

Fig. 9.7   Case demonstrating successful RCT including interappointment $Ca(OH)_2$ dressing of tooth 36, where the prognosis was deemed questionable *a priori* owing to a large distal bone lesion and a lesion in the furcal region. (a) Initial radiograph; (b) follow-up radiograph at 6 months showing almost complete resolution of the bone lesions. (Courtesy of Dr C. Reit.)

Closing the root canal system between appointments

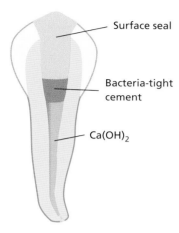

Surface seal

Bacteria-tight cement

Ca(OH)$_2$

To exclude bacterial contamination in endodontics, adequate temporary seals between appointments are required. Furthermore, canals should never be left open to the oral cavity for any extended period of time because of the risk of introducing oral organisms that are difficult to clear.

The first step is to fill the instrumented root canal space in its entirety with Ca(OH)$_2$. Application can be done following mixing of Ca(OH)$_2$ powder and sterile water to a creamy paste, which is spiraled into the canal with a lentulo spiral. This instrument is made of a fine, flexible wire spiraled in the shape of a reverse auger. It should be turned in a clockwise direction in a handpiece at slow speed and brought to the vicinity of the working length. Applying light pressure with a small cotton pellet at the canal orifice ensures the entire canal is filled. A disadvantage of this method is the risk of extruding Ca(OH)$_2$ beyond the apical foramen, and particular care should be taken when filling lower molars, which are close to the mandibular canal. While devices exist for injection of Ca(OH)$_2$, e.g. a commercially available syringe filled with Ca(OH)$_2$, the use of a lentulo spiral has been shown to be more effective (43).

After application, the excess material in the pulp chamber should be removed and blotted dry with the end of a paper point or cotton pellet. The canal orifice and adjacent part of the pulp chamber should then be sealed with a soft temporary cement (e.g. Cavit, zinc oxide–eugenol) followed by a more rigid temporary filling that withstands the wear and pressure by occlusal forces (e.g. thick mixes of zinc phosphate cement, IRM, glass ionomer). The first layer of soft cement ensures that a bacteria-tight seal is established until the second visit. At the second visit an ultrasonic scaler or spoon excavator can then easily remove the cement without running the risk of damaging the tooth structure.

Root filling

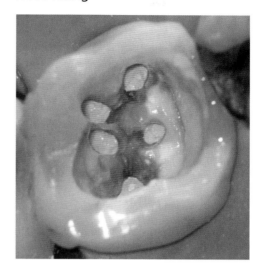

Permanent root filling of teeth with an infected necrotic pulp should not be carried out unless the biomechanical preparation is complete and no exudation exists in the canal that prevents adherence of the filling to the root canal walls. It is also regarded good clinical practice to postpone permanent root filling until the tooth is free from pain and other clinical symptoms of root canal infection. An objective means which helps the clinician to decide when bacterial elimination is complete is not readily available. It was once believed that a bacterial sample would be able to provide guidance in this respect. Hence, a positive sample taken after biomechanical preparation would indicate that it should be continued, whereas a negative culture would signal successful disinfection. The methodology is currently not commonly practiced as a treatment control as many residual organisms may escape detection by sampling and laboratory processing (see also Advanced concept 9.2).

Clinical and radiographic follow-up

Patients subjected to RCT should be asked to return for a check-up appointment within a period of 6–12 months (15). The purpose of that appointment is to ensure, by clinical and radiographic examination, that healing is complete or in progress. Signs of a successful outcome are that no clinical symptoms (pain, fistulae, tenderness and swellings) prevail or have appeared (Core concept 9.4). Inspection, palpation and percussion tests and examination of periodontal pocket probing depths (to search for fistulae along the periodontal ligament) can confirm such a condition.

Radiographic examination reveals the extent to which a preoperative radiolucency has disappeared (Fig. 9.3). By 4–6 months, radiographs may already reveal signs of bone

> ### Advanced concept 9.2 The use of bacteriological sampling in RCT
>
> There are situations when bacterial sampling of root canals is a valuable tool. One is when RCT does not result in elimination of clinical symptoms. Such problems may be associated with the presence of unusual pathogens, i.e. *Pseudomonas*, *Proteus* and *Staphylococcus aureus*. In other instances, the lack of therapeutic effect may be due to a severe contamination problem. In medically compromised patients on immunosuppressive therapy and in patients at very high risk of endocarditis or with multiple heart valve prostheses, a sample at the initial appointment is warranted to determine antimicrobial susceptibility in case a flare-up or a systemic complication ensues. This precaution may be undertaken in spite of the facts that patients are prescribed antimicrobial prophylaxis and that not all microorganisms may be susceptible to the prescription given. If possible, it is normally wise to refer these patients to an endodontic specialist.
>
> Collecting a sample from root canals requires access to a laboratory that can process it. Some dental schools and large hospitals offer a mail-in service and provide culture materials, including sampling fluid and transport media.
>
> Taking a sample requires effective rubber dam isolation and proper disinfection to avoid inclusion of contaminating organisms. This precaution is absolutely essential, otherwise the information is worthless. In line with these measures, all subsequent procedures must be undertaken with sterile instruments and proper aseptic technique. Prior to sampling, canals should have been emptied of paste medicaments for several days to allow the accumulation of a sufficient number of organisms to be collected. Following the opening of the canal, any exudate present is first collected onto an absorbent point. The point is then transferred to a vial containing transport medium. If the canal is dry, sampling fluid is added and a root canal instrument, preferably a Hedström file, is used to shave off dentin debris from the root canal walls along the canal length. Paper points are used to transfer the suspension of dentin filings and sampling fluid to the transport medium. The sample, along with a completed referral form, should be mailed to the laboratory within 1 day. The result can usually be received within 1 week.

> ### Core concept 9.4 Evaluation criteria
>
> Root canal therapy is considered successful when there is:
>
> - No pain to apical palpation.
> - No pain or tenderness to percussion.
> - No sinus tract.
> - No swelling.
> - Complete bone healing.
> - Halted root resorption.

healing in progress (Fig. 9.7). Although some lesions take longer to heal, most healing lesions are likely to resolve with complete bone fill within 1 year (see also Chapter 18). In cases with a large lesion, where a self-sustaining and expanding cyst or other pathological lesion may be suspected, it is recommended to carry out the recall by 4–6 months. If healing is obviously not in progress, a surgical procedure may be considered (Chapter 18).

Considerations in complex cases

Canal anatomy may be such that cleaning and disinfection of the root canal system can be conducted only with great difficulty, depending on partial or total obstruction due to previous injury by trauma or operative procedure (Fig. 9.5a), severe canal curvature (Fig. 9.5b) and developmental anomaly (Fig. 9.5d–h). It is therefore very important to identify carefully any potential difficulties prior to initiation of RCT (8, 46) (Fig. 9.8) and consider referral to an endodontic specialist or experienced colleague in especially challenging cases.

Nevertheless, conservative management of what appears to be a hopeless case, for example teeth with only partially negotiable canals, may still be successful by conventional RCT (1) (Fig. 9.8). The prognosis is unpredictable, however, and should be regarded as guarded. If

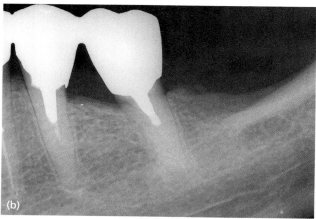

(a) (b)

Fig. 9.8 (a) Instrumentation was not possible over the entire length of the distal root in a lower molar owing to obliteration. (b) At recall 2 years later the lesion nevertheless reduced in size. Clinically, the tooth remained asymptomatic.

a permanent cast restoration is planned for the tooth in question, it is sensible to postpone restoration until there are clear signs of healing in progress.

Effects of root canal therapy on the intracanal microbiota

As described in Chapter 6, the microbiota of infected necrotic pulps is normally dominated by anaerobes, whereas facultatives usually occupy a minor portion of the root canal flora. However, there is great variation and a large number of individual species and combinations of species can be associated with the development and continuance of apical periodontitis. Therefore, and because of the potential for organisms to prevail in biofilm structures on the root canal walls (Chapter 6), there is little support for treatment approaches that selectively focus on specific organisms. Findings of a dominance of facultatives, especially therapy-resilient enterococci in retreatment cases (cases where lesions have appeared or failed to heal subsequent to endodontic therapy; 35, 60), suggest that RCT is normally effective in combating the anaerobes. On this basis, one may reason that RCT, if not effective, may select for the most robust segment of the root canal microbiota (11). Surviving microorganisms exposed to antimicrobial measures in RCT may also adapt their physiology to the changed environmental conditions set by the treatment (9). For example changes in pH by calcium hydroxide medication may trigger the release of stress proteins making surviving organisms more resistant to further treatment attempts (10). Consequently, it can be regarded as important that the best possible effort to eradicate microorganisms should be taken at the initial treatment session. It seems reasonable, therefore, to caution against a procedure whereby instrumentation and chemical disinfection is carried out only half-way, and to postpone completion of biomechanical instrumentation to a later session.

Management of symptomatic lesions

Most lesions associated with an infected necrosis of the pulp prevail without acute signs of inflammation (pain, tenderness, fistulae, swellings). Nevertheless symptomatic lesions may develop spontaneously or be initiated in conjunction with RCT (Fig. 9.9) (Chapter 7). This section of the chapter is devoted to measures to be undertaken in such cases.

Painful cases prior to RCT

Symptomatic lesions may be associated with or without a distinct soft-tissue swelling. In some of these lesions,

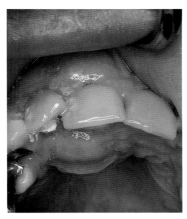

Fig. 9.9   A case with both buccal and palatal swellings due to an acute flare-up of apical periodontitis associated with tooth 12.

cellulitis or a periapical abscess may have already matured and manifested itself as a subperiosteal or submucosal abscess with distinct intraoral or extraoral swellings, or both. To alleviate the condition, RCT is still the treatment of choice. However, in these instances patients often visit the dentist for an unscheduled appointment, and time may therefore set limits for what it is possible to do. There may also be a variety of other circumstances that makes proper RCT impossible to carry out at the time the patient seeks treatment. Some of these are technically related and include the presence of obstructions in the root canal that require substantial time to remove before the rest of the canal(s) can be accessed. Examples are hard-tissue obliterations, previous root fillings and crowns with posts. Thus, by its very nature, emergency treatment will often have to be a compromise, where the primary objective is to get the patient out of pain. Consequently, although a complete instrumentation and medication of the tooth is highly desirable to combat the infecting microbiota, it is only a secondary objective at this point and RCT may have to be put on hold until the patient can be seen at a regularly scheduled appointment.

General procedure

An emergency procedure includes several critical steps:

1. Establishment of a correct diagnosis of the condition.
2. Assessment of the severity and a decision as to whether an invasive RCT and/or incision and drainage procedure is needed or if the condition can be managed by analgesics.
3. Emergency treatment.
4. Rescheduling for completion of RCT or endodontic surgery, if needed.

Any emergency treatment must take into account the management of both the root canal system and the periapex. If canals are accessible, opening the root canal(s)

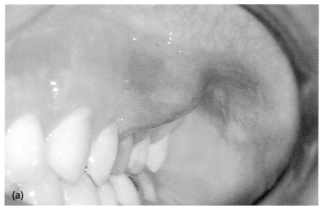

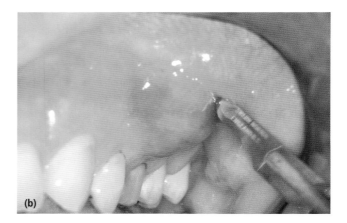

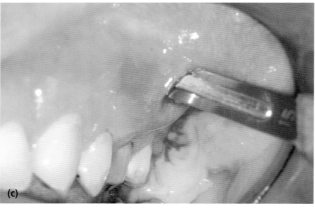

Fig. 9.10 Drainage of submucosal abscess is obtained by the use of a scalpel. (a) Fluctuant swelling in the upper premolar/molar region, (b) scalpel in place to make a ca. 1 cm cut into the abscess whereupon (c) pus is released.

gives an opportunity to obtain drainage of exudate or pus (see further below) and to combat the infecting microbiota by biomechanical instrumentation (RCT). The emergency procedure may also include an attempt to drain off an abscess by surgical incision (Fig. 9.10). If canals are not accessible and if drainage by incision is not deemed possible, the emergency treatment may have to be limited to prescription of a strong analgesic and postponement of further measures until a more suitable time is available within a couple of days.

Emergency RCT

In teeth that hurt because of a painful manifestation of apical periodontitis, even the slightest pressure may cause pain and therefore the root canals of such teeth should be accessed with high-speed burs and light pressure. Occasionally it may be necessary to give local anesthesia. In all other aspects the RCT is no different to that performed in routine non-symptomatic cases.

In spreading inflammatory processes (cellulitis, subperiosteal abscess), drainage of exudate or pus under pressure may be possible along the root canal space. Sometimes it occurs directly in conjunction with access to the pulpal chamber (Fig. 9.11). In other instances drainage may be obtained by careful bypassing of the

apical foramen using a thin root canal instrument. If such drainage does occur, there is often immediate pain relief. It is highly important that the apical foramen is not pierced with instruments of sizes larger than ISO 10–20, otherwise one runs the risk of causing an apical overpreparation and zipping of the apical foramen, thus making subsequent RCT difficult (see above). Thereafter, it is sufficient to clean the root canal system properly and close it up with a dressing of $Ca(OH)_2$ and temporary cement in the access opening.

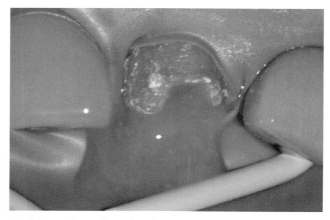

Fig. 9.11 Drainage of pus along the root canal upon access of an upper lateral incisor with a necrotic pulp and painful apical periodontitis.

Ledermix a corticosteroid–tetracycline-containing paste, has also been advocated for intracanal medication in these cases. In a clinical trial, it gave better control of pain associated with acute apical periodontitis than that experienced by patients who had received a dressing of calcium hydroxide or no intracanal dressing at all (14). The advantage of using this compound, however, must be weighed against the risk of sensitizing the patient to the antibiotic. To be effective Ledermix needs to be spun into root canal(s) with a lentulo needle so that the material makes direct contact with the periapical tissue, thus enhancing that risk.

With an abundant drainage of pus that does not halt immediately, it is advisable to let the patient sit for a while before closing the canal system, in order to equilibrate the apical tissue pressure. One should not leave canals open to the oral environment because this may cause a severe contamination problem. Leaving root canals open without a surface seal may contribute to the establishment of a microbiota, including enteric bacteria and yeasts, which may be difficult to eradicate (65).

If drainage of an abscess can be obtained by either root canal instrumentation or incision and drainage, prescribing antibiotics is redundant and undesirable.

If there is a lack of time and there is no drainage on careful piercing of the apical foramen after creating access, one has to close the canal system and postpone further biomechanical instrumentation until a more suitable occasion can be found. On many occasions pain relief can be obtained by such a drainage technique, but pain may not be alleviated immediately following emergency RCT, and the patient must be made aware of this (Core concept 9.5).

Pulp necrosis with a localized fluctuant swelling

With a localized, fluctuant, soft-tissue swelling indicating a submucosal abscess, an incision and drainage procedure should be attempted (Fig. 9.10). It is not possible to state categorically whether this should be done before or after accessing the root canal system, but as a rule of thumb it is recommended to carry out the procedure first, if there is an obvious fluctuation.

With a non-fluctuant tissue swelling it is advisable not to incise the tissue because of the concern of worsening

---

Core concept 9.5 Pain relief after emergency RCT

Pain may not disappear immediately after emergency RCT, therefore it is essential to:

- Explain the situation to the patient.
- Adjust the occlusal contacts.
- Prescribe a suitable analgesic.
- Be available to the patient if severe pain continues.

---

the condition and causing the spread of the process. Controlling the pain with analgesics until fluctuation occurs is normally the best choice of treatment because the administration of antibiotics may not be effective (see below).

Occasionally, localized intraoral swellings are accompanied by some extraoral distension resulting in an elevated cheek, swollen lips and sometimes even swollen eyelids. Usually, these symptoms do not require additional treatment or medication unless the swelling rapidly diffuses.

Pulp necrosis with diffuse swelling

In the presence of diffuse swelling that has rapidly progressed and is accompanied by systemic signs including fever (>39°C) and general malaise, patients should be referred to a hospital where intravenous antibiotics are usually given. In these cases it is not advisable to try to control the infection by oral antibiotics prescribed by the general practitioner.

Use of antimicrobials (antibiotics)

In general the systemic use of antibiotics is a valuable adjunct to the treatment of infectious diseases. However, the risk of causing bacterial resistance makes it necessary to restrict their use in endodontics to those cases in absolute need. Such cases are primarily those where symptoms of endodontic infection suggest marked progression or systemic involvement, or both. The purpose of an antibiotic prescription is then to help to contain the process and to avoid possible serious systemic consequences (see also Chapter 8). This means that antibiotic therapy is not appropriate for the treatment of localized swellings where drainage and debridement can be successfully conducted.

In the exceptional case when antibiotics are to be prescribed, an adequate drug and accurate dosage should be given. Because there is no way of knowing which specific organisms are causing the lesion, the prescription must be initiated on an empirical basis. Thus, seeing the patient on a daily basis until the infectious process is contained should allow careful monitoring of the result of therapy. If a satisfactory response does not occur within the next few days, one may consider changing the antimicrobial. For drug selection, a careful history of allergy and drug reaction is necessary and one should consult the appropriate background literature for possible side-effects.

Management of postoperative pain – endodontic flare-up

Although painful conditions are normally prevented or cured by RCT, the RCT *per se* may also cause pain and swelling. This may occur even in teeth that were free of pain prior to treatment. The incidence of such conditions has been reported to be as high as 20–40% of treated cases (18), whereas the incidence of severe pain conditions appears to be <5% (26, 61, 66).

The primary cause is to be sought in the treatment procedure itself, whereby bacteria and bacterial elements have been extruded into the periapical tissue compartment and caused an exacerbation of the inflammatory lesion. An exacerbation may also follow inadvertent extension of the apical foramen, which allows an enhanced nutritional supply to bacterial organisms that survived the initial treatment. Normally these so-called endodontic flare-ups have a sudden onset, but may not emerge until 1–2 days after the procedure. Improper use of irrigants and root canal dressings may also cause a painful condition. If used correctly, root canal dressings and irrigation do not trigger more postoperative pain than the use of saline as an irrigant (26).

Management aspects

Research has shown that in over 50% of patients who experience pain after treatment the pain disappears within 1 day. After 2 days 90% were relieved of pain, whereas for only 3% pain lasted for longer than 1 week (19) (Key literature 9.1). This means that most painful conditions do not need active treatment and can be managed by analgesics, although a number of patients experience severe pain and need to be seen again for assessment or active treatment.

If pain is not severe (can be suppressed with a mild analgesic) it is best to abstain from further treatment, reassure the patient and prescribe a mild analgesic if no analgesic is being used already. Adjustment of occlusion also provides comfort. If pain is severe, the therapy depends on whether or not the previous canal preparation was complete or if the canal was permanently filled:

- If pain develops after *incomplete instrumentation*, then opening the canal and completing the RCT is appropriate.

Key literature 9.1

Genet *et al.* (19) carried out a clinical follow-up study of 443 teeth in 443 patients, reporting the association between preoperative and operative factors and the incidence of postoperative factors after the first visit. Postoperative pain occurred in 27% of the cases, of which 5% was severe. A positive correlation was seen between the incidence of postoperative pain and: the presence of preoperative pain in cases of teeth with necrotic pulps; the presence of a radiolucency >5 mm in diameter; and the number of root canals treated. Women more frequently reported pain than men. When each of these factors was analyzed independently they remained statistically significant, suggesting that the effects were cumulative.

Core concept 9.6   Patient information and advice

Patients may be greatly upset or concerned about the development or continuance of pain after RCT, especially when they have not received proper prior information that such complications may emerge. It is crucial that patients are told that an asymptomatic tooth treated for an infected pulp necrosis may become sensitive or even painful. It is also necessary to advise the patient about which measures to undertake, e.g. to call and get an emergency appointment. Good explanation and advice prevent considerable concern and may make pain more tolerable (58).

- If pain persists or occurs in spite of *complete biomechanical preparation*, then reopening the tooth to attempt to drain off pus or exudates may alleviate the condition. After proper isolation with a rubber dam, gently instrument the canal with a thin ISO 20 instrument. If pus is discharged, then usually the pain is greatly reduced or disappears. The procedure is then to leave the tooth alone until pus stops discharging and then irrigate, dry and close up the access opening. The problem may not invariably resolve by such a measure, particularly if no pus is noticed, therefore a decision to reopen a properly instrumented and medicated root canal should be taken after careful assessment of the case and consideration of prescribing strong analgesics instead (13). The patient should be informed that the pain is expected to subside within the next few days (Core concept 9.6). If the condition continues to be severe, a surgical procedure may have to be carried out.

- Filling of the root canal seldom results in severe postoperative pain (26, 63) although discomfort may be experienced after overfilling (21). If a painful condition appears, the case is best managed by pain medication, because the root canal is blocked for possible drainage. Furthermore, removal of the root canal filling may cause extrusion of root filling material and inadvertent overpreparation of the foramen. In the case of subperiosteal or submucous abscess, an incision may result in the necessary drainage. Apical surgery or extraction may have to be carried out if the condition persists. An experienced colleague or endodontic specialist may be consulted prior to deciding on a possible unnecessary removal of the tooth.

References

1. Åkerblom A, Hasselgren G. The prognosis for endodontic treatment of obliterated root canals. *J. Endod.* 1988; 14: 565–7.

   Clinical follow-up study of cases not possible to instrument further than one-third of the root length. It was reported that complete periapical healing occurred in 10/16 teeth with preoperative periapical radiolucency.

2. Baumgartner JC, Cuenin PR. Efficacy of several concentrations of sodium hypochlorite for root canal irrigation. *J. Endod.* 1992; 18: 605–12.

3. Byström A, Sundqvist G. Bacteriologic evaluation of the efficacy of mechanical root canal instrumentation in endodontic therapy. *Scand. J. Dent. Res.* 1981; 89: 321–8.

4. Byström A, Sundqvist G. Bacteriologic evaluation of the effect of 0.5 per cent sodium hypochlorite in endodontic therapy. *Oral Surg. Oral Med. Oral Pathol.* 1983; 55: 307–12.

5. Byström A, Claesson R, Sundqvist G. The antibacterial effect of camphorated paramonochlorophenol, camphorated phenol and calcium hydroxide in the treatment of infected root canals. *Endod. Dent. Traumatol.* 1985; 1: 170–75.

6. Byström A, Sundqvist G. The antibacterial action of sodium hypochlorite and EDTA in 60 cases of endodontic therapy. *Int. Endod. J.* 1985; 18: 35–40.

7. Caliskan MK. Prognosis of large cyst-like periapical lesions following nonsurgical root canal treatment: a clinical review. *Int. Endod. J.* 2004; 37: 408–16.

8. Caplan DJ, Reams G, Weintraub JA. Recommendations for endodontic referral among practitioners in a dental HMO. *J. Endod.* 1999; 25: 369–75.

9. Chávez de Paz LE. Redefining the persistent infection in root canals: possible role of biofilm communities. *J. Endod.* 2007; 33; 652–62.

10. Chávez de Paz LE, Bergenholtz G, Dahlén G, Svensäter G. Response to alkaline stress by root canal bacteria in biofilms. *Int. Endod. J.* 2007; 40: 344–55.

11. Chávez De Paz LE, Dahlén G, Molander A, Möller A, Bergenholtz G. Bacteria recovered from teeth with apical periodontitis after antimicrobial endodontic treatment. *Int. Endod. J.* 2003; 36: 500–8.

12. Chong BS, Pitt Ford TR. The role of intracanal medication in root canal treatment. *Int. Endod. J.* 1992; 25: 97–106.

13. Cooper SA. Treating acute pain: do's and don'ts, pros and cons. *J. Endod.* 1990; 16: 85–91.

14. Ehrmann EH, Messer HH, Adams GG. The relationship of intracanal medicaments to postoperative pain in endodontics. *Int. Endod. J.* 2003; 36: 868–75.

15. European Society of Endodontology. Consensus report of the European Society of Endodontology on quality guidelines for endodontic treatment. *Int. Endod. J.* 2006; 39: 921–30.

16. Fabricius L, Dahlén G, Sundqvist G, Happonen RP, Möller ÅJ. Influence of residual bacteria on periapical tissue healing after chemomechanical treatment and root filling of experimentally infected monkey teeth. *Eur. J. Oral Sci.* 2006; 114: 278–85.

17. Fava LR, Saunders WP. Calcium hydroxide pastes: classification and clinical indications. *Int. Endod. J.* 1999; 32: 257–82.

18. Genet JM, Wesselink PR, Thoden van Velzen SK. The incidence of preoperative and postoperative pain in endodontic therapy. *Int. Endod. J.* 1986; 19: 221–9.

19. Genet JM, Hart AAM, Wesselink PR, Thoden van Velzen SK. Preoperative and operative factors associated with pain after the first endodontic visit. *Int. Endod. J.* 1987; 20: 53–64.

20. George S, Kishen A. Photophysical, photochemical, and photobiological characterization of methylene blue formulations for light-activated root canal disinfection. *J Biomed. Opt.* 2007; 12: 34029–38.

21. Gesi A, Hakeberg M, Warfvinge J, Bergenholtz G. Incidence of osteolytic lesions and clinical symptoms after pulpectomy – a clinical evaluation of one *versus* two-session treatment. *Oral Surg., Oral Med. Oral Pathol. Endod.* 2006; 101: 379–88.

22. Gilbert DB, Germaine GR, Jensen JR. Inactivation by saliva and serum of the antimicrobial activity of some commonly used root canal sealer cements. *J. Endod.* 1978; 4: 100–5.

23. Goldman LB, Goldman M, Kronman JH, Lin PS. The efficacy of several irrigating solutions for endodontics: a scanning electron microscopic study. *Oral Surg. Oral Med. Oral Pathol.* 1981; 52: 197–204.

24. Haapasalo HK, Sirén EK, Waltimo TM, Ørstavik D, Haapasalo MP. Inactivation of local root canal medicaments by dentine: an *in vitro* study. *Int. Endod. J.* 2000; 33: 126–31.

25. Haapasalo M, Qian W, Portenier I, Waltimo T. Haapasalo M, Qian W, Portenier I, Waltimo T. Effects of dentin on the antimicrobial properties of endodontic medicaments. *J. Endod.* 2007; 33: 917–25.

26. Harrison JW, Baumgartner JC, Zielke DR. Analysis of interappointment pain associated with the combined use of endodontic irrigants and medicaments. *J. Endod.* 1981; 7: 272–6.

27. Hasselgren G, Olsson B, Cvek M. Effects of calcium hydroxide and sodium hypochlorite on the dissolution of necrotic porcine muscle tissue. *J. Endod.* 1988; 14: 125–7.

28. Hülsmann M, Hahn W. Complications during root canal irrigation – literature review and case reports. *Int. Endod. J.* 2000; 33: 186–93.

29. Kerekes K, Tronstad L. Long-term results of endodontic treatment performed with a standardized technique. *J. Endod.* 1979; 5: 83–90.

30. Kvist T, Molander A, Dahlén G, Reit C. Microbiological evaluation of one- and two-visit endodontic treatment of teeth with apical periodontitis: a randomized, clinical trial. *J. Endod.* 2004; 30: 572–6.

31. Lamers AC, Van Mullem PJ, Simon M. Tissue reactions to sodium hypochlorite and iodine potassium iodide under clinical conditions in monkeys' teeth. *J. Endod.* 1980; 6: 788–92.

32. Lewis B. Formaldehyde in dentistry: a review for the millennium. *J. Clin. Pediatr. Dent.* 1998; 22: 167–77.

33. Lin L, Langeland K. Innervation of the inflammatory periapical lesions. *Oral Surg. Oral Med. Oral Pathol.* 1981; 51: 535–43.

34. Messser HH, Chen RS. The duration of effectiveness of root canal medicaments. *J. Endod.* 1984; 10: 240–5.

35. Molander A, Reit C, Dahlén G, Kvist T. Microbiological status of root filled teeth with apical periodontitis. *Int. Endod. J.* 1998; 31: 1–7.

36. Molander A, Warfvinge J, Reit C, Kvist T. Clinical and radiographic evaluation of one- and two-visit endodontic treatment of asymptomatic necrotic teeth with apical peri-

odontitis: a randomized clinical trial. *J. Endod.* 2007; 33: 1145–8.

This randomized clinical trial presented evidence that equally good healing results may be obtained regardless of one- and two-visit antimicrobial treatment of cases with infected pulp necrosis. Teeth treated with a 10 min application of 5% iodine–potassium iodide following biomechanical instrumentation were compared with teeth receiving Ca(OH)$_2$ medication over two treatment sessions. Although not reaching a statistically significant difference, culture-negative root canals fared better than culture-positive.

37. Molven O, Olsen I, Kerekes K. Scanning electron microscopy of bacteria in the apical part of root canals in permanent teeth with periapical lesions. *Endod. Dent. Traumatol.* 1991; 7: 226–9.

38. Moorer WR, Wesselink PR. Factors promoting the tissue dissolving capability of sodium hypochlorite. *Int. Endod. J.* 1982; 15: 187–96.

39. Nair PN, Henry S, Cano V, Vera J. Microbial status of apical root canal system of human mandibular first molars with primary apical periodontitis after "one-visit" endodontic treatment. *Oral Surg. Oral Med. Oral Pathol. Oral Radiol. Endod.* 2005; 99: 231–52.

40. Nair PNR, Sjögren U, Krey G, Kahnberg K-E, Sundqvist G. Intraradicular bacteria and fungi in root filled, asymptomatic human teeth with therapy-resistant periapical lesions: a long-term light and electron microscopic follow-up study. *J. Endod.* 1990; 16: 580–8.

41. Ørstavik D, Haapasalo M. Disinfection by endodontic irrigants and dressings of experimentally infected dentinal tubules. *Endod. Dent. Traumatol.* 1990; 6: 142–9.

42. Ørstavik D, Kerekes K, Molven O. Effects of extensive apical reaming and calcium hydroxide dressing on bacterial infection during treatment of apical periodontitis: a pilot study. *Int. Endod. J.* 1991; 24: 1–7.

43. Peters CI, Koka RS, Highsmith S, Peters OA. Calcium hydroxide dressings using different preparation and application modes: density and dissolution by simulated tissue pressure. *Int. Endod. J.* 2005; 38: 889–95.

44. Peters LB, Wesselink PR. Periapical healing of endodontically treated teeth in one and two visits obturated in the presence or absence of bacteria in the root canal. *Int. Endod. J.* 2002; 35: 660–7.

45. Peters LB, Wesselink PR, Buijs JF, van Winkelhoff AJ. Viable bacteria in root dentinal tubules of teeth with apical periodontitis. *J. Endod.* 2001; 27: 76–81.

46. Ree MH, Timmerman MF, Wesselink PR. An evaluation of the usefulness of two endodontic case assessment forms by general dentists. *Int. Endod. J.* 2003; 36: 545–55.

47. Ringel AM, Patterson SS, Newton CW, Miller CH, Mulhern JM. *In vivo* evaluation of chlorhexidine gluconate solution and sodium hypochlorite solution as root canal irrigants. *J. Endod.* 1982; 8: 200–4.

48. Rosenfeld EF, James GA, Burch BS. Vital pulp tissue response to sodium hypochlorite. *J. Endod.* 1978; 4: 140–6.

49. Safavi KE, Spångberg LS, Langeland K. Root canal dentinal tubule disinfection. *J. Endod.* 1990; 16: 207–10.

50. Shabahang S, Torabinejad M. Effect of MTAD on *Enterococcus faecalis*-contaminated root canals of extracted human teeth. *J. Endod.* 2003; 29: 576–9.

51. Shuping GB, Ørstavik D, Sigurdsson A, Trope M. Reduction of intracanal bacteria using nickel–titanium rotary instrumentation and various medications. *J. Endod.* 2000; 26: 751–5.

52. Sim TPC, Knowles JC, Ng Y-L, Shelton J, Gulabivala K. Effect of sodium hypochlorite on mechanical properties of dentine and tooth surface strain. *Int. Endod. J.* 2001; 34: 120–32.

53. Siqueira Junior JF, Lopes HP. Mechanisms of antimicrobial activity of calcium hydroxide: a critical review. *Int. Endod. J.* 1999; 32: 361–9.

54. Sirén EK, Haapasalo MP, Ranta K, Salmi P, Kerosuo EN. Microbiological findings and clinical treatment procedures in endodontic cases selected for microbiological investigation. *Int. Endod. J.* 1997; 30: 91–5.

55. Sjögren U, Sundqvist G. Bacteriologic evaluation of ultrasonic root canal instrumentation. *Oral Surg.* 1987; 63: 366–70.

56. Sjögren U, Hägglund B, Sundqvist G, Wing K. Factors affecting the long-term results of endodontic treatment. *J. Endod.* 1990; 16: 498–504.

In this clinical follow-up study over 8–10 years, 86% of the treated cases with pulp necrosis and periapical radiolucency showed complete healing. If mechanical instrumention and disinfection procedures as well as filling could be carried to the full length of the root canals a significantly better outcome was noticed than if roots were instrumented and filled short of or through the apex.

57. Sjögren U, Figdor D, Persson S, Sundqvist G. Influence of infection at the time of root filling on the outcome of endodontic treatment of teeth with apical periodontitis. *Int. Endod. J.* 1997; 30: 297–306.

58. Sjöling M, Nordahl G, Olofsson N, Asplund K. The impact of preoperative information on state of anxiety, postoperative pain and satisfaction with pain management. *Patient Educ. Couns.* 2003; 51: 169–76.

59. Spångberg L, Rutberg M, Rydinge E. Biologic effect of endodontic antimicrobial agents. *J. Endod.* 1979; 5: 166–75.

60. Sundqvist G, Figdor D, Persson S, Sjögren U. Microbiologic analysis of teeth with failed endodontic treatment and the outcome of conservative re-treatment. *Oral Surg.* 1998; 85: 86–93.

61. Trope M. Flare-up rate of single-visit endodontics. *Int. Endod. J.* 1991; 24: 24–6.

62. Trope M, Bergenholtz G. Microbiological basis for endodontic treatment: can a maximal outcome be achieved in one visit? *Endod. Topics* 2002; 1: 40–53.

63. Trope M, Delano EO, Ørstavik D. Endodontic treatment of teeth with apical periodontitis: single vs. multivisit treatment. *J. Endod.* 1999; 25: 345–50.

64. van der Sluis LW, Versluis M, Wu M-K, Wesselink P. Passive ultrasonic irrigation of the root canal: a review of the literature. *J. Endod.* 2007; 40: 415–26.

65. Waltimo TM, Sirén EK, Torkko HL, Olsen I, Haapasalo MP. Fungi in therapy-resistant apical periodontitis. *Int. Endod. J.* 1997; 30: 96–101.

66. Walton R, Fouad A. Endodontic interappointment flare-ups: a prospective study of incidence and related factors. *J. Endod.* 1992; 18: 172–7.

67. Weiger R, Rosendahl R, Löst C. Influence of calcium hydroxide intracanal dressings on the prognosis of teeth with endodontically induced periapical lesions. *Int. Endod. J.* 2000; 33: 219–26.

68. Wu M-K, Fan B, Wesselink PR. Leakage along apical root fillings in curved root canals. Part 1: effects of apical transportation on seal of root fillings. *J. Endod.* 2000; 26: 210–16.

69. Wu M-K, Wesselink PR. A primary observation on the preparation and obturation of oval canals. *Int. Endod. J.* 2001; 34: 137–41.

70. Yusuf H. The significance of the presence of foreign material periapically as a cause of failure of root treatment. *Oral Surg. Oral Med. Oral Pathol.* 1982; 54: 566–74.

71. Zehnder M. Root canal irrigants. *J. Endod.* 2006; 32: 389–98.
    Valuable overview of irrigating solutions for root canal disinfection is attained in this article.

Part 3
Endodontic Treatment Procedures

Chapter 10
The surgical microscope

Pierre Machtou

Introduction

The desire to see better in order to address the complexity of the root canal system of teeth by endodontics has naturally led to the use of optical aids. Simple magnifying glasses (conventional Galilean optics) or magnifying glasses mounted on spectacles make it possible to achieve magnification up to 5×. Beyond these enlargements, optical systems become too heavy and cumbersome for them to be used for long periods without discomfort. If a source of light is fitted, the weight of the device increases even further. Although these measures for magnification are distinct improvements beyond the naked eye, the surgical microscope offers a stereoscopic, three-dimensional, enlarged image under bright illumination at a comfortable working position that will greatly enhance the precision of endodontics (Fig. 10.1). Thereby root canal orifices can be more easily found (Figs 10.2 and 10.3a–c), cracks and fractures revealed (Fig. 10.4), and instrumentation and filling procedures in both conventional (Fig. 10.3d–f) and surgical endodontics (Fig. 10.5) facilitated. This short chapter describes the principal uses and applications of the surgical microscope in endodontic therapies.

Components

The optical system

The surgical microscope intended for dental operations consists of three key components: an ocular head (viewing tube) holding two eyepieces, intermediate magnification lenses and the main objective lens (Fig. 10.6).

The focal length of the eyepieces lies between 100 mm and 160 mm, with magnification values from 10× to 12.5×. The eyepieces comprise an adjustment ring with settings to compensate for visual defects. The distance between the eyepieces is adjustable in order to match the appropriate interpupillary distance of the eyes. To be functional in most clinical situations it should be possible to tilt the ocular head in the frontal plane.

The magnification lenses placed between the eyepieces and the main objective make it possible to have several magnifications (generally from 5× to 25×). They are optical blocks mounted on a turret, from which, with the aid of a ring, the magnification most appropriate to the sequence of the operation can be selected. On the most sophisticated models this variation is controlled via a zoom lens.

The lens nearest to the object to be examined, the main objective lens, may have a varying focal length, chosen depending on the height and the working habits of the operator. It can vary from 200 mm to 300 mm and determines the working distance (distance from object observed to the objective lens). See Advanced concept 10.1.

The mechanical system

A suspension system is provided to ensure stability and balance inherent movements of the microscope away from the position in which it is originally placed, otherwise major operating difficulties would ensue. The system of arms is either mounted on a movable floor stand or fixed either to the wall or to the ceiling of the surgery. On purchasing an operating microscope the flexibility and ability of this mechanical system to offset

---

Advanced concept 10.1

The total magnification (G_t) of an operating microscope can be determined by the Serafin and Georgiade formula:

$$G_t = (F_{oc}/F_{ob}) \times G_{oc} \times G_i$$

where F_{oc} is focal length of the eyepiece, F_{ob} is the focal length of the objective, G_{oc} is magnification of the eyepiece and G_i is magnification of the system of intermediate lenses (magnification prisms). The total magnification values suitable for endodontics range from 4× to 40×. When one knows that the resolving power of the eye is 200 μm and that it can attain 5 μm at a magnification of 40×, one can readily understand the quantum leap in terms of precision the surgical microscope can provide.

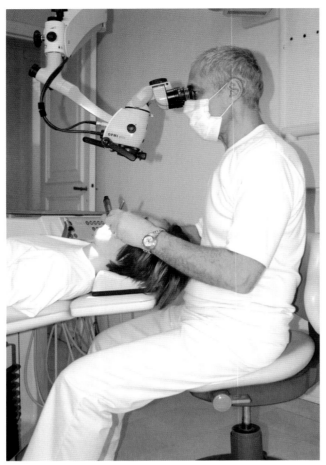

Fig. 10.1 Working position with the surgical microscope.

beam with no shadow effects. A video camera is a useful accessory, which not only makes it possible to record sequences for patient demonstration and teaching purposes, but also enables the operating assistant to follow the work and increases his or her involvement in it.

Ergonomics and working techniques

Contrary to the work carried out with no optical aids, or use of magnifying glasses, it is only exceptional that operations with the microscope can take place in direct vision. Therefore one must realize that a learning period is required to become proficient in use of the surgical microscope, the length of which depends on whether or not one is accustomed to working in indirect vision. The microscope is a new tool and, to make the mastery of its use simpler and quicker, it is of prime importance to restrict oneself to working in indirect vision during the training period.

The use of mirrors

For use of the microscope in indirect vision it is important to position the mirror as far as possible away from the teeth to be treated in order to limit spray and scatter of debris. This is especially significant when operating on maxillary teeth. Two mirrors may be used, so that one can be cleaned while the other is in use for rapid exchange. Small mirrors are sufficient and sensible to limit congestion of the working area, as endodontics does not require a view of the adjacent teeth (not the case in other operative procedures such as prosthodontics).

Working positions

The placement of the microscope and the patient determines the achievement of a comfortable position when working with a microscope. To ensure precision of the hand movements required, the thighs and the forearms of the operator must be parallel to the floor, the feet firmly placed and the back straight while the eyes are at

movements is a determining factor. Where the working conditions allow, a ceiling mount is the preferred choice.

The illumination system

The light system consists of either a 150 watt halogen lamp or a xenon arc lamp, which gives comfortable cold, white light. The light is conducted by fiber optics and generates a luminous beam parallel to the optical

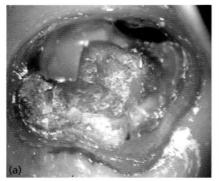
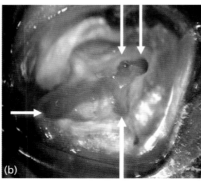

Fig. 10.2 Indistinct positions of canal orifices in a severely broken down upper molar (a) cleared by ultrasonic preparation under the use of the surgical microscope (b). (Courtesy of Dr Claes Reit.)

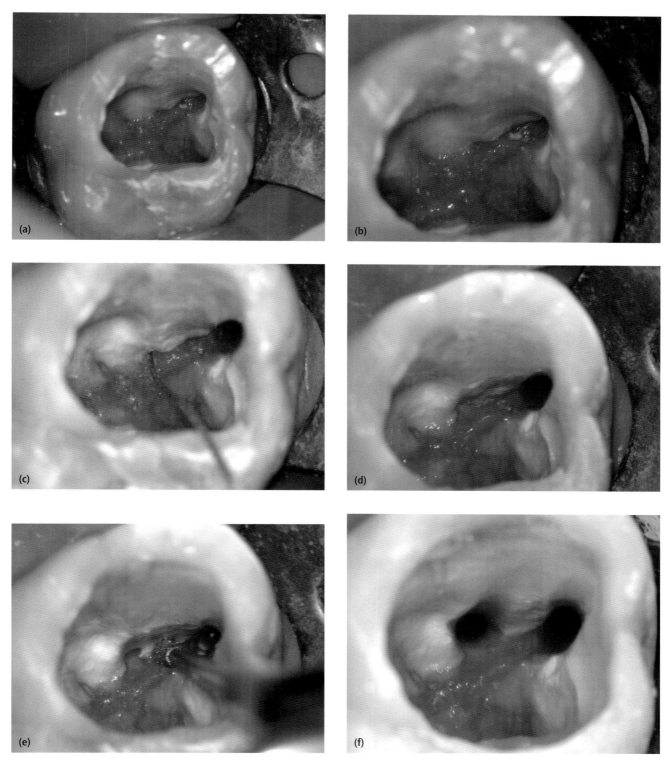

Fig. 10.3 Series of images demonstrating by the use of the surgical microscope the exploration (a–c) and initial preparation (d–f) of a second canal (MB2) in the mesiobuccal root of an upper molar.

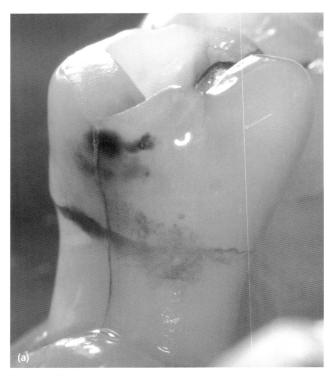
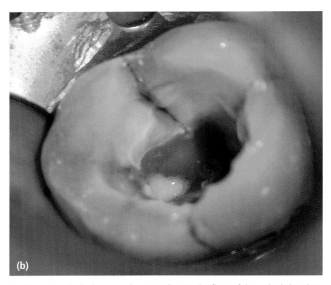

Fig. 10.4 Observation of cracks (a) at the distal aspect of a lower premolar, (b) in the lingual wall of a lower molar extending to the floor of the pulpal chamber. (Courtesy of Dr Dominique Martin.)

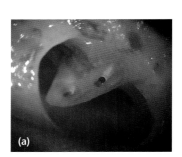
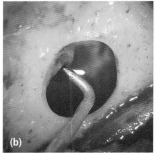
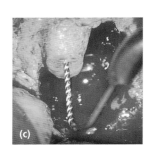
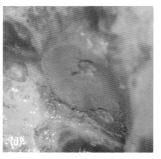

Fig. 10.5 Illustrations of various phases in surgical endodontics: (a) after resection of root tip, (b) root-end preparation with diamond-coated ultrasonic tip, (c) root-end preparation by hand instrument, (d) canals filled with MTA. (Courtesy of Dr Stéphane Simon.)

the oculars. For this reason, a chair with an armrest improves operating comfort. The operator should be positioned between 11 o'clock and 12 o'clock in relation to the patient (Fig. 10.1).

The area to be treated governs the position of the patient. In the anterior mandibular sector where direct vision may be possible, the patient is seated with the back at 120° or 180° if indirect vision is used. In lateral mandibular areas for indirect vision the patient is placed at 180° with the head hyperextended and the body of the microscope angled at 90–120° (from back to front) (Fig. 10.7a). Indirect vision of upper maxillary teeth requires the patient to be recumbent at 150–180° and the body of the microscope angled at 60–90° (from front to back) (Fig. 10.7b).

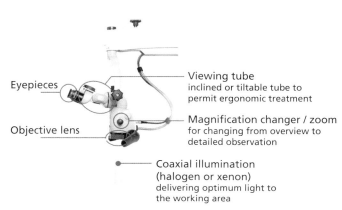

Eyepieces

Viewing tube
inclined or tiltable tube to permit ergonomic treatment

Objective lens

Magnification changer / zoom
for changing from overview to detailed observation

Coaxial illumination
(halogen or xenon)
delivering optimum light to the working area

Fig. 10.6 Essential components of a surgical microscope.

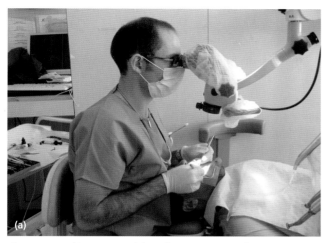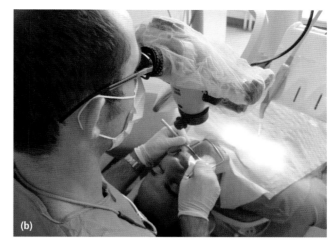

Fig. 10.7   Working position while exploring root canals of posterior teeth of (a) the lower jaw and (b) the upper jaw.

Working under the microscope can be conceived as a job for four hands. While taking care of aspiration and keeping the mirror and the working area clear, the assistant is best placed to the left of the patient with a right-handed operator. The use of a video camera and a control screen enables the assistant to anticipate the operator's needs and improves the efficiency of the support.

Microinstrumentation

Miniaturized tools have been produced to promote and assist the use of the operating microscope in endodontics. Some of these tools are mentioned as they greatly can facilitate the operations:

- micro-tips for irrigation (Stropko) producing a fine air-jet (Fig. 10.8);
- long-handle mounted K and H files to locate canal orifices without obstruction of vision (Fig. 10.9);

- micro-mirrors of varying sizes (2–5 mm) and shapes (circular or rectangular) to be used in endodontic surgery procedures (Fig. 10.10);
- sonic or ultrasonic micro-cutters for searching root canal orifices and for root preparation of canals in surgical endodontics (Fig. 10.11).

Critical steps

A series of steps is to be taken in order to set up an efficient operation with the surgical microscope:

1. Position the patient with the angle of the backrest adjusted in accordance with the area to be treated.
2. Be comfortably seated with the back straight: the height of the dental chair and the chair for the operator should be adjusted to achieve this.
3. Position the microscope.
4. Set up the illumination using a potentiometer in order to avoid thermal shock that can damage the bulb.

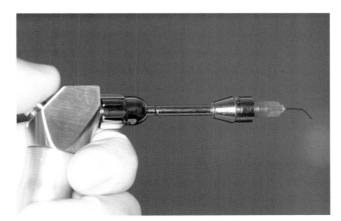

Fig. 10.8   The Stropko irrigator instrument to be used with the surgical microscope for precise control of irrigation or drying.

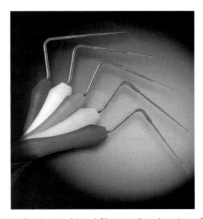

Fig. 10.9   Specially designed hand-files to allow location of canal orifices without obstruction.

5. Set proper interpupillary distance of the eyepieces, which is recorded.
6. Set the diopters to adapt to the individual operator's vision.

7. Adjust the position of the microscope using the halo reflected by the mirror positioned on the tooth to be treated.
8. Focus with the aid of the fine focus knob.

The treatment can now be initiated. Prior to the root canal work *per se* first check and adjust the sealing of the rubber dam around the tooth. Then carry out access opening, locate canal orifices and search for supernumerary, hidden or malformed canals; in maxillary molars for MB2 (Fig. 10.3). Upon completion of the instrumentation and disinfection procedures examine the canal, place interappointment dressing or fill the canal system under visual control.

Concluding remarks

With illumination and adjustable magnification the surgical microscopic has become a most useful adjunct to both orthograde and surgical endodontics. In conventional endodontic therapy it benefits not only the treatment procedures but also the ability to reveal craze lines, cracks and fractures that normally escape detection by the naked eye; these observations may impact upon the decision to continue treatment. The surgical microscope enhances the potential to carry out effective retreatment procedures by aiding in the detection of untreated root canals, perforations of the pulp chamber floor and stripping of the canal walls. It also helps in bypassing ledges and carrying out controlled removal of root filling material and intracanal obstacles, such as broken instruments and insoluble sealers.

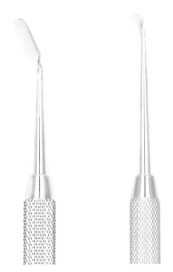

Fig. 10.10 Small micro-mirrors designed for use during surgical endodontics.

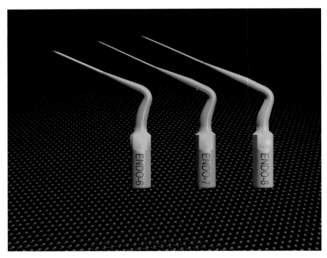

Fig. 10.11 Ultrasonic micro-cutters for use during orthograde endodontics.

References

1. Buhrley LJ, Barrows MJ, BeGole EA, Wenckus CS. Effect of magnification on locating the MB2 canal in maxillary molars. *J. Endod.* 2002; 28: 324–7.
2. Kinomoto Y, Takeshige F, Hayashi M, Ebisu S. Optimal positioning for a dental operating microscope during non-surgical endodontics. *J. Endod.* 2004; 30: 860–2.
3. Rubinstein R. The anatomy of the surgical operating microscope and operating positions. *Dent. Clin. North Am.* 1997; 41: 391–413.

Chapter 11
Root canal instrumentation

Lars Bergmans and Paul Lambrechts

Introduction

Accurately prepared root canals that allow effective elimination of soft and hard-tissue elements, disinfection and obturation of the canal system are critical to successful endodontic treatment. The procedure, which often is referred to as "cleaning and shaping" (34), is often a difficult and time-consuming task. Root canal instrumentation therefore requires a systematic approach to avoid underpreparation and iatrogenic injury, errors that may cause a poor prognosis for the treatment. In this chapter concepts for effective root canal instrumentation are reviewed. Materials and guidelines for clinical use are described, based on root canal system anatomy and final shaping objectives.

Principles of root canal instrumentation

Root canal instrumentation is accomplished by the use of endodontic instruments and (antimicrobial) irrigants under aseptic working conditions. A primary objective of this chemomechanical preparation, in teeth with either vital or non-vital pulps, is shaping the root canal space. It is generally accepted that the most appropriate final root canal shape is a tapered (conical) preparation with the smallest diameter at the end-point near the root tip, and the widest at the canal entrance. Special attention should therefore be paid to the apical level and the original path of the canal. As a general rule, the removal of root dentin should be centered, i.e. with respect to the initial root canal anatomy. In the process existing soft-tissue elements, serving as potential substrate for growth of remaining microorganisms, will be removed as well.

Root canal instrumentation may be carried out using hand-held or machine-driven (rotary) instruments. These instruments come in many configurations but are conventionally grouped according to ISO (International Organization for Standardization) and ANSI (American National Standards Institute) standards. The quality, sizing and physical properties of endodontic instruments and the materials used for their manufacture are therefore well defined. Instrument properties (e.g. stiffness) relate to type of alloy (stainless steel versus nickel–titanium), degree of taper (conicity) and cross-sectional design.

Stainless steel files have a high inherent stiffness that increases with increasing instrument size. As a result, restoring forces attempt to return the instrument to its original shape when preparing a curved root canal, especially when using a filing motion. An instrument that is too stiff will cut more on the convex (outer) side than on the concave (inner) side, thereby straightening the curve (Fig. 11.1). The resulting "hour-glass shape" and canal aberrations (e.g. ledge, zip and perforation) leave an important portion of the root canal wall uninstrumented and create an irregular canal shape that is difficult to clean, disinfect and fill properly.

Over time, researchers and clinicians have found a variety of methods to deal with the stiffness of stainless steel instruments. As a result, various movements for the manipulation of these files and approaches to shape the canal were proposed. While skillful operators can handle these techniques, shaping a curved root canal with stainless steel hand files remains a time-consuming and most challenging exercise.

Besides adaptations in file design and use, the problem of instrument stiffness has been answered by the use of nickel–titanium (Ni–Ti) rather than stainless steel (44). Nickel–titanium's unique property of super-elasticity may allow hand (and rotary) files to be placed in curved canals with less lateral force exerted. Conceptually, all such files are made from Nitinol,[1] an equiatomic Ni–Ti alloy (using about 55 wt% Ni and 45 wt% Ti, and substituting some Ni with less than 2 wt% Co) with a low modulus of elasticity and a greater resistance to plastic deformation.

Recent advances in the field of endodontics have led to the use of Ni–Ti *rotary* files in general and specialized dental practice. The idea behind this development is the belief that Ni–Ti rotary file design and the adopted

---

1 The symbols of the metals were combined with the place of invention (Naval Ordnance Laboratory, Silver Springs, MD, USA), creating the acronym NiTiNOL.

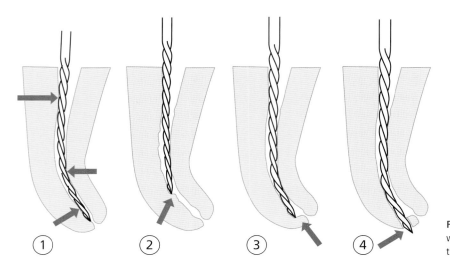

Fig. 11.1 The stiff instrument tends to straighten within the curved root canal (1), causing ledge formation (2), zipping (3) or perforation (4).

crown-down sequence (see further below) could improve both quality and efficacy of root canal preparation. For instance, owing to the existence of a greater taper design, these files could easily provide sufficient shape at the transition between the middle and apical one-thirds of root canals. However, innovation rarely comes without its own set of challenges. Before entering the exciting field of Ni–Ti rotary instrumentation, some basic preparation concepts such as straight-line access and shaping objectives in relation to tooth anatomy should be completely understood. Purely commercially driven use, on the other hand, may cause procedural errors (e.g. high incidence of instrument fracture) and frustration.

Root canal system anatomy

Root canal(s) versus root canal system

The specific features and complexity of the internal anatomy of the teeth have been thoroughly studied. Using a replica technique on thousands of teeth, Hess (15) made clear as early as 1917 that the internal space of dental roots is often a complex system composed of a central area (root canals with round, oval or irregular cross-sectional shape) and lateral parts (fins, anastomoses and accessory canals). In fact, this lateral component may represent a relatively large volume, which challenges the cleaning phase of the instrumentation procedure in that tissue remnants of the vital or necrotic pulp as well as infectious elements are not easily removed in these areas. Thus, the image of root canal(s) having a smooth, conical shape is generally too idealistic and underestimates the limited reach of root canal instrumentation.

In dental practice, complete visualization of the lateral component of the root canal system is normally not possible. Common radiographic techniques, both conventional and digital, have limited resolution and pro-

vide only two-dimensional (2D) projection views. Even though the paralleling technique with orthogonal and eccentric projections improves our understanding, part of the lateral anatomy, especially in the buccolingual (or buccopalatal) plane, will remain invisible (Fig. 11.2a–d). Limited perception of root canal system anatomy may cause procedural difficulties and may invite the clinician to follow a 2D-based approach in a routine-like fashion, where instrumentation to the final working length early in the shaping procedure often causes procedural mishaps.

A new 3D technique for *in vitro* dental research, called microfocus computed tomography (micro-CT), has provided detailed and accurate visualizations of the external and internal anatomy of teeth, which are useful for scientific and educational purposes (Fig. 11.2e, f) (5). In addition, the "typical or average anatomy", as presented for each type of tooth in many textbook tables, has given way to individual appearance being the key to achieving high success of endodontic treatment. Apart from the varying complexity of the lateral component, the anatomy of root canals also differs in terms of curvature, cross-sectional shape, diameter, apical configuration and the extent to which changes have been induced by physiological and pathological processes.

Root canal curvature

Most root canals are curved instead of straight. In addition, curved root canals are relatively narrow when compared to their straight counterparts. Root canals typically accelerate in curvature and exhibit their greatest anatomical complexity towards their apical terminus (Fig. 11.3). Root canal curvature can be described by level (coronal, middle or apical), angle and radius (29). Most curvatures are multiplanar and are thus expressed in both the mesiodistal and buccolingual (or buccopalatal) plane (Fig. 11.4).

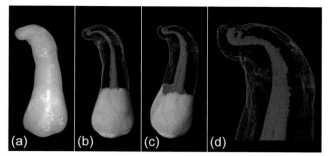

Fig. 11.3 (a) Digital photograph of an upper premolar with a single root that is severely curved towards its terminus. (b, c) Micro-CT images showing the internal anatomy of the root. (d) A detailed view on the anatomical complexity of the apical part.

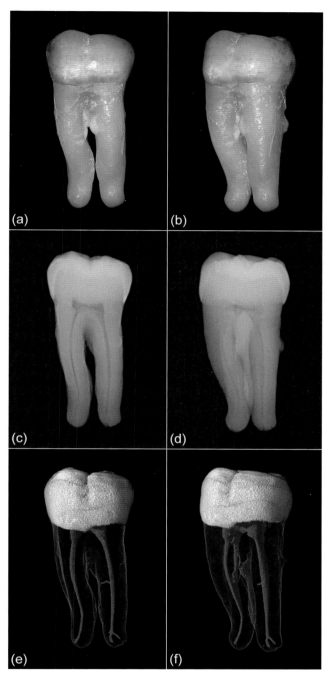

Fig. 11.2 (a, b) Digital photographs of an extracted lower molar. (c, d) Digital radiographic images of the same tooth providing a limited perception of root canal anatomy. (e, f) Micro-CT images showing the system with its lateral components.

The fact that root canals are curved and narrow in mature teeth makes it difficult to clean them of tissue and infectious elements as well as to shape. The risk of canal straightening and the creation of errors are related to the level and severity of the curvature. Abrupt apical curvatures and double curvatures (the S-shape) can be

especially difficult to negotiate and shape. In addition, canals that join or diverge always deviate from their initial path. It is important to realize that the resulting angle is often different for the canals involved (Fig. 11.5).

Besides complicating the process of instrumentation, root canal curvature results in several other procedural challenges. For example, needle placement and irrigant exchange for the removal of debris are more difficult beyond the curve. Related to visual aids, inspection with the operating microscope is restricted to the straight part of the root canal (above the curve). The creation of straight-line access, the use of flexible endodontic instruments and proper file bending and use are essential measures to prepare curved canals (see further below).

Cross-sectional shape and diameter

Root canals are round, oval or irregular (ribbon-shaped) on cross-sectional view. Oval and irregular shapes are common in the coronal two-thirds of root canals, whereas the round variant is often restricted to the apical part (Fig. 11.6). Oval cross-sectional shapes are often found in the distal root canals of mandibular molar teeth and in mandibular premolar and incisor teeth. In an investigation of 180 teeth representing all tooth types, Wu and co-workers (46) detected oval root canal shapes in 25% of the specimens investigated. When two or more canals are present in the same root, anastomoses and fins (lateral extensions) are frequently observed (Fig. 11.7). Some root canals may present with extreme cross-sectional shapes. This applies especially to the C-shaped canal (Fig. 11.8), which is more prevalent in certain ethnic groups (16). Oval and irregular cross-sectional shapes certainly do challenge root canal cleaning and shaping. Parts of the lateral anatomy are often out of reach because most endodontic instruments are designed to stay centered.

Root canal diameter is related to the concept of conicity or "taper". When looking at the root canal diameter at consecutive levels along the root, an idea of the overall conical shape is obtained. The exact value for diameter

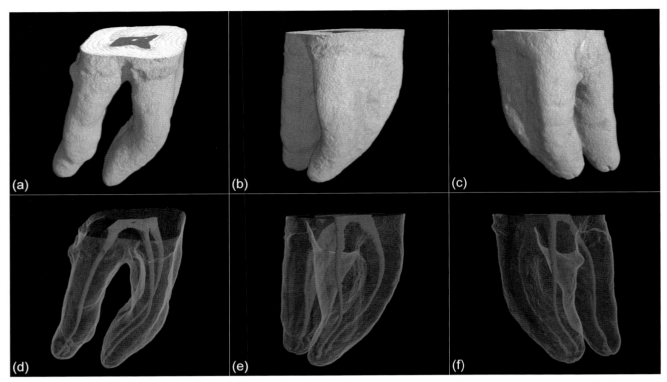

Fig. 11.4 Micro-CT data of a lower first molar. (a–c) Renderings of the outer surface of the roots. (d–f) Visualizations of the root canal system in relation to the outer root surface. Notice that most curvatures are multiplanar, thus expressed in both the mesiodistal and buccolingual plane.

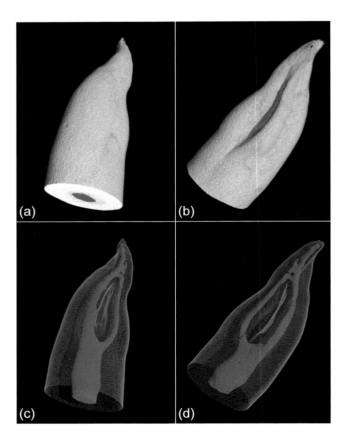

Fig. 11.5 Micro-CT data of an upper premolar. (a, b) Renderings of the outer root surface with a mesial invagination. (c, d) Visualizations of the inner root anatomy. Notice that the root canals that join or diverge deviate from their initial path, while the resulting angle is different for the canals involved.

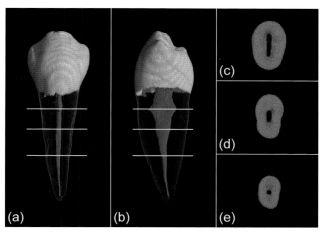

Fig. 11.6 (a, b) Visualizations of a lower premolar scanned with micro-CT. (c–e) Corresponding slices at different horizontal levels (indicated by the yellow lines) reveal the ribbon (c), oval (d), and round (e) cross-sectional shape of the canal.

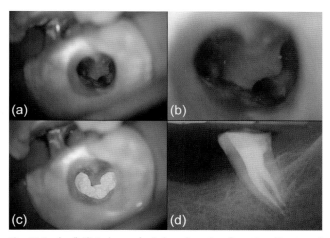

Fig. 11.8 (a–d) Clinical case of a C-shaped canal configuration. (Courtesy of Dr J. Berghmans.)

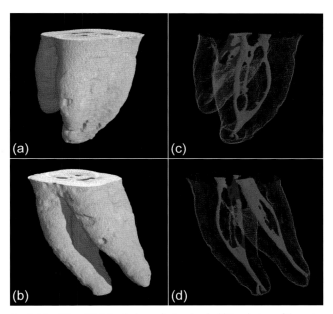

Fig. 11.7 Micro-CT data of a lower first molar. (a, b) Renderings of the outer surface of the roots. (c, d) Corresponding visualizations of the root canal system anatomy. Anastomoses and fins (lateral extensions) are present in both roots.

and taper will, however, vary for each point along the central axis. Usually root canals are wide in the coronal part and relatively narrow apically. Immature teeth and roots that are liable to some type of resorption may appear different. Also, deposition of reparative dentin may alter root canal diameter generally or locally (i.e. at sites of prior pulpal irritation).

Apical configuration

In their apical one-third, root canals are often narrow and more or less curved. Their "portals of exit" can have

the typical appearance of a foramen apicale (with or without accessory canals) (Fig. 11.9) or the sporadic appearance of an apical delta. Classical work carried out by Kuttler (21) demonstrated that, on average, the narrowest point of the canal (i.e. the apical constriction) is situated 0.48 mm (young group) and 0.60 mm (older group) from the root tip (radiographic apex). Yet there is great variation (9) (Key literature 11.1). The distance from the apical constriction to the foramen apicale is approximately 0.5 mm in the younger group and 0.8 mm in the older group for all tooth types (9, 21). In elderly patients, large amounts of secondary cementum formation may have caused the foramen apicale to move coronally, at a distance of up to 3 mm from the root tip (21). Because of this complex anatomy, the apical one-third of the root canal is prone to procedural errors such as ledges, zips and perforations, making infection control and apical seal difficult.

Key literature 11.1

Dummer et al. (9) examined 270 extracted human teeth of unknown age for evaluation of apex to foramen and apex to constriction distances; in addition the topography of the apical portion of the root canal was studied under 20× magnification. The mean apex to foramen (A–F) distance was 0.38 mm and the mean apex to constriction (A–C) distance 0.89 mm. It must be stressed that a wide range of values was observed. Four distinct types of apical constriction were routinely found, whilst a proportion of canals were apparently blocked. The study confirms the view that it is impossible, with complete certainty, to establish the position of the apical canal constriction during root canal therapy. Results of the study indicate that a combination of methods might be more successful than reliance on one method.

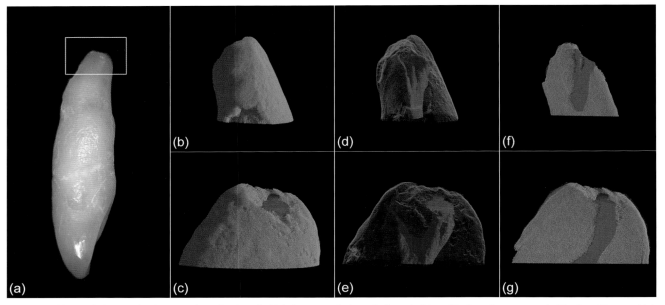

Fig. 11.9   (a) Digital photograph of an upper lateral incisor of which the most apical part (indicated with a white frame) was scanned with micro-CT at very high resolution (pixel size of 1.74 μm × 1.74 μm). (b, c) Renderings of the outer root surface. (d, e) Visualizations of the complex apical anatomy. (f, g) 3D renderings with cut-out to reveal the apical constriction and foramen apicale.

Physiologically and pathologically induced changes

Throughout the life of a tooth with a vital pulp, obliteration and narrowing of parts of the root canal system can occur owing to physiological aging and reparative processes. Low-grade irritation, such as slowly advancing dental caries, root surface exposure due to periodontal disease and acute or chronic trauma (e.g. accidents involving teeth, cavity and crown-related restorative procedures, traumatic occlusion and bruxism) may evoke such pulpal responses. In teeth with a loaded history (e.g. in elderly individuals) the deposition of reparative dentin can be particularly substantial.

The mineralization process usually begins in the coronal part of the root canal system and proceeds apically. Thus, there may eventually be generalized accumulations of hard tissue on the wall of the root canal, narrowing the lumen to such an extent that the canal appears obliterated (Fig. 11.10). Mineralizations may also take the form of pulp stones that are free within the root canal system or attached to the root canal wall. In the pulp chamber of molars the hard tissue tends to form on the roof to shorten the chamber size in a vertical dimension making it difficult to localize root canal orifices upon access preparation. Besides hampering exploration of root canals, canal negotiation is a real challenge in these cases and the creation of a ledge, and subsequent root perforation constitutes a distinct risk.

Procedural steps

Preassessment

After clinical examination and diagnosis, preassessment of the case is imperative, including the construction of a mental image of the tooth to be treated. The preoperative radiographs are carefully examined and the external root surface is palpated or probed. Special attention is paid to:

- a possible inclination of the tooth;
- the cervical contour of the (residual) tooth crown;
- the size of the pulp chamber;
- the amount of obliteration and narrowing of the root canal system;
- the integrity and course of the periodontal ligament;
- the number of roots (and root canals);
- length and diameter of the root(s);
- the degree of root canal curvature (as far as possible).

Field isolation

Asepsis is a strict requirement for non-surgical endodontic treatment. Bacterial contamination of the operation field (the tooth crown and root canal system) is avoided by using rubber dam isolation and disinfection techniques, sterilized instruments and decontaminated materials (see Chapter 4). Every experienced clinician will confirm

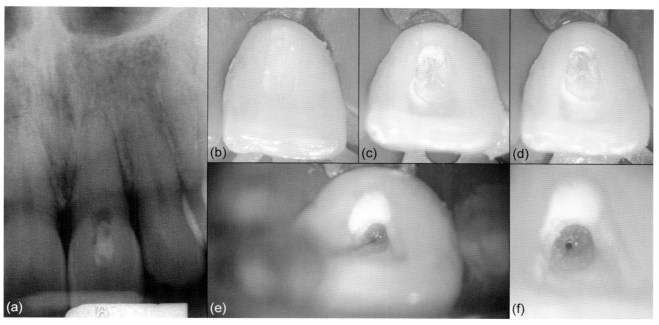

Fig. 11.10 (a) Clinical case of an upper central incisor showing an apparently calcified root canal system. (b–f) Gradual exploration in apical direction towards the deeply situated canal lumen. (Courtesy of Dr J. Berghmans.)

the view that the use of rubber dam facilitates rather than complicates endodontic treatment. Well-informed patients will accept the use of rubber dam and will appreciate the effort for quality and comfort.

Access opening

Proper access is the key to successful cleaning and shaping of root canals. While the entire roof of the pulp chamber often has to be removed, the outline of the access cavity is dictated by the number and position of the root canal orifice(s) (Fig. 11.11 and Table 11.1).

Initial penetration into the pulp chamber should be undertaken using a bur in a water-cooled high-speed handpiece. Normally a safe direction to avoid misalignment and excessive damage to the crown is towards the widest root canal (e.g. palatal root in upper molars and distal root in lower molars). Once into the pulp chamber, overhanging margins must be removed. One may then shift preparation technique to a slow-speed handpiece without water coolant in order to enhance visualization. Useful burs in this phase of the access preparation are long-shanked round burs. In cases where localization of the pulp chamber appears challenging, rubber dam placement may be delayed until an opening has been found. The advantage of this measure is to get indications on root inclinations and furcation grooves by probing the external root surface. Root surface probing can be especially useful in cases of premolars with multiple

canals in the buccal root, and in cases of preparation through a metal crown.

Complete removal of the existing coronal restoration is advised in most cases because it:

- allows better radiographic interpretation of the anatomy of the coronal part of the root canal system;
- allows complete inspection of the residual crown (e.g. for the detection of possible fractures);
- solves marginal leakage;
- detects hidden caries;
- provides a better view of the pulp chamber in the presence of more refracted light;
- prevents inconsistent readings when using electronic apex locators;
- prevents metal filings from entering the canal.

Once uncovered, the floor of the pulp chamber can be examined like a map in order to explore the root canal system anatomy. Care should be taken to avoid damaging the floor of the pulp chamber as the root canal orifices are to be sought along the groove system. A straight sharp-tipped explorer is handy here. In cases of gross depositions of mineralized tissue, exploration of the connecting grooves can be done using ultrasonically powered instruments (used at low power settings and with a light touch) or with long-shanked round burs in a slow-speed (800–1000 rpm) handpiece. Slight differences in color between the walls of the pulp chamber and the floor assist in finding the root canal entrances (Fig. 11.12).

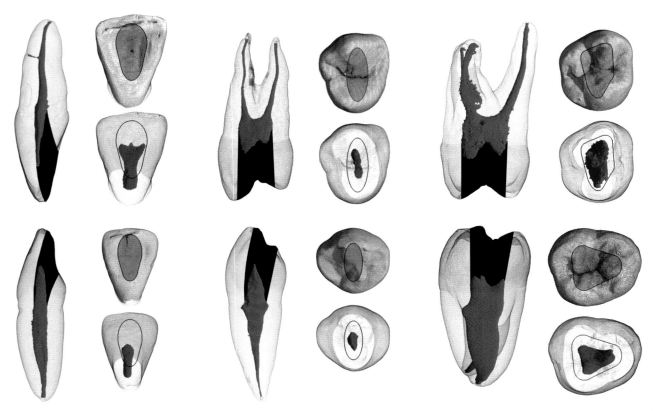

Fig. 11.11 Images of the upper (top) and lower (bottom) dentition generated with micro-CT. The outline of the access cavity (i.e. the black area that was added to the image) is dictated by the position of the root canal orifice(s), while the entire roof of the pulp chamber has to be removed.

Cavity walls are adjusted to reflect the operating light and to allow straight-line entry to the root canal(s). For example, in order to locate the MB2 (second canal in the mesiobuccal root) in maxillary molars, the access cavity should be created with a clear extension towards the mesial side (Fig. 11.13). All cavity walls are then smoothed and connected with the orifice(s) of the respective canal(s). The latter simplifies re-entry into the canal, especially when irrigants are present, without buckling the tip of small files. Of course, access cavity preparation should be performed after careful examination of the undistorted preoperative radiograph(s) and with respect for the integrity of the crown.

Initial root canal preparation (coronal preflaring)

As a general rule, the removal of root dentin should be centered, i.e. with respect to the initial root canal anatomy. In the coronal one-third of a curved root canal, however, this concept is intentionally ignored. Indeed, by carefully relocating the root canal orifice (using for instance Gates–Glidden burs), the degree of mid-root curvature is decreased without weakening the tooth (Fig. 11.14). The creation of a "straight-line access" is

mandatory to avoid obstruction of the intracanal view, root canal straightening and instrument separation.

Regarding the adopted technique for instrumentation, one makes a distinction between file movement and shaping approach. The latter is related to the instrument sequence and file insertion depth. In general, a coronal-to-apical approach is advised because:

- coronal preflaring allows more control during subsequent preparation of the middle and apical one-thirds;
- the risk of canal blockage, ledge formation and instrument fracture is reduced;
- working length determination is more precise after coronal preflaring.

In the modified double flared approach, for instance, the coronal portion of the root canal is flared first (from orifice to curvature) (see Clinical procedure 11.1). In cases of curved and narrow canals, the root canal is gradually explored and flared first, and care is taken not to overload any specific instrument as it may create a ledge. An error that is commonly made during this initial procedure is to overuse files, especially the smaller sizes. Instead of wasting one file after the other, sizes 06–10 K-files should be used in combination with flexible

Table 11.1   Root canals in teeth of maxilla and mandible.

Maxilla

Central incisor	1 canal 100%
Lateral incisor	1 canal 100%
Canine	1 canal 100%
1st premolar	2 roots 57% Single root, 2 canals 16% Single root, 2 canals, 1 foramen 12% 3 roots, 3 canals 6%
2nd premolar	1 canal 53% 2 canals, 1 foramen 22% 2 canals, 1 foramen 13% 2 roots, 2 canals 11% 3 roots, 3 canals 1%
1st molar	3 roots, 3 canals 38% 4 canals 60% Mesiobuccal canal: 2 canals 60% 2 foramina 20% 1 foramen 80%
2nd molar	3 roots 60% 1 mesiobuccal canal 70% 2 mesiobuccal canals: 1 foramen 15% 2 foramina 10% 2 roots 25% 1 root 10%

Mandible

Central incisor	1 canal 70%
Lateral incisor	1 canal 55% 2 canals, 2 foramina: central 5% lateral 15% 2 canals, 1 foramen: central 25% lateral 30%
Canine	1 canal 70% 2 canals, 1 foramen 20% 2 canals, 2 foramina 10%
1st premolar	1 canal, 1 foramen 74% Branching canal: 1 foramen 4% 2 foramina 25% 2nd premolar 1 canal, 1 foramen 97% Branching canal: 1 foramen 12% 2 foramina 3%
1st molar	2 mesial canals 60%, 1 foramen 40% 1 distal canal 70% Distal canal: 2 canals, 1 foramen 35% 2 canals, 2 foramina 10%
2nd molar	2 mesial canals 40%, 1 foramen 35% 1 canal 25% 1 distal canal 92% 2 canals, 1 foramen 5% 2 canals, 2 foramina 3% Can have a C-shaped distal canal

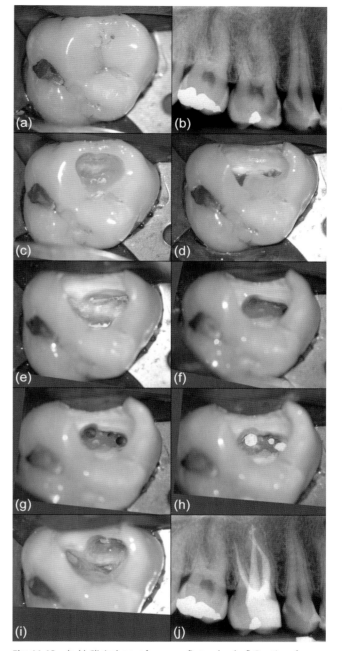

Fig. 11.12   (a, b) Clinical case of an upper first molar. (c–f) Creation of access and exploration of three canal orifices within the mesio-buccal root. (g–j) Root canal preparation, filling and radiographic control. (Courtesy of Dr J. Berghmans.)

K-files sizes 15–30 to cut more coronal shape in big increments (i.e. the "serial step-back negotiation"). The smaller-sized K-file, which was resisting further advancement, may then advance deeper into the root canal because the shank portions are released from binding. In all situations, the act of recapitulation represents a safe and effective strategy for root canal negotiation.

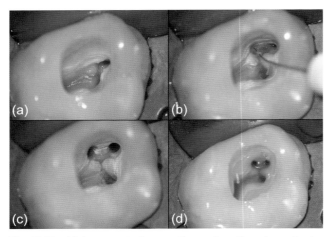

Fig. 11.13 (a) Access cavity in a maxillary molar with a clear extension towards the mesial side. (b–d) Root canal negotiation and preparation. (Courtesy of Dr J. Berghmans.)

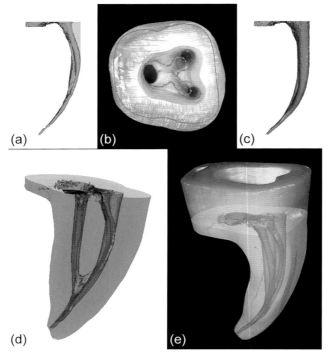

Fig. 11.14 Micro-CT data showing the mesial root canals of a lower molar (a) before (green) and (c) after (red) instrumentation with ProTaper. (b) Micro-CT generated contours layered on a digital photograph of the pulp chamber floor. Straight-line access is created by relocating the root canal orifices (i.e. from the green to the red contour line). (d, e) 3D renderings of the outer root surface and internal anatomy after registration of both datasets. (Preparation by Dr C. Ruddle.)

Clinical procedure 11.1 The modified double flared approach

(1) Pre-assessment of the case.
(2) Field isolation with rubber dam.
(3) Creation of straight-line access.
(4) Irrigation of the pulp chamber.
(5) Localization of root canal orifices and penetration with a size 15 flexible K-file (watch-winding) (if necessary start with smaller files).
(6) Careful shaping of the straight coronal portion (preflaring) with the alternating use of flexible K-files sizes 15–40 (if necessary start with smaller files) and Gates–Glidden burs (sizes 2–4). To avoid ledge formation:
   - use only light apical force;
   - work at different depths;
   - vary between different file sizes;
   - recapitulate with a small instrument.
(7) Reconfirm straight-line access (thus no strain on the file when placed coronally from the curve).
(8) Keep using irrigants; do not work in dry conditions.
(9) Working length (WL) determination: size 15 flexible K-file (if necessary start with smaller files) with balanced force motion to the apical constriction (use an electronic apex locator).

Option A: ISO-sized hand files (2% taper)
- Apical preparation to size 30–35 (balanced force motion; irrigation and recapitulation).
- Traditional step-back (from apical to coronal; steps of 0.5 mm per increase in tip size).
- Removal of small steps with apical file size 30–35 (filing motion with small amplitude).
- Apical gauging (if necessary proceed with larger files).
- Final irrigation.

Option B: GT hand files (6–12% taper)
- Work with flexible K-file size 20 to the WL (balanced force motion).
- Reconfirm patency and work with size 25 flexible K-file to the WL (balanced force motion).
- Select a GT hand file and work to the WL (*reverse* balanced force; recapitulation).
- Apical gauging (if necessary proceed with a GT hand file little beyond the constriction to achieve a preparation larger than tip size 20).
- Final irrigation.

In Ni–Ti rotary instrumentation, stainless steel 10–20/.02 K-files (hand-held, flexible) are used – first pre-curved, then straight – to scout (explore) a portion of the overall length of the canal and to create or confirm a smooth, reproducible glide path. Subsequently, Ni–Ti rotary files can be used in a crown-down sequence (coronal-to-apical) over this length (expanded upon further below).

Methods to establish working length

Determination of the apical limit for preparation of root canals (working length) is a most critical procedural step; canals should be instrumented neither too short nor too long. Instrumentation short of the canal exit risks leaving inflamed tissue and infectious elements in the root canal space, while instrumentation beyond the apical foramen may force infectious debris into the periapical tissue compartment and cause an endodontic flare-up (Chapter 7). Overpreparation may also pave the way for overfilling with lingering foreign body reaction and incomplete regeneration of the supporting tissues as a result (31). Generally, it is believed that the apical termination of the intervention should be at the apical constriction because this location indicates the junction between the periodontal and pulpal tissues (9). The working length may be determined in a number of ways but, whatever method is used, it must be accurate, repeatable and carried out easily.

Measuring working length by radiography

Undistorted periapical radiographs taken with a film-holder and the paralleling technique prior to treatment allow only for an approximate *estimation* of the length of canal preparation to be taken. For more exact measurements a precurved instrument with a silicone stop on the shaft is placed into the root canal short of the inspected length. If coronal preflaring of the root canal has been done prior to working length measurement then tactile sensation can be used to feel for the apical constriction. However, there will be no proper tactile feedback if the apical constriction has been destroyed (e.g. root resorption), if there is immature development of the root end, or if the root canal is narrow along most of its length. The root canal under exploration needs to be widened to a size 10–15 for the instrument tip to be seen clearly on the working length radiograph.

If the radiographic image shows the tip of the instrument to be more than 2 mm short of the radiographic apex, then the silicone stop should be readjusted and another film exposed. If the instrument tip exits the radiographic root contour, then the silicone stop should be adjusted accordingly and a further radiograph taken. The working length is recorded in the patient's progress notes together with the coronal reference point from which the measurement was taken. Cusp tips are not very useful for this exercise and judicious flattening will help to provide a more positive landmark.

The radiographic method is far from accurate when:

- the root canal exit deviates in the buccolingual (or buccopalatal) plane;
- the position of the apical constriction is far from the radiographic apex;

- oblique external root resorption affects the tip of the root;
- the radiographic apex is indiscernible owing to over-projection of (anatomical) structures.

For these reasons electronic apex locators (EALs) are used to supplement the radiographic method.

Measuring working length by electronic apex locators

Suzuki (40) discovered in dog experiments in 1942 that the electrical resistance between the periodontal ligament and the oral mucosa was a consistent value of 6.5 kΩ. The same observation was made in humans by Sunada (39) in 1962, thus leading to the introduction of the *resistance-type* apex locators. Unfortunately these early devices often yielded inaccurate results when electrolytes, excessive moisture, vital pulp tissue, exudates or excessive bleeding were present in the root canal (43). With the introduction of the *impedance-type* EALs in the late 1980s and especially the *frequency-dependent* EALs in the early 1990s, a more accurate canal length measurement was obtained in these various canal conditions (13).

Frequency-dependent EALs use more advanced technology and measure the impedance difference between two frequencies or the ratio of two (or more) electrical impedances. Using EALs, one side of the electrical circuit is connected to the root canal instrument and the other electrode to a lip clip that connects with the oral mucosa (Fig. 11.15). As the instrument moves towards the apex, the impedance difference (or ratio) becomes greater and shows the greatest value at the apical constriction, allowing for a measurement at this location. Some devices need to be calibrated when the instrument is inserted into the coronal portion of the canal. The accuracy of contemporary EALs is very high (approximately 90%) with a tolerance level of 0.5 mm (13). For that reason, EALs are currently used as an important adjunct to radiography to determine working length.

It should be realized that when the canal lumen of a curved canal is gradually enlarged, the instrument that is used to measure working length will follow a straighter course than initially. As a result the working length (i.e. the distance between the reference point and the intended apical level of instrumentation) will change throughout the canal preparation. By determining working length after coronal preflaring, one will minimize the risk for overinstrumentation. In addition, an EAL can be connected to each file of the series to continuously monitor file insertion relative to the working length.

Paper point evaluation

A paper point placed into a dried canal and extended beyond the working length will absorb tissue fluid at the

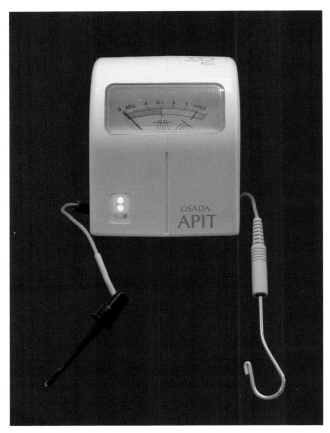

Fig. 11.15 Electronic apex locator.

apex and, if withdrawn immediately, will allow measurement of the dry portion of the point, thereby providing some indication of the working length.

Final canal preparation

As outlined in Chapters 4 and 9 a primary objective of root canal instrumentation is to physically remove pulpal tissue and infectious elements. An important objective is also to prepare root canals in such a way that optimal disinfection can be carried out and a final filling be properly placed. The instrumentation process therefore aims to attain a tapered canal. There is no firm guidance, based on biological evidence, on the amount of taper that is needed for an optimal root canal preparation. It should be noted that sufficient shape for cone fit with gutta-percha does not necessarily imply that enough preparation has been done for effective cleaning and disinfection. There is always a delicate balance between the need to remove sufficient amounts of hard tissue and the threat of fracture from weakening the tooth structure. It should also be noted that shaping teeth in a pulpectomy procedure should not be kept more restricted than that for teeth with non-vital, infected pulps; soft-tissue elimination and filling in such cases is as demanding.

The amount of preparation to be carried out in the apical one-third of root canals is the subject of controversy. Some people believe that it is unnecessary to widen the apical preparation because coronal preflaring and apical patency confirmation will allow the irrigant to reach and clean the apical part of the root canal. Most clinical experts, however, advocate rather large (size 35 or higher) but centered preparations in order to remove infected dentin in the apical few millimeters of the root canal (18–20). Certainly the widening of the apical part of the root canal to a reasonable size and taper after preparation of the coronal and middle sections allows easier placement of the needle for irrigation (47) and also of the gutta-percha cone for obturation.

Various techniques may be applied. In the modified double flared approach the second flare is obtained with a step-back sequence. This step-back means the smallest instrument is used to the working length first, and then instruments with increasing tip diameters are used more coronally in fixed increments (see Clinical procedure 11.1, Option A). Instead of this step-back sequence with 2% tapered instruments, GT hand files can be selected for a crown-down sequence to flare the apical portion more easily (see Clinical procedure 11.1, Option B).

In Ni–Ti rotary instrumentations, stainless steel 10–20/.02 K-files (hand-held, flexible) are first used to create a glide path to the working length to minimize the stress on the subsequent Ni–Ti rotary files. These files can then be used safely in a crown-down sequence (see further below).

For the final file selection, *apical gauging* is advised since the initial diameter of the apical constriction varies for different canals. This procedural step means the insertion of an instrument to the working length after coronal and apical flaring (to avoid interference of the upper part). The gauging file is then fitted to the apical constriction (without rotation) to note any resistance. If so, the diameter for the final preparation is thought to have been defined. In most cases, one selects a few sizes larger because the cross-sectional shape of the root canal can be oval with the smallest diameter measured.

Endodontic instruments

Traditional systems

For decades, instrumentation of root canals was solely performed using stainless steel (and nickel–titanium) hand files in various forms. All these files have cutting flutes 16 mm long and for each millimeter of shaft the diameter increases by 0.02 mm (2% taper), so the final cutting part of the instrument (known as D16) is 0.32 mm wider than the first part of the tip (known as D1) (Fig. 11.16). Hand files series are color-coded and increase in diameter in set increments, the smallest diameter

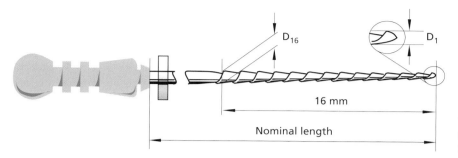

Fig. 11.16 Drawing showing a hand file (ISO-sized; 2% taper) with the distances D1 and D16 marked.

being 0.06 mm (at D1) and increasing to 1.40 mm. The length of the shaft of the instrument from the tip to the handle may be 21 mm, 25 mm (regular) or 31 mm.

One differentiates between reamers and files based on the production process of hand files, and thus on longitudinal and cross-sectional shape. The essential difference between these instruments is that reamers are used in rotation while files can also be used in a push–pull (filing) motion.

Reamers made from stainless steel may be square or triangular in cross-section. A tapered wire is twisted to create sharp cutting flutes that are present every 0.5–1.0 mm along the working part of the instrument (Fig. 11.17). When these instruments are used in rotation, the flutes cut into the dentin and remove it from the canal walls. The use of hand, stainless steel ISO-sized reamers has declined in popularity because of their lack of flexibility (especially in larger sizes), their inability to prepare canals with anything other than a round cross-section, and their lack of cutting efficiency when compared with other instruments.

Files come in a number of configurations within the standard of a 2% taper. There are three main types: K-files, flexible K-files and Hedström files. K-files are manufactured in a similar manner to reamers except that the cutting spirals produced by twisting are much tighter (Fig. 11.17). The cross-section can be triangular or square

in shape. *Flexible* K-files are essentially similar to K-files except that the cross-sectional design is such that the instrument is able to flex more than the conventional K-file (Fig. 11.17). They may be made from stainless steel alloys or nickel–titanium. Hedström files are manufactured by grinding a tapered blank that has a round cross-section (Fig. 11.17). Machining produces a spirally tapered series of cones with cutting edges at the base of each cone. The instrument is designed for a filing motion and cuts only when being withdrawn from the root canal. If used in rotation it may break relatively easily because of the small core diameter. The use of Hedström files is mainly for flaring root canals, especially oval-shaped canals. They can also be used for removal of fractured instruments and gutta-percha in retreatment cases. Hedström files in larger sizes are more rigid and may cause ledges or strip perforations within curved root canals and should therefore be used with great caution (1).

Gates–Glidden burs are, in effect, engine-driven reamers. These burs come in various sizes from ISO 050 (size 1) to ISO 150 (size 6) and are available in 15 mm and 19 mm lengths (Fig. 11.18). The tip of the instrument is elliptically shaped with short cutting flutes and a non-cutting tip. The instruments are designed so that if stressed they will fracture at the junction of the shank and the shaft. Gates–Glidden burs are used to relocate the root canal orifice and to flare the coronal straight portion of the root canal. Because they are relatively aggressive, care must be taken to avoid overuse coronally as this may weaken the tooth structure and lead to strip perforation. These instruments should be used at 800 rpm to ensure adequate control. Gates–Glidden burs generate considerable debris and preferably should be used when the pulp chamber and root canal(s) are filled with an irrigant in order to avoid canal blockage.

Nickel–titanium rotary systems

Nickel–titanium: a super-elastic alloy

The super-elasticity of Ni–Ti is based on stress-induced martensitic transformation (see Advanced concept 11.1). The application of outer stress causes martensite to form at temperatures higher than the transition temperature

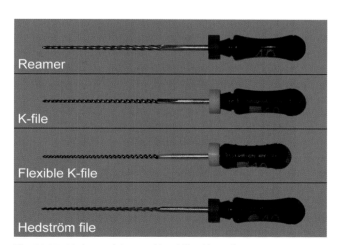

Reamer

K-file

Flexible K-file

Hedström file

Fig. 11.17 Various stainless steel hand files (size 40).

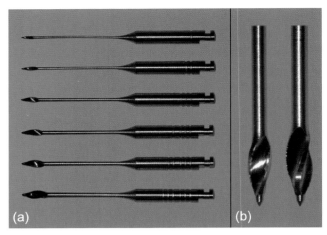

Fig. 11.18 (a) Gates–Glidden burs sizes 1 to 6. (b) A detailed view of the tip design.

Advanced concept 11.1

Nickel–titanium "shape memory metal alloy" can exist in two different temperature-dependent crystal structures called martensite (lower temperature or daughter phase) and austenite (higher temperature or parent phase). The crystal lattice structure can be altered by either temperature or stress (Fig. 11.22). This is important because several properties of both forms are notably different. From the practical point of view, Ni–Ti can have three different forms: martensite, stress-induced martensite (super-elastic) and austenite. When the material is in its martensite form, it is soft and ductile, and it can be easily deformed. Super-elastic Ni–Ti is highly elastic (rubber-like), while austenitic Ni–Ti is quite strong and hard.

(i.e. the martensitic start temperature). When the outer stress is released, the martensite transforms back into austenite and the specimen returns back to its original shape. As a result, super-elastic Ni–Ti can be strained several times more than ordinary metal alloys without being plastically deformed, and with relatively light force (low elastic modulus).

File design: the concept of greater taper

Because the super-elasticity of nickel–titanium diminishes the connection between instrument diameter and stiffness, the use of rotary files with a two- to six-fold taper (and large diameter) has become possible. These Ni–Ti rotary files are mainly manufactured for use in a torque-controlled handpiece at constant speed (rpm).

Besides variation in taper, the existing Ni–Ti rotary files have various designs for instrument shaft (including blades and grooves). The shaft design is adapted to be used in continuous rotation. Most systems flatten, modify or shorten the cutting edges and vary the depth of the groove, helical angle, pitch or taper to prevent the instrument from screwing and binding in the canal wall. The original ProFile instruments were some of the first Ni–Ti rotary instruments on the market (Fig. 11.19). Their cross-sectional shape is made by machining three equally spaced U-shaped grooves around the shaft of a tapered Ni–Ti wire. For this "classical" design, a space remains without being ground between each groove, providing a "radial land area". Without a blade projecting outwards from the middle of the shaft, this flat area prevents the file from locking in the dentin, while cutting occurs through a planing (acting passively) action. By contrast, some of the latest systems show sharp cutting edges (acting actively) resulting from a triangular cross-sectional design. Such an instrument, the so-called ProTaper, also combines multiple progressive tapers within the same shaft (Fig. 11.19).

The existing rake angle can be verified in accordance with shaft design. The rake angle can be seen as the angle between the leading edge of a cutting tool and a perpendicular to the surface being cut. A rake angle can be negative, neutral or positive (Fig. 11.20). In general, conventional endodontic instruments have a slightly negative rake angle and most Ni–Ti rotary files have a slightly negative or neutral rake angle.

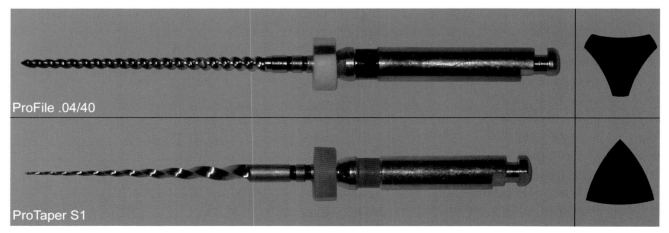

ProFile .04/40

ProTaper S1

Fig. 11.19 Design of two nickel–titanium rotary files (lengthwise and cross-sectional view).

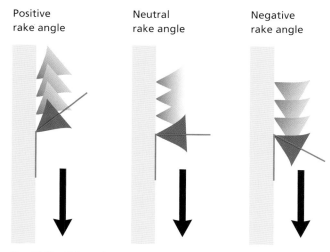

Positive
rake angle

Neutral
rake angle

Negative
rake angle

Fig. 11.20   Rake angles.

Regarding the instrument tip, one could summarize that most contemporary files, both hand-held and engine-driven, have an acceptable non-aggressive tip design and there should be little concern over tip geometry in the selection of files (ISO/ANSI guidelines). Most Ni–Ti rotary files have rounded non-cutting tips that serve as a guide within the canal. Unlike the tip, the instrument shaft retains its cutting action; only the transition angle at D1 is modified. Concerning size of the tip, most manufacturers of Ni–Ti rotary instruments make use of real increments (in 50 μm), equal to the standard guidelines used for the production of stainless steel hand files.

The file design of the Lightspeed system deserves attention. These instruments are modified so that a short cutting zone remains apically, the so-called apical action design (45) (Fig. 11.21). The files are used for apical preparation and do not cut over most of the canal length because of the existence of a smooth small-diameter shaft that also enhances instrument's flexibility. Apical action designed instruments prepare the apical portion with less transportation and less dentin removal than other instruments (12). Nevertheless, as with other Ni–Ti instruments there are risks for instrument fracture and special training is needed (23).

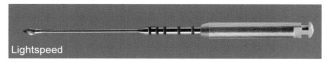

Lightspeed

Fig. 11.21   Lightspeed file design.

> ### Advanced concept 11.2   Cutting efficiency of Ni–Ti rotary files
>
> Ni–Ti *rotary* files are as effective as or better than stainless steel *hand* files in machining dentin owing to the continuous reaming motion (42). The rake angle of the cutting blades plays a central role in determining the cutting efficiency. Nearly all of the latest Ni–Ti rotary files have a neutral or slightly negative rake angle for maximum effectiveness.
>
> *Alloy hardness* is far less than that for stainless steel hand files (8) (Vickers hardness number ca. 300–350). Nevertheless, the surface of Ni–Ti instruments is not homogeneous and Serene and co-workers (35) found that the cutting edges were softer than the core of the instruments.
>
> As with stainless steel files, Ni–Ti files wear significantly upon use on dentin (49). Sterilization also has a negative effect. Repeated cycles under autoclave decrease the performance of Ni–Ti files by altering their structure underneath the surface (30). On the other hand, the presence of sodium hypochlorite around the instrument shaft for less than 30–60 min did not cause any corrosion or difference in cutting efficiency (14).
>
> Cutting efficiency also depends on the shape of the grooves. A deep groove allows more debris transportation during action of the file. In this way, cutting efficiency is related to cleaning effectiveness. The removal of cut dentin chips is therefore important to reduce clogging of the cutting blades and eventually the root canal itself. During the continuous reaming motion, macroscopic debris is taken out by the rotating grooves while existing radial land areas push microscopic debris deep into dentinal tubules. In this context, most studies indicate that Ni–Ti rotary systems are as good as or better than stainless steel hand instrumentation in removing superficial debris (2). However, Ni–Ti rotary files seem to produce a thicker smear layer, particularly in the apical one-third (28).

Instrumentation techniques

Hand instrumentation

The modified double flared approach

As a result of the 2% taper standardization for hand files, a final shaping objective with greater (4% or higher) taper can only be achieved using a series of files with different tip diameter at various levels in the root canal (see Clinical procedure 11.1, Option A). Besides the shaping approach, how the selected instruments are moved is also critical to the result. Well-known file movements include the filing (or push–pull) motion and the reaming motion (rotation).

File manipulation: the filing and reaming motions

The filing motion is especially suitable to the Hedström file. It removes dentin from the root canal wall when the instrument is inserted to a given length and then pressed against the canal walls at the same time as it is drawn coronally. This action is performed and resumed with certain amplitude. There are difficulties with this method, including the tendency to grooving into the dentinal canal wall, without a conscious effort being made to move the file circumferentially, and packing of debris ahead of the instrument tip, which may block the root canal. The push–pull motion is also possible with K-files but should be restricted to size 15 (or less) as rasping with larger instruments may cause iatrogenic damage.

The reaming motion denotes a clockwise or counter-clockwise rotation of the instrument in the root canal. It is the preferred method for reamers and (flexible) K-files.

Watch-winding is a clockwise/counter-clockwise rotation of the instrument through an arc of 30–90° while advancing the instrument into the canal. The reciprocating back and forth rotational movement alternately pulls the instrument into the canal (clockwise), and then (counter-clockwise) cuts the engaged dentin. At a certain point watch-winding will not advance the instrument further into the canal. In many cases, three to five push–pull filing strokes will loosen the shaft and allow watch-winding to advance the instrument further apically. The watch-winding method is less aggressive than the original "quarter turn–pull" and should be used with light apical pressure. With precurved stainless steel instruments this technique is extremely useful for initial negotiation of root canals, especially those that are severely curved or narrow (see Core concept 11.1).

The *balanced force motion* was devised by Roane and co-workers (32) and endorsed by Charles and Charles (7) on the basis of a mathematical model. This technique is essentially a reaming action using clockwise movement to insert the file and counter-clockwise movement to remove dentin. The file is placed into the root canal until it binds against the wall. The file is then rotated through 60–90° with light apical pressure. This creates threads within the dentin. The instrument is moved counter-clockwise through 120–360° with mild apical pressure, which crushes and breaks off the dentin threads and enlarges the root canal. A final clockwise rotation allows

flutes to be loaded with debris and removed from the root canal. This technique has been shown to be efficient and less prone to cause iatrogenic damage (36). The technique must be used with flexible K-files that are not precured. A technique of *reverse* balanced force instrumentation has been developed for use with GT hand files where the flutes of the shaft are machined in an opposite thread to normal files (see Clinical procedure 11.1, Option B).

Nickel–titanium rotary instrumentation

The crown-down sequence

In general, Ni–Ti rotary systems advocate preflaring of the coronal portion of the root canal and relocation of the canal orifices with Gates–Glidden burs prior to deeper instrumentation (22). Preflaring can also be carried out with Ni–Ti rotary files such as orifice openers or accessory files from the system. These instruments for initial shaping tend to produce centered preparations, however; anti-curvature relocation of the canal orifice is more difficult to obtain. Some of the newest systems (e.g. ProTaper) seem to behave differently. Their active cutting design, lacking radial land areas, removes dentin more selectively and allows coronal relocation (Fig. 11.14). Meticulous manipulation of this file is, however, essential to get the particular effect and to avoid strip perforations (33).

After coronal preflaring, Ni–Ti rotary files are used in a crown-down sequence (coronal to apical) up to 3–4 mm from the working length as estimated on well-angulated radiographs (NB: do not forget to create and confirm glide path first). A first concept therefore adopts the use of a constant taper (typically .06) while reducing tip size throughout the sequence, whereas the variably tapered file concept changes this taper in the sequence of canal instrumentation with or without changing tip size (see Clinical procedure 11.2). The latter maximizes cutting efficiency by increasing the force per unit area of the file against the canal wall, whereas the former runs the risk of a taper-lock (see Core concept 11.2). Proceeding further on this idea, the ProTaper was introduced, a Ni–Ti file design that combines multiple progressive tapers within the same shaft (Fig. 11.19).

Once the working length determination is complete and a glide path established, the delicate preparation of the apical portion is continued with Ni–Ti rotary files at the working length. Some systems promote the use of tapers up to 8% or 10%, while confining tip size (e.g. size 20 for small canals). Most concepts, however, begin with 4% tapered files, while gradually increasing tip size up to the final apical preparation diameter. Next, the body of the preparation is finished with 6% tapered files at the working length.

Core concept 11.1

The trick of prebending is compatible with the filing motion and the watch-winding motion. Prebending of relatively small files is required in cases of abrupt root canal curvature or branching, or to bypass ledges. Files that are bent to negotiate severely curved canals must be smoothly curved to the last flute. The prebending of larger instruments, however, is discouraged because it may cause canal straightening. If precured, more rigid files are used in full rotation, an "hour-glass shape" will occur (i.e. small preparation at the curve; large above and beyond).

Clinical procedure 11.2   Variable tip variable taper sequence

- (Orifice openers)
- Ni–Ti rotary file 40/.04
- Ni–Ti rotary file 35/.06
- Ni–Ti rotary file 30/.04
- Ni–Ti rotary file 25/.06 and 20/.04
- In the majority of cases, the 25/.06 or the 20/.04 will reach the desired working length. If not, the sequence is repeated from the beginning.

Core concept 11.2

The location of debris in the flutes provides some information on the part of the shaft that has been engaged. If the instrument is cutting along most of its total length, another file should immediately be selected to prevent taper lock and file fracture.

In general, all Ni–Ti rotary systems follow a comparable approach (see Clinical procedure 11.3). As important differences do exist it is advisable to follow the specific instructions given by the manufacturer. The Lightspeed system, however, needs further consideration. As mentioned before, this system incorporates a smooth flexible shaft with a short cutting head. As a result of the no-taper design, flare can be achieved only using a step-back sequence with numerous instrument sizes or another file with increased taper to refine the root canal walls before obturation (41).

Continuous reaming motion

The advantageous qualities of the Ni–Ti alloy are maximally exploited if the instruments are continuously rotating over 360°. As mentioned before, Ni–Ti rotary files exist in an austenitic phase that transforms to a martensitic structure on stressing at a constant temperature. In this stress-induced martensitic phase only a light force is required for bending (Fig. 11.22). Limited and constant stress is needed for optimal performance. This is accomplished by using constant speed (rpm) and light apical pressure. In this way, the Ni–Ti rotary file will operate in the horizontal part of the stress/strain curve, showing little restoring forces and no plastic deformation. Ni–Ti rotary systems have a speed range (rpm) and torque limits (N/cm²) for optimal performance that are specified by the manufacturer for each file separately. Above the allowed torque, plastic deformation and instrument fracture may occur. If the torque-limit value is set too low, the file will stop cutting even when safe. Increased speed (higher rpm) seems to increase shaft stiffness (27). For that reason, a lower rpm may be required to instrument small curved canals.

Clinical procedure 11.3   Treatment sequence for most Ni–Ti rotary systems

(1) Preassessment of the case.
(2) Field isolation with rubber dam.
(3) Creation of straight-line access.
(4) Irrigation of the pulp chamber (2.5–5% NaOCl).
(5) Localization of root canal orifices and penetration with flexible K-files size 15–20 (watch-winding) (if necessary start with smaller files).
(6) Careful shaping of the straight coronal portion (preflaring) with the alternating use of hand files, Gates–Glidden burs and Ni–Ti rotary files (if preferred). To avoid ledge formation:
   – use only light apical force;
   – work at different depths;
   – vary between different file sizes;
   – recapitulate with a small instrument.
(7) Reconfirm straight-line access (thus no strain on the file when placed coronally from the curve).
(8) Crown-down clearance up to 3–4 mm from the estimated working length (create and confirm glide path first).
(9) Keep using irrigants; do not work in dry conditions.
(10) Working length determination: size 15 flexible K-file (if necessary start with smaller files) with balanced force motion to the apical constriction (use an electronic apex locator).
(11) Create and confirm glide path (flexible K-file size 15–20).
(12) Apical preparation to size 30–35 (6% taper).
(13) Apical gauging (if necessary proceed with larger files).
(14) Final irrigation.

The use of automated handpiece systems for root canal preparation has accelerated since the introduction of Ni–Ti rotary files. In the past, some stainless steel files were used in engine-driven (reciprocal) rotation, but the incidence of canal aberrations is high (6). Although variations exist, Ni–Ti rotary files are generally used in a high-quality air reduction handpiece (with or without torque control) or, better (as the flow of air can hardly be controlled and the reported wear for air reduction

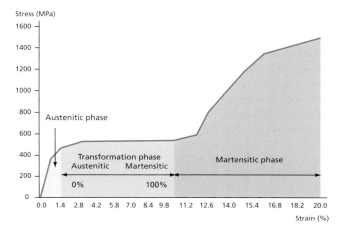
Fig. 11.22 Tensile strength curve of nickel–titanium.

handpieces is high), an electric motor whereby a feed-back circuitry compensates for torque to maintain a constant speed, and a suitable speed-reducing handpiece with a small head. The settings of the manufacturer are preprogrammed, and can be regularly updated or changed. The use of all-in-one systems (i.e. an electric motor with an integrated apex locator) should be discouraged because such devices operate on batteries and do not allow coupling with hand files.

In addition to the continuous reaming motion, the operator should follow the specific method of use (e.g. brushing motion, "pecking" movement, smooth steady pressure, etc.) and observe the recommended sequencing of files. All file types must be used with a light touch and minimal apical pressure. In addition, one must not rotate the file for too long in the canal and during this period of time, the instrument must not stop rotating. The use of an irrigating solution while cleaning and shaping the root canal system is an accepted practice. Irrigation plays an important role in lubricating the canal and in facilitating chip and debris removal. Some irrigants also serve the very important purpose of root canal disinfection.

Limitations of root canal instrumentation

Nickel–titanium rotary versus stainless steel hand files

The use of nickel–titanium under continuous rotation enables innovative design features, and it may eliminate some traditional difficulties that are associated with conventional root canal instrumentation (12). Certainly, Ni–Ti rotary instruments, if used properly, can achieve a final root canal preparation that conforms to the general shape and direction of the original canal (Fig. 11.12g–j). Because of the reduced restoring forces developed by Ni–Ti rotary instruments, it has been reported that more centered root canal preparations are created than with hand instrumentation (12, 26). The magnitude of transportation caused by Ni–Ti rotary files is small with a similar direction at the end-point of the preparation to that found with stainless steel hand files (i.e. the outer aspect of the curve). At the mid-curvature level, transportation has been reported towards the inner and outer aspect. In general, root canals with more severe curvature are wider after instrumentation with the main difference being a greater amount of dentin removal at the outer (convex) aspect of the curve. The differences between Ni–Ti rotary and stainless steel hand preparation are more pronounced if the apical preparation diameter is larger than size 30 (10, 36). There are only small discrepancies among the various Ni–Ti rotary systems at different horizontal levels.

Using stainless steel hand files in narrow and curved canals, a size 30 preparation reflects what most clinicians regard as an instrumentation end-point. Using Ni–Ti rotary instruments, the more desired size 40 preparation has become common, since the super-elasticity of Ni–Ti diminishes the connection between instrument diameter and stiffness. The instrumentation of the apical matrix to a larger size incorporates more anatomical irregularities and provides more irrigant exchange in the apical one-third (47).

Ni–Ti rotary instrumentation is faster (shorter preparation times) than stainless steel hand instrumentation and operator's fatigue is reduced (12, 36). Differences between various Ni–Ti rotary systems are more likely the result of variations in preparation technique than any differences between instrument performances. Greater taper systems that are used by moving up and down the numerical sequence in a crown-down manner to flare the canal until the smaller files reach working length have the widest percentage variation in time. The anatomy of some root canals requires moving up and down the sequence several times while in other canals working length is reached very quickly (17). In addition, the frequency of irrigation also influences preparation time. Occasionally, Ni–Ti rotary systems speed up the treatment considerably, so that the effective time for the irrigant is strongly reduced. If unnoticed, this fact may undermine the extent of chemical cleaning and disinfection. Regarding the direct efficacy in removal of bacteria it is important to notice that no difference was found between hand and rotary instruments (37).

With the launch of Ni–Ti rotary systems, too much credit was given to these systems as being a solution for root canal preparation on their own. Since then, a combined approach of Ni–Ti and stainless steel preparation has been advocated. The combined approach is especially needed in difficult cases and in most retreatment cases. In this way only, procedural errors can be avoided and the aberrations that are present can be corrected. More than ever, mental awareness is needed. Much of the result will depend on the clinician's experience (the "feel"), visualization facilities (radiography as well as direct, magnified and illuminated vision), and sound concepts, rather than on ready-for-use recipes. Indeed, the "one magical sequence" does not seem to exist. Those who have gained some experience in the use of Ni–Ti rotary files will confirm that each file system has its own special advantages and disadvantages, and that particular rules for its usage need to be followed. Eventually, instruments of different file systems can be combined using different instrumentation sequences to manage individual clinical situations according to a hybrid concept.

Besides its biocompatibility and excellent corrosion resistance, Ni–Ti is, however, an expensive alloy that is difficult to manufacture and mill. Machining the original Ni–Ti wire should be conducted with carbide burs or silicone carbide wheels under active highly chlorinated cutting oil involving light feeds and slow speeds. The surface of early Ni–Ti files was rough with grooves and irregularities, which could lead to accelerated wear, fatigue and breakage. Nowadays, most manufacturers have overcome this problem, and they perform metal treatment such as cryogenics or electropolishing. Given the high price per instrument, the incorporation of Ni–Ti as used in modern endodontics has increased the procedure costs dramatically. Therefore, patients should be informed and the highest possible level of care should be provided.

Limited reach versus unwanted dentin removal

Root canals following Ni–Ti rotary instrumentation for the most part show an oval or round preparation with most of the contours prepared. Nevertheless, specimens can present with unprepared areas in all thirds of their root canal system when a round preparation is produced in the center or at one side, leaving the remaining root canal walls uninstrumented (24). Especially flexible and passively cutting Ni–Ti rotary systems have deficiencies in the preparation of oval root canals because their super-elasticity and planing action do not allow controlled preparation of the buccal and lingual extensions. For these systems, canal preparation characteristics may be dictated more by anatomy (i.e. cross-sectional shape and curvature) than by the difference in instrumentation method (4, 24).

For the ProTaper system, which is more actively cutting, a special instrument motion called brushing has been recommended to deal with oval canals and to relocate the root canal orifice (33). In the middle and apical one-thirds of the root canal, the use of this triangular design does not seem to negatively affect centering abilities (3, 25) (Fig. 11.14d, e). However, care should be taken not to instrument the apical foramen with more actively cutting blades to avoid zipping. Furthermore, the finishing files of the ProTaper system should not be used with an extended pecking movement to avoid root canal transportation (33).

Risk of instrument fracture

Instruments may fracture as a result of misuse or overuse. Before and during treatment, files should be checked carefully to ensure that the cutting flutes are not damaged (Fig. 11.23). Regarding Ni–Ti rotary instruments, fracture can occur without any visible signs of previous permanent deformation, apparently within the elastic limit of the instrument (49). Visible inspection of the file,

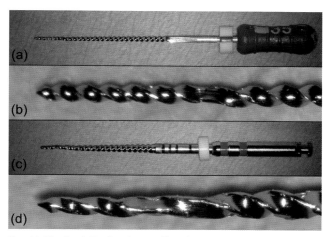

Fig. 11.23 (a, c) Hand and rotary files showing unwinding of the flutes. (b, d) A detailed view on the area with deformation.

therefore, is not always a reliable method for evaluating used Ni–Ti instruments.

Theoretically, the phenomenon of repeated cyclic (metal) fatigue may be the most important factor in separation of Ni–Ti rotary files (29). When instruments are placed in curved canals, they deform and stress occurs within the instrument. The half of the instrument shaft on the outside of the curve is in tension and the half on the inside is in compression. Consequently, each rotation causes the file to undergo one complete tension–compression cycle. Obviously, stress levels are the greatest in the area of curvature. A more severe bend (i.e. a smaller radius with an abrupt curve) creates greater stress and larger instruments will experience greater stress than smaller instruments when confined to the same curved root canal shape. Considering cycle fatigue as a contributor to instrument fracture, *larger instruments (size, taper or core) should not be considered safer or stronger in practice.* Preflaring and relocating the root canal orifice, thus creating straight-line access, can decrease the severity of curvature.

Torsional loading during rotational use is another variable to consider. The amount of torque applied to the instrument mainly depends on the manipulation of the file (e.g. the amount of apical pressure) and its shaft design. The crown-down sequence generates lower torque and lower vertical forces, although these elements also depend on the shape of the individual canals. In this regard, radius of root canal curvature is the most important factor in determining the torque value. If two canals have the same angle of curvature but have a different radius, then the one with smaller radius has the more abrupt canal deviation and results in higher torque on the file. Shaft design itself has an influence on torsional loading because cutting blades could act as stress concentrators, potentially resulting in more rapid crack initiation. On the contrary, radial land areas contribute to the strength of the instrument by the relatively large peripheral mass. The same remark can be made on the diameter of the central core. Adequate resistance to torque failure is also obtained by increasing instrument taper and size.

The introduction of the operating microscope and ultrasonically powered tips allows dentin to be removed precisely so that in many cases fractured instruments may be freed and subsequently removed. Unfortunately the canal is often overprepared during this procedure. If an instrument fractures during root canal treatment, the patient must be informed and the progress notes suitably annotated.

Preventing procedural mishaps

Blockage

If an instrument stops making progress into the root canal (i.e. if one experiences fixed or loose resistance), different reasons may include:

- the canal lumen may be truly blocked (e.g. packed with debris or vital pulp tissue);
- flutes on the cutting part of the instrument shaft may be fully loaded;
- friction on the instrument is too high (e.g. dry conditions, taper lock);
- root canal anatomy (e.g. narrow canals, abrupt curvatures and canals that converge or diverge);
- canal aberrations (e.g. ledges and broken instruments).

To avoid mishaps, it is important to figure out what is happening and to take proper action. Above all, one must not increase force on the file as this will most probably result in ledge formation or separation of the tip.

Blockage that is caused by the compaction of vital pulp tissue frequently happens with a size 15 K-file after negotiating the root canal with sizes 06–10 K-files. The tip diameters of the latter are smaller than the initial apical dimensions of most canals, allowing them to disrupt apical pulp tissue. When this happens in dry conditions, the sliced tissue can subsequently readhere to itself and meld into a solid mass of collagen if it is pushed by the tip of a larger file (e.g. a size 15 K-file in narrow canals). To prevent this from happening, *root canals should never be negotiated without the presence of an irrigant* (with or without lubricant) in the pulp chamber. When a rubber-band sensation is felt, vital pulp tissue is present and must be broached.

Especially with Ni–Ti, not all curves can be taken with all instruments, even if the files are brand new. Our mental image of root canal curvature (level, angle and radius) is, however, seldom complete and, therefore, the exploration of curves with stainless steel instruments

should compensate for the reduced tactile feedback from Ni–Ti rotary files. Based on this information and literature reports, a sound file selection should be made. In some cases, the use of GT hand files will solve the problem because these instruments combine the greater taper design with the safety of manual instrument use.

Stripping

Eccentric or excessive root canal preparation will often result in overpreparation of the inner wall, known as stripping. This is a particular problem on the distal surface of the coronal part of the mesial roots of mandibular molars (Fig. 11.24). Indiscriminate removal of tooth structure in this area may cause strip perforation. To avoid such an occurrence, shaping must be carried out with regard to the anatomy of the tooth and overenlargement must be avoided; removal of root canal wall should achieve a suitable shape and diameter to allow efficient delivery of irrigant and subsequent obturation. Using hand files in a rasping action or the injudicious use of Gates–Glidden burs increases the likelihood of stripping in the furcation region.

Ledging

A ledge may result from the use of excessive apical force, repeated insertion of the same file to a fixed level in the root canal, inappropriate file movement (e.g. filing motion with inflexible files) or a bad shaping approach (e.g. the insertion of a relatively large file to a particular

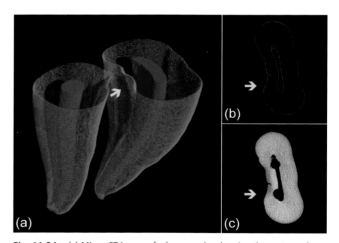

Fig. 11.24 (a) Micro-CT image of a lower molar showing the root canal system in relation to the outer root surface. The distal surface of the furcation region of the mesial root (yellow arrow) is particularly prone to stripping. (b) Micro-CT data of another sample showing registered contours before (green) and after (red) instrumentation. Notice the eccentric preparation in one of the canals (yellow arrow). (c) Corresponding micro-CT slice of the same tooth after preparation showing overpreparation of the inner wall (yellow arrow) that eventually may lead to strip perforation (not shown).

level in the root canal, which is usually at the beginning of the curve, early in the procedure) (Fig. 11.1).

The resulting ledge makes subsequent preparation apically very difficult or impossible. In an attempt to bypass a ledge, a twist (30° or more) is placed in the apical 1–2 mm of a size 10–15 K-file and this instrument is passed down the canal with an exploration motion. If the ledge can be bypassed then a gentle push–pull motion (small amplitude) with successively larger files (or GT hand files) may remove the ledge.

Zipping

Root canal zipping is caused by transportation (straightening) of the apical one-third towards the outer aspect of the curve (Fig. 11.1). Zipping results in the destruction of the apical constriction and the creation of a relatively large root canal exit with an irregular cross-sectional canal shape that is difficult to clean, disinfect and obturate.

Perforation

Perforation may occur at any time during the shaping of the root canal system but is more prevalent during the access preparation and when undertaking instrumentation in curved canals. Sudden bleeding from the root canal system is indicative of a perforation. Injudicious use of large burs in the floor of the pulp chamber may cause furcal perforation, which is difficult to repair (Fig. 11.25). As mentioned before, roots with a pronounced concavity on cross-sectional view (e.g. the mesial roots of mandibular molars) are prone to strip perforation (Fig. 11.26). Early detection and immediate treatment of an iatrogenic perforation are most important for a good prognosis. Radiography often hinders accurate detection of the perforation, particularly when it occurs in the buccolingual (or buccopalatal) plane. The use of EALs makes early detection of a root perforation possible (13).

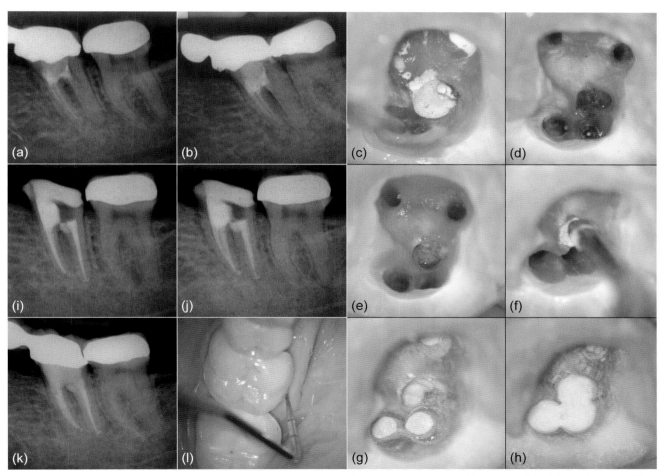

Fig. 11.25   (a–d) Clinical case of a lower molar showing an iatrogenic perforation of the pulp chamber floor. (e–h) Treatment of the defect with MTA and filling of the prepared root canals with gutta-percha. (i, j) Immediate postoperative radiographs. (k, l) One-year follow-up shows complete healing. (Courtesy of Dr J. Berghmans.)

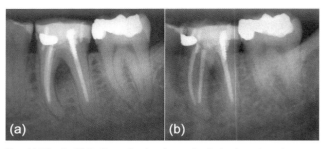

Fig. 11.26 (a, b) Radiographs showing periradicular bone loss due to an existing strip perforation within the mesial root of a lower first molar (later verified with intracanal view).

> **Core concept 11.3**
>
> Each Ni–Ti-based instrument will have a mean number of cycles to failure that is determined by angle and radius of the root canal curvature and instrument diameter (29). A higher speed (rpm) will consume the useful life of the instrument faster than a lower speed. The separation of unbound instruments in the area of the most severe canal curvature should always be considered a result of cyclic fatigue with any system. In abrupt and severe angles, discarding the instrument after a single use is the safest measure.

Instrument fracture

Automated handpiece systems with torque control reduce the mechanical stress on Ni–Ti rotary instruments. The torque value for an individual file is set just below the limit of elasticity, and these data are pre-programmed in the device. The values range between the martensitic start clinical stress and the martensitic finish clinical stress, which is dependent on design and dimensions of the individual instrument. If the motor is loaded up to the torque limit, the motor stops momentarily or rotates anticlockwise to avoid permanent deformation and file breakage (11). Torque control may reduce the incidence of fracture but does not offer complete protection. In addition, a unit with auto-reverse function may lead the instrument to repeatedly move in a forward and reverse motion, resulting in increased cyclic fatigue.

Initially all electric motors were high-torque. Some time later, low-torque motors came on the market. While the first are successfully used by experienced endodontists, the latter are valuable and safe for the beginner. Indeed, for an inexperienced operator the use of a low torque-control unit significantly reduces the incidence of intracanal breakage (48). For instruments with a taper of 6% or higher it becomes difficult, however, to determine a torque that is sufficient to rotate the larger, more coronal part of the instrument efficiently while not endangering the more fragile apical part of the file. Accordingly, it has been advocated that the creation of a glide path (see above) should allow the tip of the instrument to act as a passive pilot and thus protect the instrument from breakage even with high torque.

The number of times that one should use a particular instrument (i.e. the amount of root canals that can be prepared safely) is an issue under debate. Even though cumulative damage by the mechanism of cyclic fatigue is theoretically important, Spanaki-Voreadi and co-workers (38) confirmed that a single overloading event causing ductile fracture of the file is a most common fracture mechanism. This failure mechanism denotes that certain factors (e.g. difficulty of the case, handling parameters, root canal anatomy, instrumentation technique and operator's experience), which may increase the stresses during instrumentation, play the most crucial role in causing separation of these (and probably other) instruments (see Core concept 11.3) The "number of times question" is also related to the high costs of these instruments. In some countries, an additional fee can be asked when Ni–Ti rotary files are used, to promote single use. On the other hand, the process of sterilization is also costly and it decreases the cutting efficiency of Ni–Ti files (30). In addition, retrieval of broken instruments is an expensive burden; from an economic point of view, therefore, the risks of file separation should be minimized.

References

1. al-Omari MA, Dummer PM, Newcombe RG, Doller R. Comparison of six files to prepare simulated root canals. Part 2. *Int. Endod. J.* 1992; 25: 67–81.
2. Bechelli C, Zecchi Orlandini S, Colafranceschi M. Scanning electron microscope study on the efficacy of root canal wall debridement of hand versus Lightspeed instrumentation. *Int. Endod. J.* 1999; 32: 484–93.
3. Bergmans L, Van Cleynenbreugel J, Beullens M, Wevers M, Van Meerbeek B, Lambrechts P. Progressive versus constant tapered shaft design using NiTi rotary instruments. *Int. Endod. J.* 2003; 36: 288–95.
4. Bergmans L, Van Cleynenbreugel J, Beullens M, Wevers M, Van Meerbeek B, Lambrechts P. Smooth flexible versus active tapered shaft design using NiTi rotary instruments. *Int. Endod. J.* 2002; 35: 820–8.
5. Bergmans L, Van Cleynenbreugel J, Wevers M, Lambrechts P. A methodology for quantitative evaluation of root canal instrumentation using microcomputed tomography. *Int. Endod. J.* 2001; 34: 390–8.
6. Campos JM, del Rio C. Comparison of mechanical and standard hand instrumentation techniques in curved root canals. *J. Endod.* 1990; 16: 230–4.
7. Charles TJ, Charles JE. The "balanced force" concept of instrumentation in curved canals revisited. *Int. Endod. J.* 1998; 31: 166–72.

8. Craig RG, Peyton FA. The microhardness of enamel and dentin. *J. Dent. Res.* 1958; 37: 661–83.

9. Dummer PM, McGinn JH, Rees DG. The position and topography of the apical canal constriction and apical foramen. *Int. Endod. J.* 1984; 17: 192–8.

10. Esposito PT, Cunningham CJ. A comparison of canal preparation with nickel–titanium and stainless steel instruments. *J. Endod.* 1995; 21: 173–6.

11. Gambarini G. Rationale for the use of low-torque endodontic motors in root canal instrumentation. *Endod. Dent. Traumatol.* 2000; 16: 95–100.

12. Glosson CR, Haller RH, Dove SB, del Rio CE. A comparison of root canal preparations using Ni–Ti hand, Ni–Ti engine-driven and K-Flex endodontic instruments. *J. Endod.* 1995; 21: 146–51.

13. Gordon MPJ, Chandler NP. Electronic apex locators. *Int. Endod. J.* 2004; 37: 425–37.

14. Haikel Y, Serfaty R, Wilson P, Speisser JM, Allemann C. Cutting efficiency of nickel–titanium endodontic instruments and the effect of sodium hypochlorite treatment. *J. Endod.* 1998; 24: 736–9.

15. Hess W. Zur Anatomie der Wurzelkanäle des menschlichen Gebisses mit Berücksichtigung der feineren Verzweigungen am Foramen apicale. *Schweiz Vierteljahrschr. Zahnheilkd.* 1917; 27: 1.

16. Jerome CE, Hanlon RJ Jr. Dental anatomical anomalies in Asians and Pacific Islanders. *J. Calif. Dent. Assoc.* 2007; 35: 631–6.

17. Kavanagh D, Lumley PJ. An *in vitro* evaluation of canal preparation using .04 and .06 taper instruments. *Endod. Dent. Traumatol.* 1998; 14: 16–20.

18. Kerekes K, Tronstad L. Morphometric observations on root canals of human anterior teeth. *J. Endod.* 1977; 3: 24–9.

The theoretical possibility of using a standardized endodontic preparation and obturation technique in anterior teeth was investigated by measuring the widths of the roots and root canals of 100 teeth. Providing the canals were not too curved, circular-shaped preparations might be made with acceptable frequency in the apical 5 mm of maxillary central incisors and canines, and in the apical 3 mm of mandibular canines. A circular canal might be prepared in maxillary lateral incisors and mandibular incisors only at the 1 mm level from the apex.

19. Kerekes K, Tronstad L. Morphometric observations on root canals of human premolars. *J. Endod.* 1977; 3: 74–9.

The theoretical possibility of using a standardized endodontic preparation and obturation technique in premolars was investigated by measuring the widths of the roots and root canals of 80 teeth. Providing the canals were not too curved, circular-shaped preparations might be made with acceptable frequency in the apical 2–3 mm of maxillary second premolars and mandibular premolars. Theoretically, this technique is not generally applicable in maxillary first premolars.

20. Kerekes K, Tronstad L. Morphometric observations on root canals of human molars. *J. Endod.* 1977; 3: 114–18.

The theoretical possibility of using a standardized endodontic preparation and obturation technique in molars was investigated by measuring the widths of the roots and root canals of 40 teeth. Providing the canals were not too curved, circular-shaped preparations might be made with acceptable frequency only in the apical 1–3 mm of the buccal roots of maxillary molars and at the 1 mm level from the apex in the distal roots of mandibular molars. Theoretically, this technique is not generally applicable in molars.

21. Kuttler Y. Microscopic investigation of root apices. *J. Am. Dent. Assoc.* 1955; 50: 544–52.

22. Leeb J. Canal orifice enlargement as related to biomechanical preparation. *J. Endod.* 1983; 9: 463–70.

23. Massa GR, Nicholls JL, Harrington GW. Torsional properties of the Canal Master instrument. *J. Endod.* 1992; 18: 222–7.

24. Peters OA, Laib A, Göhring TN, Barbakow F. Changes in root canal geometry after preparation assessed by high-resolution computed tomography. *J. Endod.* 2001; 27: 1–6.

25. Peters OA, Peters CL, Schönenberger K, Barbakow F. ProTaper rotary root canal preparation: assessment of torque and force in relation to canal anatomy. *Int. Endod. J.* 2003; 36: 93–9.

26. Portenier I, Lutz F, Barbakow F. Preparation of the apical part of the root canal by the Lightspeed and step-back techniques. *Int. Endod. J.* 1998; 31: 103–11.

27. Poulsen WB, Dove SB, del Rio CE. Effect of nickel–titanium engine driven instrument rotational speed on root canal morphology. *J. Endod.* 1995; 21: 609–12.

28. Prati C, Foschi F, Nucci C, Montebugnoli L, Marchionni S Appearance of the root canal walls after preparation with NiTi rotary instruments: a comparative SEM investigation. *Clin. Oral Invest.* 2004; 8: 102–10.

29. Pruett JP, Clement DJ, Carnes DL. Cyclic fatigue testing of nickel–titanium endodontic instruments. *J. Endod.* 1997; 23: 77–85.

30. Rapisarda E, Bonaccorso A, Tripi TR, Guido G. Effect of sterilization on the cutting efficiency of rotary nickel–titanium endodontic files. *Oral Surg. Oral Med. Oral Pathol. Oral Radiol. Endod.* 1999; 88: 343–7.

31. Ricucci D, Langeland K. Apical limit of root canal instrumentation and obturation. Part 2: a histological study. *Int. Endod. J.* 1998; 31: 394–409.

32. Roane JB, Sabala CL, Duncanson MG. The "balanced force" concept for instrumentation of curved canals. *J. Endod.* 1985; 11: 203–11.

33. Ruddle CJ. The ProTaper technique. *Endod. Topics* 2005; 10: 187–90.

34. Schilder H. Cleaning and shaping the root canal. *Dent. Clin. North Am.* 1974; 18: 269–96.

35. Serene TP, Adams JD, Saxena A. *Nickel–Titanium Instruments. Application in Endodontics.* St. Louis, MO: Ishiyaku Euro-America, 1995.

36. Short JA, Morgan LA, Baumgartner JC. A comparison of canal centering ability of four instrumentation techniques. *J. Endod.* 1997; 23: 503–7.

37. Siqueira JF Jr, Lima KC, Magalhaes FA, Lopes HP, de Uzeda M. Mechanical reduction of the bacterial population in the root canal by three instrumentation techniques. *J. Endod.* 1999; 25: 332–5.

38. Spanaki-Voreadi AP, Kerezoudis NP, Zinelis S. Failure mechanism of ProTaper Ni–Ti rotary instruments during clinical use: fractographic analysis. *Int. Endod. J.* 2006; 39: 171–8.

39. Sunada I. New method for measuring the length of the root canal. *J. Dent. Res.* 1962; 41: 375–8.

40. Suzuki K. Experimental study on iontophoresis. *J. Jpn. Stomatol.* 1942; 16: 411–17.
41. Thompson SA, Dummer PMH. Shaping ability of Lightspeed rotary nickel–titanium instruments in simulated root canals. Part 1. *J. Endod.* 1997; 23: 698–702.
42. Tucker DM, Wenckus CS, Bentkover SK. Canal wall planing by engine-driven nickel–titanium instruments, compared with stainless steel hand instrumentation. *J. Endod.* 1997; 23: 170–3.
43. Ushiyama J. New principle and method for measuring the root canal length. *J. Endod.* 1983; 9: 97–104.
44. Walia HM, Brantley WA, Gerstein H. An initial investigation of the bending and torsional properties of Nitinol root canal files. *J. Endod.* 1988; 14: 346–51.
45. Wildley WL, Senia ES. A new root canal instrument and instrumentation technique: a preliminary report. *Oral Surg. Oral Med. Oral Pathol.* 1989; 67: 198–207.
46. Wu MK, Roris A, Barkis D, Wesselink PR. Prevalence and extent of long oval shape of canals in the apical third. *Oral Surg. Oral Med. Oral Pathol. Oral Radiol. Endod.* 2000; 89: 739–43.
47. Wu MK, Wesselink PR. Efficacy of three techniques in cleaning the apical portion of curved root canals. *Oral Surg. Oral Med. Oral Pathol.* 1995; 79: 492–6.
48. Yared GM, Sleiman P. Failure of ProFile instruments used with air, high torque control, and low torque control motors. *Oral Surg. Oral Med. Oral Pathol. Oral Radiol. Endod.* 2002; 93: 92–6.
49. Zuolo ML, Walton RE. Instrument deterioration with usage: nickel–titanium versus stainless steel. *Quintessence Int.* 1997; 28: 397–402.

Chapter 12
Root canal filling materials

Gottfried Schmalz and Preben Hørsted-Bindslev

Introduction

Purpose

To prevent bacteria and bacterial elements from spreading from (or through) the canal system to the periapical area, the fully instrumented root canal has to be provided with a tight and long-lasting obturation. Furthermore, any bacteria that could not be fully removed during cleaning and shaping procedures should be sealed ("entombed") and thus rendered harmless by being deprived of nutrients. A root canal filling material should, therefore, prevent infection/reinfection of treated root canals. Together with an acceptable level of biocompatibility (inert material) this will provide the basis for promoting healing of the periodontal tissues and for maintaining healthy periapical conditions.

In addition to this traditional concept of the purpose of a root canal filling material, it has recently been put forward that a root canal filling material should be able to actively stimulate tissue regeneration, especially after a sometimes aggressive treatment procedure or after apical pathosis. Relevant materials may be osteoconductive (serving as a scaffold for the ingrowth of precursor osteoblasts) or osteoinductive (inducing new bone formation by differentiation of pluripotent local connective tissue cells into bone-forming cells).

Classification

Root canal filling materials may be divided into three types:

- cones;
- sealers;
- combinations of the two.

Cones are prefabricated root canal filling materials of a given size and shape (taper). Sealers are pastes and cements that are mixed and hardened by a chemical setting reaction after a given amount of time. Setting time varies between the various preparations, from minutes up to days. Owing to several reasons outlined later, combinations of cones and sealers are currently recommended. Thermoplastic materials prepared from gutta-percha are gaining increasing interest and are heated for better adaptation to the root canal wall. They may also be melted and injected into the root canal in a liquid state and then hardened by cooling. Again, it is usually recommended to use these materials together with a sealer.

Limitations

As will be shown in this chapter, all materials recommended for root canal filling have advantages and disadvantages and there is no material/method yet available that fulfills all the requirements. Therefore clinicians are well advised to observe new developments and the relevant scientific literature carefully. It also should be kept in mind that clinical properties of root canal filling materials depend substantially upon the treatment technique: e.g. the amount of sealer used may determine the tissue reaction and the amount of leakage of some materials, due to factors such as shrinkage during setting, the formation of pores and enhanced solubility (45). Therefore, the selection and the use of a root canal filling material must be part of a whole treatment concept. Finally, there is no magic material by which the tedious work of correct diagnosis and chemomechanical preparation of the root canal system can be avoided.

Selection

Root canal filling materials should be selected on the basis of a critical evaluation of the presented evidence (preferably reports in scientific journals) in relation to the requirements, which will be mentioned below. Sometimes, however, contradicting results are reported for the same material. This may be due to the particular circumstances of both the test method used and the preparation of the specimens (tested freshly after mixing or in a set state). Thus, the clinician should ask for a set of tests preferably performed in a comparative (i.e. controlled) way, testing the new product against one or more currently accepted preparations. Selection of a suitable root canal filling material is a challenge for the clinician regarding both his or her level of updated information and his or her ability to critically assess presented information.

Requirements

Root canal filling materials may be considered as implants and thus should fulfill the requirements of such materials concerning technical, biological and handling properties (Core concept 12.1).

Technical properties

Technical properties are mainly related to sealing aspects, taking into account that the success of a root canal filling significantly depends upon the prevention of infection/ reinfection of the apical and lateral periodontal ligament and the adjacent bone. In cases of material extrusion beyond the apex, which is associated with elevated rates of clinical failure (79), resorption of the material would be desirable. However, this is in contradiction to the required insolubility. Therefore utmost care must be taken to avoid overfilling.

Core concept 12.1   Requirements for an ideal root canal filling material

Technical
- No shrinkage
- No solubility in tissue fluids, undisturbed setting in the presence of moisture
- Good adhesion/adaptation to dentin or combining materials (cones, sealers)
- No pores and water absorption
- No tooth discoloration

Biological
- No general health problems or allergies for patients and dental personnel
- No irritation of local tissues
- Sterile
- Antimicrobial – no enhanced bacterial growth
- Stimulation of the periapical healing process

Handling
- Radiopaque: ISO 6876 (76) requires >3 mm aluminum (dentin has 0.6–0.7) (radiopacity of dental materials is measured as mm aluminum equivalent)
- Setting in an adequate time, allowing sufficient time for obturation and radiographic control
- Easy to apply and easy to remove (e.g. for post placement or revision) using solvents, heat or mechanical instrumentation

---

Biological properties

Biological properties are related to preventing systemic and local tissue irritation for both the patient and the dental personnel and providing the potential for regeneration of the apical tissues. The risk (frequency and severity of adverse effects) for general health impairment as a consequence of the use of root canal filling materials is generally low. Single cases of allergic reactions of patients and medical personnel have been reported. Local effects are more dramatic, especially in the context of overfilling beyond the apex and eventually into the mandibular canal (see below).

There are some inherent contradictions between the requirements for a root canal filling material that have to be weighed against each other, e.g. antibacterial properties versus local toxicity. Bacteria in the root canal should be removed by chemomechanical debridement. However, the complex anatomy of the root canal system (e.g. lateral canals) makes debridement difficult, especially in the apical delta region (see Chapter 11). Furthermore, bacteria have been shown to invade dentinal tubules and thus they may not be removed totally by chemomechanical debridement. Thorough cleaning, shaping and irrigation with disinfectants may not, therefore, result in a completely sterile root canal system. Owing to the fact that leakage cannot be totally prevented by any material/method available today, percolation of nutrient-rich fluid followed by bacterial regrowth may occur. Antimicrobial activity of root canal sealers may compensate for these imperfections, although this is not supported by direct scientific evidence.

It should be recognized that sealers with high antimicrobial activity, especially formaldehyde-releasing ZnOE (zinc oxide–eugenol), are also toxic to cells and tissues. Furthermore, sealers that release antimicrobial substances may disintegrate at the same time. Therefore, antibacterial properties of a root canal filling material based on the release of antibacterial substances from the sealer should not compromise its physical properties (such as stability and sealability) or biological properties. Some materials (e.g. epoxy resin sealers) are only antimicrobially active during the setting period, which is an interesting approach. For a short period residual bacteria may be killed (toxicity is accepted); in the long run, the material is not toxic, leaving time for the surrounding tissues to heal (Fig. 12.1).

Handling properties

Handling properties will facilitate the actual use of the material and the control of the technique/treatment result. The length of the root canal filling is of utmost importance for clinical success and a sufficient radiopacity is needed for radiographic control. Setting conditions must be adjusted to the particular clinical situation the

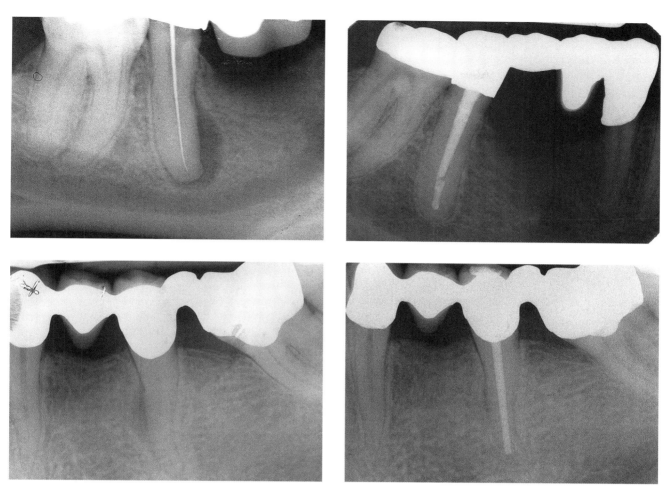

Fig. 12.1   Lateral and apical regeneration of an osteolytic process in two cases after shaping and cleaning the root canal and filling with cones and a sealer of temporary toxicity (gutta-percha with an epoxy resin sealer).

root canal filling techniques are aimed at and relevant requirements may be different for regular root canal fillings (slow setting allowing for condensation and eventual correction after radiographic control) and retrograde fillings (fast setting for better moisture control during the operation).

The ideal root canal filling material has not been developed yet. Compromises have to be made between the different requirements in relation to the individual clinical situation. New formulations, however, should be checked *critically* against the list of requirements (Core concept 12.1).

Biocompatibility

An acceptable level of biocompatibility is an essential requirement for a suitable root canal filling material. According to EU regulations (Medical Device Directive 93/42 EEC) valid within the EU and in Switzerland, Iceland, Liechtenstein and Norway, root canal filling materials have to successfully pass a clinical risk assessment procedure before they are allowed to be marketed.

The CE sign on the package (Fig. 12.2) shows that the material conforms with the essential requirements of this directive: namely safety, efficacy and quality. In other parts of the world (e.g. the USA, Japan, Australia, South America) similar regulations are in effect. Although for this process the term "clinical risk assessment" is used, it should be noted that a new root canal filling material

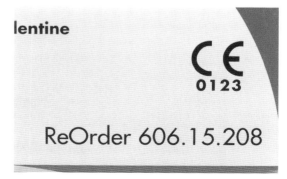

Fig. 12.2   The CE sign on the package shows that the material has passed a risk assessment procedure; note the number that identifies the supervising body ("Notified Body").

does not necessarily have to pass clinical testing if the manufacturer assumes that the material is both safe and effective from preclinical and other data (e.g. so-called "historic" data from similar/identical materials that are on the market already and/or have been tested in the past). The dentist should therefore ask the manufacturer for clinical data (see below), because he or she is finally responsible for the selection of the material in the individual patient situation and the patient relies on his or her independent expertise (71). There are so far no official regulations concerning recommended periods for a clinical test of root canal filling materials. In analogy to restorative materials, a time of 1 year for excluding catastrophic failures and a time span of 3–5 years for the final testing may be advisable. Products without a CE mark must not be used in those countries where the aforementioned EU Directive is in effect.

Root canal filling materials come into close and prolonged contact with living tissue (e.g. bone, connective tissue, sinus maxillaris, nervus alveolaris inferior) and of dental personnel (e.g. skin of hands). Possible adverse reactions are of a systemic toxic, allergenic (immunological) or local toxic nature. Accordingly, many different methods have been designed to test the different aspects of the biocompatibility of root canal filling materials. Relevant test methods have been included in international standards (ISO 10993 or ISO 7405) (71).

The clinical relevance of *in vitro* test methods (cell and bacterial cultures) is limited, because they do not take the complex clinical situation of the apical region of a tooth into account (Fig. 12.3). Data from such tests provide basic information on the material and can be used to explain certain clinical reactions, e.g. in relation to extrusion of root canal material over the apex. In isolation, they are not sufficient to show biocompatibility of a material (70).

In vivo biocompatibility test methods are mainly performed on laboratory animals. Relevant tests involve the implantation of a material into the subcutaneous/muscle tissues of rats, mice or rabbits (Fig. 12.4). These tests are mainly designed to test the potential for local toxicity. Of special interest are endodontic usage tests, in which the material is applied as used in the patient, i.e. for filling root canals. With such an approach, special aspects such as apical repair (e.g. new cement formation) or the formation of hard tissue after treatment of teeth with open apices (root-end closure) can be studied, because this requires the interaction of different specialized cell types that so far cannot be simulated in *in vitro* tests or in implantation studies. Although endodontic usage tests are closer to the clinical situation than *in vitro* tests, again they have disadvantages. For example the results of endodontic usage tests depend strongly on the treatment method and there are indications that these tests do not provide a sensitive discrimination between endodontic materials of widely different chemical composition (58).

The allergic potential of dental materials is tested preclinically mainly on guinea pigs, which provides a rough estimate. Patients who show clinical symptoms of an allergic reaction to a dental material may be subjected to special allergy tests, which apply a series of materials to the skin (e.g. patch test). Positive patch test results together with corresponding clinical symptoms (e.g. swelling, redness, itching) are indicative of a material-related allergy. For allergy testing and for avoiding relevant allergenic products in the sensitized patient, the composition of the material to be used must be known.

None of the test models described so far for assessing the biological properties of root canal filling materials is identical to the clinical situation under which the material is to be used. Therefore clinical trials are essential; clinical

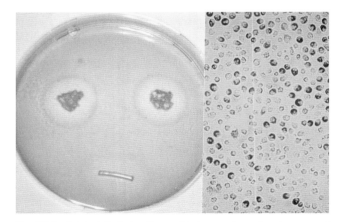

Fig. 12.3 Cytotoxicity test with a polyketone root canal sealer: zone of decoloration around the test specimen (left) indicates moderate toxicity; the partial loss of dye (neutral red) from the cells (right) indicates moderate cell damage.

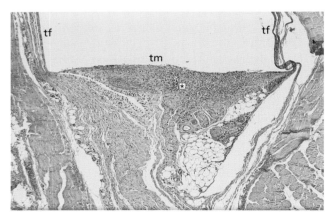

Fig. 12.4 Tissue reaction 14 days after subcutaneous implantation (rat) of a set polyketone root canal sealer filled into a Teflon tube: accumulation of inflammatory cells (mainly polymorphonuclear neutrophilic granulocytes) at the contact area (*) with the test material indicates moderate toxicity; no tissue reaction at the contact area with the Teflon tube. tm = test material; tf = Teflon tube (negative control and material carrier).

trials seldom allow for histological evaluation, however. This means that the biocompatibility of a new root filling material cannot be evaluated by one test alone (68).

Leakage/sealing

It is generally believed that the main cause for failure of endodontic treatment is the lack of seal of the root canal filling (apical and coronal leakage), facilitating bacterial growth. Many studies (about 25% of the current endodontic literature) are devoted to leakage and sealability. Leakage mainly occurs between the root canal filling and the root canal wall, although there are some reports showing leakage between sealer and core material (gutta-percha) and throughout the sealer. Leakage is influenced by the root canal filling material itself and by a number of other factors (Core concept 12.2). The penetration of a sealer into the dentinal tubules is considered to improve the seal (51).

Results reported in the literature on leakage depend greatly upon the test methods being used. Tests most often are performed *in vitro* and include dye penetration, with additional pressure, centrifugation or vacuum; bacterial penetration and fluid transport are also used (97). The clinical relevance of *in vitro* studies is questionable and contradictory results have often been reported for the same material using different methods (5). Therefore these tests are – at best – valid in a comparative manner whereby a new material is compared with a clinically established one. *In vivo* usage tests (e.g. on experimental animals) reveal more relevant results but are more difficult to perform and more uncontrollable variables (e.g.

Core concept 12.2   Factors influencing leakage

(1) *Root canal anatomy and preparation.* Oval, C-shaped and key-hole-shaped profiles of the root canals and unsuitable cleaning and shaping impede the correct application of the root canal filling material.

(2) *Access cavity.* Bacteria may penetrate an obturated root canal within a few days/weeks if the access cavity is not sufficiently sealed (coronal leakage).

(3) *Smear layer.* Removal using citric acid (10–50%) or EDTA (ethylenediaminetetraacetic acid) (17%) may influence leakage, although results are equivocal. The effect depends apparently upon the sealer used (Fig. 12.5).

(4) *Hemostasis/dryness of the root canal.* The wall of the root canal must be clean and dry for tight adaptation of the sealer to the wall.

(5) *Root canal filling material.* Stability, adhesion to dentin and lack of pores.

(6) *Sealer thickness and obturation technique.* Thick layers of root canal sealers (e.g. a ZnOE sealer or a calcium hydroxide sealer) showed more leakage than a thin one (40), which may be due to the fact that most sealers contain pores or dissolve faster in thick layers. A thin layer of root canal sealer is therefore generally recommended.

(7) *Rinsing regimen.* Marginal adaptation and setting of (resin-based) sealers may depend upon the rinsing solution; e.g. by the removal of the smear layer allowing for better penetration of the sealer into the dentinal tubules and the formation of an interdiffusion zone between the sealer and dentin collagen fibers (51).

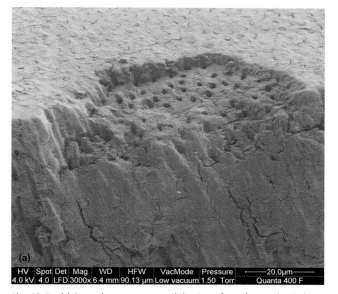
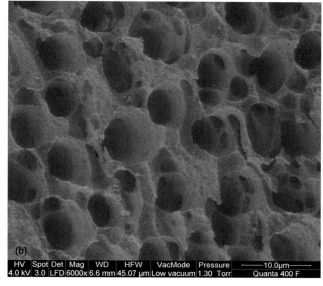

Fig. 12.5   (a) Smear layer on root canal dentin surface after mechanical instrumentation: smear layer partially lost due to fracture of the specimen. (b) Removal of smear layer and erosion of dentin surface after rinsing with 10% citric acid and 5.25% NaOCl.

application technique) are included. Again, a set of different test methods is necessary to evaluate the leakage properties of a new root canal filling material. Leakage data reported in the literature for root canal filling materials therefore should be regarded with caution. As with data on other properties (e.g. biological), they are only mosaic tiles that need other information to determine the clinical value of the new material. At present, there is no root canal filling material available which can prevent leakage. Therefore, a bacteria-tight coronal restoration is of critical importance to ensure the success of root canal treatment (99).

Gutta-percha cones

Gutta-percha is the most common cone material used for root canal filling. Silver was used in the past but has been abandoned because of the mediocre sealing qualities, even when used together with sealers, and because of high corrosion leading to tooth discoloration and local tissue reactions (Fig. 12.6). Titanium cones are available and have good biocompatibility, but they show low radiopacity and poor adaptation to the root canal wall where the cross-sectional shape of the root canal is not circular. This requires a comparatively high amount of sealer and therefore endangers the seal of the filling. These cones may be considered for use in narrow and curved canals, where the application of gutta-percha points is difficult. Thermoplastic polyester or resin-coated gutta-percha cones have been marketed together with new methacrylate-based sealers (see also Methacrylate-based sealers).

Gutta-percha cones are the material of choice for filling the major part of the canal volume. Gutta-percha cones (even standardized ones) do not fit optimally to the shaped root canal and therefore must be compacted

and used together with sealer; the less sealer necessary, the better.

Composition

Gutta-percha is a natural product that consists of the purified coagulated exudate of mazer wood trees (*Isonandra percha*) from the Malay archipelago or from South America. It is a high-molecular-weight polymer. Two forms of gutta-percha are relevant for dental products: the α- and the β-form. The β-form is used in most gutta-percha cones (less brittle than the α-form) but the α-form is used for injectable products because of its better flow characteristics.

The composition of gutta-percha cones (Table 12.1) varies considerably between manufacturers. This and the fact that gutta-percha is a natural product may be the reasons for the different properties reported for different brands. Formerly, cadmium (Cd)-based dyes were added to provide a yellow color, which should facilitate removal (if necessary, e.g. for revision). Modern gutta-percha preparations use other colorants and do not contain any *intentionally* added Cd compounds. Some gutta-percha preparations contain calcium hydroxide or chlorhexidine, with the aim of enhancing their antibacterial activity (temporary root canal dressing) and thereby stimulating apical healing. Clinical experience of such additions is so far limited.

Gutta-percha cones are supplied by the manufacturers in different sizes (length, diameter, taper; Table 12.2). Standardized cones are frequently used and the idea of having a cone that corresponds closely to the shape and the dimensions of the prepared root canal is striking. However, there are discrepancies between the shapes of the cones and the shaping instruments (Fig. 12.7), and the actual dimensions of the gutta-percha cones may show considerable variation. Therefore, it is advisable to check the dimensions of each cone, e.g. by a suitable gauge, prior to use (Fig. 12.8). Some manufacturers offer gutta-percha cones with a color coding according to the ISO system for the different sizes (ISO 10–ISO 140) (Fig. 12.9). Cones with a 4% or 6% (and up to 12%) taper are offered in sizes using the ISO numbering system (i.e. 10–140); gutta-percha cones with the same dimensions as special root canal shaping instruments with varying taper are available.

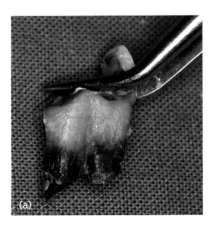
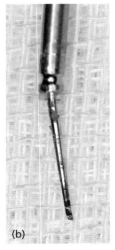

Fig. 12.6 (a) Discoloration of a root after root canal filling with a silver cone. (b) Removed silver cone showing signs of severe corrosion.

Table 12.1 Typical composition of gutta-percha cones.

Components	Composition (%)
Zinc oxide	66
Metal sulfates (radiopacity)	11
Gutta-percha	20
Additives like colophony (rosin, mainly composed of diterpene resin), pigments or trace metals	3

Table 12.2   Dimensions of gutta-percha cones.

Type of cone	Size
Standardized cones	Corresponds in diameter and taper (2%) to root canal shaping instruments according to ISO 6877. The sizes of the gutta-percha cones range from ISO 10 to ISO 140 (Fig. 12.9)
Accessory cones	Larger taper, descriptive size, may be used for lateral compaction
Greater taper cones	Cones with a 4% or 6% (and up to 12%) taper or cones with varying taper used together with special engine-driven root canal shaping instruments (see Chapter 11)
Compaction cones	Taper corresponds to the taper of finger-spreaders

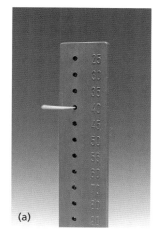
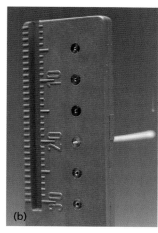

Fig. 12.8   (a) Gauge for controlling the size of the actual gutta-percha cone. (b) The actual cone is too thin, because it reaches out of the gauge.

Gutta-percha may be used cold in combination with a sealer. Owing to its thermoplastic properties, gutta-percha may be used also in a heated state, which allows closer adaptation to the canal walls (Fig. 12.10). The products consist of a plastic core (carrier) coated by α-form gutta-percha for improved flow characteristics and to reduce shrinkage after cooling. Gutta-percha also may be liquefied at 70°C (Ultrafil) or 160/200°C (Obtura II) and injected directly into the root canal (see Chapter 13).

Technical properties/leakage

Gutta-percha cones are flexible (elastic) at room temperature, become plastic at about 60°C and are volume constant under mouth conditions. Heating leads to expansion (and cooling to contraction), a fact that reduces

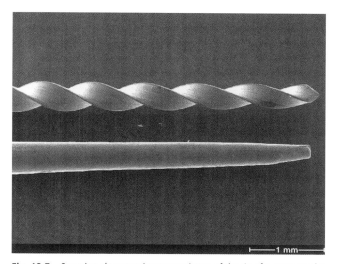

Fig. 12.7   Scanning electron microscope picture of the tip of a gutta-percha cone and the corresponding root canal file; note the discrepancies in shape.

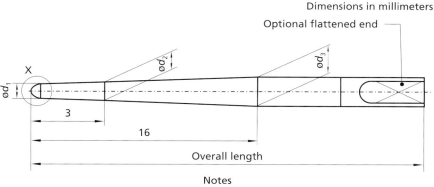

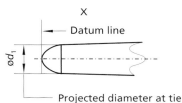

Dimensions in millimeters

Optional flattened end

$\varnothing d_1$ $\varnothing d_2$ $\varnothing d_3$

X

3

16

Overall length

X

Datum line

$\varnothing d_1$

Projected diameter at tie

Notes

1. The diameters are expressed in hundredths of millimeters. ISO-table gives the values of d_1, d_2 and d_3 for each size.
2. The taper of standardized cones is 0.02 mm per 1 mm length, therefore $d_3 = d_1 + 0.32$ mm.
3. In detail X, the exact shape of the tip is left to the manufacturer.

Fig. 12.9   Scheme for the dimensions of a standardized gutta-percha cone according to ISO 6877; $d_1 \times 100 =$ size designation of gutta-percha cone (ISO 10–ISO 140).

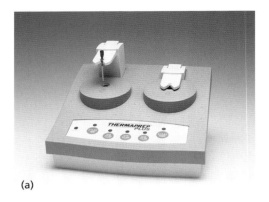 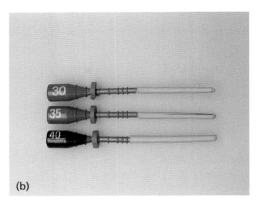

Fig. 12.10 (a) Oven for warming gutta-percha cones; (b) and the corresponding cones.

the sealing quality of warm or liquid gutta-percha application (when used without a sealer). Gutta-percha is soluble in organic solvents such as eucalyptus oil.

Gutta-percha does not adhere to the canal walls, regardless of the filling technique applied, resulting in the potential for marked leakage. Therefore, it is generally recommended that gutta-percha (used cold or heated) is used together with a sealer. For an optimal seal the sealer layer should generally be as thin as possible, therefore the skill of the operator plays an important part in the success of the treatment by correctly compacting gutta-percha; it is apparently of minor importance which method of compaction is used.

Biological properties

No systemic toxic reactions toward gutta-percha have been reported in the literature. Allergic reactions to gutta-percha are extremely rare. One case was reported of a suspected allergic reaction during a root canal treatment with a patient who was sensitized to natural latex. No latex gloves were worn during treatment, but pain, swelling of lips and diffuse urticaria developed after treatment. After 4 weeks the gutta-percha cone was removed and the symptoms abated. The allergy was attributed by the authors to the fact that pure gutta-percha and natural latex are fabricated from natural substances derived from trees of the same botanical family (11). No further cases have been reported. Cones made from synthetic gutta-percha are available.

Depending on the product, several cell culture studies have demonstrated gutta-percha to have little or no cytotoxicity (Fig. 12.11). Generally, gutta-percha is well tolerated by animal tissues (e.g. rat and mouse connective tissue); it induces the formation of a collagenous capsule with no or almost no inflammation (Fig. 12.12).

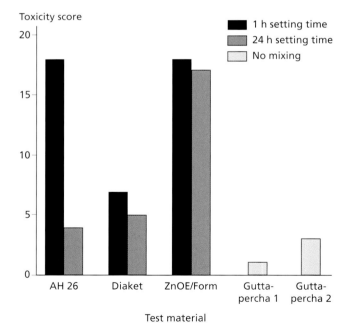

Fig. 12.11 Cytotoxicity of different root canal filling materials; human cells were exposed to eluates of the materials and the effect upon cell growth was measured; high scores indicate strong cytotoxicity. For sealers, effects of freshly mixed materials and set materials were measured; for gutta-percha, two brands were tested. ZnOE/Form = formaldehyde-containing ZnOE sealer (69).

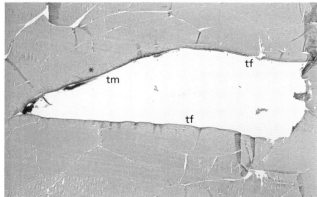

Fig. 12.12 Tissue reaction 7 days after intramuscular implantation of gutta-percha: no inflammatory cells can be observed at the contact area with the test material (*), which indicates good biocompatibility. tm = test material; tf = Teflon tube (negative control and material carrier).

The elevated temperatures involved in the application of injectable liquefied gutta-percha or of heat-mediated condensation/compaction techniques have been the motive for several investigations into the involved risk for adverse clinical effects. Intracanal temperatures have been measured, the highest being for the thermo-mechanical condensation technique (see Chapter 13) (Table 12.3). Interestingly, for liquefied gutta-percha (Obtura II), which is heated to more than 160°C, the intracanal temperature shows a maximum of only 61°C, which reflects the cooling process during application (94).

However, the main target tissue (the periodontal ligament) is separated from the heated gutta-percha by dentin, which, owing to its low thermal conductivity, acts as a thermal isolator. Its effectiveness depends on the dentin thickness. Therefore temperature measurements at the surface of the root are clinically more relevant. It is generally accepted that a temperature rise of approximately 10°C above normal body temperature is critical if maintained over 1 min; over 5 min bone damage will occur (23). Again, the highest temperatures were measured on the root surface with the thermomechanical compaction technique, with differences depending on the rotational speed of the compacting instrument. After stopping compaction, heat dissipated in 15–30 s for an elevation of less than 10°C (66).

The reaction of the target tissues (periodontal ligament) after injection of heated gutta-percha into the root canals of a dog showed no evidence of inflammation. In the case of overfilling, an acute inflammatory reaction was observed briefly after insertion and a chronic/foreign body reaction was found in long-term experiments (46). The classical warm vertical condensation or the warm lateral condensation technique did not cause any heat-related periodontal damage in monkeys and miniature pigs. Contrary to these data, thermomechanical compaction of gutta-percha with a sealer caused tissue damage (see Key literature 12.1).

In conclusion, for melted injectable gutta-percha, no tissue damage is expected due to rapid cooling during application and the isolating capacity of the dentin layer. If this layer is not present, e.g. after overfilling, a tissue reaction may occur. No such risks exist for the classical

Table 12.3 Temperature measurements for liquefied gutta-percha.

Technique	Intracanal temperature (°C)	Tooth surface temperature rise (°C)
Ultrafil	70	
Obtura II	Max. 61	Max. 8.9
Warm vertical condensation	45–80	3–7
Thermomechanical compaction	55–100	14–35

Key literature 12.1

Saunders (67) studied histologically the effect of thermomechanical compaction (10 000 rpm) of gutta-percha with a calcium hydroxide sealer upon the cementum of ferret teeth. Twenty days after root filling, 20% of the experimental teeth showed signs of surface resorption of cementum in the central section of the root with no signs of inflammation. After 40 days, 28% showed resorption and, of these, 22% exhibited ankylosis of alveolar bone to cementum. Controls with lateral condensation showed no resorption or ankylosis. The author concluded that heat generation by this method is sufficient to stimulate surface resorption and ankylosis in the longer term.

warm condensation technique, with the use of heated instruments or with the prewarming of gutta-percha cones. The use of sealers further reduces temperature rises. However, with the thermomechanical compaction technique elevated temperatures on the root surfaces have been recorded, as well as tissue damage with cementum resorption and ankylosis.

Antimicrobial properties

Gutta-percha provides some antimicrobial properties, with the active substance being ZnO from which zinc ions (Zn^{2+}) are mobilized by hydrolysis. Some brands of gutta-percha are active against anaerobically cultivated isolates from root canals. The occurrence and the size of the inhibition zones varied with the bacteria used for testing and the brand of the gutta-percha cone (93).

Handling properties

Gutta-percha cones are usually supplied by the manufacturer in a non-sterile form. Storage in commonly used disinfectants may have a negative influence on the mechanical properties of the cones and should be avoided, unless evidence is presented that the cones are not damaged. Instead, an effective surface disinfection (e.g. with 5.25% NaOCl) immediately prior to use is advisable; afterwards the cones should be rinsed in 70% alcohol to prevent NaOCl crystals forming on the gutta-percha cone. Recently, gutta-percha cones that are "free of living germs" (declaration of the manufacturer) have been marketed (Fig. 12.13). Gutta-percha cones should be stored in cool and dark conditions in order to prevent hardening and brittleness due to further crystallization and/or oxidation. A technical problem with the use of heated gutta-percha is the higher frequency of extrusion of root canal sealer.

Owing to its comparatively soft consistency, gutta-percha can be removed mechanically by conventional hand file or by rotary instruments (see Chapter 20). Gutta-percha preparations using a plastic carrier can be

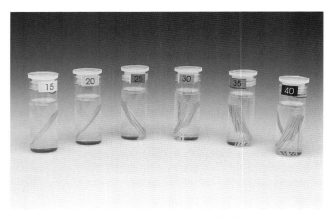

Fig. 12.13 Gutta-percha cones delivered ("germ-free") in an aqueous solution of ethanol and hexetidine.

removed using organic solvents, e.g. eucalyptus oil. The carrier can be bypassed by endodontic instruments. The radiopacity of gutta-percha was measured to be between 6.14 and 8.8 mm Al (76) and this is considered to be sufficient.

Sealers

Sealers are used to fill voids and minor discrepancies of fit between the gutta-percha cones and the root canal wall. Without a cone, leakage increases significantly, probably owing to the fact that sealers may shrink during setting, pores may develop and the solubility of the sealers is enhanced when used in thick layers; the net effect is volume dependent, which is the main reason for using no more sealer than is absolutely necessary. Therefore, the use of sealers without any cone, as was recommended in the past, is obsolete today. Sealers comprise a heterogeneous group of materials with different compositions (Core concept 12.3).

One polyketone sealer has been marketed for some decades. It has good mechanical and sealing properties and no effects on general health are to be expected. On the other hand, the comparatively short period for setting may be a problem, especially when complicated compaction techniques are used and teeth with more than one root canal are to be treated. However, this may be advantageous in a root-end filling situation. The material is only moderately toxic and apparently does not actively stimulate the healing of apical tissues.

Glass ionomer cements (GICs) have also been recommended as root canal sealers. The main problems of the GIC sealer are related to leakage, which may be due to moisture sensitivity during setting. The formation of pores may be another problem. On the other hand, these materials may offer the possibility of strengthening the root due to chemical binding to dentin, therefore further test results and/or material improvements should be monitored. These sealers are not in widespread use. Sealers commonly used will be discussed in more detail in the following paragraphs.

Zinc oxide–eugenol sealers

Zinc oxide–eugenol (ZnOE) sealers have been used for many years and ample clinical experience exists with these materials. However, sealing ability and biological properties are, in general, inferior compared with other root canal sealers. Because of its tendency for disintegration ZnOE is still recommended as a root canal filling material for deciduous teeth. However, it has not been shown that disintegration of the material occurs parallel to tooth resorption. Formaldehyde-releasing ZnOE root canal sealers should not be used any more because of their inherent toxic potential. The European Society of Endodontology discourages the use of these materials (26).

Composition

These sealers comprise a fairly large group of different preparations. In addition to the standard composition of ZnOE sealers (Grossman sealer, Table 12.4), some preparations contain thymol or thymol iodide for increasing the antimicrobial effects. Also, hydroxyapatite or calcium hydroxide has been added to improve apical healing. In some sealers eugenol is partially or totally replaced by oil of cloves, Peru balsam or eucalyptol. Oil of cloves is a natural product that contains 60–80% eugenol. The ZnOE sealers may contain colophony (a rosin, mainly diterpene resin acids) to give body, to impart adhesiveness to the sealer and to reduce the solubility/disintegration of the sealer. Some ZnOE-based sealers contain paraformaldehyde (e.g. 7% of the powder), with the claim of long-term disinfection by the release of formaldehyde.

The ZnOE preparations harden in a humid environment by forming a ZnOE chelate compound. The mix sets within 24 hours but the speed can be regulated by

---

Core concept 12.3 Classification of root canal sealers

Sealers commonly used are based on:
- Polyketone
- Glass ionomer cement
- Zinc oxide and eugenol (ZnOE)
- Epoxy resin
- Calcium hydroxide
- Methacrylate resins
- Mineral trioxide aggregate (MTA)
- Silicone

Table 12.4   Typical composition of a ZnOE sealer.

Powder	Liquid
Zinc oxide (42%)	Eugenol (4-allyl-2-methoxyphenol)
Staybelite resin (27%)	
Bismuth subcarbonate (15%)	
Barium sulfate (15%)	
Sodium borate, anhydrous (1%)	

the addition of resins, calcium phosphates or zinc acetate. The setting reaction is reversible, releasing eugenol and zinc ions under hydrolytic conditions.

Technical properties/leakage

Several studies showed *apical* leakage around ZnOE sealers that increased with storage time (measured up to 2 years) in thick layers more than in thin layers (45). Sealing properties of ZnOE sealers were inferior in comparison to other sealers (epoxy resin or calcium hydroxide sealers). Adhesion of ZnOE sealers to gutta-percha cones is sufficient. Also, *coronal* leakage was greater for a ZnOE sealer (when used with a lateral condensation technique) than for a calcium hydroxide sealer, probably due to the relatively high solubility of the ZnOE sealer (4). It can be concluded that the sealing properties of ZnOE sealers in general are somewhat inferior to most other available materials. Removal of the smear layer improves the seal.

Biological properties

Eugenol, a phenol derivative, has attracted prime interest from a biological point of view. Systemic toxicity was evaluated to be low and eugenol is an accepted nutrition additive. However, eugenol is a known contact allergen, as are colophony and Peru balsam. Eugenol and its derivatives are used in fragrances, and allergies to fragrances may be related to eugenol. Cases of allergic reactions toward ZnOE-containing temporary filling materials have been reported (38), but apparently not for root canal sealers. Formaldehyde, which is released from certain ZnOE sealers, is also a known allergen. A female patient, a few hours after the application of a high formaldehyde-containing root canal paste, reported urticaria of the lower jaw that rapidly cleared with oral corticosteroids. In a skin test, the patient reacted positively to the formaldehyde-containing liquid of the root canal paste (21).

Eugenol is cytotoxic and the same has been shown frequently for ZnOE with different cell culture systems, especially after mixing but also in a set state. Even higher cytotoxicity was observed with formaldehyde-containing ZnOE sealers, which were classified as highly/extremely cytotoxic (Fig. 12.14) (3) and reveal strong cytotoxic effects (Fig. 12.11) even after several elutions of the hardened specimens (31).

Some components of ZnOE sealers have neurotoxic effects. Eugenol inhibited nerve conductance *in vitro* in experiments with different nerve tissues. Furthermore,

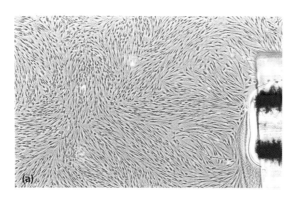
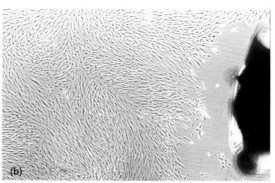
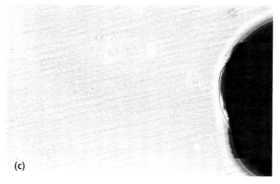

Fig. 12.14   (a) An empty polytube, (b) a tube filled with a ZnOE sealer, and (c) a tube filled with a formaldehyde-releasing ZnOE sealer were transferred, immediately after obturating, to tissue culture flasks containing cultures of human oral fibroblasts. Toxicity was evaluated after 5, 10 and 15 days. The illustration shows the results after 15 days. In (a), the control group, the fibroblasts proliferate close to the test tube (right). In (b) a narrow inhibition zone persists adjacent to a ZnOE-containing tube. In (c), where the tube contained a formaldehyde-releasing sealer, no vital cells are seen (3).

eugenol has both local and general anesthetic effects. Taking into consideration the concentrations involved, a possible neurotoxic effect of eugenol may be reversible *in vivo* (14). On the contrary, formaldehyde irreversibly suppressed nerve conduction in concentrations that may be reached in patients with formaldehyde-containing root canal sealers owing to the high solubility of formaldehyde in water (14). The results with the formaldehyde-containing sealers suggest permanent damage of the nerve *in vivo* (14, 15).

ZnOE sealers have a moderate local toxicity that is strongly enhanced by the addition of paraformaldehyde (40) (Key literature 12.2, Fig. 12.15). There are reports indicating favorable clinical results using sealers containing formaldehyde. However, as mentioned, clinical outcome depends on many variables and is by itself no proof of acceptable biological properties.

ZnOE sealers with paraformaldehyde were reported to induce aspergillosis of the sinus maxillaris if the material is overfilled into the sinus. A typical radiograph shows a homogeneously clouded antrum with one or more round-to-oval radiodense objects (Fig. 12.16). Clinical symptoms are inconclusive: most patients report intermittent pain and tenderness of the cheek. Other patients have no clinical symptoms and aspergillosis may be detected incidentally at an X-ray examination (6).

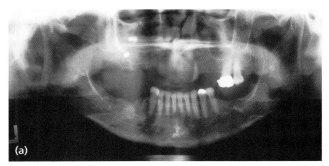

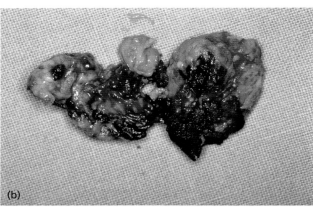

Fig. 12.16 Radiograph of a maxillary sinus with suspected aspergillosis from an overfilled root canal in the right sinus: round to oval radiodense objects in the right sinus indicate aspergillosis; the responsible tooth was extracted (a) and the tissue was removed from the sinus (b). (Courtesy of Dr Härle.)

Key literature 12.2

Hong *et al.* (40) performed experiments on the incisors of monkeys. They deliberately overfilled the root canals (thus simulating a worst-case situation) with two ZnOE sealers, one releasing formaldehyde and the other not. The tissue reaction was evaluated histologically. The formaldehyde-releasing ZnOE sealer caused severe periapical inflammation even after 6 months; the formaldehyde-free sealer evoked milder alterations. Under the same experimental conditions a calcium phosphate sealer (experimental material) produced only minimal tissue reactions and even new bone was formed. Based on their results the authors recommend materials that alter periapical tissues as little as possible, to prevent severe and chronic tissue reactions after inadvertently overfilling the root canal.

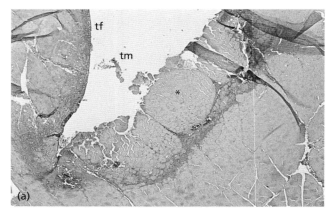

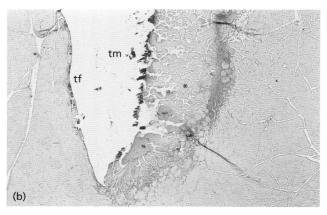

Fig. 12.15 Tissue reaction 7 days after intramuscular implantation of a formaldehyde-releasing ZnOE sealer: extended area of inflammatory cells and necrotic tissue at the contact area with the test material (*) indicates strong toxicity for the material (a) after mixing and (b) after 7 days of setting. tm = test material; tf = Teflon tube (negative control and material carrier).

Antimicrobial properties: ZnOE sealers have demonstrated antimicrobial properties on a variety of microorganisms, including *Enterococcus faecalis* suspensions and anaerobic bacteria even 7 days after mixing. This effect was stronger than the effect produced with calcium hydroxide products but less than an effect from an epoxy resin sealer (Fig. 12.17). Apparently, eugenol is the main antimicrobial agent. Ørstavik (57), in an experimental model of contaminated dentinal tubules, has shown that a ZnOE sealer in the pulp chamber disinfected the dental tubules to a depth of 250 μm (Fig. 12.18). Formaldehyde-releasing ZnOE sealers show extensive antimicrobial properties (Fig. 12.17). This activity lasts longer than that of formaldehyde-free sealers but also decreases with time.

Handling properties

ZnOE-based sealers are easy to handle. They can be mixed to a smooth paste, which allows enough time for obturation and control radiography before setting. Removal can be performed with organic solvents. The radiopacity of different ZnOE sealers was 5.16–7.97 mm Al (76) and thus can be regarded as sufficient.

Epoxy resin sealers

Epoxy resin sealers have comparatively good mechanical and sealing properties. No effects on general health are expected and allergic reactions are apparently rare. Antimicrobial properties are good, especially in a freshly mixed state. Cytotoxicity is moderate to low (set state). Mutagenicity is mainly observed shortly after mixing and no unacceptable risk is expected for the patient. For dental personnel, a "no touch technique" is recommended.

Composition (Table 12.5)

The original preparation (AH26), although still on the market in some countries, has been replaced by a follow-up product (AHPlus, Topseal). Because the silver in AH26 may lead to tooth discoloration due to the formation of black silver sulfides, preparations are available

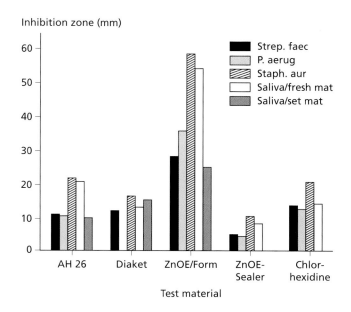

Fig. 12.17 Antimicrobial properties: distance of growth inhibition zone for several root canal sealers and different bacterial strains. Large zones indicate extensive antimicrobial properties. ZnOE/Form = formaldehyde-containing ZnOE sealer (56).

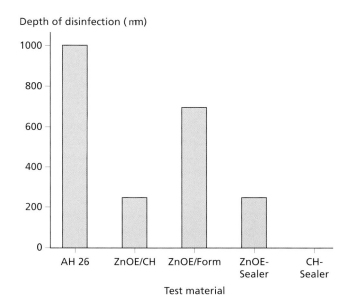

Fig. 12.18 Antimicrobial properties: depth of dentin at which bacteria (*Enterococcus faecalis*) were killed by the root canal sealers. ZnOE/Form = formaldehyde-containing ZnOE sealer; ZnOE/CH = calcium hydroxide-containing ZnOE sealer (57).

Table 12.5 Composition of epoxy sealer.

Powder	Liquid
Bismuth (III) oxide (60%)	Bisphenol-A-diglycidylether (BADGE)
Hexamethylene tetraamine (25%)[a]	
Silver (10%)[b]	
Titanium dioxide (5%)	

[a] For a follow-up product adamantane amine, *N,N′*-dibenzoyl-5-oxanonane-diamine-1,9-TCD-diamine is used as a catalyst.
[b] Sealers with bismuth oxide instead of silver are on the market.

without silver, and bismuth oxide is added for radiopacity. A newly developed preparation (AHPlus) is also based on an epoxy resin (BADGE) but contains a different catalyst.

The setting reaction of AH26 takes about 1–2 days (at body temperature) and is a polymerization process during which formaldehyde is released, but the concentration is more than 300-fold less than that of a formaldehyde-releasing ZnOE formulation (82). AHPlus sets in about 8 hours. There are indications that AHPlus does not release formaldehyde.

Technical properties/leakage

Epoxy-based sealer shows comparatively good mechanical properties and adhesion/adaptation to dentin. After initial volumetric expansion, the sealer shows some shrinkage when tested at longer intervals. In general, *in vitro* and *in vivo* studies with the material showed better sealing properties than with any other sealer tested, although it was far from perfect because an increasing storage time (up to 2 years) decreases the sealing quality (45). Studies on the sealing properties of AHPlus compared with AH26 show inconsistent results. If the smear layer is removed from the root canal walls, AH26 is able to flow into the orifices of the dentinal tubules (Fig. 12.19), which is the reason for the comparatively good adhesion of AH26 to dentin. The adhesion to the gutta-percha cone is sometimes not as good (Fig. 12.20).

Biological properties

Epoxy resins are biologically active molecules but no reports are available in the literature on systemic toxic reactions caused by epoxy-based sealers. One case of allergic reaction to AH26 was reported after root canal filling, characterized by erythema of the face and the neck and a positive skin test (Fig. 12.21) (41). Positive

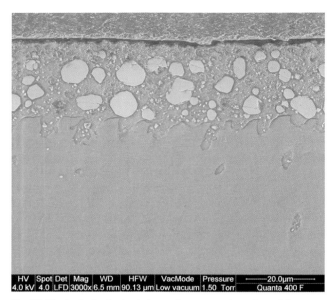

HV | Spot | Det | Mag | WD | HFW | VacMode | Pressure | ———20.0μm———
4.0 kV | 4.0 | LFD | 3000x | 6.5 mm | 90.13 μm | Low vacuum | 1.50 Torr | Quanta 400 F

Fig. 12.20 Lack of adhesion between the epoxy resin sealer and the gutta-percha point.

reactions to AH26 have also been observed in the guinea pig maximization test (37).

The cytotoxicity of AH26 is related to the setting reaction: freshly mixed, the material is cytotoxic, but after setting it is not toxic or only slightly toxic (Fig. 12.11) (69). Cytotoxicity was related to the initial release of formaldehyde during setting. *In vitro* AH26 showed some inhibition of nerve conductance, which was partially reversible (15).

In both *in vitro* and *in vivo* experiments AH26 was mutagenic (24, 35), especially in a freshly mixed state (73, 75). The cause of the mutagenic reaction may be formaldehyde formed during the setting reaction or the epoxy monomer (BADGE). AHPlus (which also contains BADGE) was also shown to be mutagenic, but only immediately after mixing (74). Because the set material in

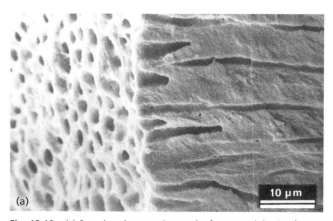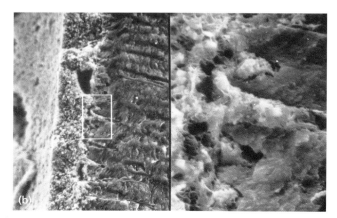

Fig. 12.19 (a) Scanning electron micrograph of root canal dentin after smear layer removal with citric acid. (b) AH26 used as a sealer on a smear-layer-free dentin surface: the sealer enters the dentinal tubules. (Courtesy of Dr A. Petschelt.)

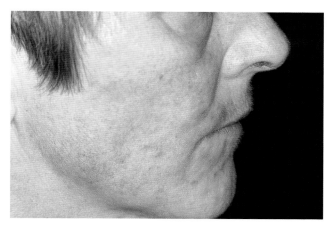

Fig. 12.21 Allergic reaction to an epoxy resin sealer. A couple of hours following root filling of tooth 46 the patient developed swelling and erythema of the right side of the face and neck. Redness of the oral mucosa around tooth 46 was experienced and the tooth became tender to percussion. The symptoms subsided after a couple of days. The root filling was removed and the canals were later obturated without complications using gutta-percha points and ZnOE cement. Before obturation a strong positive patch test reaction to bisphenol-A-ethyldimethacrylate (BISEMA), bisphenol-A-glycidyldimethacrylate (BISGMA) and epoxyacrylate was demonstrated. The patient recalled that almost similar symptoms had arisen 6 months previously when another tooth was root filled. However, the previous reactions were not as serious.

most studies was non-mutagenic, it was concluded that it can be used in the patient situation but care should be taken by the dental personnel, who may come into frequent contact with the unpolymerized material. Therefore, a "no touch technique" is recommended.

After implantation or root canal filling in different small laboratory animals, the epoxy sealers proved to be toxic initially but the reaction resolved partially or even totally with prolonged postoperative observation periods (Fig. 12.22). Overfilled AH26 was solubilized and phagocytosed or surrounded by fibrous tissue.

Antimicrobial properties: AH26 has antimicrobial properties (Fig. 12.17). Similar to local toxicity, the antimicrobial effect decreases with increasing setting time. Compared with ZnOE, calcium hydroxide and GIC sealers on the model of infected root dentin, AH26 showed the strongest antimicrobial effect (Fig. 12.18) (36), probably due to the initial release of formaldehyde.

Handling properties

Epoxy-based sealers have been used for more than 40 years worldwide and their handling properties are usually considered to be good. Radiopacity is sufficient (6.6 mm Al). However, the materials set to a hard mass that, in a clinically relevant time, is virtually insoluble even for organic solvents. Therefore, this material must be used together with gutta-percha cones.

Calcium hydroxide sealers

Calcium hydroxide sealers have inferior technical properties compared with polyketone or epoxy resin preparations. Leakage studies show inconsistent results, with a tendency for poorer sealing quality compared with other sealers. From a biological point of view, calcium hydroxide sealers are very favorable materials and they exhibit – at least in a freshly mixed state – considerable antimicrobial activity. Furthermore, they belong to the few materials that apparently support apical healing and hard-tissue formation (root-end closure).

Composition

These sealers were introduced in an attempt to stimulate periapical healing with bone repair through the release of calcium hydroxide (Table 12.6). The setting reaction is based on the salicylate compounds. Calcium hydroxide

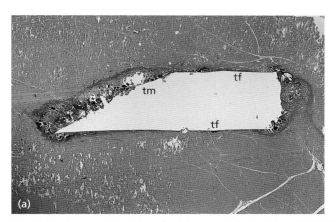
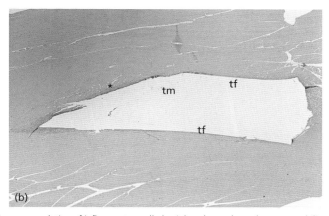

Fig. 12.22 Tissue reaction 7 days after intramuscular implantation of AH26: (a) an accumulation of inflammatory cells (mainly polymorphonuclear neutrophilic granulocytes) at the contact area between the test material and the tissue (*) indicates moderate toxicity of the material directly after mixing; (b) the tissue in contact with the set material shows no inflammatory cells (*) so the set material is therefore virtually non-toxic. tm = test material; tf = Teflon tube (negative control and material carrier).

Table 12.6 Main components of a calcium hydroxide sealer.

Base paste	Catalyst paste
Calcium hydroxide (32%)	Disalicylates (36%)
Colophony (32%)	Bismuth carbonate (18%)
Silicon dioxide (8%)	Silicon dioxide (15%)
Calcium oxide (6%)	Colophony (5%)
Zinc oxide (6%)	Tricalcium phosphate (5%)
Others (16%)	Others (21%)

sealers release OH^- and Ca^{2+} ions. The amount varies between different brands, but the clinical significance of this difference is not known. Release of these ions is markedly higher when suspensions are used. Calcium hydroxide sealers evoked an increase of pH to between 9.5 and 11.5 when placed in distilled water (48 hours after setting); under the same conditions pure calcium hydroxide paste increased pH to 12.5. When calcium hydroxide sealers are used together with lateral condensation of gutta-percha, the outer dentin surface does not become alkaline, in contrast to the use of calcium hydroxide suspensions (25).

Technical properties/leakage

Mechanical properties of calcium hydroxide sealers are inferior compared with polyketone-, epoxy- or GIC-based sealers. The desired release of OH^- ions may be associated with degradation of the sealer, enhancing leakage. Degradation of salicylate-based materials is known from their application as pulp capping agents. Studies clearly indicate significant volumetric expansion, disintegration and high solubility of a calcium hydroxide sealer following long-term observations. Apparently, some calcium hydroxide sealers dissolve at a relatively high rate, especially when used in a thick layer (Fig. 12.23) (98). The bond to dentin is weak (95). One calcium hydroxide sealer (Sealapex) showed comparatively good sealing capability when used alone in primary teeth and was recommended for this indication (42).

Biological properties

There are no reports available in the literature about systemic–toxic, allergic or mutagenic effects of calcium hydroxide sealers (24). Their cytotoxicity is reported to be generally low (compared with other commonly used sealers) when tested in different cell culture systems (13, 31). However, both a calcium hydroxide sealer and a calcium hydroxide-containing ZnOE sealer tested *in vitro* induced a fast and complete inhibition of nerve conductance when in direct contact with the nerve. After 30 min of contact, the nerve conduction was irreversibly blocked by both materials (8).

After implantation in rats and guinea pigs, calcium hydroxide sealers initially caused a severe reaction that diminished after several months and was finally lower than with a ZnOE sealer. A calcium hydroxide sealer applied in root canals evoked an extensive apical hard-tissue formation (81).

Antimicrobial properties: Antimicrobial properties have been shown for calcium hydroxide-based sealers in several *in vitro* experiments, and the activity may even increase over time along with partial disintegration of the sealer. The mechanism is related to the high pH. However, the buffer capacity of body fluid will reduce the antimicrobial effect, which may explain why ZnOE sealers exhibit a stronger antimicrobial effect than calcium

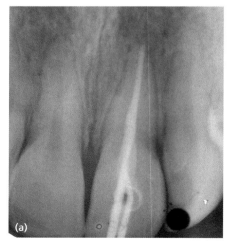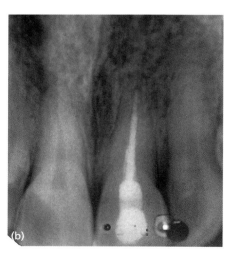

Fig. 12.23 Resorption of sealer: (a) root filling with gutta-percha points and a calcium hydroxide sealer after pulpectomy; (b) resorption or dissolution of the most apical part of the root filling after 10 months. (Courtesy of Dr A. Burhart.)

hydroxide products regardless of the microorganisms tested (1). In accordance with the latter study, the calcium hydroxide sealer did not disinfect the dentinal tubules infected with *Enterococcus faecalis* after 4 hours (Fig. 12.18) (57). This is in line with the observation that enterococci, which are frequently isolated from persistent root canal infections, resist calcium hydroxide.

Root-end closure

A "root-end closure" is the induction of calcified tissue formation to obturate the dental apical foramen; it was first reported in 1960. In several experiments with monkeys, osteocementum/cementoid substances at and around the open root apices were developed after the application of a calcium hydroxide suspension for 3 and 6 months. Clinical success rates are in the range of 74–100% (Fig. 12.24).

The mechanism by which calcium hydroxide preparations provide for hard-tissue formation is not yet elucidated. It is apparently related to the high pH and the released calcium ions from the material, which promote a state of alkalinity of the adjacent tissues – a condition that arrests root resorption and favors repair, due to inhibition of osteoclastic activities. It has been postulated further that Ca^{2+} acts on the process of cell differentia-

tion and on macrophage activation and that acids produced by osteoclasts are neutralized and calcium phosphate complexes are formed. It was suggested that activation of ATP, which accelerates bone and dentin mineralization, and the induction of TGFβ (transforming growth factor beta), which represents a group of signaling molecules, play a central role in biomineralization. A further factor is the antimicrobial activity of calcium hydroxide sealers.

Handling properties

Handling properties of calcium hydroxide sealers are adequate; the radiopacity is regarded as sufficient. The material can be removed from the root canal with common rotary instruments.

Methacrylate-based sealers

In order to reduce leakage, methacrylate-based materials used in adhesive coronal dentistry were transferred to the root canal system. As in a coronal cavity, in the root canal a smear layer is present on the dentin after instrumentation. However, in contrast to the dentin surfaces in cavities, the anatomy of the root canal is more irregular with lateral canals and a decreasing number of

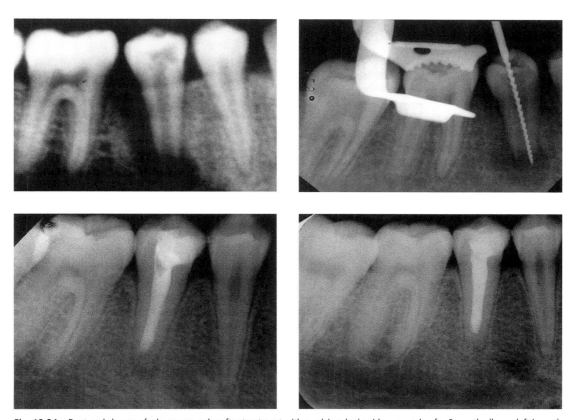

Fig. 12.24   Root-end closure of a lower premolar after treatment with a calcium hydroxide suspension for 6 months (lower left image). For the final root canal filling (lower right image) an epoxy sealer with gutta-percha was used. (Courtesy of Dr B. Thonemann.)

Table 12.7 Composition of resin-based root canal filling systems (68); information from the literature (36, 81, 100) and from material safety data sheets.

Epiphany system®*			RC – Sealer®#		EndoRez®	
Primer	Sealer	Point (Resilon)	Sealer	Point	Sealer	Point
AMPS* and hydrophilic monomers solution Camphorquinone *2-Acrylamido-2-methylpropane sulfonic acid	UDMA PEGDMA EBPADMA Bis-GMA Amines Peroxide Photo-initiator Stabilizers Silane-treated barium-borosilicate glasses Barium sulfate Silica Calcium hydroxide Bismuth oxychloride Pigments	Copolymer of polycaprolactone and urethane methacrylate Bioactive glass Radiopaque fillers Coloring agent	**Liquid:** 4-META HEMA Dimethacrylates **Powder:** Polymethylmethacrylate Zirconium dioxide Amorphous silica TBB (tri-n-butylborane) partially oxidated Polymerization initiator	Resilon or gutta-percha	2,2'-(p-Tolylimino) diethanol TEGDMA DUDMA Benzoylperoxide Zinc oxide Barium sulfate Pigments	Resin-coated (polybutadien-diisocyanat-methacrylate) gutta-percha

Materials of similar or identical composition: * = Real Seal® (primer, sealer, points); # = Hybrid Root Seal® and MetaSEAL®.
Bis-GMA = bisphenol A-glycidyldimethacrylate; UDMA = 1,6-bis(methacrylyloxy-2-ethoxycarbonylamino)-2,4,4-trimethylhexane; PEGDMA = polyethylene glycol dimethacrylate; EBPADMA = ethoxylated bisphenol A dimethacrylate; HEMA = 2-hydroxyethyl methacrylate; 4-META = 4-methacrylolyloxyethyl trimellitate anhydride; TEGDMA = triethylene glycol dimethacrylate; DUDMA = diurethane dimethacrylate.

dentinal tubules in the apical area. Furthermore, the apical canal wall is partially covered with calcified appositions. Therefore, the transfer of adhesive dentistry to the root canal is not unproblematic. *In vitro* studies report conflicting results and clinical experience is limited. Methacrylate-based sealers materials are in an early state of development. They have a great potential, although there is no clear proven clinical advantage so far (72).

Composition

Methacrylate-based sealers are used as such or together with a self-etching primer. The main components of currently used preparations (Table 12.7) are methylmethacrylate derivatives, which are mainly known from restorative dentistry. The sealers are self- or dual-curing. The latter sealers (e.g. Epiphany) are exposed to standard polymerization light, as in composite technology, in order to cure the coronal part of the sealer. Complete setting varies from 20 min to 7 days (10).

Some resin-based sealers are recommended to be used together with conventional gutta-percha cones. However, as these sealers may not adhere to gutta-percha, special points have been developed (see Table 12.7). Resilon is a thermoplastic copolymer of polycaprolactone and urethane methacrylate (10, 77). This material can be thermocompacted similarly to gutta-percha. A chemical bond to

the methacrylate-based sealers is looked for through the inclusion of dimethacrylates. Together with the corresponding sealer (Epiphany) a solid "mono-block" has been advertised. The formation of the mono-block is, however, questioned (72). Alternatively, resin-coated gutta-percha has been recommended to be used with such sealers (see Table 12.7).

Technical properties/leakage

The technical properties of methacrylate-based sealers are mainly in accordance with relevant standards but one sealer (Epiphany) was outside the acceptable range for solubility and dimensional stability (91). Furthermore, the polyester cone material is susceptible to alkaline and enzymatic degradation via ester bond cleavage (86). In a clinical study, an apically extruded sealer (EndoREZ) was observed to be resorbed within 5 years; this shows a certain level of solubility, which may be advantageous in the case of overfilling but disadvantageous for canal sealing.

For sealers with and without separate primers, resin tags in dentinal tubules and a hybrid layer were found rather consistently (Fig. 12.25) (47). However, such tubule penetration was even deeper with an epoxy resin sealer (Fig. 12.19) (51). Fewer tags were observed in the apical area compared to the middle or the coronal part of the root canal probably because of the smaller number of

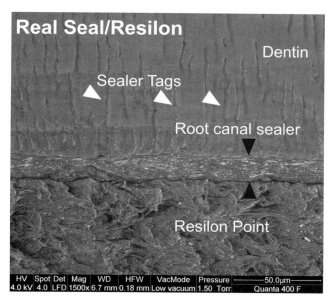

Fig. 12.25 Tag formation in the root dentin after the application of a methacrylate-based sealer, but gap formation between the sealer and the polyester point.

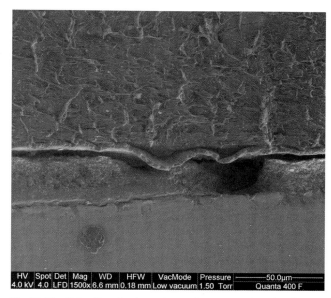

Fig. 12.26 Dislocation of resin coating on the gutta-percha point after root canal obturation.

tubules in this area. Interestingly, the presence of tags did not exclude the existence of gaps (7).

The tight bonding of the sealer with the two relevant interfaces (dentin and the cone) is challenged by several factors, one of them being the polymerization shrinkage of methacrylates during setting. This becomes even more problematic because the filler content, which partially compensates for monomer shrinkage, is comparatively low in order to guarantee adequate flow properties. Furthermore, in the root canal the amount of available free surface is very low. With an unfavorable ratio between free surface and bonded surface (configuration factor) (85) stress on the interface increases and may result in debonding and leakage (85). This may be compensated for by the slow polymerization time (72).

Hydrolysis of the collagen fibrils may also challenge the stability of the bond between the sealer and the dentin. Owing to the long setting time of the sealers, the materials are prone to absorption of fluids from the dentin (e.g. through the hydrophilic primer). This moisture contamination may lead to the breakdown of the bond (72). Substances used for canal rinsing may also compromise the bond, e.g. NaOCl and H_2O_2, because polymerization is inhibited through the formation of an oxygen-rich dentin layer (72). Conflicting data are reported for chlorhexidine. Calcium hydroxide dressings have apparently no effect on the bond strength or on leakage (92).

Although scanning electron microscopy studies initially suggested a better seal of methacrylate-based sealers together with the respective cones (77), other studies showed gaps both between the sealer and the cone and the sealer and dentin (72). The amount of dimethacrylates incorporated in the polyester cone may not be sufficient for an optimal coupling to the methacrylate sealer (84).

Although initial leakage studies have been very promising, in later bacterial (*E. faecalis*) and dye penetration studies methacrylate sealers leaked the same as or even more than AH26 used with gutta-percha for different application techniques; e.g. single cone or lateral condensation (30, 47). Coating gutta-percha with resin or the use of special cones (polyester material) did not prevent gap formation or leakage (72). The resin coat may be dislocated by condensing techniques (Fig. 12.26). Some authors speculate that the application technique may play a major role (33), but conclusive information is not available.

A reduced root fracture susceptibility after the application of these sealers/cones was shown *in vitro* compared to gutta-percha and AH26 (87). Again, this could not be supported by other studies (62) and the bond strength was inferior compared to AH26 (push-out test) (72). It was concluded that such sealers with the respective cones are unlikely to reinforce root canal strength (72).

Biological properties

In cell culture experiments and in implantation studies some sealers (Epiphany primer, sealer, EndoRez) and the Resilon points were severely cytotoxic (more cytotoxic than AH26 and silicone-based sealers (48)); other preparations (RC sealer) were only slightly cytotoxic (22). Toxicity of Epiphany decreased with increasing setting time (52). There are no data available on allergic reactions after the application of methacrylate-based sealers. However, it is known that patients may have developed an allergy to methacrylates. Obviously, such sealers must not be used in patients with a known allergy to one of the components of these sealers. There are data indicating that one sealer (EndoREZ) is well tolerated in the periapical tissues of subhuman primates (49) and clinical results in a non-controlled study over 5 years were in the range of other sealers (99). However, the amount of available data is limited. The antibacterial properties of these materials are rather limited (72, 78).

Handling properties

Uniform application of a primer or an adhesive in root canals and removal of solvent are considered to be difficult, especially in the apical third (72). Massive air blowing into the canal should generally be avoided and the use of paper point is not very effective (72). Special delivery systems (e.g. microbrushes) are recommended for application of primers and sealers.

Root canal fillings with methacrylate sealers and respective cones can mechanically be removed just as root canal fillings with gutta-percha and epoxy sealers. The removal speed can be improved by heat or solvents (72). Flow, film thickness and radiopacity are sufficient.

Mineral trioxide aggregate (MTA)

This cement was introduced in 1993, as a root-end filling material for sealing of communications between the root canal system and the periapical tissue (88). The cement, similarly to calcium hydroxide, supports hard-tissue repair at root ends as well of pulpal exposures and has therefore also been used for apexification in root-open teeth and for pulp capping and pulpotomy procedures (see also Chapters 4, 5 and 15).

Composition

MTA is based on Portland cement, which primarily consists of tricalcium silicate, dicalcium silicate, tricalcium aluminate and tetracalcium aluminoferrite (16). Sulfates in various amounts regulate working and setting time. The particles of MTA are smaller than in Portland cement and bismuth oxide is added to increase radiopacity. Variations in the composition of MTA cement have been marketed. A white formula of the original gray MTA has been developed because of claims of tooth discoloration when gray MTA (ProRoot original) was used for pulp capping and pulpotomy in anterior teeth of young people. The white MTA and another more recent formu-

lation (MTA-Angelus) set slightly faster than the original gray MTA. When the cement powder is mixed with sterile water a silicate–hydrate gel is formed which sets to a hard mass releasing nascent calcium hydroxide. The pH is high during and shortly after setting, which for the original MTA takes about 3 hours (89). The long setting time may be disadvantageous in some situations because of the risk of washing out. On the other hand it may be advantageous in other situations as the material is able to set properly in moist environments (and needs moist environments in order to set properly).

Technical properties/leakage

The compressive strength of MTA is about 40 MPa after 24 hours in contrast to the 52 MPa of IRM, 60 MPa of super EBA and 313 MPa of amalgam (89). After 3 weeks the compressive strength is similar to that of fortified ZnOE cements. The sealing efficacy against penetration of bacteria in microspaces between cement and tooth substance has shown better adaptation and less leakage of MTA compared to amalgam, IRM and SuperEBA (28). The initial high sealing ability may be caused by a slight expansion during setting and it has been shown that an apical barrier of MTA can resist displacement during gutta-percha condensation (83). Three millimeters of MTA is suggested as the minimum amount for protection against microleakage in most cases, while 5 mm has been suggested in the treatment of immature apices (63).

Biological properties

Biocompatibility of MTA has been studied in cell culture, implantation in connective tissue or bone of animals and in some clinical and histological studies on humans (for review see 16, 63). In general MTA was less toxic than ZnOE preparations and freshly mixed material was more toxic than set. No significant difference was found between MTA and Portland cement. Results from all the *in vitro* and *in vivo* animal studies conclude that set MTA is well tolerated by the various cells and tissues. Similar results have been found in the moderate number of human studies of rather short duration. Thus, a high success rate has been demonstrated after root resections (17, 19) and root perforations (50). Following direct pulp capping a more solid bridge has been described with MTA compared to calcium hydroxide in a limited number of studies on healthy pulps (53, 55).

In primary teeth better outcomes after pulpotomies with MTA were found than following formocreosol treatment (61). Finally, in teeth with immature apices promising results with formation of an apical barrier have been reported (39). The hard-tissue inducing effect is not fully understood but the property may be attributed to a stimulating effect on biological molecules important for hard-tissue formation. Mutagenicity of MTA has not been shown (63) and reports of allergic reactions have so far not been published.

Handling properties

The material is rather difficult to place and the working time may be short. Special MTA Endo Carriers have been developed to facilitate placement and condensation. If the cement starts to harden during placement and if it is difficult to manipulate more water can be added to obtain a feasible plasticity.

Silicones

Silicone was introduced in 1984 as a basis for root canal sealers. Recent preparations based on A-silicones show comparatively little leakage, are virtually non-toxic, but display no antibacterial activity. Clinical data are few but promising.

Composition

The first of those materials was based on C-silicones (condensation cross-linking silicones); newer materials are based on A-silicones (addition cross-linking). Recently, gutta-percha powder with a particle size of less than 30 μm has been introduced into a silicone matrix (polydimethylsiloxane). Silver particles have been added as preservative (10). Working time is 15 min and setting time is 25–30 min.

Technical properties/leakage

A gutta-percha containing silicone sealer expands slightly and thus leakage was reported to be less than for AH26 with gutta-percha over a period of 12 months (43). Furthermore, this sealer allowed less fluid movement along a filled straight root than AH26 (9). However, other studies reported sealing of a silicone sealer to be equal to or even worse than for AH26 and not as effective as Grossman's sealer for filling simulated lateral canals (12, 59). The wettability of AH26 is better than that of hydrophobic silicone sealers. Thus, more load is needed for sufficiently wetting gutta-percha and dentin (44).

Biological properties

No data for systemic toxicity and allergy are available. However, based on the composition of the material, neither of these adverse type reactions is to be expected. In contrast to older preparations based on C-silicones, those based on A-silicones were only slightly toxic or non-toxic in different cell culture and in implantation tests (Fig. 12.27) (10, 32). No antibacterial properties were found, e.g. on infected dentin (65). Current clinical experience with silicone-based sealers is limited.

Handling properties

Silicone sealers are supplied in capsules and after mixing can easily be injected into the canal followed by the insertion of gutta-percha. The filling can be removed as with other sealers.

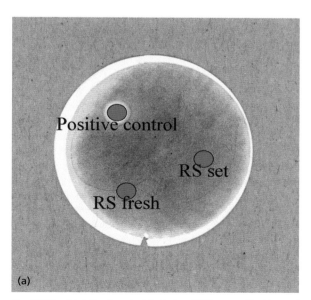 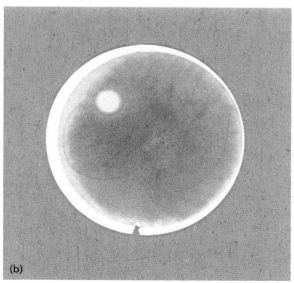

Fig. 12.27   (a) Cell culture toxicity test on L929 mouse fibroblasts of an "A-silicone" root canal sealer. The cells are growing beneath the filter (circular gray area). A positive control (5% phenol), the freshly prepared sealer and the set sealer are placed on top of the filter in three different rings. (b) The cells beneath fresh and set material are not damaged, whereas all cells beneath the control are dead. RS = root sealer. (Courtesy of Dr D. Ørstavik.)

Materials for retrograde fillings (root-end fillings) and replantation

It is normally agreed that placement of a retrograde filling is necessary after root resection to create an apical seal and to permit regeneration of the periodontal ligament apparatus (19). Contrary to conventional root canal filling therapy, these materials are used in a surgical environment characterized by early moisture access and a bony defect.

Several different materials have been used for root-end fillings, such as gutta-percha, composite resins, glass ionomers, amalgams, modified ZnOE cements and a polyketone sealer. MTAs and calcium phosphate cements are potentially applicable. Preformed titanium inlays in combination with standard ultrasonic preparation were recommended (cemented with a modified ZnOE cement), as well as ceramic inserts. Because of the potential to release metallic components, especially mercury, into the surrounding tissue the classical material for root-end filling – amalgam – has been gradually abandoned and in a few countries it is not allowed to be used for this indication. Modified ZnOE cements, a polyketone sealer (thick consistency) used with or without metallic/ceramic inserts or a light-cured GIC were successfully used instead. However, reports on cementum deposition are equivocal. A resin composite has shown promising results in the hands of a single group and MTAs apparently have the potential to stimulate further apical healing and thus may – after further clinical experience is gained – replace other materials for this purpose.

Composition

Most materials are the same as used for orthograde root filling and have been described previously in this chapter. A few materials are modifications and will be described briefly below.

Modified and fortified ZnOE preparations are composed of: 60% zinc oxide, 34% alumina and 6% natural resin (powder); or 62.5% *ortho*-ethoxy benzoic acid and 37.5% eugenol (liquid). Another frequently used cement contains 80% ZnO and 20% PMMA (polymethylmethacrylate) in the powder, and the liquid is eugenol. These materials are preferably used for temporary fillings of the access cavity and for root-end fillings.

Technical properties/leakage

The good mechanical properties of amalgams were the reason for their widespread use in the past. Data reported on the marginal seal of amalgams are, however, controversial. A polyketone sealer and a GIC sealer were reported to produce a better seal than various amalgams.

Good sealing ability of a light-cured GIC was reported, probably due to the fast setting and little moisture sensitivity. Modified ZnOE cements have also been shown to produce a good seal, as well as a composite resin. Mineral trioxide aggregate produced a better seal than amalgam, being the most effective root-end filling material against bacterial penetration in comparison with amalgam and two modified ZnOE sealers (28).

Biological properties

The group of materials used for root-end filling is rather heterogeneous. Much literature is available on real or claimed systemic–toxic effects, especially for composite resins and amalgams. The same is true for allergies. The reader is referred to textbooks on the subject (68). However, in general, there is no contraindication for the use of any of the mentioned materials due to systemic toxic or allergenic effects. In the single patient situation, materials must not be used that contain a substance to which the patient is sensitized.

Cell culture experiments for local toxic effects show consistently that all setting materials used for root-end filling are cytotoxic immediately after mixing. In the set state, cytotoxicity decreases to different levels characteristic of each material. MTA is less cytotoxic than amalgam, ZnOE or epoxy sealers (60). Implantation studies are available for all root-end filling materials, because they are used for other applications (e.g. filling technique). In parallel with cell culture experiments, the local inflammatory reaction decreases with increased aging of the material. The same is basically true for antimicrobial properties. For details, see the paragraphs on the specific materials above.

Of special clinical relevance are usage tests. Poor sealing properties, measured in animal experimentation (Key literature 12.3), are in line with the poor clinical

---

Key literature 12.3

In a study in dogs by Harrison and Johnson (34), root canals were obturated with a ZnOE material (IRM) or amalgam and then the root ends were resected. Orthograde fillings with gutta-percha/ZnOE sealer were used as controls. The test materials evoked no inhibition of osseous wound healing and cementum was present in contact with all materials after a 45-day observation period. However, Chong *et al.* (18) modified this test method: after artificial infection of root canals *before* the root resection and application of the root-end filling, amalgam caused persistent inflammation in the apical area at up to 8 weeks. Better results were observed with a ZnOE material and a light-cured GIC. It was concluded that the poor sealing properties of amalgam were the main reasons for the negative test result and that in a corresponding clinical situation a ZnOE material or a light-cured GIC is recommended.

long-term prognosis of amalgam root-end fillings, as was reported by some authors (29).

A polyketone sealer with and without tricalcium phosphate (TCP) showed a preosteoid/cementoid-like matrix in direct and intimate approximation to the root-end filling material in dogs after 60 days (96). A dentin-bonded resin composite (BIS-GMA/TEGDMA mixture) used in animals for root-end fillings without intentionally infected canals evoked cementum coverage, indicating optimal tissue tolerance. However, if the root canal was infected, less favorable results were observed. The resin material hardly entered the apical cavity and thus provided only a superficial seal (2).

Root-end fillings with MTA in animal teeth showed cementum coverage over the filling, whereas amalgam produced inflammation and no cementum layer on the material. MTA stimulates cytokine release from bone cells with the potential of actively promoting hard-tissue formation (90).

Clinical data indicated inferior clinical success rates when amalgam was used compared with other materials (29). Further disadvantages are the potential of staining of the mucosa, scattering of particles during placement and corrosion. For modified ZnOE cements, good clinical results are reported over a period of up to 14 years (20). For composite resins only a few clinical studies have been published, but a clinical success rate of about 90% was reported recently (64).

Handling properties

Owing to the special surgical environment mentioned above, good handling properties are important. Whereas ZnOE, MTA (and amalgam) harden in a moist environment, conventional GIC is susceptible to moisture and desiccation. Light-cured products may have certain advantages in this respect because of fast setting. It had been reported also that it is not easy to apply dentin bonding agents and a resin devoid of voids into a rather small apical cavity. Root-end filling materials should have a radiopacity greater than that of root canal filling materials.

Mandibular nerve injuries

These injuries after root canal filling therapy occur rather seldom in daily practice but they are dramatic in each case. At least four different pathogenic mechanisms have been proposed:

- Instrumentation beyond the apex and mechanical severance.
- Combined effect of regional analgesia and mechanical nerve damage.

- Degeneration of the nerve due to the mechanical compression caused by filling the materials in the nerve canal.
- Toxicity/neurotoxicity of the root canal filling material.

Irreversible sensory nerve damage may involve frequent paresthesia, which constitutes altered sensation of pain, touch or temperature. Symptoms are the sensation of warmth, cold, burning, aching, prickling, tingling, pins and needles, numbness, itching and formication (feels as if ants are crawling on the skin) (54). In the endodontic literature most cases have resulted from overfill of paraformaldehyde-containing sealers in the vicinity of the inferior alveolar nerves. Long-term paresthesia of up to 13 years has been described. A survey of the literature in 1988 (14) showed that more than 40 cases of root canal cements associated with paresthesia of the inferior alveolar nerve had been reported in the previous two decades. Most of these patients had been treated with materials that contained (para)formaldehyde. The reaction of ZnOE sealers with the addition of formaldehyde was irreversible unless surgical treatment was performed. This is in line with data from *in vitro* experiments on different nerve tissues described above, which have shown an irreversible effect on nerve conductance from formaldehyde-releasing root canal sealers. Thus, there are indications that the material and especially the release of formaldehyde may play a major role in these injuries (14).

There are also case reports on paresthesia after overfill of AH26, which was attributed to the short-term release of formaldehyde during setting. A 4-month paresthesia was reported to be eugenol induced. Another case caused by ZnOE was reversible. Six cases of paresthesia after overfill of gutta-percha/chloroperca were reported and the symptoms resolved after a maximum of 3 months (54).

Single cases were reported for other root canal filling materials/techniques. Melted gutta-percha (thermomechanical compaction used with a calcium hydroxide-based sealer) was extruded into the mandibular canal causing severe nerve injury with persistent local paresthesia (numbness and intermittent bouts of pins and needles in the lip and chin). A few days later the area of paresthesia was replaced by anesthesia. After surgical removal from the periapical area and from the nerve canal, anesthesia was replaced by paresthesia. The authors assume that the reason for this adverse reaction was the elevated temperature by which the gutta-percha was extruded out of the root canal (27).

It can be concluded that with most of the currently used root canal filling materials, detrimental effects on local nerve tissues were observed when the root canals were dramatically overfilled and the local nerve fibers were involved. However, most cases are described in connection with formaldehyde-releasing sealers with long-lasting/irreversible damage to the nerve tissues. The clinician should be aware of this situation and be familiar with preventive measures when choosing the root canal filling material. These are:

- *Appropriate treatment technique*: to reduce the risk that the filling material is displaced beyond the apex and into the vicinity of the nerve.
- *Appropriate material selection*: use root canal filling materials with the fewest possible (neuro)toxic effects.

References

1. Abdulkader A, Duguid R, Saunders EM. The antimicrobial activity of endodontic sealers to anaerobic bacteria. *Int. Endod. J.* 1996; 29: 280–3.
2. Andreasen JO, Munksgaard EC, Fredebo L, Rud J. Periodontal tissue regeneration including cementogenesis adjacent to dentin-bonded retrograde composite fillings in humans. *J. Endod.* 1993; 19: 151–3.
3. Arenholt-Bindslev D, Hørsted-Bindslev P. A simple model for evaluating relative toxicity of root filling materials in cultures of human oral fibroblasts. *Endod. Dent. Traumatol.* 1989; 5: 219–26.
4. Barnett F, Trope M, Rooney J, Tronstad L. *In vivo* sealing ability of calcium hydroxide-containing root canal sealers. *Endod. Dent. Traumatol.* 1989; 5: 23–6.
5. Barthel CR, Moshonov J, Shuping G, Ørstavik D. Bacterial leakage versus dye leakage in obturated root canals. *Int. Endod. J.* 1999; 32: 370–5.
6. Beck-Mannagetta J. Zinc and aspergillus. *Oral Surg. Oral Med. Oral Pathol. Oral Radiol. Endod.* 1996; 81: 138–40.
7. Bergmanns L, Moisiadis P, De Munck J, Van Meerbeek B, Lambrechts P. Effect of polymerization shrinkage on the sealing capacity of resin fillers for endodontic use. *J Adhes. Dent.* 2005; 7: 321–9.
8. Boiesen J, Brodin P. Neurotoxic effect of two root canal sealers with calcium hydroxide on rat phrenic nerve *in vitro. Endod. Dent. Traumatol.* 1991; 7: 242–5.
9. Bouillaguet S, Shwa L, Barthelemy J, Krejci I, Wataha JD. Long term sealing ability of pulp canal sealer, AH-Plus, GuttaFlow and Epiphany. *Int. Endod. J.* 2008; 41: 219–26.
10. Bouillaguet S, Wataha JC, Tay FR, Brackett MG, Lockwood PE. Initial *in vitro* biological response to contemporary endodontic sealers. *J. Endod.* 2006; 32: 989–92.
11. Boxer MB, Grammer LC, Orfan N. Gutta-percha allergy in a health care worker with latex allergy. *J. Allergy Clin. Immunol.* 1994; 93: 943–4.
12. Brackett MG, Martin R, Sword J, Oxford C, Rueggeberg FA, Tay FR, Pashley DH. Comparison of seal after obturation techniques using a polydimethylsiloxane-based root canal sealer. *J. Endod.* 2006; 32: 1188–90.
13. Bratel J, Jontell M, Dahlgren U, Bergenholtz G. Effects of root canal sealers on immunocompetent cells *in vitro* and *in vivo. Int. Endod. J.* 1998; 31: 178–88.
14. Brodin P. Neurotoxic and analgesic effects of root canal cements and pulp-protecting dental materials. *Endod. Dent. Traumatol.* 1988; 4: 1–11.
15. Brodin P, Roed A, Aars H, Ørstavik D. Neurotoxic effects of root canal filling materials on rat phrenic nerve *in vitro. J. Dent. Res.* 1982; 61: 1020–3.
16. Camilleri J, Pitt Ford TR. Mineral trioxide aggregate: a review of the constituents and the biological properties of the material. *Int. Endod. J.* 2006; 39: 747–54.
17. Chong BS, Pitt Ford TR, Hudson MB. A prospective clinical study of mineral trioxide aggregate and IRM when used as root-end filling materials in endodontic surgery. *Int. Endod. J.* 2003; 36: 520–6.
18. Chong BS, Pitt Ford TR, Kariyawasam SP. Tissue response to potential root-end filling materials in infected root canals. *Int. Endod. J.* 1997; 30: 102–14.
19. Christiansen R, Kirkevang L-L, Hørsted-Bindslev P, Wenzel A. Randomized clinical trial of root-end resection followed by root end filling with mineral trioxide aggregate or smoothing of the orthograde gutta-percha root filling – 1-year follow up. *Int. Endod. J.* 2009; 42: 105–14.
20. Dorn SO, Gartner AH. Retrograde filling materials: a retrospective success–failure study of amalgam, EBA, and IRM. *J. Endod.* 1990; 16: 391–3.
21. El-Sayed F, Seite-Bellezza D, Sans B, Bayle-Lebey P, Marguery MC, Bazex J. Contact urticaria from formaldehyde in a root canal dental paste. *Contact Dermatitis* 1995; 33: 353.
22. Eldeniz AU, Mustafa K, Ørstavik D, Dahl JE. Cytotoxicity of new resin-, calcium hydroxide- and silicone-based root canal sealers on fibroblasts derived from human gingival and L929 cell lines. *Int. Endod. J.* 2007; 40: 329–37.
23. Eriksson AR, Albrektson T. Temperature threshold levels for heat-induced bone tissue injury: a vital-microscopic study in the rabbit. *J. Prosthet. Dent.* 1983; 50: 101–7.
24. Ersev H, Schmalz G, Bayirli G, Schweikl H. Cytotoxic and mutagenic potencies of various root canal filling materials in eukaryotic and prokaryotic cells *in vitro. J. Endod.* 1999; 25: 359–63.
25. Esberard RM, Carnes DL Jr, del Rio CE. Changes in pH at the dentin surface in roots obturated with calcium hydroxide pastes. *J. Endod.* 1996; 22: 402–5.
26. European Society of Endodontology. Quality guidelines for endodontic treatment: consensus report of the European Society of Endodontology. *Int. Endod. J.* 2006; 39: 921–30.
27. Fanibunda K, Whitworth J, Steele JG. The management of thermomechanically compacted gutta percha extrusion in the inferior dental canal. *Br. Dent. J.* 1998; 184: 330–2.
28. Fischer EJ, Arens DE, Miller CH. Bacterial leakage of mineral trioxide aggregate as compared with zinc-free amalgam, intermediate restorative material, and Super-EBA as a root-end filling material. *J. Endod.* 1998; 24: 176–9.
29. Frank AL, Glick DH, Patterson SS, Weine FS. Long-term evaluation of surgically placed amalgam fillings. *J. Endod.* 1992; 18: 391–8.
30. Gernhardt CR, Krüger T, Bekes K, Schaller HG. Apical sealing ability of 2 epoxy resin-based sealers used with root canal obturation techniques based on warm gutta-percha compared to cold lateral condensation. *Quintessence Int.* 2007; 38: 229–34.

31. Geurtsen W, Leyhausen G. Biological aspects of root canal filling materials – histocompatibility, cytotoxicity, and mutagenicity. *Clin. Oral. Invest.* 1997; 1: 5–11.

32. Gorduysus MO, Etikan I, Gokoz A. Histopathological evaluation of the tissue reactions to Endo-Fill root canal sealant and filling material in rats. *J. Endod.* 1998; 24: 194–6.

33. Gulsahi K, Cehreli ZC, Onay EO, Tasman-Dagli F, Ungor M. Comparison of the area of resin-based sealer and voids in roots obturated with Resilon and gutta-percha. *J. Endod.* 2007; 33: 1338–41.

34. Harrison JW, Johnson SA. Excisional wound healing following the use of IRM as a root-end filling material. *J. Endod.* 1997; 23: 19–27.

35. Heil J, Reifferscheid G, Waldmann P, Leyhausen G, Geurtsen W. Genotoxicity of dental materials. *Mutat. Res.* 1996; 368: 181–94.

36. Heling I, Chandler NP. The antimicrobial effect within dentinal tubules of four root canal sealers. *J. Endod.* 1996; 22: 257–9.

37. Hensten-Pettersen A, Ørstavik D, Wennberg A. Allergenic potential of root canal sealers. *Endod. Dent. Traumatol.* 1985; 1: 61–5.

38. Hensten-Pettersen A, Jacobsen N. Perceived side effects of biomaterials in prosthetic dentistry. *J. Prosthet. Dent.* 1991; 65: 138–44.

39. Holden DT, Schwartz SA, Kirkpatrick TC, Schindler WG. Clinical outcomes of artificial root-end barriers with mineral trioxide aggregate in teeth with immature apices. *J. Endod.* 2008; 34: 812–17.

40. Hong YC, Wang JT, Hong CY, Brown WE, Chow LC. The periapical tissue reactions to a calcium phosphate cement in the teeth of monkeys. *J. Biomed. Mater. Res.* 1991; 25: 485–98.

41. Hørsted P, Söholm B. Overfölsomhed overfor rodfyldningsmaterialet AH26. *Tandlaegebladet* 1976; 80: 194–7.

42. Kielbassa AM, Uchtmann H, Wrbas KT, Bitter K. *In vitro* study assessing apical leakage of sealer-only backfills in root canals of primary teeth. *J. Dent.* 2007; 35: 607–13.

43. Kontakiotis EG, Tzanetakis GN, Loizides AL. A 12-month longitudinal *in vitro* leakage study on a new silicon-based root canal filling material (Gutta-Flow). *Oral Surg. Oral Med. Oral Pathol. Oral Radiol. Endod.* 2007; 103: 854–9.

44. Kontakiotis EG, Tzanetakis GN, Loizides AL. A comparative study of contact angles of four different root canal sealers. *J. Endod.* 2007; 33: 299–302.

45. Kontakiotis EG, Wu MK, Wesselink PR. Effect of sealer thickness on long-term sealing ability: a 2-year follow-up study. *Int. Endod. J.* 1997; 30: 307–12.

46. Langeland K, Liao K, Costa N, Pascon EA. Efficacy of Obtura and Ultrafil root filling devices. *J. Endod.* 1987; 13: 135.

47. Lin ZM, Jhugroo A, Ling JQ. An evaluation of the sealing ability of a polycaprolactone-based root canal filling material (Resilon) after retreatment. *Oral Surg. Oral Med. Oral Pathol. Oral Radiol. Endod.* 2007; 104: 846–51.

48. Lodiene G, Morisbak E, Bruzell E, Ørstavik D. Toxicity evaluation of root canal sealers *in vitro*. *Int. Endod. J.* 2008; 41: 72–7.

49. Louw NP, Pameijer CH, Norval G. Histopathological evaluation of a root canal sealer in subhuman primates. *J. Dent. Res.* 2001; 80: 654.

50. Main C, Mirzayan N, Shabahang S, Torabinejad M. Repair of root perforations using mineral trioxide aggregate: a long term study. *J. Endod.* 2004; 30: 80–3.

51. Mamootil, K, Messer, HH. Penetration of dentinal tubules by endodontic sealer cements in extracted teeth and *in vivo*. *Int. Endod. J.* 2007; 40: 873–81.

52. Merdad K, Pascon AE, Kulkarni G, Santerre P, Friedman S. Short term cytotoxicity assessment of components of epiphany resin-percha obturating system by indirect and direct contact millipore filter assays. *J. Endod.* 2007; 33: 24–7.

53. Min KS, Park HJ, Lee SK, Park SH, Hong CU, Kim HW, *et al.* Effect of mineral trioxide aggregate on dentin bridge formation and expression of dentin sialoprotein and heme oxygenase-1 in human dental pulp. *J. Endod.* 2008; 34: 666–70.

54. Morse DR. Endodontic-related inferior alveolar nerve and mental foramen paresthesia. *Compend. Contin. Educ. Dent.* 1997; 18: 963–78.

55. Nair PNR, Duncan HF, Pitt Ford TR, Luder HU. Histological, ultrastructural and quantitative investigations on the reponse of healthy human pulps to experimental capping with mineral trioxide aggregate: a randomized controlled trial. *Int. Endod. J.* 2008; 41: 128–50.

56. Ørstavik D. Antibacterial properties of root canal sealers, cements and pastes. *Int. Endod. J.* 1981; 14: 125–33.

57. Ørstavik D. Antibacterial properties of endodontic materials. *Int. Endod. J.* 1988; 21: 161–9.

58. Ørstavik D, Mjör IA. Usage test of four endodontic sealers in *Macaca fascicularis* monkeys. *Oral Surg. Oral Med. Oral Pathol.* 1992; 73: 337–44.

59. Ozok AR, van der Sluis LW, Wu MK, Wesselink PR. Sealing ability of a new polydimethylsiloxane-based root canal filling material. *J. Endod.* 2008; 34: 204–7.

60. Osorio RM, Hefti A, Vertucci FJ, Shawley AL. Cytotoxicity of endodontic materials. *J. Endod.* 1998; 24: 91–6.

61. Peng L, Ye L, Tan H, Zhou X. Evaluation of the formocresol versus mineral trioxide aggregate primary molar pulpotomy: a meta-analysis. *Oral Surg. Oral Med. Oral Pathol. Oral Radiol. Endod.* 2006; 102: 40–4.

62. Ribeiro FC, Souza-Gabriel AE, Marchsan MA, Alfredo E, Silva-Sousa YT, Sousa-Neto MD. Influence of different endodontic filling materials on root fracture susceptibility. *J. Dent.* 2008; 36: 69–73.

63. Roberts HW, Toth JM, Berzin DW, Charlton DG. Mineral trioxide aggregate material use in endodontic treatment: a review of the literature. *Dent. Mat.* 2008; 24: 149–64.

64. Rud J, Rud V, Munksgaard EC. Periapical healing of mandibular molars after root-end sealing with dentine-bonded composite. *J. Endod.* 2001; 34: 285–92.

65. Saleh IM, Ruyter IE, Haapasalo M, Ørstavik D. Survival of *Enterococcus faecalis* in infected dentinal tubules after root canal filling with different root canal sealers *in vitro*. *Int. Endod. J.* 2004; 37: 193–8.

66. Saunders EM. *In vivo* findings associated with heat generation during thermomechanical compaction of gutta-percha.

Part I. Temperature levels at the external surface of the root. *Int. Endodont. J.* 1990; 23: 263–7.

67. Saunders EM. *In vivo* findings associated with heat generation during thermomechanical compaction of gutta-percha. Part II. Histological response to temperature elevation on the external surface of the root. *Int. Endod. J.* 1990; 23: 268–74.
68. Schmalz G, Arenholt-Bindslev D. *Biocompatibility of Dental Materials.* Berlin: Springer Heidelberg, 2009.
69. Schmalz G. *Die Gewebeverträglichkeit zahnärztlicher Materialien – Möglichkeiten einer standardisierten Prüfung in der Zellkultur.* Stuttgart: Georg Thieme Verlag, 1981.
70. Schmalz G. Use of cell cultures for toxicity testing of dental materials – advantages and limitations. *J. Dent.* 1994; 22 (Suppl. 2): S6–11.
71. Schmalz G. Biological evaluation of medical devices: a review of EU regulations, with emphasis on *in vitro* screening for biocompatibility. *ATLA* 1995; 23: 469–73.
72. Schwartz RS. Adhesive dentistry and endodontics. Part 2: Bonding in the root canal system – the promise and the problems: a review. *J. Endod.* 2006; 32: 1126–34.
73. Schweikl H, Schmalz G. Evaluation of the mutagenic potential of root canal sealers using the salmonella/microsome assay. *J. Mater. Sci. Mater. Med.* 1991; 2: 181–5.
74. Schweikl H, Schmalz G, Federlin M. Mutagenicity of the root canal sealer AHPlus in the Ames test. *Clin. Oral. Invest.* 1998; 2: 125–9.
75. Schweikl H, Schmalz G, Stimmelmayr H, Bey B. Mutagenicity of AH26 in an *in vitro* mammalian cell mutation assay. *J. Endod.* 1995; 21: 407–10.
76. Shah PM, Chong BS, Sidhu SK, Ford TR. Radiopacity of potential root-end filling materials. *Oral Surg. Oral Med. Oral Pathol. Oral Radiol. Endod.* 1996; 81: 476–9.
77. Shipper G, Ørstavik D, Teixeira FB, Trope M. An evaluation of microbial leakage in roots filled with a thermoplastic synthetic polymer-based root canal filling material (Resilon). *J. Endod.* 2004; 30: 342–7.
78. Sipert CR, Hussne RP, Nishiyama CK, Torres SA. *In vitro* antimicrobial activity of Fill Canal, Sealapex, mineral trioxide aggregate, Portland cement and EndoRez. *Int. Endod. J.* 2005; 38: 539–43.
79. Sjögren U, Hägglund B, Sundqvist G, Wing K. Factors affecting the long-term results of endodontic treatment. *J. Endod.* 1990; 16: 498–504.
80. Sjögren U, Figdor D, Persson S, Sundqvist G. Influence of infection at the time of root filling on the outcome of endodontic treatment of teeth with apical periodontitis. *Int. Endod. J.* 1997; 30: 297–306.
81. Sonat B, Dalat D, Günhan O. Periapical tissue reaction to root fillings with Sealapex. *Int. Endod. J.* 1990; 23: 46–52.
82. Spångberg LS, Barbosa SV, Lavigne GD. AH26 release formaldehyde. *J. Endod.* 1993; 19: 596–8.
83. Stefopoulos S, Tsatsas DV, Kerezoudis NP, Eliades G. Comparative *in vitro* study of the sealing efficiency of white vs grey ProRoot mineral trioxide aggregate formulas as apical barriers. *Dent. Traumatol.* 2008; 24: 207–13.

84. Tay FR, Hiraishi N, Pashley DH, Loushine RJ, Weller RN, Gillespie WT, Doyle MD. Bondability of Resilon to a methacrylate-based root canal sealer. *J. Endod.* 2006; 32: 133–7.
85. Tay FR, Loushine RJ, Lambrechts P, Weller RN, Pashley DH. Geometric factors affecting dentin bonding in root canals: a theoretical modeling approach. *J. Endod.* 2006; 32: 85–6.
86. Tay FR, Pashley DH, Yiu CK, Yau JY, Yiu-fai M, Loushine RJ, *et al.* Susceptibility of a polycaprolactone-based root canal filling material to degradation. II. Gravimetric evaluation of enzymatic hydrolysis. *J. Endod.* 2005; 31: 737–41.
87. Teixeira FB, Teixeira EC, Thompson JY, Trope M. Fracture resistance of roots endodontically treated with a new resin filling material. *J. Am. Dent. Assoc.* 2004; 135: 868.
88. Torabinejad M, Watson TF, Pitt Ford TR. Sealing ability of mineral trioxide aggregate when used as a root end filling material. *J. Endod.* 1993; 19: 591–5.
89. Torabinejad M, Hong CU, McDonald MS, Pitt Ford TR. Physical and chemical properties of a new root-end filling material. *J. Endod.* 1995; 21: 349–53.
90. Torabinejad M, Pitt Ford TR, McKendry DJ, Abedi HR, Miller DA, Kariyawasam SP. Histologic assessment of mineral trioxide aggregate as a root-end filling in monkeys. *J. Endod.* 1997; 23: 225–8.
91. Versiani MA, Carvalho JR, Padilha MI, Lacey S, Pascon EA, Sousa-Neto MD. A comparative study of physicochemical properties of AH Plus and Epiphany root canal sealants. *Int. Endod. J.* 2006; 39: 464–71.
92. Wang CS, Debelian GJ, Teixeira FB. Effect of intracanal medicament on the sealing ability of root canals filled with Resilon. *J. Endod.* 2006; 32: 532–6.
93. Weiger R, Manncke B, Löst C. Antibakterielle Wirkung von Guttaperchastiften auf verschiedene, endodontopathogene Mikroorganismen. *Dtsch. Zahnärztl. Z.* 1993; 48: 658–60.
94. Weller RN, Koch KA. *In vitro* radicular temperatures produced by injectable thermoplasticized gutta-percha. *Int. Endod. J.* 1995; 28: 86–90.
95. Wennberg A, Ørstavik D. Adhesion of root canal sealers to bovine dentine and gutta-percha. *Int. Endod. J.* 1990; 23: 13–19.
96. Williams SS, Gutmann JL. Periradicular healing in response to diaket root-end filling material with and without tricalcium phosphate. *Int. Endod. J.* 1996; 29: 84–92.
97. Wu MK, Wesselink PR. Endodontic leakage studies reconsidered: Part I. Methodology, application, and relevancy. *Int. Endod. J.* 1993; 26: 37–43.
98. Wu MK, Wesselink PR, Boersma J. A 1-year follow-up study on leakage of four root canal sealers at different thicknesses. *Int. Endod. J.* 1995; 28: 185–9.
99. Zmener O, Pameijer CH. Clinical and radiographical evaluation of resin-based root canal sealer: a 5-year follow-up. *J. Endod.* 2007; 33: 676–9.
100. Zmener O, Banegas G, Pameijer CH. Bone tissue response to a methacrylate-based endodontic sealer: a histological and histometric study. *J. Endod.* 2005; 31: 457–9.

Chapter 13
Root filling techniques

Paul Wesselink

Introduction

Filling the instrumented root canal is the final step in the completion of an endodontic treatment. Regardless of whether the treatment was undertaken to remove a vital pulp (pulpectomy), a necrotic and/or infected pulp (root canal therapy) or a previous root canal filling (retreatment), the prime objective of the root filling is to prevent microbial organisms from entering, growing and multiplying in the empty space that resulted from the instrumentation procedure (Fig. 13.1). Root filling also serves as a wound dressing against which healthy periapical tissue can be laid down.

Specific objectives

After pulpectomy a wound surface remains that will not heal with epithelium as wounds do in other body sites. Such a wound surface is therefore constantly vulnerable to infection. Wound infection may be induced inadvertently in conjunction with the treatment procedure, e.g. from improper rubber dam isolation or by bringing chips of carious dentin to the apical region of the root canal. It may also develop from entry of bacterial organisms from the oral environment after completion of the filling. The latter is known as *coronal leakage* and occurs along incompletely sealed canal spaces. Therefore, a hermetic and permanent seal of the wound surface is essential to allow proper healing after pulpectomy and to prevent bacterial elements from later accessing the periapical tissue if, for any reason, the coronal restoration breaks down. Core

concept 13.1 summarizes the overall functions of a root filling.

In the treatment of a tooth with an infected, non-vital pulp (i.e. root canal therapy), instrumentation and irrigation with a disinfecting solution will not always eliminate the microbial organisms. If such a root canal is left unfilled or improperly filled, residual organisms may continue to grow and multiply (Chapter 9). It needs to be recognized that microbial organisms require both space and nutrition for growth, therefore in root canal therapy the root filling has two additional objectives:

1. To prevent nutritional elements from accessing the pulpal space along any entrance to the root canal, including apical foramina, accessory canals and the oral access cavity.
2. To eliminate space for further growth of microorganisms that may have survived the biomechanical preparation.

Usually it is sufficient to block the portal of exit to the periapical tissue. However, lateral or accessory canals may also allow egress of bacterial elements to the periodontium. Therefore it is essential that the entire length of the instrumented canal becomes completely filled. If properly done this means that all portals of exit to the periodontal tissue will be sealed. The quality of root fillings in general is assessed from this aspect (see further below).

Selecting a root canal filling material

A variety of factors determines the choice of a root canal filling material. Although a primary requirement is to allow a complete fill of the instrumented root canal(s), it should also be biologically compatible because it will often be in direct contact with vital tissue. In other words, beside a variety of technical and physical demands, a root filling material should also satisfy the requirements that are requested from implant materials (Chapter 12).

The most critical technical and physical requirements of a root filling material are:

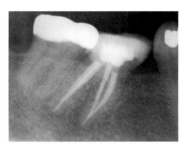

Fig. 13.1 Radiograph depicting optimal root canal fillings of a lower molar. (Courtesy of Dr A. Braun.)

Core concept 13.1

The overall function of a root filling is to occupy the instrumented root canal space to allow proper healing of the periapical tissue. Specifically it attempts:

(1) To prevent leakage of bacterial organisms, bacterial elements and nutritional elements from the oral environment to the root canal (coronal leakage).

(2) To restrain growth of any surviving bacteria in dentinal tubules and uninstrumented parts of the root canal space.
(3) To prevent release of bacterial elements in the other direction, i.e. from the root canal to the apical environment (apical leakage).
(4) To prevent leakage of nutritional elements from the periapical tissue to the canal space.

1. Stops coronal leakage
2. Entombs surviving bacteria
3. Stops influx of periapical tissue fluid and release of bacterial elements

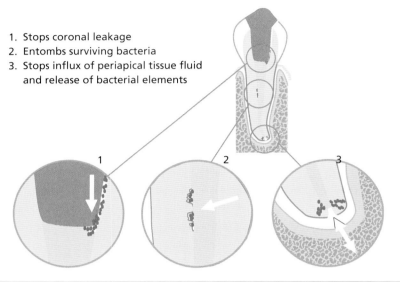

- *Ability to adapt to the shape of the canal.* After cleaning and shaping, root canals may still harbor various irregularities that can allow space for bacterial growth. It has been shown that in many cases it is impossible to create a round and smooth root canal without removing so much of the inner root canal wall that the root structure is critically weakened. Therefore, to provide a seal, a root canal filling material should be able to fill these irregularities.
- *Length control.* A root canal filling material should allow a technique that keeps the entire material within the canal space. Extrusion of material to the periapical tissue compartment is undesirable because it may cause both cytotoxic and neurotoxic effects (7, 29, 40). It may also produce a foreign body reaction (40). Furthermore, results of clinical outcome studies indicate that extrusion and overextension of root filling material negatively influence the healing of the periapical tissue (12, 32).
- *Safety.* The material and the technique used for its application should be safe for the patient. The demand for biocompatibility has already been stated (see Chapter 12), but the technique should also not pose risks for root fracture, require overzealous instrumentation or cause damage to the periodontal ligament by, for example, detrimental temperature increases or extrusion of material.

- *Insoluble.* Because of the risk for coronal leakage and the fact that root filling material may be exposed to percolation of tissue fluid at the apical foramen, it is important that it is not affected by moisture. Therefore, after setting, a root filling material should be insoluble in both saliva and tissue fluid.
- *Removable.* A root filling may not be performed perfectly at the first attempt or may turn out to be defective at a follow-up. The outcome of a treatment may also be such that one suspects ongoing root canal infection. In these instances, retreatment and refilling of the root canal may be necessary (Chapter 20). The material used should, therefore, be removable by simple means without involving the risk of damaging the root structure or the apical tissue.
- *Radiopaque.* In order to judge whether the root canal has been adequately filled, a most important requirement is that the root filling is discernible in a radiograph, i.e. it should be radiopaque.

Hardly any root filling material so far developed has been able to satisfy all these demands. Yet a formulation based on gutta-percha as one of the principal ingredients has stood the test of time and has been widely used since the end of the 19th century. Although new core materials are under exploration it is still the material of choice in most countries. By pressure or by softening with heat or organic solvent, gutta-percha is suitable for application in instrumented root canals using a variety of techniques (see further below). Combined with a sealing agent, the material can be adapted to the shape of root canals and serve as a reasonably insoluble and non-porous core of filling. At the same time, it is fairly easy to remove if necessary. Gutta-percha-based formulations also satisfy

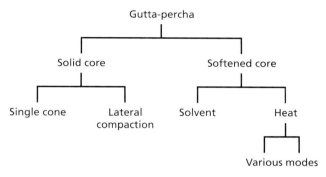

Fig. 13.2   Outline of techniques to fill root canals with gutta-percha.

biological demands (Chapter 12). Because of the universal use of gutta-percha in endodontics, techniques that are based on this material will mainly be considered in this chapter.

Root filling techniques for gutta-percha

There are various methods for delivering and packing gutta-percha in root canals and they can be divided into solid core and softened core techniques (Fig. 13.2). Solid core techniques imply that unsoftened gutta-percha cones are fitted to the instrumented canal(s) (Fig. 13.3a) and cemented to the canal walls with a root canal sealer. Techniques exist whereby either a single cone or multiple cones are placed in the root canal space (Fig. 13.4). In softened core techniques gutta-percha is plasticized either prior to or after insertion in the root canal by solvent or heat. These techniques also often make use of a sealing agent to supplement the filling.

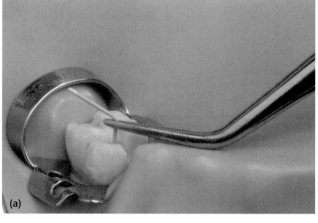
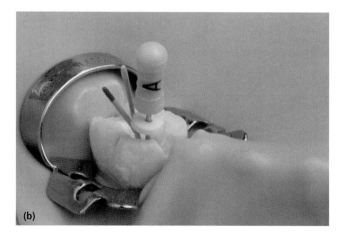
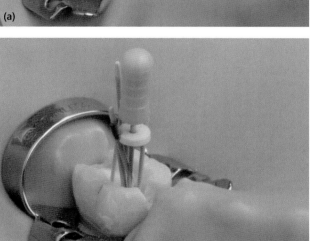
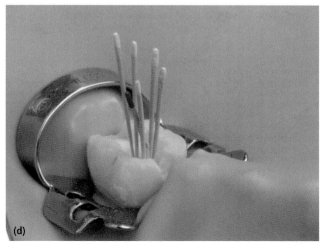

Fig. 13.3   Outline of the lateral compaction technique. (a) Master cone fit. (b) Lateral compaction with spreader following addition of one accessory cone. (c) Continued lateral compaction. (d) Further addition of accessory cones. Root filling is complete when it is not possible to place another accessory cone further than 2 mm into the root canal.

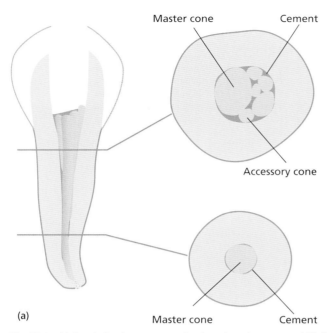

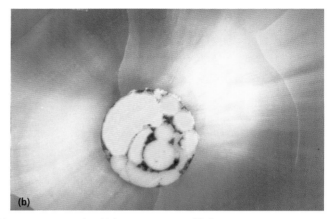

Fig. 13.4 (a) Sketch showing a cross-sectional cut through a root canal filled with a master cone and multiple accessory cones. (b) The cross-sectional cut shows a true filling where the sealer (black material) unites the cones and fills out space laterally to the root canal wall.

Gutta-percha cones

For solid core techniques, gutta-percha cones of different lengths, sizes and shapes may be obtained. In general, cones are round and have a tapered form so they gradually increase in size from the tip. So-called "standardized" cones were designed to match the size and taper of the root canal instruments used to shape the canal at its apical end. In early days these cones had a rather small taper of 2%, corresponding to the ISO standard of root canal instruments. Nowadays there are cones standardized to fit canals prepared with differently tapered instruments. Hence, there are cones with 4% and 6% tapers. "Conventional" cones are also available; these are not standardized and are classified as fine, medium and large.

Root canal sealers

Unsoftened gutta-percha does not adhere to dentin and softened gutta-percha may shrink after cooling as a result of being heated or from evaporation of the solvent used, thus leaving gaps between the material and the root canal walls (50). Naturally such defects may allow either coronal or apical leakage, or both, to cause or maintain apical periodontitis. It is, therefore, considered necessary to use a cement or sealer that forms a tight connection between the gutta-percha and the root dentin. In general, it is believed that this layer should be as thin as possible because, upon setting, sealers may shrink and dissolve in a moist environment (20).

This has led to the development of gutta-percha techniques that aim to create a filling consisting of a well-adapted mass of gutta-percha with a thin layer of root canal sealer between the gutta-percha and the root dentin. In this respect, consideration is similar to that with cast restorations, where well-fitting margins are created to leave as little cement as possible between the metal and the tooth structure.

As a general trait, but to a varying extent, root canal sealers in the initial setting phase are cytotoxic and bacteriotoxic. Although most sealers become substantially less bioactive thereafter (29, 45), as little contact as possible with the apical pulp tissue or periapical tissue is desirable. In particular overfilling of sealer material should be avoided. There are several reasons for this view:

1. As well as being initially cytotoxic, all root canal sealers may potentially elicit allergic reactions (15). Although animal and clinical observations indicate that sensitization via the root canal occurs rarely, it is occasionally reported (13, 19, 21).
2. Root canal cements in contact with nerve tissue, e.g. when inadvertently extruded into the mandibular canal, may cause anesthesia and long-lasting paresthesia as well as severe and long-lasting pain (7, 27, 41).
3. Although sealer material may be dissolved and resorbed over time (25), components of sealer material may be found in the periapical tissue many years after filling, where it causes ongoing phagocytic reac-

tions (32). Root filling material also may be found in several peripheral organs (11).

Currently used root canal sealers may be divided into four groups:

- zinc oxide–eugenol based;
- resin based;
- dentin-adhesive materials;
- materials to which medicaments have been added.

The benefits, uses and problems of each are discussed below and summarized in Core concept 13.2. For a more detailed description of these materials, the reader is referred to Chapter 12.

Zinc oxide–eugenol-based sealer

Once zinc oxide–eugenol materials set, they form a weak porous product that is decomposed in tissue fluids over time (25, 44, 46). Nonetheless, these materials are regarded to be clinically satisfactory (28). Practically all zinc

---

Core concept 13.2   Properties of different sealers

Zinc oxide–eugenol-based sealers
- Reasonable seal
- Dissolve in fluids
- Long-lasting cytotoxicity
- Sensibilization

Resin-based sealers
- Good seal
- Initial cytoxicity
- Once set, biocompatible
- Allergenic

Gutta-percha-based sealers
- Moderate seal
- Initial cytotoxicity
- Shrinkage
- Plasticize gutta-percha

Dentin-adhesive sealers
- Good seal
- Set very quickly
- Good biocompatibility
- Difficult to remove

Formaldehyde-containing sealers
- Zinc oxide–eugenol based
- Severe long-lasting cytotoxicity
- Sensibilization

Calcium hydroxide-containing sealers
- Release calcium hydroxide, which may result in disintegration
- Once set and integrity is maintained, no calcium hydroxide leaches out and no effect can be expected
- Initial antibacterial effect
- Risk of dissolution over time

---

oxide–eugenol sealers are cytotoxic and the response may be more long lasting compared to that of most other sealers owing to release of free eugenol upon gradual hydrolysis (29). Potential for sensitization exists (13, 15). Zinc oxide–eugenol cements are commercially available as Hermetic, Tubliseal, Procosol, Roth's sealer and Kerr pulp canal sealers, and form the basis of many medicament-containing sealers.

Resin-based sealers

Well-known resin-based materials are AH26, AHPlus and Diaket. Both AH26 and AHPlus consist of an epoxy resin. They are thin fluid materials that set slowly. The long setting time may sometimes be an advantage because it gives sufficient time to correct deficiencies in the root canal filling that were noticed at the postoperative radiographic check. Diaket is a mixture of vinylpolymerizates that sets rapidly within minutes, which makes it less suitable in techniques that require some working time.

These resin-based sealers elicit an initial severe inflammatory reaction that subsides in subsequent weeks and thereafter becomes well tolerated by the periapical tissues (28, 29). However, the sealer AH26 has been shown to have both a strong allergenic and a mutagenic potential (15, 26) and contact allergy to this material has been reported (16).

Sealer based on silicon, e.g. RSA Roekoseal, GuttaFlow, is a recent development. The advantage of this material is volume stability and biocompatibility. One product, RSA Roekoseal, a polydimethylsiloxane, appeared to seal straight canals well *in vitro* with a single gutta-percha cone even after a long-term exposure to water (51). Another product, GuttaFlow, has the same composition as RoekoSeal except for additions of gutta-percha (<30 μm) and nanosilver particles for radiographic contrast. It has been introduced to the market as the first non-heated, flowable gutta-percha that, unlike heated gutta-percha, does not shrink. A recent evaluation of its sealing capacity seemed not very favorable (30) but its toxicity appeared low (6).

Dentin-adhesive materials

Adhesive cements have been tested as root canal filling material in an attempt to improve the sealing quality of sealers. Cyanoacrylate, calcium phosphate, polycarboxylate and glass ionomer cements have all been explored. Of these, only glass ionomer cements have been widely marketed (Ketac-Endo, Endion). Although appearing favorable in biocompatibility tests and in long-term clinical follow-up studies, the materials have never gained great popularity. Likely reasons are short setting time (20) and difficulty of removal for retreatment.

Recently, new dentin-adhesive root canal cements have been introduced to enhance the bond between the core material of gutta-percha and the root canal walls. Examples are Endo-Rez and Epiphany, which are resin-based materials with hydrophilic properties. Epiphany may also be combined with a synthetic polymer-based root canal filling material (Resilon) in the Epiphany–Resilon system. Resilon mainly consists of polymers of polyesters (polycaprolacton) and bioactive glass, giving this material physical properties similar to those of gutta-percha. This means that it can be used cold or plasticized by heat. While a promising development, research documentation has so far primarily been based on *in vitro* and animal studies observing sealing capability (1, 37–39) and biocompatibility aspects (5, 6). Independent clinical research has yet to show superiority of these materials to traditional products with gutta-percha as the core material.

Materials to which medicaments have been added

These materials may be divided into two groups:

1. Materials based on the inclusion of strong disinfectants and/or antiphlogistic agents to suppress possible postoperative pain.
2. Materials based on calcium hydroxide.

In the first group the added disinfectant is paraformaldehyde and the anti-inflammatory component is often a corticosteroid. Examples of brands in this category of sealers are Endomethasone, N2, Spad and Rocanal. If deposited in the periapical tissue, these filling materials may give rise to severe inflammatory reactions and thus do not satisfy the requirement for biocompatibility (24, 31). Paraformaldehyde also elicits allergic reactions (10) and, as mentioned above, strong neurotoxic effects, if extruded near the mandibular nerve.

Calcium hydroxide is known to incite the formation of hard tissue at the foramen and therefore has been incorporated as an active component in several root canal sealers. The most popular commercial calcium-hydroxide-based cements are calciobiotic root canal sealer (CRCS, a zinc oxide–eugenol-based sealer), Sealapex (a polymeric resin-based sealer) and Apexit (a colophonium-based salicylate resin).

In vitro leakage studies have shown their sealing ability to be similar to that of zinc oxide–eugenol cements or slightly less favorable in the long run (20). The latter observation supports the concern that during long-term exposure to tissue fluid, calcium hydroxide may leach out of the cement, which may result in a loss of root filling integrity (43, 52).

Root filling techniques employing gutta-percha and sealer

Techniques for filling root canals with gutta-percha can be divided into solid core and softened core techniques (Core concept 13.3).

Core concept 13.3   Root filling techniques

Solid core techniques
- Single cone
  - Simple
  - Quick
  - Good length control
  - Round standard preparation required
- Lateral compaction
  - Good length control
  - Not one compact mass of gutta-percha
  - Time-consuming technique
  - Supposed risk of root fracture

Softened core techniques
- Warm lateral compaction
  - Moderate length control
  - Time-consuming technique
  - Heat may damage periodontium
- Warm vertical compaction
  - Poor length control
  - Sealer extrusion
  - Heat may damage periodontium

- Injection-molded gutta-percha
  - Quick technique
  - Poor length control
  - Heat may damage periodontium
- Thermomechanical compaction
  - Quick technique
  - Poor length control
  - Heat may damage periodontium
  - Instrument fracture risk
- Core carrier
  - Quick technique
  - Sealer extrusion
  - Gutta-percha may be stripped off carrier in curvature
  - Difficult to remove for retreatment
  - In combination with posts, inconvenient technique
- Chloroform–resin
  - Quick technique
  - Potential health hazard effects on dental personnel with long-term use

Solid core techniques

Whether a single cone or multiple cones (lateral compaction; Fig. 13.3a–e) are used, the most important step in solid core methods is to select and fit a cone (point) of gutta-percha to the apical 3–4 mm of the canal walls. This cone is often referred to as the *master cone*. It is critical that the fitting procedure is given considerable attention, because the cone should fit tightly to the apical portion of the root canal.

Single cone

The single-cone technique consists of matching a cone to the prepared canal. For this technique a type of canal preparation (Chapter 11) is advocated so that the size of the cone and the shape of the preparation are closely matched. When a gutta-percha cone fits the apical portion of the canal snugly, it is cemented in place with a root canal sealer.

Although the technique is simple, it has several disadvantages and cannot be considered as one that seals canals completely. After preparation, root canals are seldom round throughout their length, except possibly for the apical 2 or 3 mm. Therefore, the single-cone technique, at best, only seals this portion. *In vitro* research has shown that the single-cone technique permitted significantly more dye penetration than other techniques (2, 4) (see also Advanced concept 13.1).

Lateral compaction

In lateral compaction techniques additional secondary points are inserted and compacted laterally around the master cone to reduce the thickness of the sealer layer (Figs 13.3 and 13.4). In this technique, after cementing the master cone in position, specially designed spreaders – long, tapered, pointed instruments – are placed in the canal as far apically as possible and the master cone is laterally compacted against the wall. Next, the spreader is removed and the first auxillary point forced fully into place. The canal is filled in this way until it is not possible to place another accessory cone further than 2–3 mm into the root canal. Excess gutta-percha is then removed with a heated instrument at the canal orifice and final compaction is completed by vertical pressure with a plugger or condensor – an instrument with a flat apical tip.

The advantage of the lateral compaction technique in comparison with the single-cone technique is that it reduces the amount of sealer left in the canal. Because the relation between the butt end of the cones and the reference point of the preparation can be monitored during the filling procedure, the length control of the filling is quite good and usually no filling material is extruded beyond the foramen. The seal is good in comparison with other techniques (47).

The disadvantage of the lateral compaction method is that the root filling consists not of a homogeneous mass of root filling material but rather of a large number of individual points tightly pressed together and joined by the frictional grip of the cementing substance (Fig. 13.4b). In spite of this criticism, the technique has been used for many years with considerable success and appeared clinically to be an improvement over the single-cone technique (17).

Softened gutta-percha techniques

In an attempt to overcome the deficiencies of the cold lateral compaction technique, heat and solvents have been applied to render gutta-percha plastic. Gutta-percha is then compacted to create a homogeneous root canal filling of greater density throughout the canal than solid-core techniques can provide.

In recent years several modes of utilizing heat have been developed to soften gutta-percha. In principle, heat softening can be carried out inside the root canal or outside: the latter in the form of injecting preheated gutta-percha and the former by applying heat after insertion of unsoftened cones. These techniques will be described in some detail.

Techniques employing heat inside the canal

Warm lateral compaction: This technique evolved as a compromise between lateral compaction of cold gutta-percha and the vertical compaction of warm gutta-percha (see below). The technique is similar to lateral compaction of cold gutta-percha but here a heated spreader is initially advanced into the mass of gutta-percha cones placed in the canal (Fig. 13.5). Following its removal a cold spreader is inserted, and the space thus obtained is filled up with accessory cones. The process is repeated until the canal is completely filled. Originally, it was advised to insert a heated spreader after every accessory cone. In practice, the gutta-percha mass is usually heated after every three to four accessory cones and the compaction is continued. There are devices in which the spreader is heated electrically in a few seconds and thereafter quickly cools down again (e.g. Touch 'n Heat, System B). The advantage of warm lateral compaction is that it leads to a homogeneous mass that, *in vitro*, permitted significantly less leakage than cold lateral compaction (19). A distinct disadvantage is that the softening of the gutta-percha may lead to overextension of root filling material.

Warm vertical compaction: The objective of this technique is to obliterate the canal with a filling material softened by heat and packed with sufficient vertical pressure to

Advanced concept 13.1   Leakage tests

Randomized, controlled, clinical studies that compare the efficacy of various root filling materials and techniques as to their ability to promote a successful outcome of endodontic therapy are virtually lacking. Therefore, to select the material and method, results of *in vitro* leakage tests are often claimed. Although having limited clinical value *per se*, they contribute important information alongside biocompatibility testing (Chapter 12). A common denominator for these methods, which are described below, is that extracted teeth are employed that have been instrumented and filled with the materials and techniques to be tested.

Dye penetration
After filling, either the coronal portion or the root tip is exposed to a dye that will penetrate any voids in and around the root filling. After the dye exposure, either transverse or longitudinal sections of the roots are cut at different levels, or the teeth are demineralized and cleared with chemicals. The length of dye penetration along the root filling is a measure of leakage around the filling.

An advantage of this technique is that it is a relatively simple and inexpensive way to acquire preliminary evaluation of the sealing quality of a root filling. A disadvantage is that it does not provide a quantitative evaluation because it gives no information about the volume of leakage and the size of the void. Entrapped air in the voids, furthermore, may hinder penetration of dye into the void, giving an underestimation of its length (49). Also, the method leads to destruction of the specimens studied, making an evaluation of the same root filling at several time periods impossible. Some filling materials may discolor the dye, resulting in an underestimation of the leakage.

Microbial penetration
A coronal and an apical reservoir are attached to the tooth containing the root filling. The coronal reservoir is filled with a bacterial suspension and the apical container holds culture medium. If bacteria or microorganisms pass along the root filling, they will reach the apical reservoir and result in growth turbidity of the medium (42, 48). An advantage of this technique is that bacterial leakage is measured, which may seem more relevant biologically than small dye particle leakage. The disadvantage is that this system requires considerable attention in order to prevent contamination. It is not quantitative because even one bacterium will result in growth. Whether a bacterium passes along a filling in 10 or 20 days does not really give an indication about the difference in quality of these fillings. Only complete voids from crown to apex can be detected.

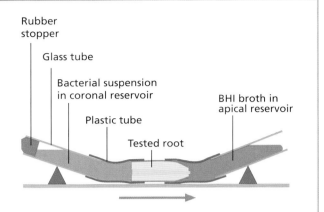

Fluid transport
Tubes filled with water are attached at both ends. At one end the water is applied under pressure. At the other end, a fine glass capillary tube is attached that contains a small air bubble to measure fluid transport, if any, as indicated by movement of the air bubble. The method is simple and inexpensive. It gives quantitative data and allows the leakage pattern to be followed over time, because the specimen is not destroyed during the evaluation process (48). The disadvantage is that it only detects voids that run from crown to apex, with dead-end tract or cul-de-sac voids not being detected.

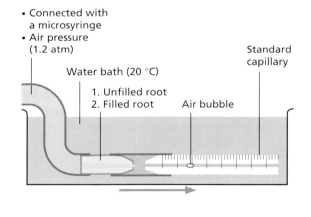

force it to flow into the root canal system, including accessory and lateral canals. A non-standardized master cone is selected and adjusted so that it is loose in the coronal and the middle third, fits to the apical terminus of the preparation and is snug in its apical extent. The canal is lightly coated with sealer. The cone is plasticized with a hot instrument. Next, the soft gutta-percha is compacted with a cold plugger in an apical and lateral direction.

Devices such as the System B Heat Source are available to simplify the down-pack of gutta-percha. This system, often described as the *continuous wave technique* (23), has the advantage that the tip of the instrument acts as a heat carrier and cold plugger at the same time. The tip of the plugger maintains a temperature of 200°C throughout the down-pack procedure, permitting a smooth continuous progression of the plugger to a depth just shy of the apical terminus. The coronal portion of the canal is then backfilled with small segments of warmed gutta-percha, or an additional cone is compacted with the System B. Backfilling is facilitated by using a gutta-percha injection technique. For this a special instrument has been designed in which the instrument to plasticize gutta-percha in the canal is combined with a gutta-percha injection syringe (e.g. BeeFill 2in1).

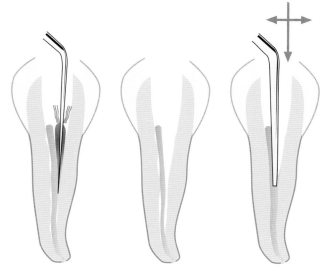

Fig. 13.5 Demonstration of gutta-percha compaction with a hot instrument.

The advantage of the warm vertical compaction technique is that it results in a homogeneous mass of gutta-percha, well-adapted to the canal wall, that requires a minimum of sealer. The disadvantage is that the technique almost consistently leads to extrusion of filling material.

Thermomechanical compaction: In this technique gutta-percha is plasticized by frictional heat and inserted by means of a compactor that forces the material apically. The compactor is an engine-operated instrument resembling a Hedström file, but with the blades directed toward the blunt-tipped end, and operates on the principle of the reverse turning screw (Fig. 13.6). The technique with which this method gives best results is different from the original one suggested, where only one cone slightly larger than the master apical file and a compactor of the same size as the master apical file were used. To improve the reliability of the technique, thermomechanical compaction has been used following lateral compaction of the apical part of the canal (hybrid technique).

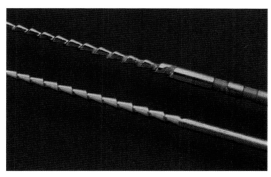

Fig. 13.6 Profiles of a compactor (top) and a Hedström file (bottom).

The advantage is that it is a very fast technique leading to a compact mass of gutta-percha that, in wide canals, resulted in less leakage than lateral compaction (18). The disadvantage is that the technique requires a lot of practice to get consistent results. In inexperienced hands, instrument fracture, extensive extrusion or poorly compacted fillings may occur. If the instrument is used by accident, when rotating clockwise it may perforate the foramen and fracture, leaving part of the instrument in the periapex.

Techniques employing heat outside the canal

Injection technique: Gutta-percha is thermoplastically molded and ejected out of a needle into the canal. The Obtura system (Fig. 13.7) uses a pressure syringe in which the gutta-percha is warmed to 200°C and expressed into the canal through a needle as fine as 25 gauge (0.5 mm diameter). The gutta-percha leaves the needle at approximately 70°C.

Pluggers are prefitted to ensure that they match the middle portion of the canal while not contacting the dentin wall. A small amount of root canal cement is wiped along the canal wall and gutta-percha is passively injected into the root canal. In 5–10 s the softened gutta-percha will fill the apical segment and begin to push the needle out of the root. During this lifting by the softened, flowing mass, the middle and the coronal portions of the canal are continuously filled until the needle reaches the canal orifice. Compaction of the material follows to adapt the gutta-percha to the canal walls.

A slightly different delivery system, BeeFill 2in1 (Fig. 13.7), has a cartridge with gutta-percha is heated in a specially designed heating device. The injection technique is used as the sole technique to fill the canal but is also frequently applied for the so-called back-pack phase of vertical compaction once the apical fill has been properly compacted.

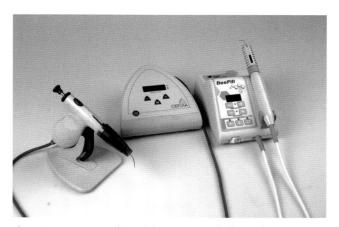

Fig. 13.7 Two commonly used devices to provide thermoplastic gutta-percha for injection: Obtura system (left) and BeeFill 2in1 (right).

Advantages of the injection technique are similar to those of warm vertical compaction. It also is useful in wide canals with an apical stop (Fig. 13.8) and in cases of internal resorption (Fig. 13.9).

The disadvantage is the difficulty of controlling the level of the root filling, with a possible under- or overfill as a result. Shrinkage of the gutta-percha during cooling may cause voids, which may make it necessary to use continuous compaction with pluggers during the cooling phase. For this reason a segmental filling technique where small portions are injected and compacted with pluggers is advocated.

Core carrier technique: A metal or resin core coated with gutta-percha is used (Thermafil, Soft core) (Fig. 13.10). After root canal preparation the correct size of the cone is selected and heated in a special oven for 45 s. After heating, the cone is pushed with pressure into the canal that is coated with sealer. Next, the coronal part is removed from the core that remains in the canal and the gutta-percha is then compacted in the canal orifice with a hand plugger.

The advantage of this technique is that, once the cone is properly heated in the oven with this system, the canal can be well obturated in all its dimensions within a short time. So far, this system has been evaluated only *in vitro* and it seems reasonable to assume that at least in straight canals the technique is about as good as lateral compaction of gutta-percha (3).

The disadvantage of the system is that, especially in curved canals, there is a risk for gutta-percha to be stripped off, thus, the core material will only become cemented apically (14). In almost all studies it appeared that, just as with most of the other warm gutta-percha techniques, sealer is extruded beyond the apical foramen (3).

Warm gutta-percha techniques – concluding remarks

Although dentin is a good insulator, concern exists as to whether the high temperatures generated with warm gutta-percha techniques are damaging to the periodontal ligament. *In vitro* the temperature rise at the root surface may be as high as 15–30°C (23). In animal experiments root resorption and ankylosis have been observed with these techniques (34).

The warm gutta-percha techniques have much to commend them and undoubtedly the resultant root filling appears to be homogeneous and, from radiographs, seems to fill the root canal space well. Yet there is no evidence to show that these techniques result in higher clinical success than, for example, cold lateral compaction. So far, *in vitro* studies have not answered the question as to which of these techniques results in the least leakage (47).

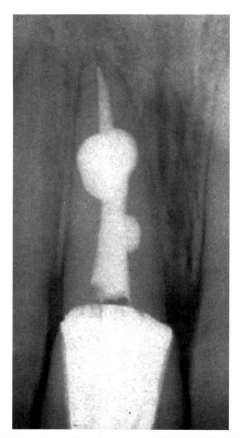

Fig. 13.9   Internal resorption of a root canal filled with injectable thermoplasticized gutta-percha.

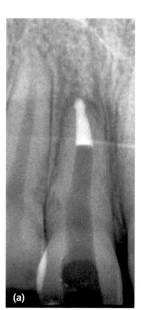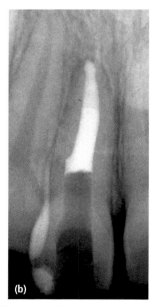

Fig. 13.8   (a) MTA filling carried out to obtain an apical stop in a traumatized incisor. (b) The remaining coronal canal space has been filled with injectable thermoplasticized gutta-percha.

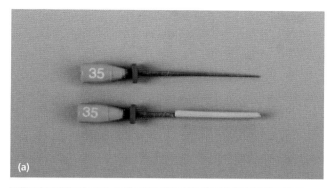

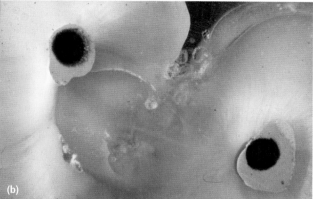

Fig. 13.10 The principle for the core carrier technique: (a) uncoated and gutta-percha-coated cores; (b) a cross-sectional cut of two filled canals with the core material in the middle.

Techniques employing solvent

Chloroform–resin technique: This is a method based on softening the master gutta-percha cone in chloroform for a few seconds prior to insertion. The master cone then should be cut approximately 2 mm short of the working length and is moved to length by a slight pumping movement. Six percent resin in chloroform is used as a sealing agent in the canal. This technique is not commonly practiced any longer, primarily owing to the alleged risk for shrinkage of the root filling after evaporation of the softening agent and the potential carcinogenecity of chloroform (Chapter 12).

Procedures prior to root canal filling

Smear layer removal

The instrumented dentin surface of the root canal interior will be covered with a debris layer that sticks to its underlying structure and consists of (pre)dentin, pulpal remnants and, in previously infected root canals, microbial elements. Its presence may jeopardize a proper seal of the root canal space.

Although it is reasonable to see the smear layer as a weak link, which should be removed to allow better adherence of the root filling to the root canal walls (35), studies are contradictory as to whether removal of the smear layer reduces leakage of fluid and bacterial elements along the root filling (33, 36, 37). To remove the smear layer, irrigation with EDTA (15%) or citric acid followed by a sodium hypochlorite flush seems to be effective (35, Chapter 9).

Drying canal

It is critical that, prior to root filling, the canal is completely evacuated of irrigation solution to allow good adaptation of the filling material. This is accomplished most easily by aspiration with a syringe, followed by drying with one or two paper points to the full working length. It may be necessary to measure up the paper points so that they are not extruded into the apical tissue, where they may cause bleeding or where fragments may be left to cause a foreign body reaction. The last point should not show signs of fluid present after its removal. It is important to note that if tips continue to be wet by bleeding or exudation, root filling should be postponed and the canal dressed temporarily (Chapter 9). To eliminate moisture 90% alcohol is often used but the efficacy of this extra procedure has not been confirmed.

Sealer placement

Because a thin layer of sealer between the gutta-percha and canal wall is preferred, it seems desirable to coat the complete canal wall with sealer prior to applying the core material. Generally, it is recommended that a file be used that is one size smaller than the last instrument used for enlargement and set just short of the working length. A small amount of sealer is gathered on the blades of the instrument, which is carried up by rapidly "twirling" the handle counter-clockwise. The procedure is repeated until the canal appears to be coated liberally with cement. The point itself is "buttered" in cement and slowly passed into the root canal, allowing time for the cement to flow back in a coronal direction. Sealers may also be placed with a lentulo needle or bidirectional spiral whereupon a dry paper point removes excess sealer from the canal. Sealer extrusion occasionally occurs with this technique.

Assessing root filling quality

After completion of the root filling procedure the quality of the fill should be checked radiographically with regard to the extent the instrumented canal was filled. An acceptable fill should reach the working length, as indicated by the trial file, and completely fill the canal space over its entire length (Core concept 13.4). Proper assessment is often difficult in an orthogonal view, therefore an angulated view is essential (Fig. 13.1), not least to be able to observe the quality of fills in two- and multirooted teeth. If the root filling does not fill the canal properly, i.e. if there is a short fill or if the fill displays obvious voids, the filling should be adjusted (see Core concept 13.4). Often, complete removal and reinsertion of a new filling is the best strategy in such cases rather than adjustment by compaction. An overextended filling normally cannot be corrected owing to the diffuse spreading of sealer material.

Filling of the pulp chamber and coronal restoration

Because of the potential presence of accessory canals near the floor of the pulp chamber of multirooted teeth and the fact that exposure of the root canal filling to saliva and bacteria seriously deteriorates the quality of the seal, application of a well-sealing, colored dentin-adhering cement is recommended (8, 22, 42). In case of retreatment, this material should have a color distinct from dentin so that the canal can be located again, but not to the extent that it discolors the crown of the tooth.

Considering the negative effect of the oral fluids on the quality of the root canal filling, it is not surprising that the quality of the coronal restoration may also influence the outcome of endodontic treatment, particularly if the root canal is not perfectly sealed. It is recommended that a good coronal restoration be placed immediately after root canal filling. Therefore, the root filling material should be removed at or just apical to the canal orifice, and in single-rooted teeth just apical to the cemento-enamel junction, because root canal cements may stain dentin to cause tooth discoloration. In cases where a cast restoration is indicated, a core material is placed. This procedure is omitted if a post and core are indicated shortly after filling the canal. In that case, space for a post may be created right after filling the root canal, leaving at least 3–4 mm of gutta-percha in the canal (9).

Core concept 13.4   Assessment of root filling quality

(1) Good-quality root filling after a pulpectomy procedure. Length of the filling is to an appropriate working length (a). The canal space is densely filled in its entirety (b).

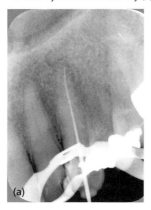 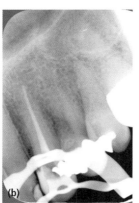

(2) Redo case because of short fill of upper canine.

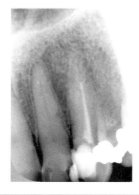

(3) Redo case because of incomplete fill of palatal root canal in upper first molar.

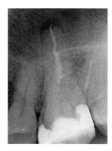

(4) Overextended root filling on both the mesial and distal canals. Canal space appears to have been filled properly. No retreatment because of the limited potential to remove the excess root filling material.

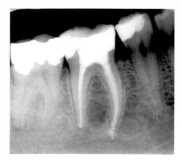

Conclusions and recommendations

Insufficient research has been carried out to determine which technique under certain given conditions (root canal anatomy, apical constriction, preparation shape) is the most appropriate (47). However, there are indications that the risk for leakage of bacteria and bacterial elements is larger when the single-cone technique is used than with the use of other techniques (2, 4). Therefore, the clinician is advised to make him or herself confident with one or two of the techniques described. It needs to be recognized that no root filling technique can compensate for an improper root canal preparation.

References

1. Adanir N, Cobankara FK, Belli S. Sealing properties of different resin-based root canal sealers. *J. Biomed. Mater. Res. B. Appl. Biomater.* 2006; 77: 1–4.
2. Beatty RG. The effect of standard or serial preparation on single cone obturations. *Int. Endod. J.* 1987; 20: 276–81.
3. Becker TA, Donnelly JC. Thermafil obturation: a literature review. *Gen. Dent.* 1997; 45: 46–50.
4. Beer VR, Gängler P, Beer M. In-vitro Untersuchungen unterscheidlicher Wurzelkanalfülltechniken und -materialien. *Zahn-. Mund-. Kieferheilk.* 1986; 74: 800–6.
5. Bouillaguet S, Wataha JC, Lockwood PE, Galgano C, Golay A, Krejci. Cytotoxicity and sealing properties of four classes of endodontic sealers evaluated by succinic dehydrogenase activity and confocal laser scanning microscopy. *Eur. J. Oral Sci.* 2004; 112: 182–7.
6. Bouillaguet S Wataha JC, Tay FR, Brackett MG, Lockwood PE. Initial in vitro biological response to contemporary endodontic sealers. *J. Endod.* 2006; 32: 989–92.
7. Brodin P, Roed A, Aars H, Ørstavik D. Neurotoxic effect of root filling materials. *J. Dent. Res.* 1982; 61: 1020–3.
   The neurotoxic effects of some commonly used root canal sealers were evaluated in in vitro experiments employing action potentials evoked by electrical stimulation of isolated rat phrenic nerves. The formaldehyde-releasing zinc oxide–eugenol-containing cements, Endomethasone and N2 Normal, completely and irreversibly inhibited conductance, while a similar cement, ProcoSol, lacking this component, caused complete but reversible inhibition.
8. Chailertvanitkul P, Saunders WP, Saunders EM, MacKenzie D. An evaluation of microbial coronal leakage in the restored pulp chamber of root canal treated multirooted teeth. *Int. Endod. J.* 1997; 30: 318–22.
9. De Cleen MJH. The relationship between the root canal filling and post space preparation. *Int. Endod. J.* 1993; 26: 53–8.
10. Fehr B, Huwyler T, Wütrich B. Formaldehyd- und Paraformaldehyd-allergie. *Schweiz. Monatsschr. Zahnmed.* 1992; 102: 94–6.
11. Feiglin B, Reade PC. The distribution of ^{14}C leucine and ^{85}Sr labeled microspheres from rat incisor root canals. *Oral. Surg.* 1979; 47: 277–81.
12. Friedman S. Treatment outcome and prognosis of endodontic therapy. In: *Essential Endodontology* (Ørstavik D, Pitt Ford TR, eds). Oxford: Blackwell Munksgaard, 2008; 408–69.
13. Grade AC. Eugenol in Wurzelkanalzementen als mögliche Ursache für eine Urtikaria. *Endodontie* 1995; 2: 121–5.
14. Gutmann JL, Saunders WP, Saunders EP, Nguyen L. An assessment of the plastic Thermafil obturation technique. Part 2. Material adaptation and sealability. *Int. Endod. J.* 1993; 26: 179–83.
15. Hensten-Pettersen A, Ørstavik D, Wennberg A. Allergenic potential of root canal sealers. *Endod. Dent. Traumatol.* 1985; 1: 61–5.
16. Hørsted P, Søholm B. Overfølsomhed overfor rodfyllnings materialet AH26. *Tandlaegebladet* 1976; 80: 194–8.
17. Kerekes K, Tronstad L. Long-term results of endodontic treatment performed with a standardized technique. *J. Endod.* 1979; 5: 83–90.
18. Kersten HW, Fransman R, Thoden van Velzen SK. Thermomechanical compaction II. A comparison with lateral condensation in curved canals. *Int. Endod. J.* 1986; 19: 134–40.
19. Kersten HW. Evaluation of three thermoplasticized guttapercha filling techniques using a leakage model *in vitro. Int. Endod. J.* 1988; 21: 353–60.
20. Kontakiotis EG, Wu M-K, Wesselink PR. Effect of sealer thickness on long-term sealing ability: a 2-year follow-up study. *Int. Endod. J.* 1997; 30: 307–12.
21. Longwill DG, Marshall FJ, Creamer RH. Reactivity of human lymphocytes to pulp antigens. *J. Endod.* 1982; 8: 27–32.
22. Madison S, Wilcox LR. An evaluation of coronal microleakage in endodontically treated teeth. Part III. *In vivo* study. *J. Endod.* 1988; 14: 455–8.
23. McCullagh JJ, Setchell DJ, Gulabivala K, Hussey DL, Biagioni P, Lamey PJ, Bailey G. A comparison of the infrared thermographic analysis of temperature rise on the root surface during the continuous wave of condensation. *Int. Endod. J.* 2000; 33: 326–32.
24. Negm MM. Biologic evaluation of SPAD II. A clinical comparison of Traitement SPAD with the conventional root canal filling technique. *Oral. Surg.* 1987; 63: 487–93.
25. Ørstavik D. Weight loss of endodontic sealers, cements and pastes in water. *Scand. J. Dent. Res.* 1983; 91: 316–19.
26. Ørstavik D, Hongslo JK. Mutagenicity of endodontic sealers. *Biomaterials* 1985; 6: 129–32.
27. Ørstavik D, Brodin P, Aas E. Paraesthesia following endodontic treatment: survey of the literature and report of a case. *Int. Endod. J.* 1983; 16: 167–72.
28. Ørstavik D, Kerekes K, Eriksen HM. Clinical performance of three endodontic sealers. *Endod. Dent. Traumatol.* 1987; 3: 178–86.
29. Ørstavik D, Mjör IA. Histopathology and x-ray microanalysis of the subcutaneous tissue response to endodontic sealers. *J. Endod.* 1988; 14: 13–23.
30. Özok AR, van der Sluis LW, Wu MK, Wesselink PR. Sealing ability of a new polydimethylsiloxane-based root canal filling material. *J Endod.* 2008; 34: 204–7.
31. Pitt Ford TR. Tissue reactions to two root canal sealers containing formaldehyde. *Oral. Surg.* 1985; 60: 661–4.
32. Ricucci D, Langeland K. Apical limit of root canal instrumentation and obturation. Part II. *Int. Endodont. J.* 1998; 31: 394–409.

33. Saleh IM, Ruyter IE, Haapasalo M, Ørstavik D. Bacterial penetration along different root canal filling materials in the presence or absence of smear layer. *Int. Endod. J.* 2008; 41: 32–40.

34. Saunders EM. *In vivo* findings associated with heat generation during thermo-mechanical compaction of gutta-percha. Part II. Histological response to temperature elevation on the external surface of the root. *Int. Endod. J.* 1990; 23: 258–64.

35. Sen BH, Türkün M, Wesselink PR. The smear layer: a phenomenon in root canal therapy. *Int. Endodont. J.* 1995; 28: 141–8.

36. Shahravan A, Haghdoost AA, Adl A, Rahimi H, Shadifar F. Effect of smear layer on sealing ability of canal obturation: a systematic review and meta-analysis. *J. Endod.* 2007; 33: 96–105.

37. Shemesh H, Wu M-K, Wesselink PR. Leakage along apical root fillings with and without smear layer using two different leakage models: a two-month longitudinal *ex vivo* study. *Int. Endod. J.* 2006; 39: 968–76.

38. Shipper G, Ørstavik D, Texeira FB, Trope M. An evaluation of microbial leakage in roots filled with a thermoplastic synthetic polymer-based root canal filling material (Resilon). *J. Endod.* 2004; 30: 342–7.

39. Shipper G, Texeira FB, Arnold RR, Trope M. Periapical inflammation after coronal microbial inoculation of dog roots filled with gutta-percha or resilon. *J. Endod.* 2005; 31: 91–6.

40. Sjögren U, Sundqvist G, Nair PR. Tissue reaction to gutta-percha particles of various sizes when implanted subcutaneously in guinea pigs. *Eur. J. Oral. Sci.* 1995; 103: 313–21.

41. Teeuwen R. Schädigung des Nervus alveolaris inferior durch überfülltes Wurzelkanalfüll-material. *Endodontie* 1999; 8: 323–36.

42. Torabinejad M, Ung B, Kettering JD. *In vitro* bacterial penetration of coronally unsealed endodontically treated teeth. *J. Endod.* 1990; 16: 566–9.

43. Tronstad L, Barnett F, Flax M. Solubility and biocompatibility of calcium hydroxide-containing root canal sealers. *Endod. Dent. Traumatol.* 1998; 4: 152–9.

44. Von Fraunhofer JA, Branstetter J. The physical properties of four endodontic sealers and cements. *J. Endod.* 1982; 8: 126–30.

45. Weiss EI, Shallav M, Fuss Z. Assessment of antibacterial activity of endodontic sealers by a direct contact test. *Endod. Dent. Traumatol.* 1996; 12: 179–84.

46. Wilson AD, Clinton DJ, Miller RP. Zinc oxide-eugenol cements. IV. Microstructure and hydrolysis. *J. Dent. Res.* 1973; 52: 253–60.

47. Wu M-K, Wesselink PR. Endodontic leakage studies reconsidered. Part I. Methodology, application and relevance. *Int. Endod. J.* 1993; 26: 37–43.

48. Wu M-K, De Gee AJ, Wesselink PR, Moorer WR. Fluid transport and bacterial penetration along root canal fillings. *Int. Endod. J.* 1993; 26: 203–8.

49. Wu M-K, De Gee AJ, Wesselink PR. Fluid transport and dye penetration along root canal fillings. *Int. Endod. J.* 1994; 27: 233–8.

50. Wu M-K, Fan B, Wesselink PR. Diminished leakage along root canal fillings filled with gutta-percha without sealer over time: a laboratory study. *Int. Endod. J.* 2000; 33: 121–5.

51. Wu M-K, Tigos E, Wesselink PR. An 18-month longitudinal study on a new silicon-based sealer, RSA RoekoSeal: a leakage study *in vitro*. *Oral Surg. Oral Med. Oral Pathol. Oral Radiol. Endod.* 2002; 94: 499–502.

52. Zmener O, Guglielmotti MB, Cabrini RL. Biocompatibility of two calcium hydroxide-based endodontic sealers. A quantitative study in the subcutaneous connective tissue of the rat. *J. Endod.* 1988; 14: 229–35.

Part 4
Diagnostic Considerations and Clinical Decision Making

Chapter 14
Diagnosis of pulpal and periapical disease

Claes Reit and Kerstin Petersson

Introduction

Diagnosing disease conditions of the pulp and the periapical tissues is often a demanding and sometimes also a frustrating procedure, e.g. when patients are in severe pain. Because the tissue reactions mostly take place in a concealed part of the body, the disease picture frequently must be made "visible" by indirect methods and tests. The clinician must also learn to navigate with a limited diagnostic armamentarium. In this situation, besides personal experience and intuition (which cannot be learnt from a textbook), the accuracy and correct interpretation of diagnostic information are all important. Evaluation and re-evaluation of data have to be carried out in a continuous process.

From textbooks, students normally learn about diagnosis through studying the traits of various diseases. Expected symptoms, signs and test results of, for example, pulpal inflammation, are presented, the diseases are given and their clinical, radiographic and laboratory expressions discussed. However, such a learning procedure is the reverse of what happens in the clinical situation. Patients rarely know what they suffer from. Instead they present with certain symptoms, signs and test results. While suspicions often can be raised in several directions, the task of the clinician is to carefully weigh the collected information to find the right signal or diagnosis. This chapter therefore will start with a discussion on how diagnostic information may be evaluated before the specific measures that may be taken to identify the endodontic disease conditions are reviewed.

Evaluation of diagnostic information

Making the right diagnosis is often a complex task and clinicians may easily arrive at different conclusions. Many studies have demonstrated how physicians and dentists vary in the way they practice their profession, regardless of whether they are defining a disease, making a diagnosis or selecting a therapeutic procedure. For example, in a study on microscopic investigation of

biopsy specimens from the uterine cervix, 13 pathologists were asked to read 1001 specimens and to repeat the readings at a later point in time. On average, each pathologist agreed with him or herself only 89% of the time (intraobserver agreement) and with a panel of "senior" pathologists only 87% of the time (interobserver agreement). Looking only at patients who actually had cervical pathology, the intraobserver agreement was only 68% and the interobserver agreement was 51% (34).

Many similar studies on various signs and symptoms have been carried out and the literature on observer variation has been growing for a long time (8) (Key literature 14.1). From a diagnostic point of view it has been found that, in general, observers looking at the same attribute will disagree with each other or even with themselves 10–50% of the time (10). Many authors have regarded the diagnostic process more as an act of art than of science: "Traditionally, the process of diagnosis was left undefined, a natural art, or explained as a process of intuition. Despite recent advances, this is still too often the case" (12). In *Dorland's Medical Dictionary* (7) "diagnosis" is defined as "The *art* of distinguishing one disease from another". During recent years clinical reasoning has been the subject of substantial research, and both descriptive and normative models have been proposed (22).

Diagnostic accuracy

Let us assume that the question of whether or not a patient has a certain disease D in a clinical situation can be determined only by a test T. It is possible to obtain two test results: one indicating that the patient has D (a positive test, T+) and one suggesting that the patient does not have D (a negative test, T–) (see Core concept 14.1). Unfortunately, T has the drawback (which it shares with almost all tests and procedures) that it cannot completely separate persons who have D and those who have not. Two types of error are then possible. A person who has D can be informed that he or she has not (a false-negative diagnosis) and another person can receive

> **Key literature 14.1   Observer variation in periapical radiographic diagnosis**
>
> In a study by Reit and Hollender (37) the radiographs of 119 endodontically treated roots were examined by six observers. Each root was visible on two separate radiographs. Three of the examiners were specialists in endodontics and three in oral radiology. The observers were asked to distinguish between "normal periapical conditions", "increased width of the periodontal membrane space" and "periapical radiolucency". In the opinion of one or more observers, 82 of the 119 roots presented normal periapical conditions. However, only at 33 (37%) of these roots was the decision shared by all six. The diagnosis of "increased width of the periodontal membrane space" was made in agreement in only 9% of 65 recorded cases. Periapical radiolucency was reported at 37 of the roots, and at ten of these (27%) all observers agreed. This study serves as an illustration of the difficulties in defining and maintaining criteria in radiographic evaluation of the periapical tissues.

> **Core concept 14.1   Measures of diagnostic accuracy**
>
> | | | Test results | |
> | --- | --- | --- | --- |
> | | | T+ | T− |
> | Actual state | D+ | TP (True positive) | FN (False negative) |
> | | D− | FP (False positive) | TN (True negative) |
>
> T+ = positive test result
> T− = negative test result
> D+ = disease present
> D− = disease absent
>
> **Sensitivity** = the proportion of diseased patients (D+) correctly identified as positive (TP/TP + FN).
>
> **Specificity** = the proportion of non-diseased patients (D−) correctly identified as negative (TN/TN + FP).
>
> **Positive predictive value** = the proportion of positive tests (T+) that are true positive (TP/TP + FP).
>
> **Negative predictive value** = the proportion of negative tests (T−) that are true negative (TN/TN + FN).

positive test although he or she does not have D (a false-positive diagnosis). Of course there are also two types of correct outcomes of the test: true-positive and true-negative diagnoses, respectively. The proportions of these four possible outcomes can be used to express the diagnostic value attached to the test. Sensitivity – or the true-positive ratio – is a measure of the proportion of patients with D correctly identified as positive. Specificity – the true-negative ratio – is a measure of the proportion of persons without D correctly identified as negative. In order to determine the sensitivity and specificity of a

diagnostic test a comparison with some sort of ideal "gold standard" has to be made. There must be some test-independent way of making a definitive diagnosis of whether the patient is diseased or not. Preferably, such a gold standard is created by means of a biopsy, but often another test normally not clinically available because of high costs or severe adverse effects may serve this purpose. In most cases investigators have to use gold standards that are below "24 carats".

In the clinical situation the most interesting questions are formulated in a slightly different way. When the test indicates that the patient is diseased (T+), what is the probability that he or she really has D? And if the patient gets a negative result (T−), what is the probability that D is not present? These probabilities are given in the so-called *positive predictive value* (PPV) and the *negative predictive value* (NPV). In contrast to sensitivity and specificity, PPV and NPV are dependent on the prevalence of the disease. Let us assume that a test has 90% sensitivity and 95% specificity for a certain disease. If the prevalence of the disease is 50%, then the PPV will reach 95%. This means that if a patient receives a positive result there is 95% probability that he or she is diseased. If the prevalence is 10%, the PPV will decrease to 67%; if the prevalence is 1%, the PPV is only 15%. This mathematical exercise tells us that tests do not work well when prevalences are low. Accordingly, in a clinical situation, tests should not be used on a routine basis. By history taking and oral examination the clinician selects patients in which a specific test may be used. What he or she actually does is to increase the prevalence of the suspected disease!

Receiver operating characteristic analysis

If rates of true-positive response (TPR) and false-positive response (FPR) are calculated for different decision criteria (cut-offs), the obtained pairs of values may be plotted in a simple graph with the TPR placed vertically and the FPR horizontally. Various cut-off points may be obtained in many ways. For example, in radiographic diagnosis of periapical lesions the level of confidence of the observer often is used. Both the TPR and the FPR are calculated for five decision critera: definitely a lesion; probably a lesion; uncertain; probably no lesion; definitely no lesion. The plotted points form what is called the receiver operating characteristic (ROC) curve (Fig. 14.1).

The position of the ROC curve will tell us how good a test is at discriminating between people (or teeth) who have the disease from those who do not. The ROC curve of the perfect test coincides with the axes, whereas the curve of the worthless test lies along the 45° diagonal. We can measure the discriminatory power of a test by how close its ROC curve is to the axes and how far it is from the diagonal. More precisely, the discriminatory power

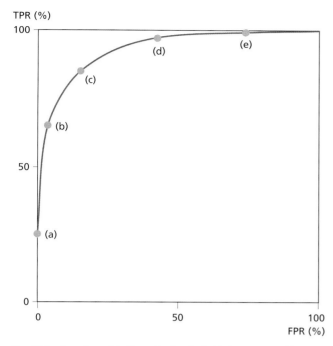

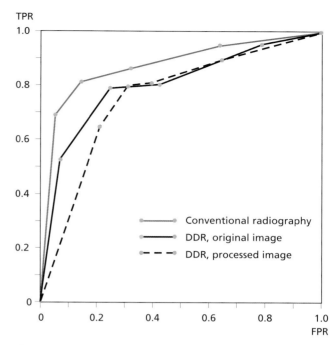

Fig. 14.1 In radiographic diagnosis of periapical lesions, true-positive rates (TPR) and false-positive rates (FPR) can be calculated for five decision criteria: (a) definitely a lesion, (b) lesion probable, (c) lesion uncertain, (d) probably no lesion, (e) definitely no lesion.

Fig. 14.2 ROC analysis of periapical radiography showing observer decisions for 59 radiographs (23).

is measured by the *area* under the curve, which is 100% for the perfect test and 50% for the worthless test. An ROC analysis demonstrates that changing the cut-off point will *not* influence the discriminatory power of a test, it just moves its position *along* the curve. However, different cut-off points can have momentous clinical consequences for those affected by the judgment, and a strategy for deciding the position to be taken on the curve must be developed (see next section).

Receiver operating characteristic analysis of periapical radiography

In a study by Kullendorff *et al.* (23) the aim was to compare the observer performance of direct digital radiography, with and without image processing, with that of conventional radiography, for the detection of periapical bone lesions. For 50 patients a conventional periapical radiograph using E-speed film was taken and then a direct digital image of the same area was made. The images of 59 roots were assessed by seven observers using a five-point confidence scale: definitely no lesion; probably no lesion; uncertain; probably a lesion; definitely a lesion. A gold standard was created by independent readings of 73 films by two experienced radiologists. Only images where they agreed (totalling 59) were included in the study. ROC curves were established and mean values of the observers' decisions are shown in Fig. 14.2.

Conventional film radiography came out slightly better from the study than direct digital radiography. Image processing did not improve the observer performance.

Diagnostic strategy

The diagnosis is not a goal in itself but only, in the words of a Scottish clinician, "a mental resting-place" for prognostic deliberation and therapeutic decisions (45). One of the main concerns for this deliberation is of course the fact that no diagnostic method has perfect sensitivity and specificity, which means that false diagnoses cannot be avoided completely. Also, from ROC analysis we learn that diagnostic decisions always have "costs". If we want to be sure that all cases treated are really diseased, we have to take a low position on the ROC curve. The cost for this will be a number of missed cases. In contrast, if we want to treat all diseased patients (or teeth), a high position on the ROC curve is needed and the cost will be a number of healthy cases being treated. If an analysis of an actual clinical situation results in a strategic decision to avoid overtreatment (low ROC position), then the clinician should signal for disease only when he or she is absolutely certain that it is present. If the problem is to avoid false-negative diagnoses, the best consequences will be obtained if disease is reported at the slightest suspicion of it (high ROC position). It is important to notice that a decrease in one type of error will lead to an increase in the other.

On which grounds should a certain strategy be chosen? This is a complex problem and an in-depth analysis is beyond the scope of this chapter. However, certain important factors may be identified: the consequences of untreated disease; risk of complications or adverse effects of instituted therapy; economic costs; and personal values.

In a situation where untreated disease will not lead to any serious complications of the patient's general health or well-being, one normally wants to avoid overtreatment. The diagnostic process will be directed towards the avoidance of false-positive diagnoses and a low position on the ROC curve is taken. If untreated disease will lead to serious complications it is important to identify and find all or most of the diseased individuals. From a strategic point of view, false-positive diagnoses must be accepted and we have to move higher up the ROC curve.

It is obvious that if the available cure also implies great risk of severe complications or serious adverse effects, one does not want to perform any unnecessary treatments. The price to pay for accepting false-positive diagnoses will then be too high. In contrast, the diagnostic position should be moved higher up the ROC curve if treatment is simple and without any considerable risk.

All medical and dental care is associated with economic costs and thus resources must be regarded as limited. Diagnosis and treatment have to be cost-effective and if the available therapy is very expensive one does not want to start a treatment on a false-positive diagnosis. For example, if a crown and post have to be removed in order to reach a root canal for retreatment, it is essential to be absolutely sure that this is the right thing to do. Accordingly, a lower position on the ROC curve has to be taken.

Personal values have to be included in a decision strategy. Faced with the same clinical situation, people will not evaluate the benefits and risks of a treatment procedure in identical ways. This means that the position of the diagnostic criterion has to be discussed with the individual patient. Will the patient take a false-positive diagnosis before a false-negative diagnosis, or the other way around? Attempts have been made to measure patients' values in order to incorporate them in various decision models (38). These possibilities are discussed in more detail in Chapter 18.

Clinical manifestations of pulpal and periapical inflammation

The clinical manifestations of inflammatory processes in the pulp and periapical tissues cover a broad range of expressions. Patients' experience of dental pain may vary from a barely noticeable discomfort to an unbearable torment, from an odd pain attack of short duration to a lingering continuous suffering. Patients may, in addition, display various signs of infection, including fistulae, swellings and raised body temperature. Discolored teeth is another patient complaint that may draw a suspicion of a diseased pulp. In Core concept 14.2 the most commom symptoms and signs associated with pulpal inflammation, pulp necrosis and periapical pathosis are collected and displayed. Strangely, however, patients are usually free of symptoms and the majority of pulpal inflammations in need of endodontic treatment are revealed during operative procedures (36). In most cases. inflammatory involvement of the periapical tissues is detected only by radiographic means.

Collecting diagnostic information

Inferences regarding disease processes in the pulp and periapical tissues have to be made with the help of a rather limited diagnostic armamentarium. The main sources of information are the patient's report on pain and other symptoms, the clinical examination of the tooth and surrounding structures, and the radiographic examination (Core concept 14.3). The problem for which the patient seeks dental care (chief complaint) is the natural point of departure for the diagnostic process. If the patient is in acute distress, the examination and diagnosis must be focused on solving that particular problem as fast as possible and a complete examination and establishment of a definitive treatment plan have to be postponed until later. A quieter situation will allow the examiner to expand on the present dental illness. The patient's report on character, intensity, frequency, localization and external influence of the symptoms will often give clues to a *tentative diagnosis*. This initial notion may be strengthened or refuted by penetrating the dental history, including information on such matters as recently placed restorations, pulp cappings and potential bruxism.

When reviewing the medical history the clinician will focus on illnesses, medication and allergic reactions. Consultation with the patient's physician is recommended when physical or mental illness is expected to interfere with diagnosis and treatment plan. There are no systemic disease conditions for which endodontic treatments are contraindicated, other than those affecting any dental procedure.

The status of the tentative diagnosis is explored further at the clinical examination. Crowns of suspected teeth are evaluated with regard to caries, defective fillings and discoloration. A fiber optic light source may be useful to disclose the presence of cracks in the enamel or dentin, and the patient may be asked to bite on a cotton roll or a firm object to confirm the diagnosis. As pointed

Core concept 14.2   Clinical manifestation of pulpal and periapical disease

Symptoms and signs of pulpal inflammation
- History of sharp pain, spontaneous or to thermal stimuli
- Pain attack may be provoked clinically by thermal stimuli (a)

Symptoms and signs of pulp necrosis (b)
- The pulp is insensitive to vitality testing
- The crown is discolored (grayish)

Symptoms and signs of periapical inflammation (c–e)
- Tooth is insensitive to vitality testing
- Dull, continuous pain
- Intra- or extraoral swelling
- Draining fistula
- Periapical radiolucency

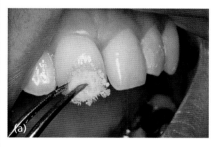
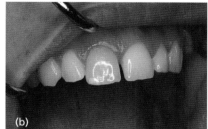
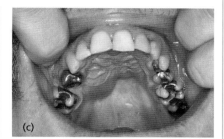
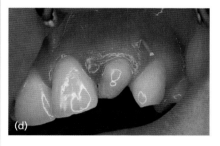
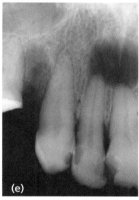

Core concept 14.3   Sources of diagnostic information

- Anamnesis
  - Chief complaint
  - Present dental illness
  - Dental history
  - Medical history
- Clinical examination
  - Evaluation of the crown
  - Evaluation of the pulp
  - Evaluation of the periapical tissues
- Radiographic examination

out in Chapter 4 the true condition of the pulp is often difficult to assess but pain provocation and pulp vitality testing are helpful. Tenderness to percussion and palpation confirms a suspicion of periapical inflammation, as of course does the presence of a fistula and swelling or a periapical radiolucency in the radiograph.

Some informative sources are more important than others. The following series of cases will demonstrate how pain report, pulp vitality testing and radiographic findings interact and come into play in the process of reaching a diagnosis in endodontics.

Diagnostic methodology: assessment of pulp vitality

Pulp vitality means that a given pulp has an intact neurovascular supply. Traditionally, pulp vitality has been determined by investigating response to painful stimuli. It needs to be recognized therefore that such methods test only for sensory nerve function and not necessarily for an intact pulpal blood supply. Yet, the presumption can most often be made that a tooth which responds to the provocation with a sharp pain sensation has a vital pulp. Because this is an indirect methodology the clinician has to work with hypotheses of the relation between the test result and the reality. Two main assumptions about this relation usually are made:

Case study 1

Pulp vitality?

A 25-year-old man visited his dentist 3 days after receiving a blow from the elbow of an opponent against his upper incisors during an ice hockey game. Immediately after the incident the teeth felt slightly mobile, but at the examination the patient had no symptoms besides slight tenderness on chewing. The incisors were stable and no cracks or fractures were found. The crowns showed normal color. Pulp vitality was investigated by means of sensitivity tests. All front teeth were sensitive to cold and electric current. Thus, the pulps of the teeth seemed to have survived the traumatic injury. Therefore no treatment was recommended, but the patient was scheduled for a future follow-up in case a pulp complication developed later.

Comment: In a clinical situation the condition of the pulp may be difficult to assess. The pulp can rarely be directly observed and whether it is vital or not has to be established by indirect methods. Evaluating the reaction to painful stimuli by sensitivity tests is among the most important tools of pulp diagnosis.

1. If the pulp is sensitive, it is vital.
2. If the pulp is sensitive and the patient has no symptoms, the pulp is healthy.

There are three types of pulp sensitivity tests:

- mechanical;
- thermal;
- electrical.

The guiding rules for the use of sensitivity tests are given in Core concept 14.4.

Mechanical tests

Directing a jet of compressed air and probing exposed dentin in a cavity or cervically at the neck of the tooth normally results in a sensitive reaction in a tooth with a vital pulp. Pulp sensitivity also may be evoked during drilling for removal of caries or defective fillings. In these procedures nociceptive mechanoreceptors at the pulp–dentin border are stimulated by hydrodynamic forces moving the fluid in the affected dentinal tubules (see also Chapter 3). Of course, a prerequisite for these tests is that the tooth in question has not been anesthetized. In ambiguous cases drilling a small test cavity can be useful, especially in teeth with full crown restorations. Such test cavities can also be used for thermal and electrical tests. While scientific data on the diagnostic accuracy of mechanical stimulation are lacking, it is a simple and effective means to test the status of the pulp. Indeed it is a good clinical routine in restorative procedures to postpone the administration of local anesthetics until a sensitive reaction is received from the tooth. Such a routine will prevent restoration of a tooth with a necrotic pulp.

Thermal tests

Cold air, water or a cold object may elicit a pain response when placed at a tooth surface. Similar to mechanical tests the temperature changes will influence the flow of dentinal fluid and a subsequent mechanical stimulation of pulpal nerves. A common method is to apply a cotton pellet soaked in a fast evaporating fluid, such as ethyl chloride or dichlorodifluoromethane or carbon dioxide snow. Ice sticks – made by filling empty cylinders with water and placing them in the freezer – can also be used but are not as efficient as the above-mentioned agents that provide lower temperatures.

Application of heat to the tooth surface is sometimes also used for vitality testing. A gutta-percha bar (temporary stopping) is heated in an open flame for a few seconds until it softens. It is then placed on the buccal surface on the tooth, away from the gingiva. The bar is removed as soon as the patient signals a pain response. Because studies indicate that the diagnostic accuracy is very low (35) (Key literature 14.2), heat should not be used as a test of pulp vitality, but can be useful for pain provocation.

Electrical test

An electric pulp tester sends a weak electric current through the tooth, which stimulates the pulpal nerves. Various technical devices are available. Studies have shown that the pain threshold is influenced by the placement of the electrode. Several authors registered the lowest threshold values when it was placed on incisal or cusp tips (4). At this part of the tooth the enamel layer usually is very thin (the enamel has greater electrical resistance than the dentin) and the concentration of sensory nerves is highest in the pulpal horns (24).

Core concept 14.4   Guiding rules for the clinical use of vitality tests

- Explain the procedures to the patient.
- Do not rely on only one test; use combinations.
- Make comparisons with other teeth, preferably contralaterals but also with neighboring teeth.
- In cases with doubtful reactions, repeat the tests in a different order, "hiding" the suspicious tooth.

Key literature 14.2   Diagnostic accuracy of thermal and electronic pulp tests

In a study by Petersson *et al.* (35), the pulpal status of 75 teeth was investigated by cold (ethyl chloride), heat (hot gutta-percha) and electricity (Analytic Technology Pulp Tester). True-positive, false-positive, true-negative and false-negative test results were calculated for each method compared with a gold standard. The gold standard was established by direct pulp inspection (59 teeth in need of end-odontic treatment) and by judging radiographs (16 intact teeth). Twenty-nine teeth (39%) were judged to be necrotic. The authors found that an insensitive reaction represented a necrotic pulp in 89% with the cold test, in 48% with the heat test and in 88% with the electrical test. A sensitive reaction was found to correspond to a vital pulp in 90% with the cold test, in 83% with the heat test and in 84% with the electrical test.

Sensitivity testing by electrical stimulation has good diagnostic accuracy (29, 35) but its use is often prohibited when restorations cover most of the tooth structure. To overcome this problem, Pantera *et al.* (33) suggested the use of a bridging technique. The tip of an explorer coated with toothpaste was placed against an exposed part of the tooth surface and the pulp tester then was placed against the explorer. For some vitality test devices extra-thin electrodes are available.

Interpretation of test results

The outcome of a sensitivity test is the result of an inter-action between the given stimulus and the patient's reaction to it. Accordingly, a failing correlation between sensitivity and vitality may be either *stimulus* or *reaction dependent*. The former situation may be illustrated by an electrical impulse that does not reach a vital pulp tissue owing to, for example, excessive amounts of reparative dentin. False recordings also may be obtained if the pulp is necrotic but the impulse reaches nerve fibers in the periodontal membrane or in a neighboring tooth. Such possibilities have been discussed in detail by several authors (16, 30). Sometimes a vital pulp cannot respond to stimulation owing to a traumatic injury having dam-aged the intradental nerves. The accuracy of the test also may be impaired by the patient's behavior. He or she may be anxious or feeling uneasy and thus have difficulty in giving a correct report (see Case study 2). Therefore, when test results are doubtful and difficult to interpret, a combination of methods must be used (Core concept 14.4).

In recent years other concepts of pulp vitality testing than eliciting painful stimuli have been suggested, includ-ing blood flow assessment. Laser–Doppler flowmetry has been developed for this purpose and recently a pulse oximeter dental probe was presented. Both methods are reported to have high diagnostic accuracy for anterior

Case study 2

Tooth-related pain

A 53-year-old woman consulted her dentist about periodic pain from the left upper molar region. The pain started a week earlier and was elicited by hot and cold food. Each period of intense penetrating pain lasted for about 30 min. Between the acute episodes the patient constantly felt a mild rather dull pain. She was convinced that the pain emanated from the *upper first molar*. The clinical examination disclosed extensive fillings in both the upper and the lower molars. No signs of caries were found. None of the teeth was tender to percussion. In the bitewing radiograph a deep amalgam filling, close to the pulp, was observed in the *lower first molar*. When cold was applied a strong and lasting pain reaction was elicit-ed only from this tooth. After a mandibular anesthetic injection the pain disappeared. When the amalgam fill-ing was removed a pulp capping area was exposed. The case was diagnosed as *symptomatic pulpitis* and the pulp was extirpated.

Comment: Painful symptoms from a pulp are most often associated with active caries but can also emerge in a number of other situations in which microorganisms reach and provoke the pulp. In this case a small part of the pulp was exposed several years ago, when caries was excavated. Over the years microorganisms might have slowly penetrated the margins of the filling and eventu-ally reached the capping area and caused the pulp response. In pain cases the patient's report of the symp-toms is very significant. However, it is important to understand that the discriminatory accuracy of the nerve system is not precise and that the patient's report might lead the clinician in a wrong direction. If symptomatic pulpitis is suspected a bitewing radiograph is preferred over a periapical radiograph because the projection more easily reveals the proximity of carious lesions and resto-rations to the pulp, and information regarding the upper as well as the lower teeth is presented in one image (see also Case study 2, Chapter 4).

---

teeth (9, 14). Yet neither methodology has gained recog-nition in clinical practice, primarily because of cost and demanding technique.

Diagnostic methodology: evaluation of reported pain

From a subjective point of view the main sign of pulpal and periapical disease is the experience of pain. Patients usually associate pathology with pain, and a pain-free condition with non-disease. However, studies have revealed low correlation between pulp pathology and patients' symptoms (1, 26, 41) and in most cases inflammatory lesions of the pulp and the periapical tissues will not give rise to pain. Thus, the sensitivity of pain as a diagnostic criterion of endodontic disease is very low.

The clinical picture is even more complicated. Studies have shown that when a patient reports spontaneous dental pain and locates the origin of symptoms to a certain tooth, the clinician cannot act on this information alone because the discriminatory power of the pulpal nerves is not perfect. When healthy teeth were stimulated electrically, Mumford and Newton (31) found that only 46% of subjects could correctly identify the right tooth being tested. In a similar experiment Friend and Glenwright (11) reported that 73% of subjects made a correct area localization (one neighboring tooth on each side included). In these studies electric pulp testers were used, which stimulate mostly A-delta fibers. When pain is elicited by pulpal inflammation, nerve impulses will originate mostly from C-fibers. Those fibers have a lesser discriminatory ability, which means that the chance of correct tooth identification will decrease further. Thus, patients may experience pain in one tooth while the pathosis in fact is to be found in another. This phenomenon is called *referred pain* (13, 42). Pain may also be referred to teeth from pathological processes elsewhere, for example in the ear, salivary glands, maxillary sinus and masticatory muscles (1, 18). Even organs outside the head may generate what appears as "toothache". Bonica (5) reported that patients with angina pectoris rather frequently referred the pain to their teeth.

Case study 3

Cracked tooth

A 46-year-old man visited his dentist for severe pain localized to the right molar area of the lower jaw. The pain started a week earlier with a twinge in one of the teeth. Since then the symptoms returned in periods. Each period lasted from 30 min to an hour. The pain became very severe and he consumed a lot of painkillers. At the clinical examination the patient was symptom free. Both left lower molars were normally sensitive to testing. No pain could be provoked but the first molar was slightly tender to percussion. The teeth were restored with occlusal amalgam fillings and no caries was detected clinically or radiographically (a). During the examination the pain suddenly returned so severely that the patient started to cry. A mandibular anesthetic injection relieved the pain. At a closer inspection small cracks were found

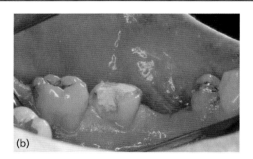

(b)

at the distal as well as lingual parts of the first molar. The amalgam filling was removed and the cracks were found to engage with the pulp chamber. Pulpectomy was then performed and a calcium hydroxide dressing placed in the root canals. When the patient return a week later he was pain free but the distolingual cusp had fractured and the fragment was lost (b).

Comment: Molars and premolars may suffer more or less complete breaks of the tooth structure due to forces of mastication. While some cracks may go outside the pulpal space and involve a cuspal area only, others may directly engage the pulp. In either case bacterial elements may reach the pulp and cause inflammation and painful symptoms. In addition to the classical pulpitis symptoms, cracked teeth may display acute pain on chewing hard food items. The diagnosis of cracked teeth is nevertheless far from clear-cut because such teeth may not always be extensively or deeply restored. The symptom complex can also be quite variable and therefore the condition may go undiagnosed for years. Eventually pulp necrosis and apical periodontitis may develop, especially if the crack has involved the pulp.

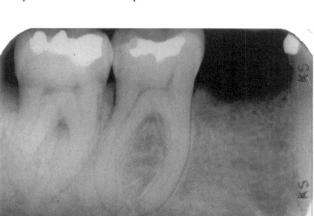

(a)

Important diagnostic information can be found in the patient's description of the pain. Pulpal pain has a wide experience range: from a slightly increased sensitivity to intraoral temperature changes, to very intense, almost unbearable pain. In a typical case the pain comes in attacks often elicited by hot or cold food (Advanced concept 14.1). Initially, with such a provoked attack a sharp pain is felt (A-delta fiber-mediated). After the stimulus is removed, the pain lingers on for varying amounts of time (seconds to hours), often described as deep, dull and throbbing (C-fiber activation). Paradoxically, in some cases, taking a solid dose of ice water into the mouth may relieve the symptoms. This observation is mostly made when pain is continuous and very intense and is held to be a sign of excessive and irreversible pulpal inflammation.

As soon as the inflammatory reaction spreads out of the pulpal space to involve the periodontal membrane, the tooth may be tender to percussion, palpation and chewing. Nociceptors and mechanoreceptors can be found in the periodontium and each terminal controls its own territory along the root. Some nerve endings are especially close to collagen fiber bundles (32). Pain associated with periapical inflammation is mostly continuous and described as dull in character. The symptoms will not be influenced by changes in the temperature and thus may not be provoked.

Diagnostic methodology: provocation/inhibition of pain

Pain is the most important symptom of pulpal inflammation, but, as discussed above, in the clinical situation the diseased tooth can be hard to determine. Pain from an inflamed pulp is often periodic and there might be a pause in symptoms at the examination. If the pain is continuous the patient often experiences that it "spreads"

Advanced concept 14.1   Temperature changes and pulpal pain

The hypothetical explanation to the phenomenon that temperature changes influence pulpal pain is that such changes influence the tissue pressure inside the pulpal chamber with its rigid dentin walls. Because of low compliance in the pulpal chamber, even modest changes in pulpal fluid volume will be reflected in the tissue pressure (28). An increased pressure in the pulpal tissue due to increased temperature, for example, would start a pain attack because the biochemical inflammatory mediators already maintain subclinical pain signals and a decreased pain threshold. Congruent to this reasoning, a significant decrease in temperature would decrease the tissue pressure and thus also the pain sensation. Tooth-related pain in patients subjected to pressure changes, called barodontalgia, is sometimes experienced by airborne or diving people and is important as an indicator of pulpal inflammation.

---

over a greater area, which makes localization difficult. In order to find the right source of the pain, the most informative diagnostic move, besides clinical and radiographic examination, is to try to provoke or extinguish the symptoms. Pulpal pain may be triggered or aggravated by applying cold or hot stimuli to the tooth, e.g. a heated gutta-percha bar (see above). In cases with continuous pain, it may be helpful to inject anesthetics systematically and the occurrence or not of pain relief will indicate the site (region, upper or lower jaw) from which the symptoms emanate.

Differential diagnosis of pulpal pain

A number of other conditions can contribute to or mimic pulpal pain. Hence, pulpal pain may be associated with teeth suffering from so-called "traumatic occlusion". Such teeth can be hypersensitve to hot and cold stimuli and may be tender to percussion due to activation of the sensory nerve system in the pulp as well as in the periodontium. If no obvious cause of a pulpal inflammation can be observed, such as a deep carious lesion, a restoration close to the pulp chamber, crack or fracture, trauma from occlusion should be considered and checked for.

Symptoms from some non-dental conditions might mimic pulpal or periapical pain. Patients with *maxillary sinusitis* frequently have symptoms which they associate with the upper premolars and the first molar. A common finding is that two to three adjacent teeth are tender to percussion and that the pain increases when the patient leans forward or shakes the head.

Trigeminal neuralgia can mimic pulpitis with its sharp pain attacks. However, the pain attacks also continue at stimulation of "trigger points" after the suspected tooth has been anesthetized, which facilitates the discrimination between pulpitis and trigeminal neuralgia.

Herpes zoster infection of the trigeminal nerve is another neurological disorder that gives sharp pain attacks similar to pain from pulpitis. Especially in its initial stage it can be hard to distinguish from pulpitis but, after some days, when small vesicles emerge along the trigeminal branches extraorally in the skin or intraorally in the mucosa, the diagnosis becomes obvious.

Temporal arteritis, inflammation of the temporal artery, and *sialolothiasis* are other conditions that can give sharp pain in the orofacial region.

Diagnostic methodology: evaluation of tooth discoloration

A *gray* or *gray–brown* discoloration is considered to be one of the major diagnostic clues in disclosing pulp necrosis after subluxation, extrusive and lingual luxation of teeth following dental trauma (20) (see also Chapter 15). In studies of primary teeth discoloration was associated

Case study 4

Internal root resorption

At a visit to a new dentist the first upper left incisor of a 45-year-old man was examined radiographically. The patient had no symptoms but the tooth had been subjected to trauma 5 years ago. The radiograph revealed signs of an intracanal dentin resorptive process as well as an apical shortening of the root (a). The pulp was sensitive to vitality testing. The case was diagnosed as internal root resorption. The pulp was extirpated and the canal was cleaned and filled with warm gutta-percha.

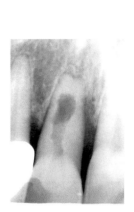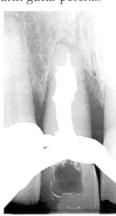

Comment: Besides pain there are few clinical signs of pulpal inflammation. Inflammatory–resorptive processes emerging inside the root canal space, as in this case, are rare and infrequently cause pain and, thus, are revealed only by radiographic examination.

with pulp necrosis in ≥97% of the cases (17, 43). No specific studies on the diagnostic accuracy of discoloration as a sign of pulp necrosis are available and a common recommendation is to test discolored teeth with suspected pulp necrosis for vitality and make a radiographic examination, as sometimes vital pulp functions may prevail.

A *yellow* discoloration of the crown can be seen after trauma, mainly luxation injuries. It is a sign of excessive dentin formation and narrowing of the pulpal space. Pulp necrosis and apical periodontitis may develop in such teeth with an increasing frequency over time (21, 40).

A *pink* discoloration of a tooth with vital pulp immediately after a full crown preparation is a sign of internal bleeding that can lead to extensive pulpal damage. Vibrations created by, for example, an eccentrically rotating bur, can cause intrapulpal bleeding with blood cells penetrating the dentin. Such an injury often leads to pulp necrosis.

Case study 5

Discolored crown

A 47-year-old man consulted his dentist about discoloration of the crown of the left upper incisor. The color change had slowly increased over the years and the patient wanted to improve the situation from an esthetic point of view. About 5 years ago one of his children had accidentally given him a blow with her small fist against the mouth. He had had almost no symptoms from the region. The dentist found that the tooth was insensitive to tests with cold and electric current. No signs of apical periodontitis were observed in the radiograph. The case was diagnosed as *pulp necrosis* and root canal treatment and bleaching of the crown were recommended.

Comment: There are several reasons for color change of a tooth crown. While internal bleeding is a common cause in trauma cases, pulp necrosis not induced by trauma can also occasionally be associated with tooth discoloration.

Case study 6

Symptomless periapical inflammation

A radiograph of a 49-year-old woman showed apical as well as interradicular radiolucencies in the first lower left molar. The patient reported to never have felt any pain or discomfort. The tooth was insensitive to pulp vitality testing. The case was diagnosed as *asypmtomatic apical periodontitis* and root canal treatment recommended. When the root canal space was opened up the pulp was found to be non-bleeding (necrotic).

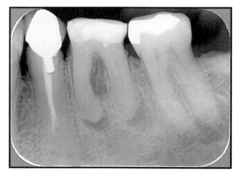

Courtesy of Dr Peter Jonasson.

Comment: As in this case apical periodontitis frequently develops without palpable clinical symptoms and is diagnosed only radiographically.

A *pink spot* on the tooth surface can also be a sign of invasive cervical resorption, an often aggressively destructive form of external root resorption. It is characterized by the invasion of the cervical region of the root by fibrovascular tissue, which progressively resorbs dentin, enamel and cementum. The dental pulp remains protected by an intact layer of dentin and predentin until late in the process (15).

Diagnostic methodology: interpretation of periapical radiographs

Because inflammatory reactions of the periapical tissues often proceed without any clinical symptoms, these conditions are frequently diagnosed by radiographic means only. Numerous investigators have studied the diagnostic sensitivity of periapical radiography and a common approach has been to create artificial bone lesions in cadavers and determine the minimum amount of bone loss that will result in a visible radiolucency. A now classic study by Bender and Seltzer (3) reported that a

bone lesion was not visible until the cortex or the interface between cortical and cancellous bone was involved. They also stated that bone destructions were always larger than that suspected from studying the radiographs. In a study of human autopsy material, Brynolf (6) compared the radiology and histology of periapical areas of upper incisors. She reported a high frequency of radiographically undetected inflammatory lesions. Several other investigators have confirmed the findings of Bender and Seltzer (3) and Brynolf (6), and pointed out the high risk of false-negative recordings, which in turn will influence the sensitivity of the test.

Clinicians arrive at false-positive diagnoses mainly by erroneous interpretation of normal anatomical structures. Major blood vessels and spaces in the bone marrow, for example, might simulate the image of an inflammatory periapical lesion. Other disease processes that might cause periapical bone lesions, such as marginal periodontitis and cementoma, also influence the specificity of radiographic diagnosis. In such cases, pulp sensitivity testing of the tooth is decisive.

Case study 7

Tooth-related pain and swelling

A 70-year-old woman appeared for emergency treament of a swelling in the area of the right lower molars. The problem started a week earlier when she noticed a slight tenderness on chewing. After a couple of days a dull, constant pain appeared. She kept the symptoms in check with painkillers. The pain disappeared but she observed that a small swelling had emerged. The radiographic examination disclosed periapical radiolucencies in the first right lower molar (a). The oral examination showed a localized small swelling close to the gingival margin (b). The swelling was soft and bled on probing. By means of a gutta-percha cone it was possible to find and explore

a sinus tract (c). When an occlusal test cavity was drilled the pulp was found to be non-sensitive. The case was diagnosed as *apical periodontitis with fistula* (synonymous to the term *chronic apical abscess* as described in Chapter 7) and root canal treatment was recommended.

Comment: Sometimes apical periodontitis is associated with symptoms like pain and swelling. The pain usually differs from painful sensations elicited from an inflamed vital pulp. It is often described as dull and continuous and it cannot be provoked by thermal stimuli. In this case the pain stopped when the apical process penetrated the bone and the buccal mucosa to create a sinus tract. Apical inflammatory processes might also drain extra-orally (Fig. 14.3).

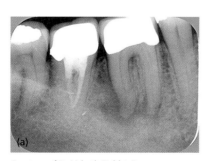
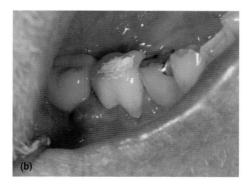
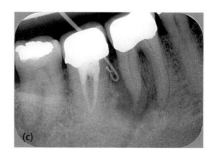

Courtesy of Dr Lisbeth Dahlström.

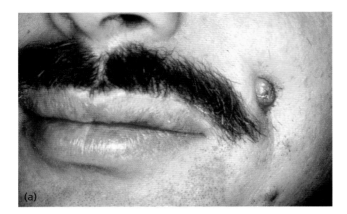

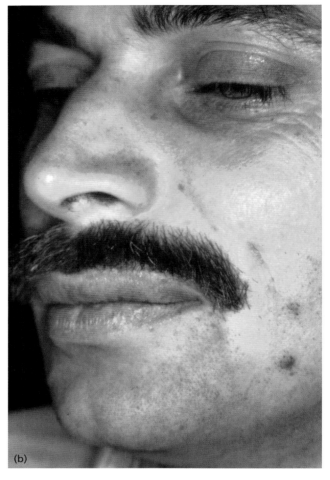

Fig. 14.3   (a) Extraoral sinus tract originating from a periapical lesion in the upper left second premolar. (b) The sinus tract healed as a result of root canal treatment.

Diagnostic methodology: clinical evaluation of the periapical tissues

The inflammatory response to root canal infection often takes place without any clinical symptoms. However, the situation may change if the ecological balance in the root canal flora changes and/or if the individual's defense against infection is impaired (see Chapters 6 and 7). The patient, who finds the tooth to be tender on chewing, might also experience dull continuous pain or swelling of the soft tissues in the area.

Tenderness is one of the cardinal signs of inflammation and is utilized to disclose teeth with pulpal and periapical lesions. Thus, a tooth with periapical inflammation might be sore when the root tip hits the inflamed area from tapping the tooth crown in the *percussion test*. Directing pressure by *palpation* over the area of periapical inflammation might elicit the same sensitive experience in the patient. Percussion and palpation examinations are low-cost tests, easy to perform and with practically no risk of complications. Their diagnostic accuracy has

not been evaluated but they are probably more useful to identify a tooth with apical periodontitis than to rule out the disease and must be combined with radiographic examination of the area.

The presence of a sinus tract is a sign of a draining periapical abscess. In order to find the origin of the tract a gutta-percha cone may be inserted and a radiograph exposed (so-called *fistulography*). In the image the cone will follow the tract and end in the inflamed area. Such an examination is often helpful to find the right tooth or to be able to distinguish between apical and marginal periodontitis.

Microorganisms originating from the root canal are not always the cause of inflammatory reactions in the periapical tissues. For example, a vertical root fracture may open an avenue for microfilaments to the periapical area and marginal periodontitis may progress and cause apically positioned radiolucent reactions. Therefore it is important to explore the *probing depth* of periodontal pockets in order to arrive at a correct diagnosis.

Case study 8

Apical radiolucencies in teeth with vital pulps

In a full-mouth radiographic survey, radiolucencies were observed around the apices of the lower central incisors in a 35-year-old woman (a). Sensitivity testing of the teeth with cold and electricity indicated vital pulps. The patient had no clinical symptoms. No carious lesions were detected and no deepened periodontal pockets were observed. The case was diagnosed as *periapical*

cemental dysplasia. The radiolucency becomes filled by coalescent radiopacities of cementum later in the process of such cases (b).

Comment: Radiolucent reactions in the periapical area are not always caused by endodontic infection and inflammation. Several differential diagnoses are possible. In particular the clinician should be observant of the combination of a sensitive reaction to vitality testing and a periapical radiolucency.

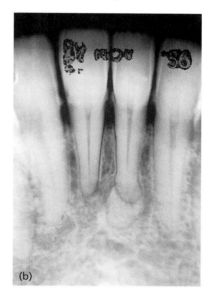

Differential diagnosis

Since apical periodontitis frequently presents without signs and symptoms the diagnosis often has to be based on the interpretation of the radiographic image. The clinician must therefore be aware of how the various anatomical structures are depicted and which non-endodontic pathological processes can be misinterpreted as apical periodontitis. There are several hazards on the diagnostic journey and a list of the most common periapical radiolucencies and radiopacities is shown in Core concept 14.5. Some case studies are presented to illustrate this particular diagnostic problem and how diagnostic reasoning can be maintained.

Diagnostic classification

The end of the diagnostic process is the formulation of a diagnosis. The collected information has to be related to a disease entity. In the literature, several classification systems have been suggested and various terms used to denote disease processes in the pulp and periapical tissues. At first glance this situation may appear confusing to the reader but a closer look will disclose that the systems express rather small variations on a common theme and "translations" between them are not difficult to carry out. It is important to recognize that a useful diagnostic system must be based on *clinically available* information only.

Diagnostic terms

Clinically healthy pulp

When a dental pulp remains within intact walls of dentin and responds normally to external stimuli without producing a lingering pain reaction, the pulp is considered to be clinically healthy. There are situations when teeth with healthy pulps are treated endodontically. The barrier function in the tooth may have been accidentally violated through operative procedures and the pulp

---

Core concept 14.5 Structures and disease processes appearing as periapical radiolucencies or radiopacities

Radiolucencies
- Anatomical structures
  - Incisive foramina and canals
  - Mental foramen
  - Greater palatine foramen
  - Maxillary sinus
- Endodontic processes
  - Granuloma
  - Radicular cyst
  - Scar/surgical defect
  - Foreign-body reaction
  - Osteomyelitis
- Non-endodontic origin
  - Periodontal disease
  - Periapical cementoma
  - Traumatic bone cyst
  - Non-radicular cyst
  - Malignant tumor

Radiopacities
- Condensing/sclerosing apical periodontitis
- Idiopathic osteosclerosis
- Hypercementosis
- Mature periapical cementoma

---

tissue exposed. Occasionally root canal retention is needed in prosthetic therapies when the possibilities for coronal retention are insufficient. Hemisection of multi-rooted teeth also initiates the need for endodontic treatment of a healthy pulp.

Pulpitis: symptomatic/asymptomatic

Pulpitis implies an inflammatory pulpal status that may or may not be associated with painful symptoms. As mentioned above and discussed in Chapter 4, findings from numerous studies indicate that the presence or absence of pain provides little information on the true condition of the pulp (2, 25, 26, 27, 41, 44). Hence, the extent of inflammatory involvement in a given pulp cannot be determined by the lead of diagnostic tests. From a practical point of view, however, it is helpful to regard excavation of caries and removal of fillings as part of the diagnostic process. Painful pulps found to be covered by dentin are provisionally regarded as being reversibly inflamed and can be treated temporarily by filling the cavity with ZnOE cement, for example, and, only if this does not curb the pain, pulpectomy may be performed.

Conversely, if pain is associated with a pulpal exposure by caries or following removal of a prior filling this is normally regarded an irreversible condition prompting radical removal of the tissue (see also Chapter 4). Thus, the diagnosis of "pulpitis" covers a broad range of pathological situations, including painful and non-painful conditions causing different clinical signs.

Although it often does not have a bearing on the therapeutic decision, it can be valuable for practical reasons to record whether or not the patient has symptoms when a treatment is started. Useful clinical diagnoses for a supposedly inflamed vital pulp therefore are *symptomatic pulpitis* when the patient has painful symptoms, and *asymptomatic pulpitis* when the patient has no symptoms. The diagnostic decision here is based on our knowledge of the etiology of pulpal inflammation, its clinical symptoms and the reaction pattern of the pulp.

Necrotic pulp

This term means that all the vital functions of the pulp are gone. A failure of reaction to a vitality test is not, however, sufficient information to act on this diagnosis. In combination with a discolored crown or periapical radiolucency, an access preparation to the pulp chamber is justified and the diagnosis confirmed with the finding of a non-bleeding pulp.

Normal periapical tissue

There are no clinical symptoms of periapical disease. The radiographic image shows normal periapical bone structure with a periodontal membrane space not more than double the width in other parts of the root.

Apical periodontitis: symptomatic/asymptomatic

Inflammatory processes of the periapical tissues caused by microorganisms in the root canal system are usually asymptomatic and the diagnosis is verified only by radiographic examination. Sometimes, in clinically acute situations, bone resorption may not have reached the level at which radiolucency is detectable in the radiograph. The clinical diagnosis of "apical periodontitis" makes no attempt to differentiate between various histological manifestations such as granulomas and cysts. For practical reasons it may be valuable to know if the patient had symptoms or not when the treatment was started. Useful clinical diagnoses therefore are *symptomatic apical periodontitis* (when the patient has overt clinical symptoms of periapical inflammation) and *asymptomatic apical periodontitis*. The latter diagnostic term is used when there are no clinical signs present (except for a sinus tract) and the supposed inflammatory reaction is disclosed only by radiographically visible apical bone destruction.

Case study 9

A sinus recess simulating apical periodontitis

The upper left second molar in this case was endodonti-cally treated (a) and thereafter used as an abutment tooth in a fixed partial denture. Two years later, at a routine check-up, the periapical radiograph showed a large radiolucent area at the apical region of the tooth (b).

Since both non-surgical and surgical retreatment in this case implied risk for complications it was considered cost effective to use the more expensive cone beam computed tomography (CBCT) (34) for a detailed image of the peri-apical area. The CBCT examination showed that a recess in the maxillary sinus mimicked a periapical bone destruction and disease could be ruled out (c).

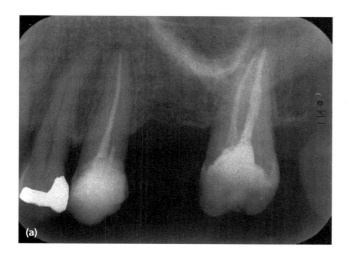
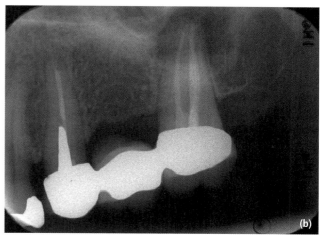
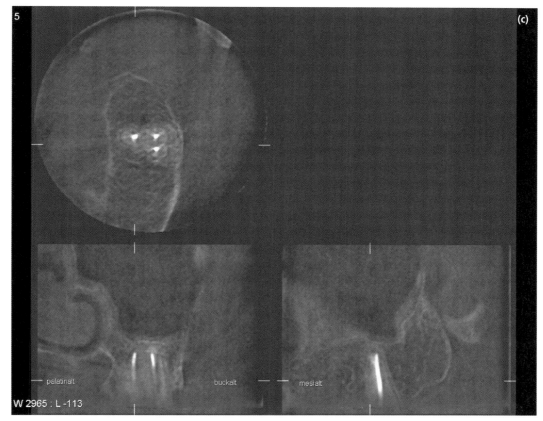

Case study 10

Periapical healing with scar tissue

A 40-year-old man presented at the clinic with a slight buccal swelling in the area of the right lateral incisor. A radiograph (a) disclosed that the tooth was root filled and apicectomized. After discussion with the patient a surgical re-entry was scheduled and a new root-end filling was placed. At a follow-up examination 2 years postoperatively (b) an apical radiolucency was still visible. However, the periodontal contour seemed to be intact and the case was examined by CBCT (c). The latter showed a "through and through" bone destruction and a continuous lamina dura was observed surrounding the tooth. The case was classified as healed with scar tissue.

Comment: Healing with scar tissue is rarely observed after non-surgical endodontic treatment. However, in cases treated surgically parts of the buccal bone plate are normally removed and if the lesion has penetrated the palatal wall a "through and through" bone cavity will be created. In such situations collagen-rich connective tissue might fill out the cavity and prevent bone replacement. The case illustrates a typical radiographic image of scar healing: an intact periodontal membrane and an apical radiolucency at a distance from the root.

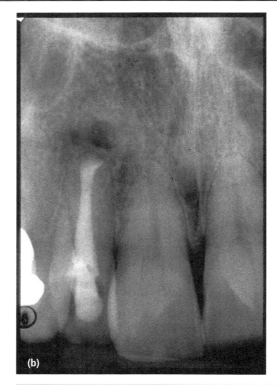

(b)

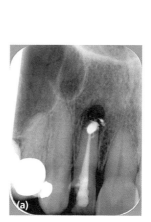

(a)

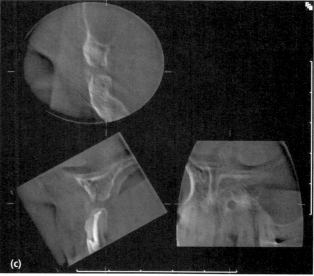

(c)

Courtesy of Dr Miguel Aranibar.

Case study 11

Differential diagnosis between granuloma and radicular cyst

There are no specific signs related to periapical bone destruction or the surrounding bone structures that can be used to differentiate between a granuloma and an apical cyst. However, the more extensive the lesion the higher the probability of a cyst. In this case a large periapical bone destruction at the right lower canine extended over the periapical area of the lower incisors (a). The diagnostic question was whether root canal infection in two or more teeth had caused the lesion, resulting in a large continuous bone cavity, or if the periapical radiolucency corresponded to an apical cyst emanating from one tooth only (the right lower canine). A CBCT examination revealed that the bone destruction enclosed the periapical region in the lower right canine end extended buccally to the periapical region of the incisors and thus probably represented an apical cyst (b).

Comment: A differential diagnosis is important only if it makes a difference for the treatment and/or the prognosis. In this case it was important to know if one or more teeth were involved in the process. In a situation like this vitality testing of the teeth is mandatory. However, if there are excessive amounts of reparative dentin there is a risk of a false test response and the interpretation of the radiograph will be all important.

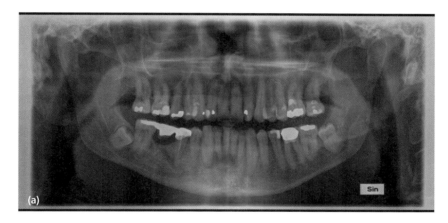

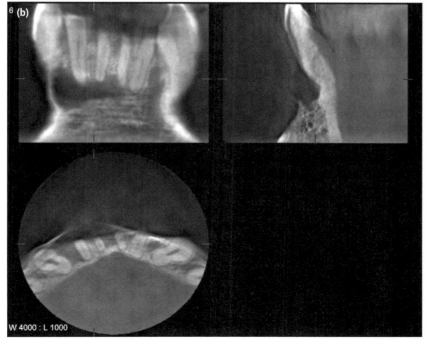

Case study 12

Condensing osteitis/sclerosing apical periodontitis

The right lower first molar was endodontically treated because of a pulp exposure. The preoperative radiograph showed a periapical radiopacity (a). The case was pulpectomized and root canals were filled (b). At an examination 6 years postoperatively, the radiopacity seemed to be resolved.

Comment: The reasons for the development of sclerosing periapical bone reactions are not clear. It is often suggested that a low-grade irritant will cause such a response (see also Chapter 7).

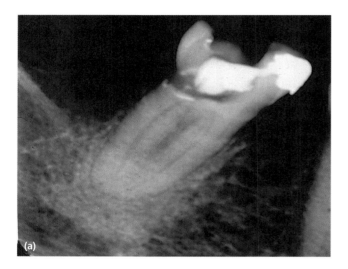

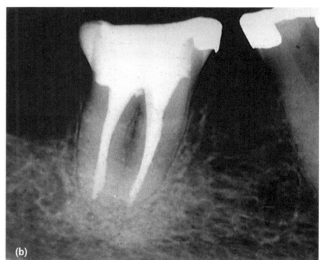

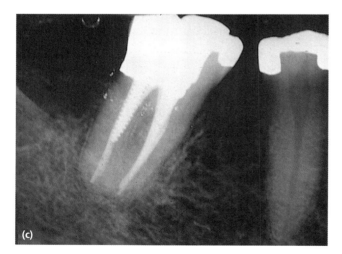

Case study 13

Malignant tumor

A 60-year-old man visited his dentist for emergency care beause of pain localized to the back teeth of the right upper jaw. At examination there were no remarkable findings either clinically or radiographically and the pain symptoms the patient reported were interpreted as pulpitis. The pain was of the character that urgent treatment was deemed necessary. Both teeth 16 and 15 had been well restored many years ago, 15 with a porcelain fused to metal crown. While both teeth were thought to be candidates for the ailment, the dentist opened tooth 16 and found a necrotic pulp and believed the right tooth had been localized. The pain condition did not resolve in spite of careful instrumentation and medication of the root canals. A few days later, the dentist therefore also decided to open tooth 15 and had the same finding of a necrotic pulp. This time the patient became asymptomatic but only for a few weeks. Although not in severe pain any longer, a swelling had emerged in the palatal mucosa and the patient now sought emergency care yet again and received an incision and drainage procedure. The swelling did not disappear and following another attempt for incision and drainage as well as treatment with antibiotic, not only did the swelling remain but another one appeared distal to the first one. At this point

in time (6 weeks after the first treatment) the patient was referred for specialist evaluation and it was eventually confirmed that the condition was not of endodontic origin but a manifestation of a primary tumor of malignant lymphoma.

Comment: While the diagnosis of endodontic disease conditions in most cases is reasonably straightforward it is important to be watchful for false leads. In this particular case there were several warning signals of a misdiagnosis. (i) It is unusual that two properly restored teeth without caries develop pulpitis and pulp necrosis simultaneously. (ii) While a periapical abscess may drain off in different directions and even towards the palate it is important that pus drainage is confirmed upon an incision and drainage procedure. This was not the case at either occasion. (iii) A comparison with a radiograph taken 10 years earlier (c) would have revealed that the lower border of the maxillary sinus was missing in the primary radiograph (a) as well as in the trial file radiograph (b). (iv) At no occasion could periapical radiolucencies be detected in the radiographs taken both at the start and during later treatment sessions. (v) The maxillary sinus appeared dense, suggesting soft-tissue presence. Collectively these observations strongly indicate a different etiology for the patient's symptoms than an inflammatory condition of endodontic origin.

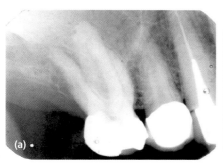 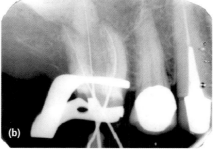 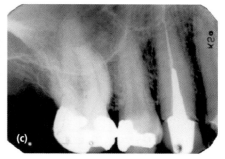

References

1. Arendt-Nielsen L, Svensson P. Referred muscle pain: basic and clinical findings. *Clin. J. Pain* 2001; 17: 11–19.
2. Baume LJ. Diagnoses of diseases of the pulp. *Oral Surg.* 1970; 29: 102–16.
3. Bender IB, Seltzer S. Roentgenographic and direct observation of experimental lesions in bone. *J. Am. Dent. Assoc.* 1961; 62: 150–60, 708–16.
4. Bender IB, Landau MA, Fonsecca S, Trowbridge HO. The optimum placement-site of the electrode in electric pulp testing of the 12 anterior teeth. *J. Am. Dent. Assoc.* 1989; 118: 305–10.
5. Bonica JJ. *The Management of Pain.* Philadelphia: Lea & Febiger, 1953.
6. Brynolf I. Histological and roentgenological study of periapical region of human upper incisors. *Odontol. Revy* 1967; 18: Suppl. 11.
7. *Dorland's Illustrated Medical Dictionary.* Philadelphia: Saunders, 1965.
8. Eddy DM. Variations in physician practice: the role of uncertainty. *Health Affairs* 1984; 3: 74–89.
9. Evans D, Reid J, Strang R, Stirrups D. A comparison of laser Doppler flowmetry with other methods of assessing the vitality of traumatised anterior teeth. *Endod. Dent. Traumatol.* 1999; 15: 284–90.

10. Feinstein AR. A bibliography of publications on observer variability. *J. Chron. Dis.* 1985; 38: 619–32.

11. Friend LA, Glenwright HD. An experimental investigation into the localization of pain from the dental pulp. *Oral Surg.* 1968; 25: 765–74.

12. Gale J, Marsden P. *Medical Diagnosis: from Student to Clinician.* Oxford: Oxford University Press, 1983.

13. Glick DH. Locating referred pulpal pain. *Oral Surg.* 1962; 15: 613–23.

14. Gopikrishna V, Tinagupta K, Kandaswamy D. Evaluation of efficacy of a new custom-made pulse oximeter dental probe in comparison with the electrical and thermal tests for assessing pulp vitality. *J. Endod.* 2007; 33: 411–14.

15. Heithersay GS. Invasive cervical resorption following trauma. *Aust. Endod. J.* 1999; 25: 79–85.

16. Himmel VT. Diagnostic procedures for evaluating pulpally involved teeth. *Curr. Opin. Dent.* 1992; 2: 72–7.

17. Holan G, Fuks AB. The diagnostic value of coronal dark-gray discoloration in primary teeth following traumatic injuries. *Pediatr. Dent.* 1996; 18: 224–7.

18. Ingle JI, Glick DH. Differential diagnosis and treatment of dental pain. In: *Endodontics* (Ingle JI, Bakland LK, eds). Philadelphia: Williams & Wilkins, 1994; 524–49.

19. Izumi T, Kobayashi I, Okamura K, Sakai H. Immunohistochemical study on the immunocompetent cells of the pulp in human non-carious and carious teeth. *Arch. Oral Biol.* 1995; 40: 609–14.

20. Jacobsen I. Criteria for diagnosis of pulp necrosis in traumatized permanent incisors. *Scand. J. Dent. Res.* 1980; 88: 306–12.

21. Jacobsen I, Kerekes K. Long-term prognosis of traumatized permanent anterior teeth showing calcifying processes in the pulp cavity. *Scand. J. Dent. Res.* 1977; 85: 588–98.

22. Kassirer JP, Kopelman RI. *Learning Clinical Reasoning.* Baltimore: Williams & Wilkins, 1991.

23. Kullendorff B, Peterson K, Rohlin M. Direct digital radiography for the detection of periapical bone lesions: a clinical study. *Endod. Dent. Traumatol.* 1997; 13: 183–9.

24. Lilja J. Sensory differences between crown and root dentine in human teeth. *Acta Odontol. Scand.* 1980; 38: 285–94.

25. Lundy T, Stanley HR. Correlation of pulpal histopathology and clinical symptoms in human teeth subjected to experimental irritation. *Oral Pathol.* 1969; 27: 187–201.

26. Michaelson PL, Holland GR. Is pulpitis painful? *Int. Endod. J.* 2002; 35: 829–32.

27. Mitchel DF, Tarplee RE. Painful pulpitis. A clinical and microscopic study. *Oral Surg.* 1960; 38: 1360–81.

28. Mjör I, Heyeraas K. Pulp–dentine and periodontal anatomy and physiology. In: *Essential Endodontology* (Ørstavik D, Pitt Ford TR, eds). Oxford: Blackwell Munksgaard, 2008; 10–43.

29. Mumford JM. Evaluation of gutta percha and ethyl chloride in pulp testing. *Br. Dent. J.* 1964; 116: 338–42.

30. Mumford JM. *Toothache and Orofacial Pain.* London: Churchill Livingstone, 1976.

31. Mumford JM, Newton AV. Convergence in the trigeminal system following stimulation of human teeth. *Arch. Oral Biol.* 1971; 16: 1089–97.

32. Nanci A. *Ten Cate's Oral Histology, Development, Structure, and Function.* St Louis: Mosby, 2003; 269–73.

33. Pantera EA, Anderson RW, Pantera CT. Use of dental instruments for bridging during electric pulp testing. *J. Endod.* 1992; 18: 37–8.

34. Patel S, Dawood A, Ford TP, Whaites E. The potential applications of cone beam computed tomography in the management of endodontic problems. *Int. Endod. J.* 2007; 40: 818–30.

35. Petersson K, Söderström C, Kiani-Anaraki M, Lévy G. Evaluation of the ability of thermal and electrical tests to register pulp vitality. *Endod. Dent. Traumatol.* 1999; 15: 127–31.

36. Petersson K, Wennberg A, Olsson B. Radiographic and clinical estimation of endodontic treatment need. *Endod. Dent. Traumatol.* 1986; 2: 62–4.

37. Reit C, Hollender L. Radiographic evaluation of endodontic therapy and the influence of observer variation. *Scand. J. Dent. Res.* 1983; 91: 205–12.

38. Reit C, Kvist T. Endodontic retreatment behaviour: the influence of disease concepts and personal values. *Int. Endod. J.* 1998; 31: 358–63.

39. Ringsted J, Amtrup C, Asklund P, Baunsgaard HE, Christensen L, Hansen L. *et al.* Reliability of histopathological diagnosis of squamous epithelial changes of the uterine cervix. *Acta Pathol. Microbiol. Immunol. Scand.* 1978; 86: 273–8.

40. Robertson A, Andreasen FM, Bergenholtz G, Andreasen JO, Norén JG. Incidence of pulp necrosis sunsequent to pulp canal obliteration from trauma of permanent incisors. *J. Endod.* 1996; 22: 557–60.

41. Seltzer S, Bender IB, Zionz M. The dynamics of pulp inflammation: correlation between diagnostic data and actual histologic findings in the pulp. *Oral Surg.* 1963; 16: 846–77.

42. Sharav Y, Leviner E, Tzukert A, McGrath PA. The spatial distribution, intensity and unpleasantness of acute dental pain. *Pain* 1984; 20: 363–70.

43. Soxman JA, Nazif MM, Bouquot J. Pulpal pathology in relation to discoloration of primary anterior teeth. *ASDC Dent. Child.* 1984; 51: 282–4.

44. Warfvinge J, Bergenholtz G. Healing capacity of human and monkey dental pulps following experimentally induced pulpitis. *Endod. Dent. Traumatol.* 1986; 2: 256–62.

45. Wulff HR, Gotzsche PC. *Rational Diagnosis and Treatment.* Oxford: Blackwell Science, 2000.
    This important book covers the theoretical foundations of diagnostic and therapeutic decision making and expands on the knowledge presented in the present chapter. It also contains reasoning on clinical research methodology and how to read scientific articles.

Chapter 15
Diagnosis and management of endodontic complications after trauma

John Whitworth

Introduction

Blows to the mouth can transmit sufficient energy to fracture teeth, displace teeth or fracture alveolar bone. The immediate consequences may appear obvious and dramatic (Fig. 15.1) or seemingly quite trivial, but in many circumstances, the true picture takes time to emerge. Complications can be serious in the long term, resulting not only in the loss of vital pulp functions, but in the gradual or rapid destruction of tooth structure by resorptive processes. Clinicians should consequently be aware that their emergency care must be followed by a structured program of review appointments, if complications are to be identified early and treated with success. The purpose of this chapter is to outline important considerations in the management of teeth which have suffered trauma. It will examine how trauma can make the pulp vulnerable to breakdown and infection, how trauma complicates pulp diagnosis and treatment planning and how pulp infection may combine with other injuries to promote secondary conditions such as root resorption. Some of the endodontic and restorative challenges presented by traumatized teeth with immature, fractured or resorbed roots will also be discussed.

Common dental injuries

Traumatic injuries to the teeth include fractures, luxations and combinations of the two. Tooth fractures may be confined to the structure of the crown or the root, or involve both. They may be classified according to their position, the degree of tooth tissue loss and whether or not they are complicated by direct exposure of pulp tissue to the oral environment (see Table 15.1 and Fig. 15.2). Intra-alveolar "horizontal" root fractures often run obliquely, but are usually classified according to their horizontal level as apical, mid-root or coronal third fractures (Fig. 15.2d). Horizontal root fractures detach the coronal part of the tooth from the remainder of the root, and may potentially disrupt the pulp's neurovascular supply at the fracture line, though they rarely expose pulp tissue to the mouth. Fractures may be undisplaced and difficult to identify with certainty (Fig. 15.2e), but if the crown is also luxated, the fracture will be displaced and more readily identified (Fig. 15.2f).

Luxation is an injury where the tooth has been loosened from its alveolus to a varying extent (see Table 15.2 and Fig. 15.3). Following minor injury, there may be no permanent dislocation of the tooth. More severe injuries

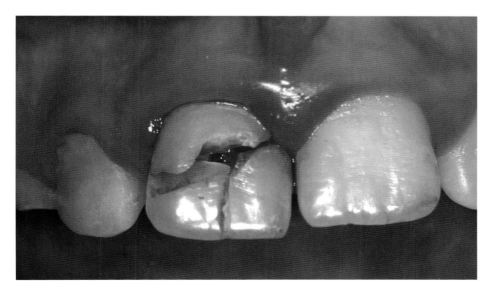

Fig. 15.1 The consequences of trauma may appear obvious, but time may reveal lesser injuries, including those in adjacent teeth, to be equally serious in the long term. (Courtesy of Dr Ben Cole.)

Table 15.1 Tooth fractures – classification, clinical features and risks of complication (see also Fig. 15.2). Percentages derived from Andreasen *et al.* (7).

Description	Definition	Presenting symptoms	Risk of pulp death	Risk of resorption-promoting root-surface injury
Uncomplicated crown fracture	Fracture of enamel and dentin with no visible pulp exposure	Exposed dentin may be sensitive	Minimal if dentin covered promptly	Minimal
Complicated crown fracture	Fracture of enamel and dentin, with visible pulp exposure	Exposed dentin and pulp tissue may be sensitive	Low if pulp capped and dentin protected promptly	Minimal
Crown/root fracture	Fracture of enamel and dentin extending onto the root of the tooth which may or may not involve the pulp	Coronal fragment may be mobile. Exposed dentin and pulp may be sensitive	Low if pulp capped and dentin protected promptly	Minimal
Root fracture	Fracture of the root at any level, usually involving the pulp	Clinical crown may be displaced or mobile	Coronal fragment: 20–40% Apical fragment: usually remains vital	Areas of coronal fragment may be crushed at points of compression against the alveolus and at risk

Low risk   Moderate risk   High risk

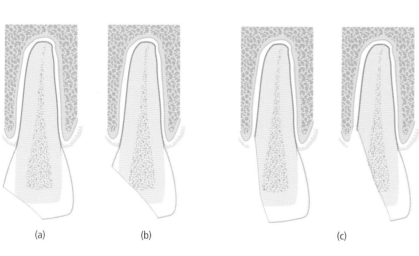

(a)   (b)   (c)

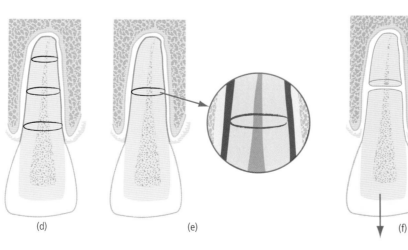

(d)   (e)   (f)

Fig. 15.2 Fractured teeth. (a) Uncomplicated crown fracture. (b) Complicated crown fracture. (c) Crown–root fractures, which may or may not directly involve the pulp. (d) Intra-alveolar "horizontal" root fractures in the coronal, middle or apical root third. Although the pulp is invariably involved in the fracture line, it may not be directly exposed to the oral environment. (e) Undisplaced intra-alveolar "horizontal" root fracture. Radiographically (inset) the fracture may be difficult to detect, or may be misinterpreted as more than one fracture line with an apparent island of tooth tissue interposed between them. (f) Displaced intra-alveolar fracture following concomitant luxation and displacement of the crown.

Table 15.2 Tooth luxation – classification, clinical features and risks of complication (see also Fig. 15.3). Percentages derived from Andreasen *et al.* (7).

Description	Definition	Presenting symptoms	Risk of pulp death	Risk of resorption-promoting root-surface injury
Concussion	Movement of a tooth within its socket which is insufficient to displace the tooth, but may damage the attachment apparatus and apical neurovascular bundle	Tooth may be tender to touch or percussion, but has no increased mobility and is not displaced	Open apex: minimal Closed apex: <5%	Minimal
Subluxation	Movement of a tooth within its socket which is insufficient for permanent displacement, but may increase mobility	Tooth may be tender and mobile to touch and under biting pressure	Open apex: minimal Closed apex: 5%	Minimal
Lateral luxation	Lateral movement of a tooth, sufficient for the tooth to be permanently displaced in a buccolingual or mesiodistal direction	Tooth may be painfully interfering with the occlusion	Open apex: 9% Mature apex: 77%	High in localized areas of root compression against the alveolus
Intrusive luxation	Vertical displacement of a tooth in an apical direction, driving the root apex through the floor of the bony socket	Tooth may have totally or partially disappeared from view	Open apex: 62% Mature apex: 100%	High risk in areas of compression against the alveolus
Extrusive luxation	Incomplete vertical displacement of a tooth in a coronal direction from its bony socket	Tooth is extruded, may be mobile or interfering with the occlusion	Open apex: 9% Mature apex: 55%	Minimal – injuries generally tear rather than crush the periodontium
Avulsion	Complete displacement of a tooth from its bony socket	Tooth may be absent or partially/completely reimplanted into its socket	Open apex: 25% Mature apex: 100%	Highly variable, depending on extra-alveolar time, extraoral dry time and handling

Low risk   Moderate risk   High risk

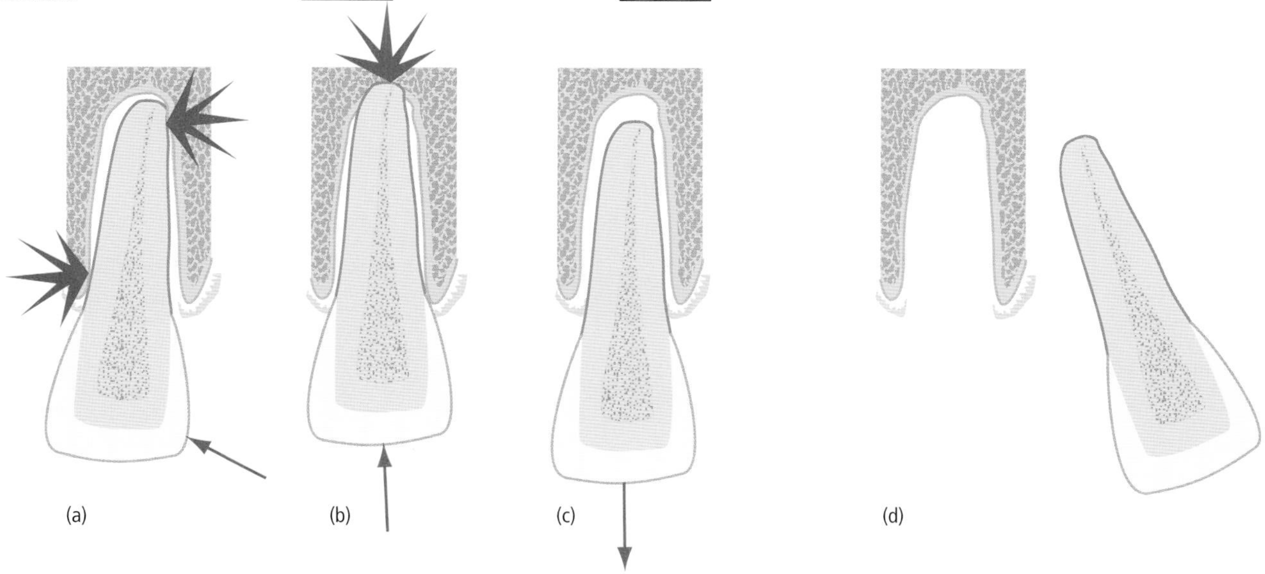

Fig. 15.3   Luxated teeth. (a) Lateral luxation – may sever the pulp's neurovascular supply and compress areas of the root against the alveolus. (b) Intrusive luxation – invariably disrupts the pulp's neurovascular supply and drives the root end into the alveolus. (c) Extrusive luxation – may disrupt the pulp's neurovascular supply; periodontal fibers are torn rather than crushed. (d) Avulsion – complete loss of the tooth from the alveolus severs the pulp's neurovascular supply and exposes the root surface to considerable risk of damage.

Table 15.3   Alveolar fracture – classification, clinical features and risks of dental complication.

Description	Definition	Presenting symptoms	Risk of pulp death	Risk of resorption-promoting root-surface injury
Alveolar bone fracture	Fracture of tooth-supporting bone	Affected teeth may be mobile or displaced singly or *en masse*	Highly variable; greatest risk in teeth with mature apices that are directly involved in the fracture line	Highly variable; greatest risk in teeth directly involved in the fracture line

Low risk   Moderate risk   High risk

can dislocate teeth in a lateral, apical or coronal direction or even displace them completely from the alveolus (avulsion) (Fig. 15.3d).

Fractures to the alveolar process may cause individual or groups of teeth to become mobile, disrupt the neurovascular supply to their pulps resulting in transient or permanent loss of pulp functions (Table 15.3), or damage the surface of their roots.

The following sections will examine in greater detail how different types of injury endanger the pulp and

integrity of the root surface, and how unwanted complications may arise.

Dental trauma and its consequences

Flow diagram 15.1 provides a schematic overview of the complications, which may follow traumatic dental injuries.

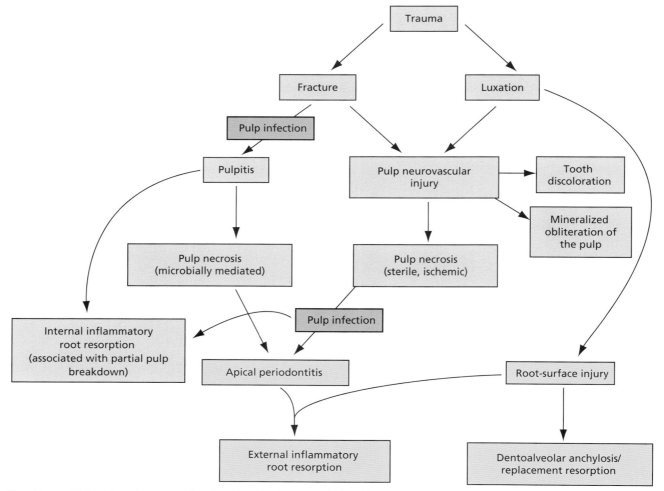

Flow diagram 15.1   Schematic representation of complications after traumatic dental injury.

Core concept 15.1

Trauma threatens pulp survival by:

(1) Exposing dentin and pulp to the mouth.
(2) Disrupting pulp blood supply.
(3) Altering pulp responses to diagnostic tests, and risking the unnecessary extirpation of a recovering pulp.
(4) Obliteration of the pulp space by mineralized tissue (contentious).

Traumatic injuries and the pulp

Both fracture and luxation injuries can have serious implications for the short- and long-term functions of the pulp (see Core concept 15.1).

Fractures

Uncomplicated crown fractures (Table 15.1, Fig. 15.2a) expose dentinal tubules to the mouth and create a potential gateway for pulp infection. The pulp is often in a healthy condition at the time of injury, and defensive mechanisms within the dentin–pulp complex protect the pulp from significant microbial invasion provided the exposed tissue is appropriately covered. More severe fractures which directly expose the pulp to the oral environment (Fig. 15.2b, c) may risk significant pulp infection and breakdown, but if properly managed by conservative non-invasive treatment (see further below and Chapter 4), there is a good chance of long-term pulp survival.

Luxations

On the other hand, luxation injuries frequently threaten the vital functions of the pulp. Neurovascular bundles are often torn when teeth are displaced or involved in fractures. At its most extreme, this may cause immediate, avascular necrosis of pulp tissue lying peripheral to the neurovascular tear (Fig. 15.4). Less severe disruption may cause only temporary ischemic injury of the pulp, but this may nevertheless reduce its defensive capacity and leave it vulnerable to otherwise trivial microbial challenges. Finally, an altered neurological response may complicate pulp diagnosis and result in the unnecessary extirpation of a healthy but non-responsive pulp (see further below, Diagnostic quandaries).

Another cause of neurovascular damage is from internal bleeding, due to rupture of the larger blood vessels in the pulp tissue *per se*. The bleeding reaction, if extensive, may result not only in reddening and later graying of the crown (38), but in breakdown of the entire tissue within a very short period of time.

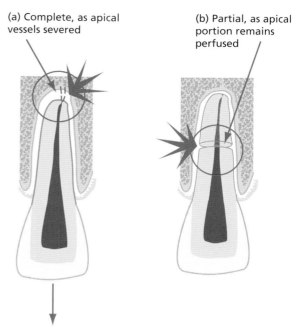

(a) Complete, as apical vessels severed

(b) Partial, as apical portion remains perfused

Fig. 15.4 Avascular necrosis after serious disruption of the pulp's neurovascular supply. (a) Complete, after displacement of a tooth with a mature apex. In teeth with open, immature apices, there is a reasonable prospect that the pulp may revascularize and recover. (b) Partial, after horizontal root fracture. Coronal pulp breakdown is not inevitable, but even if the pulp tissue in the coronal portion loses vitality, the apical fragment usually remains vital.

Only in teeth with immature, open apices can pulp revascularization be expected after significant displacement or avulsion (Table 15.2). Teeth with mature apices have limited capacity for pulp regeneration through the narrow apical foramen and complete, avascular pulp necrosis is almost certain after avulsion or intrusive luxation, and highly likely after extrusive or lateral luxation.

The prospects of pulp revascularization are generally higher in both mature and immature teeth after horizontal root fracture, and the well-perfused pulp of the apical fragment invariably remains vital even if complete pulp breakdown occurs in the coronal fragment. The level of the fracture line may have a significant bearing on outcome, with the greatest risk of coronal pulp breakdown after fractures involving the coronal third of the root (see Key literature 15.1).

Sterile, necrotic pulps may persist quietly in that state for many years, and are incapable of initiating or propagating apical periodontitis (9, 44). They do, however, provide a nutritious environment for microbial colonization, an event which will trigger the development of periapical inflammation and its consequences. In an apparently intact tooth with no obvious fractures, the likelihood of microorganisms invading the necrotic pulp may seem remote. But without a constant outflow of dentinal fluid, dentinal tubules present defenseless portals for microbial entry through exposed dentin

Key literature 15.1

Andreasen *et al.* (5, 6) reviewed 400 intra-alveolar root fractures in children and adolescents to identify factors associated with different healing patterns. Clinical and radiographic findings showed that 120 out of 400 teeth (30%) healed by hard-tissue fusion of the tooth fragments. Soft tissue (possibly periodontal ligament) alone was found in 170 teeth (43%), bone and soft connective tissue (possibly periodontal ligament) in 22 teeth (5%), and inflammatory tissue associated with necrosis of the coronal fragment in 88 teeth (22%). The preinjury and injury-related factors with the greatest influence on hard-tissue healing and pulp survival in the coronal fragment were patient age, stage of root development (i.e. the diameter of the pulp at the fracture site), mobility of the coronal fragment and the degree to which the coronal fragment had been displaced from the apical fragment.

When initial displacement of the coronal fragment was 1 mm or less, optimal repositioning and providing a splint, which allowed some degree of flexibility, promoted pulp survival and hard-tissue union. Splinting beyond 4 weeks conferred no additional benefit, and outcomes were not markedly worsened if treatment was delayed by a few days.

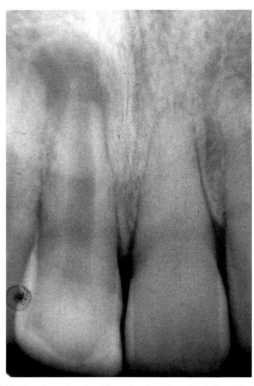

Fig. 15.5 Accelerated pulp obliteration by mineralized tissue in tooth 21 after trauma. The adjacent tooth 11 suffered pulp necrosis and arrested root development (see also Fig. 2.9).

surfaces, around restoration margins and even through microcracks in the overlying enamel (27). Direct pulp exposure allows unimpeded access for the oral flora. More contentious is the concept of anachoresis, where microorganisms gaining entry to the circulation from a variety of body sites (including the oral cavity and the gut) may be transported and seeded into areas of necrotic pulp tissue (37). It is rare for organisms other than oral residents to be recovered from infected pulp canals, suggesting that this may not be a major route of colonization (see Chapter 6).

Obliteration of the pulp space by mineralized tissue

Pulp volume diminishes throughout life by the physiological apposition of secondary dentin and by the deposition of tertiary dentin in response to localized insults. An additional and distinctive mineralized response is the accelerated formation of hard tissue after trauma; this may partially or completely obliterate the pulp space, particularly of young teeth (1). The incidence is highest after luxation injuries and changes may be identified as early as 3 months after injury, though 12 months is more common (Fig. 15.5; see also Fig. 2.9) (1). The mechanisms of this response are incompletely understood, though it has been postulated that odontoblasts, and perhaps other mesenchymal cell populations within the pulp, may lose autonomic regulatory control during neurovascular injury and regeneration, resulting in accelerated and disorganized hard-tissue deposition.

Histopathologically, the tissue often resembles osteodentin with an irregular tubular pattern and a maze of spaces and cul-de-sacs containing pulp cells which have become trapped within the rapidly deposited material (1). Clinically, the tooth may take on a yellow, or occasionally gray, hue as a result of the thickened and less translucent coronal dentin.

From a practical standpoint, it is important to understand whether pulp canal obliteration represents a degenerative change, leading ultimately to pulp breakdown and infection, and whether interventions to improve the appearance of the tooth such as orthodontic movement, veneer or crown preparation make these events more likely. A perennial question, which flows from this, is whether prophylactic root canal treatment is indicated to prevent apical periodontitis in all teeth that show signs of pulp space obliteration. A related question is whether there is any realistic hope of successfully treating pulp infection in an obliterated pulp space. As a worst-case scenario, Jacobsen and Kerekes (24) (see Key literature 15.2) observed apical periodontitis on 21% of teeth with complete pulp obliteration during a 10–23-year review period. They concluded that routine prophylactic root canal treatment could not be justified in all teeth showing signs of pulp space obliteration. Similar conclusions were drawn by Robertson *et al.* in 1996 (36); they found evidence of pulp necrosis in only 8.5% of teeth with pulp canal obliteration during a mean observation period of 16 years. This study provided

Key literature 15.2

Jacobsen and Kerekes (24) followed 122 traumatized anterior teeth with abnormal hard-tissue development in their pulp chambers for 10–23 years (mean 16 years) in order to assess the progress of hard-tissue deposition and determine the risk of pulp breakdown with apical periodontitis. Overall, 44 teeth (36%) persisted in a partially obliterated state, while 78 (64%) went on to complete obliteration. None of the partially and 16 (21%) of the completely obliterated teeth developed apical periodontitis. Significantly, 45 of the 52 teeth (86%) with severe injuries (luxation, extreme subluxation, root fracture with dislocation and deep coronal dentin fracture), compared with 26 of the 51 teeth (51%) with moderate injuries (slight subluxation, undisplaced root fracture, enamel or shallow coronal dentin fracture), developed complete obliteration. Again significantly, ten of the 52 severely injured (21%) and only two of the 51 of the moderately injured teeth (4%) developed apical periodontitis. Other risk factors for late pulp breakdown included complete root formation at the time of injury, and a relatively rapid rate of mineralization.

It was concluded that even if 21% of completely obliterated teeth developed pulp necrosis and apical periodontitis, this was insufficient justification to routinely conduct root canal treatment on all teeth with signs of pulp space obliteration.

further insight into the impact of caries, new trauma, orthodontic treatment and crown/veneer preparation on pulp survival. None of these additional insults had a significant impact on pulp survival, and it was concluded that, although the incidence of pulp necrosis increased with time in teeth with pulp canal obliteration, routine prophylactic endodontics did not seem justified (1, 36).

In the event of pulp breakdown, clinical data from the early 1980s (16) suggest that root canal treatment is possible and can result in complete healing in 80% of cases. The situation may well have improved in the light of contemporary microscope-assisted endodontic practice for canal detection, and developments in endodontic microsurgery may have created additional possibilities for the successful management of teeth which cannot be treated non-surgically.

Consequences of pulp breakdown and infection after trauma

Key endodontic consequences of pulpal necrosis and subsequent infection after trauma include inflammatory bone resorption, inflammatory root resorption and the arrest of dental development.

Inflammatory bone resorption

As described in Chapter 7, infected pulps cause inflammatory lesions in the alveolar bone adjacent to any portal of pulp–periodontal communication. It is critical to note that teeth damaged by trauma may present new path-

ways of communication which did not exist previously, such as fractures through the body of the root and tubular communications through dentinal tubules which have been made patent by the loss of root-surface cementum. Damage to the root surface is least likely when the periodontal ligament is stretched or torn, and most likely when the periodontium is crushed, dehydrated, handled or heavily soiled. Tables 15.1–15.3 present the likely risks of root-surface injury associated with different categories of trauma. Tooth avulsions, which expose the whole root surface to injury (Fig. 15.3d), and lateral and intrusive luxations which drive areas of the root against the walls of the alveolar socket (Fig. 15.3a, b) present the greatest risk. Open dentinal tubules, combined with an infected pulp, provide the conditions for periradicular inflammation in the bone adjacent to the open tubules, and for external inflammatory root resorption, a particularly damaging and unwanted complication.

Inflammatory root resorption

While alveolar bone exists in a state of constant remodeling, the intact teeth which it supports are usually unaffected. The most likely explanation is that incompletely mineralized layers of predentin and precementum cover the internal and external surfaces of teeth, respectively, and inhibit resorptive activity (47). Injuries, which cause these surfaces to be damaged, lost or mineralized make them vulnerable to resorption, as mononuclear phagocytes rapidly migrate to the area and coalesce to form multinuclear clastic cells of the monocyte lineage, termed "odontoclasts". Resorption is likely to commence soon after, but may be short-lived. The activity of clastic cells requires constant stimulation and in the absence of a propagating stimulus, the resorption will be only "transient" (46). These "surface" resorption defects arrest within 2–3 weeks and are repaired by cementum-like material. If, on the other hand, there is a propagating stimulus, such as periradicular inflammation caused by pulp–space infection (Fig. 15.6a), resorption is likely to progress: "external inflammatory root resorption". Hard tissue can be destroyed rapidly and there is great danger in watching and waiting if areas of external root resorption are identified on teeth with non-vital pulps. Removal of the propagating stimulus predictably arrests external inflammatory root resorption. Cvek (14) reported 97% success after treatment, which included an interim calcium hydroxide dressing. The need for intracanal medication with calcium hydroxide is by no means certain, however (14).

External inflammatory root resorption is usually identified on routine radiographic review as punched-out areas of hard-tissue loss from the root surface (Fig. 15.6b), associated with radiolucent areas in the adjacent alveolar bone. Lesions on the labial or lingual root surface can be

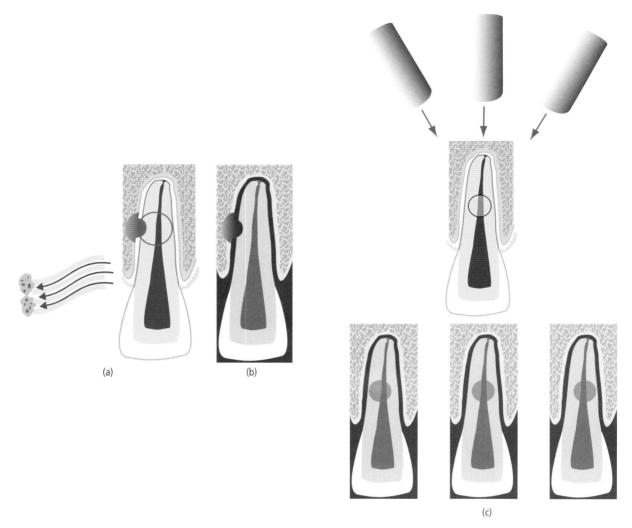

Fig. 15.6 External inflammatory root resorption. (a) Propagated by an infected, necrotic pulp. Trauma has resulted in concomitant root surface injury and pulp breakdown. Secondary infection of the pulp provides the propagating stimulus necessary for progressive resorption, microbial elements diffusing to the root surface through patent dentinal tubules. (b) A characteristically punched-out area the of root surface with an associated bone radiolucency. (c) Labially or palatally placed lesions shift with changes of radiographic angle and may be superimposed by the "tram-lines" of the pulp canal walls.

confused with internal resorption (see Fig. 15.8), but a change in the radiographic angle usually reveals that the lesion moves in relation to the root canal, and the lateral margins of the pulp canal are usually superimposed (Fig. 15.6c). Exciting developments in the diagnostic imaging of resorptive lesions (13, 33) are introduced in Advanced concept 15.1.

External inflammatory root resorption can arise at any level of the root surface and may present in the cervical region where it communicates with the oral environment: "cervical" or "extracanal invasive" resorption (Fig. 15.7a). Although the pathogenesis is incompletely understood, traumatic injury to the cervical part of the root has been suggested as a risk factor (23), and the infected pulp space may again serve as the propagating stimulus. It must, however, be borne in mind that such

lesions may also occur in teeth which have no known history of trauma and in teeth with healthy pulps. Some considerations in the clinical management of cervical resorption are outlined in Advanced concept 15.2.

Internal inflammatory root resorption

A similar process, internal inflammatory root resorption, may arise within a tooth after damage or mineralization of areas of predentin lining the pulp chamber (Fig. 15.8). This could arise after a blow which causes intrapulpal hemorrhage and localized compression with death of odontoblasts. Damaged surfaces, or surfaces which have become mineralized following direct exposure to tissue fluids, are again believed to be colonized by clastic cells derived from mononuclear phagocytes (50), which begin

Advanced concept 15.1   The potential of three-dimensional imaging

Imaging techniques are necessary to reveal the anatomical location of normal and pathological structures in three planes. The limitations of conventional plain-films are well recognized, but recent developments in three-dimensional digital imaging, including computed tomography, magnetic resonance imaging and most recently cone beam computed tomography, have opened up exciting new opportunities for diagnosis and treatment planning. Cone beam tomography is rapidly becoming established as an invaluable tool in trauma management, providing volumetric images of diagnostic resolution but without excessive cost or exposure to ionizing radiation. In the case of dental root resorption, it allows lesions to be accurately localized (external or internal, buccal or palatal), their volumetric extent to be assessed and any complications such as pulp/periodontal communications and pathological root fractures to be identified; all critical to diagnosis, treatment and prognosis (13, 33). Further developments, including flat panel volumetric computed tomography, are likely to improve image resolution and diagnostic yield in years to come, making even the visualization of vertical root fractures and cracks a realistic possibility (13).

Advanced concept 15.2   Cervical resorption

Clinically, cervical resorption may be identified during the examination of localized gingival inflammation around the neck of a tooth, or as a "pink spot" caused by invasion of the crown by vascular resorptive tissue. Careful exploration of the gingival crevice may reveal a small entry point from which the lesion may burrow extensively. Diagnosis is commonly a chance radiographic finding, with a characteristically sited radiolucency (Fig. 15.7b).

Treatment note: Cervical resorptions may be propagated by the infected contents of the pulp canal, but unlike external inflammatory resorptions, which are sited more deeply, simple root canal treatment is not enough. The resorptive tissue must be formally eliminated by a combination of physical curettage and chemical means (most commonly trichloroacetic acid) (23). On many occasions, this can be done internally, but where access is difficult, or where the area of communication with the marginal periodontium is extensive, open (surgical) debridement is indicated. The defect is then repaired with an appropriate restorative material, which seals the resorbed area from the oral environment. If the affected tooth has a vital pulp, open debridement and restoration are indicated without resorting to pulp extirpation.

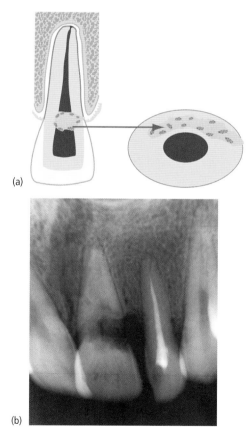

(a)

(b)

Fig. 15.7 Cervical resorption. (a) A characteristically placed lesion, which may be visible as a pink discoloration through the crown. The external entry point may be small, though the resorption burrows extensively within dentin. (b) Radiographic appearance. In this case, the lesion is extensive and has broad communication with the marginal periodontium, necessitating open debridement and restoration.

the process of transient (internal) root resorption. In many circumstances, the entire pulp will proceed to break down, denying nutrition to the clastic cells and arresting the resorptive process. In others, the pulp may recover, and in the absence of a propagating stimulus, resorption would be expected to cease within 2–3 weeks.

On rare occasions, the pulp may partially break down, with infected, necrotic pulp tissue coronally and vital pulp tissue persisting apically. Tissue at the interface persists in an inflamed state, under the influence of microbial elements within the necrotic coronal pulp. It has been postulated that branching, transverse communications between dentinal tubules may provide a pathway for microbial products to act as a propagating stimulus for progressive internal inflammatory root resorption (Fig. 15.8a) (46). This form of resorption expands the pulp canal in a characteristically symmetrical, ballooning fashion. Internal root resorptions may be detected as a chance radiographic finding, or present with painful symptoms when the lesion has perforated the root surface. Occasionally, lesions affecting the coronal third of the root may cause pink discoloration of the crown.

Internal and external inflammatory root resorptions can be confused radiographically, though it is unusual to observe the lateral margins of the pulp canal superimposed on an internal resorption. Additionally, since internal resorption represents expansion of the canal, its relationship is unlikely to change with alterations of radiographic angle (Fig. 15.8a).

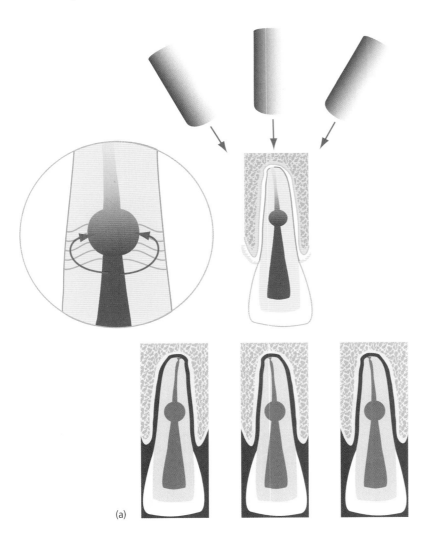

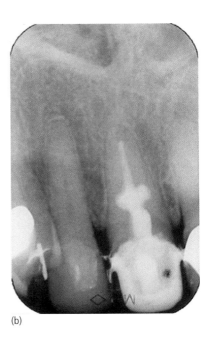

(b)

Fig. 15.8 Internal inflammatory root resorption. (a) Characteristic, symmetrical expansion of the pulp space is noted at the interface between necrotic and vital tissue. The resorbed area has a constant relationship to the pulp space with alteration of the radiographic horizontal angle. There are no superimposed "tram-lines" of the pulp chamber walls running across the resorbed area (compare with Fig. 15.6c). (b) Root canal filling with thermoplastic gutta-percha. (Courtesy of Dr Jeremy Hayes.)

The conditions which must prevail for internal resorption to develop (persistent partial pulp necrosis, suitable vertical communications through dentin) mean that this is a rare condition. Consequently, details of its pathogenesis remain unclear, and there has been some debate whether the tissue at the interface between necrotic and vital pulp simply represents typical inflamed pulp tissue. One report (51) has suggested that this tissue differs markedly from normal pulp tissue, having either been replaced by ingrowing periodontal connective tissue, or undergone metaplasia to such.

Whatever the details of its pathogenesis, internal resorption can progress rapidly and should be considered a form of irreversible pulpitis, which needs immediate treatment. It is predictably arrested if the propagating stimulus (infected pulp tissue) is removed by pulpectomy, which also severs the blood supply to the resorbing cells. Notes on its clinical management are contained in Clinical procedure 15.1.

Non-inflammatory root resorption

Traumatized teeth can also be affected by replacement resorption. This is not a condition fuelled by necrotic pulp tissue, pulp infection or periapical inflammation, but is a case of mistaken identity during healing after extensive damage to the root surface. Injuries most often associated with extensive root-surface injury are intrusive and lateral luxations, which crush the attachment apparatus against the alveolus (Fig. 15.3a, b). This type of resorption is also a common sequela to avulsions in which drying or scrubbing of the root surface, or storage of the tooth in an inappropriate solution causes significant cell death on the root surface (Fig. 15.9a).

After repositioning or reimplantation, tissues around the damaged root may heal in two distinct patterns. Ideally, a periodontal ligament is fully re-established (Fig. 15.9b) following the migration of periodontal fibroblasts to cover the areas of root which were denuded of cells. Complete re-establishment of the periodontal liga-

Clinical procedure 15.1	Clinical considerations in the management of internal inflammatory root resorption

During the root canal treatment of internally resorbed teeth:

- Access is usually to a necrotic coronal pulp, but bleeding can be torrential as instruments advance into the intensely inflamed resorptive tissue. This can be controlled by instrumenting to full working length to sever the pulp's blood supply and by copious sodium hypochlorite irrigation.
- Tissue residing in the expanded area of the canal is impossible to instrument mechanically and should be eliminated by a combination of sodium hypochlorite irrigation (often with ultrasonic activation to throw irrigant into the expanded region) and intracanal medication, traditionally non-setting calcium hydroxide. For lesions which are located coronally, and which afford good visibility, consideration may be given to chemical debridement with trichloroacetic acid (refer to Advanced concept 15.2).
- The expanded area is not amenable to filling with cold laterally condensed gutta-percha. Thermoplastic filling techniques are usually best employed (Fig. 15.8b).
- Alternative materials such as MTA or fiber posts and composite may offer new opportunities for the rehabilitation of teeth whose canals have been hollowed out by internal resorption.

ment protects the tooth from resorptive activity in the surrounding bone. Research work continues on local and systematic agents which may actively promote periodontal repair, such as enamel matrix proteins (39) and tetracyclines (in patients over 12 years of age) with their anticollagenolytic activity (12).

Alternatively, and especially if the denuded area is extensive, bone cells may grow into direct continuity with areas of root dentin, fusing the root with bone (Fig. 15.9b, c). Healing to bone without a fibrous joint is termed dentoalveolar ankylosis, and is analogous to the fusion or osseointegration of an implant with bone. Once direct contact is established, cells in the alveolar bone will involve the tooth in its remodeling activity, and gradually replace it with bone: replacement resorption (Fig. 15.9d).

Teeth with any degree of dentoalveolar ankylosis present with no physiological mobility and a characteristically bright percussion note as sound waves reverberate through the facial skeleton, rather than being dampened by a cushioning periodontal ligament. Radiographically, the periodontal ligament space in the area is not readily discerned. In time, the root will become increasingly difficult to differentiate from bone (Fig. 15.9e). The speed at which the process develops varies, however, and it may

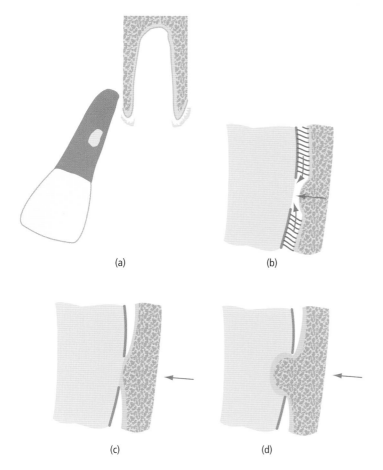

(a)   (b)

(c)   (d)

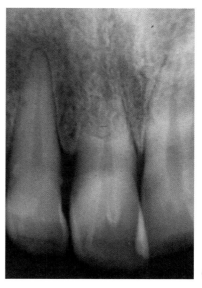

(e)

Fig. 15.9 Root surface healing after tooth avulsion. (a) Localized necrosis and loss of root surface periodontal tissues after tooth avulsion. (b) The defect may be covered by migration of periodontal fibroblasts and re-establishment of a periodontal ligament, or by migration of bone cells causing ankylosis. (c) Localized bony ankylosis will inevitably lead to progressive replacement resorption as the root becomes involved in bony remodeling. (d) Area of tooth undergoing replacement resorption. (e) Radiographic appearance of a tooth undergoing replacement resorption. There is no bony radiolucency indicative of inflammation and areas of the root are difficult to distinguish from bone.

take years or even decades for the root to be completely lost, the tooth remaining rock-solid throughout. Late complications may include gradual infraocclusion (especially in the young) as adjacent teeth and their supporting alveoli adopt mature positions, and the development of periodontal infections as replacement resorption extends to communicate with the gingival crevice.

There is no treatment to arrest or reverse replacement resorption, and all efforts should be made to minimize root surface damage and prevent it from developing in the first place.

It should be understood that ankylosed teeth can also have infected pulps and that inflammatory resorption can coexist with replacement resorption. The aggressive inflammatory resorption once again responds predictably to conventional treatment, but thought may be given to the use of a root filling material, which may resorb as the root is inevitably lost to the slowly progressing replacement resorption.

Arrest of dental development

A primary role of dentists is to preserve pulp health until tooth development is complete (see Chapter 4). If complete pulp breakdown is unavoidable, or if pulp-preserving treatment fails, a tooth with an unfavorable crown/root ratio and a root with thin, fragile walls (Fig. 15.10a) may result. A wide and often diverging root apex complicates root canal treatment and restorative considerations must focus on coronal seal as well as reinforcing the tooth against fracture.

If immature teeth lose pulp vitality and root canal treatment is required, efforts should be made to clean the canal without undue loss of structurally important dentin. Cleaning can often be accomplished with ultrasonically activated sodium hypochlorite, rather than extensive dentin removal (30). Closure of the root end has traditionally involved dressing the canal with non-setting calcium hydroxide, replaced at 3 monthly intervals for 9–24 months. Lengthy treatment of this sort tests patient compliance, and growing concerns about tooth embrittlement and cervical root fracture following long-term medication with calcium hydroxide (4, 17) have prompted a search for alternatives.

MTA, packed with or without a resorbable matrix, has become established as a one-step root-end closure procedure (Fig. 15.10b), and a recent prospective study in patients aged between 7 and 53 has validated this approach (42).

The practice of backfilling wide canals with gutta-percha has also been challenged, as bonded materials may be able to offer internal reinforcement (Fig. 15.11). Knowledge of bonding to radicular dentin is limited, and most research in this area is, as yet, laboratory based. Composite resins (25, 34), in combination with contemporary fiber post systems (10, 22), may offer real potential for the future, but accomplishing an ideally bonded restoration within the root canal space continues to present formidable challenges, including those of smear layer management, variable tubule availability for resin tag formation, adhesive application, air entrapment and polymerization contraction within resin-based materials. The theory remains simpler than the reality (45).

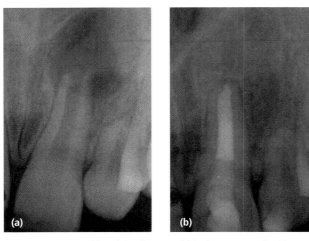

Fig. 15.10   Arrested dental development. (a) An immature tooth with arrested root development after trauma. (b) Periapical healing 12 months after orthograde root canal filling with MTA, overlaid with thermoplastic gutta-percha and sealer. (Courtesy of Dr Bader Al-Baqshi.)

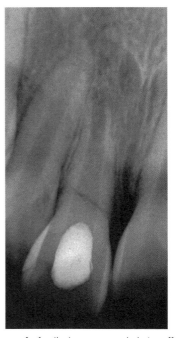

Fig. 15.11   Fracture of a fragile, immature tooth during efforts to preserve it by root canal treatment. (Courtesy of Dr Ingegerd Mejàre.)

Having now considered the key events which may arise after dental trauma, the following sections will describe the clinical management of traumatic injuries and the measures which may optimize the healing potential of the tissues involved.

General considerations in the management of dental trauma

Best trauma management is generally informed not by the outcome of randomized, controlled clinical trials, but by epidemiological surveys, retrospective surveys, case reports and expert opinion. Immediate and longer-term actions may be critical to outcome, and detailed consensus-based guidelines published by the International Association of Dental Traumatology (20, 21) provide a readily available framework for structured short- and long-term management. A downloadable version is available without charge at www.iadt-dentaltrauma.org. The reader is also referred to well-established, comprehensive textbooks of dental traumatology (7) and shorter texts for chairside reference (53).

Immediate management of patients with dentoalveolar trauma

Patients attending for emergency care are likely to be distressed not only by the incident, but also by the appearance of swollen and bleeding orofacial tissues. Care may be especially challenging for children and for adolescents and adults under the influence of drugs and alcohol. Patients should of course be managed sympathetically, but with confidence and efficiency to identify key injuries and implement necessary initial treatment.

General details of the incident should be quickly ascertained, medical history reviewed and significant maxillofacial or head injuries in need of secondary referral identified. Tetanus immunization should be checked if wounds are likely to have been contaminated with soil.

Clinical examination

Examination should commence with gentle face washing and, sometimes, mouth rinsing to improve patient comfort and clarify the position and extent of injuries.

Fractured, mobile, displaced and avulsed teeth should be identified by clinical examination. A structured dental examination is helped by the use of a standardized template (Fig. 15.12). Where possible, the baseline pulp condition of injured and adjacent teeth should be assessed by thermal (usually cold challenge with ethyl chloride) and electronic sensibility testing. Currently, the single most useful test for assessing the neurovascular status of the pulp in a traumatized tooth is the electronic pulp test (8). Output is often numerical, allowing responses to be tracked over time. Emergency care should rarely involve pulp extirpation, and sensibility data serve principally as a baseline to monitor the recovery or otherwise of vital pulp functions (see later section on Diagnostic quandaries).

Radiographic examination

The maturity of traumatized teeth, and the extent of injuries affecting the root and supporting tissues cannot be assessed on clinical parameters alone. Even teeth which appear firm and undisplaced may be associated with intra-alveolar root fractures or fractures of alveolar bone; good-quality radiographs form an essential part of

Tooth	13	12	11	21	22	23
Color						
Mobility						
Percussion tenderness						
Cold pulp test						
Electronic pulp test						
Radiograph						
Other notes						

Fig. 15.12   A standardized template such as a "trauma stamp" can provide a structured framework for initial and follow-up clinical examination and allow convenient monitoring of responses and observations over time. No single test should be taken in isolation as a picture builds of pulp and periradicular condition.

patient evaluation, diagnosis, treatment planning and monitoring in all cases of dental trauma.

In most settings, imaging is limited to plain radiographic films, and their limitations should be recognized. Root fractures, for example, may not be imaged well unless they happen to run parallel with the central radiographic beam. For this reason, exposures from more than one angle are generally recommended. The first intraoral film should be at a 90° horizontal angle, centering on the tooth in question. This may readily identify horizontal root fractures, especially those in the cervical third of the root (20), but if more apical or oblique fractures are suspected, further periapical films exposed from a mesial or distal angulation, or occlusal films may be helpful. Single intraoral views may be acceptable to confirm tooth luxations, though, again, additional films may help to rule out hitherto unsuspected injuries. Lateral soft-tissue views should be exposed if injuries to the lips raise suspicion that they may contain fragments of broken tooth or other foreign bodies, and extraoral plain and tomographic views may be considered if there is any indication of alveolar fracture (20). Three-dimensional digital imaging presents considerable advantages for the assessment of complex trauma, and may ultimately replace plain film imaging as the technology becomes more affordable and accessible (see Advanced concept 15.1).

Immediate and long-term management of patients with dental trauma

The central goals of immediate and ongoing care are summarized in Core concept 15.2.

Core concept 15.2

Immediate treatment of traumatic injuries aims to secure comfortable function and promote healing by:

(1) Covering exposed dentin and pulp.
(2) Repositioning and stabilizing displaced and mobile teeth.
(3) Providing information on general mouthcare, nutrition and analgesia.
(4) Stressing the need for follow-up.

Ongoing management of traumatic injuries aims to preserve a healthy, functional and esthetic tooth by:

(1) Monitoring pulp status.
(2) Monitoring tooth position and stability.
(3) Monitoring for signs of secondary conditions, such as root resorption.
(4) Promoting general mouthcare.
(5) Stressing the need for ongoing review.

Fractured teeth – coronal and crown–root fractures

The overriding principle when a patient appears with any form of fractured tooth, be it an uncomplicated crown fracture, a complicated crown fracture or a crown–root fracture, is to protect the exposed tissue from further microbial exposure. Ideally, fragments of tooth are re-attached with dentin/enamel adhesives, or the crown/root is rebuilt with composite resin. Often, however, a simple coverage of glass ionomer cement is the most realistic emergency care followed by an early recall for definitive coronal restoration. In the case of crown–root fracture, gingival hemostasis may be needed for proper assessment of the injury and to assist the bonding of moisture-sensitive materials.

If the pulp is not directly exposed, the risk of pulpal breakdown is minimal, provided the exposed dentin is effectively and promptly covered. It is critical that leakage potentials are limited. In crown–root fractures where moisture control is difficult, a leaky restoration may result in pulpal complications (hypersensitivity, pulpitis and pulp necrosis) at a later date. Therefore, guidelines currently recommend clinical and radiographic review of pulp status at 6–8 weeks and 1 year (20), though more frequent assessment may be deemed appropriate. Fractured teeth may also have suffered concomitantly from a luxation injury that went unnoticed. The follow-up scheme should include checks for developing pulp necrosis due to circulatory disturbance and any signs of external inflammatory root resorption (see Fig. 15.6).

When the pulp is directly exposed to the mouth, it should be borne in mind that unlike the cariously exposed pulp, the traumatically exposed pulp is rarely deeply inflamed and can resist significant infection for some time. Cvek (15) observed favorable healing responses in teeth with traumatic pulp exposures, even when the area of tissue exposure was extensive and treatment was delayed for up to 1 month. This does not provide any justification for postponing treatment, since pulp tissue which is open to the oral environment is always at risk of microbial invasion, progressive infected pulp necrosis and its consequences. It does, however, point to the considerable healing potential, particularly of young pulps, if a conducive environment is created.

Recognizing the likelihood of superficial microbial contamination and inflammation, Cvek (15) performed a superficial pulpotomy with a high-speed diamond bur under rubber dam isolation and strict asepsis. After hemostasis with physiological saline, the wound was covered with calcium hydroxide before sealing coronally. Crown–root fractures present special challenges, and in these circumstances, the entire coronal pulp was removed in order to avoid its constriction and subsequent necrosis following hard-tissue repair. Cvek's report described follow-up at 3 weeks, 3, 6 and 12 months, though current guidelines suggest clinical and radiographic review at 6–8 weeks and 12 months after treatment (20). Signs of unfavorable outcome which may indicate the need for root canal treatment include the development of:

• overt pulpits or acute symptoms of apical periodontitis;
• persistent negative responses to pulp testing;
• signs of apical periodontitis;
• in the case of immature teeth, arrest of dental development.

Further consideration of vital pulp treatments, including the potential of MTA, particularly the non-staining white version, as an alternative pulpotomy wound dressing (20, 54) can be found in Chapter 4.

Fractured teeth – intra-alveolar root fractures

Root fractures may present in any plane and at any level of the root. If the coronal portion of the tooth has not been displaced and is not mobile, the root fracture may not be identified during clinical examination, and single radiographic views, which fail to capture the fracture line, may also result in a missed diagnosis. Radiographs exposed from more than one angle are always indicated when root fractures are suspected. In many circumstances the fracture line may be oblique, or the radiographic angle may project it as such, giving the impression of two fracture lines with an interposing section of tooth tissue (see Fig. 15.2e).

Key considerations are whether the neurovascular supply to the pulp has been disrupted at the fracture line, and whether there is any likelihood that the fracture will reunite.

Andreasen and Hjørting-Hansen (3) described four patterns of tissue response following intra-alveolar root fracture (Fig. 15.13). In the first (Fig. 15.13a), the coronal and apical fragments become reunited by mineralized tissue, which may be of dentinoid or cementumoid origin. In all other categories, the fragments of root do not reunite, but the coronal portion of tooth is retained, with the fracture line occupied by soft connective tissue (possibly periodontal ligament) (Fig. 15.13b), bone and soft connective tissue (possibly periodontal ligament) (Fig. 15.13c), or granulation tissue, representing an inflammatory response to either pulp or gingival infection, and with associated expansion of the fracture line and lateral radiolucencies (Fig. 15.13d). Regardless of events in the coronal pulp or at the fracture line, the pulp in the apical fragment almost always remained vital.

In an effort to understand the factors associated with healing patterns, Andreasen and co-workers (5, 6) undertook a retrospective study of 400 intra-alveolar root fractures, correlating outcome with preinjury, injury and treatment factors. The findings are summarized in Key

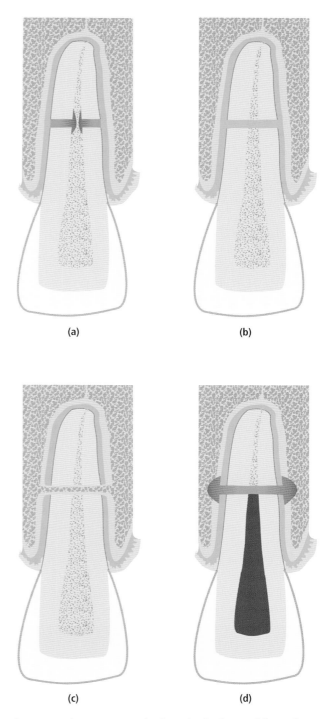

(a)   (b)

(c)   (d)

Fig. 15.13 Tissue responses after intra-alveolar fracture (after Andreasen and Hjørting-Hansen (3)). (a) Reuniting of the tooth fragments with hard tissue. (b) Fracture line occupied by healthy soft connective tissue (possibly periodontal ligament). (c) Fracture line occupied by bone and soft connective tissue (possibly periodontal ligament). (d) Fracture line occupied by chronic inflammatory tissue following pulp breakdown and infection in the coronal element. There are associated areas of inflammation in the adjacent alveolar bone.

literature 15.1. The prognosis for survival of the coronal fragment is worst when fractures involve the cervical third of the root (52). Even with prolonged or rigid splinting, the crown to supported root ratio may be hopeless and the risks of microbial infection from the mouth are considerable.

If there is no displacement and the crown is not mobile, repositioning and splinting may be unnecessary (6). If there is displacement and if it is considered that there will be sufficient bone to support the coronal fragment, it should be gently repositioned with clinical and radiographic checks to avoid traumatic occlusal contacts and ensure good approximation. Repositioned or mobile teeth should be stabilized with a flexible splint such as wire and composite resin (Fig. 15.14), or a dedicated flexible titanium "trauma splint" (49) which allows both physiological mobility and access for meticulous plaque control. Splinting is generally continued for 4 weeks to allow periodontal healing and to provide optimal conditions for the development of a hard-tissue union across the fracture line. Fractures in the cervical third may never heal properly, but may be stabilized for up to 4 months in an effort to promote tissue repair and tooth preservation (20).

The stability and pulp condition of teeth with root fractures should be further monitored at 6–8 weeks, 4 months, 6 months, 1 year and 5 years (20). Evidence of pulp breakdown in the coronal element, such as persistent negative pulp sensitivity testing or the development of radiolucency at the fracture line, is an indication for root canal treatment. During root canal treatment, instrumentation and root canal filling should be limited to the fracture line only (18) as the apical pulp usually retains vital functions. Efforts are sometimes made to develop a mineralized barrier at this level by repeated calcium hydroxide medication. A contemporary alternative is to place 3–4 mm thickness of MTA back from the fracture line (40), before filling the remainder of the canal with thermoplastic gutta-percha and sealer or with bonded

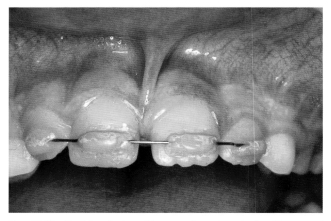

Fig. 15.14 Flexible splinting with composite resin and wire. (Courtesy of Dr Vidya Srinivasan.)

composite resin. If apical periodontitis develops on the apical fragment, it is better to remove this surgically rather than attempt root canal treatment across the fracture line (16) (Fig. 15.15).

Luxated teeth

Luxation injuries vary in severity and extent. At their most serious, they can displace teeth entirely from the mouth, move them to a position where they interfere with oral functions, or leave them unacceptably mobile. Luxation may disturb or sever the pulp's neurovascular supply, tear or crush the attachment apparatus and, in the case of avulsion, expose the root surface to any number of insults, including drying and mechanical abrasion (Table 15.2).

Emergency treatment must focus on restoring comfortable function and optimizing the conditions for re-establishment of periodontal attachment and restoration of the pulp's neurovascular supply. In practical terms, that means reimplanting avulsed teeth without delay, repositioning displaced teeth and supporting any teeth which are unstable with an appropriate splint (see Core concept 15.2). As in the case of horizontal root fractures, luxated teeth should be supported by a flexible splint, which allows some degree of physiological movement. This not only promotes periodontal healing, which after a simple tearing injury should be well established within 2 weeks and essentially complete by 8 weeks (29), but also diminishes the risks of ankylosis.

The emergency visit should also establish baseline pulp responses, which will be essential in assessing the restoration of vital pulp functions over time. Generally, teeth with open apices are more likely to recover healthy pulp functions after neurovascular injury than those with mature apices. However, after major disruption such as avulsion or intrusive luxation, even the immature tooth is at significant risk of pulp breakdown (see Table 15.2). For the mature tooth, loss of pulp vitality is all but certain after avulsion or intrusive luxation and is a greater than 50% risk after extrusive and lateral luxations. Even if avascular pulp necrosis is certain, pulpectomy is rarely performed at the emergency visit. Rather, the patient is allowed to recover from the traumatic episode and necessary interventions to preserve their tooth before returning, usually within 7–10 days, to re-evaluate pulp status and commence the root canal treatment if needed.

Concussion and subluxation

In the case of concussion and subluxation, little active treatment is needed, though teeth which are uncomfortably mobile can be supported with a splint for up to 2 weeks.

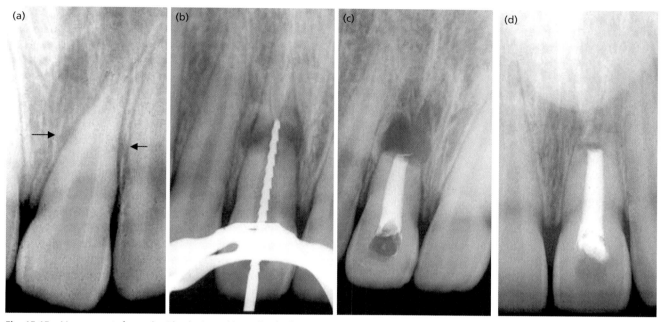

Fig. 15.15   Management of a tooth with a horizontal intra-alveolar fracture in an 11-year-old boy. (a) Radiograph taken 2 weeks after traumatic injury. Small radiolucent areas at the mid-root portion (arrows) suggest the potential of an intra-alveolar root fracture. Three months after injury the patient presents with a fistulous tract at the buccal aspect of the tooth. Radiographic examination confirms a horizontal fracture, with clear separation of the tooth fragments and a bone lesion associated with the fracture line. (b) Trial file radiograph in conjunction with endodontic treatment of the coronal fragment. Despite efforts to control the root canal infection, the lesion did not resolve. A surgical procedure was therefore carried out at which the apical fragment was removed, the area debrided and the root canal filled with gutta-percha (c). (d) 5-year follow-up. (Courtesy of Dr Gunnar Bergenholtz.)

Extrusive, lateral and intrusive luxation

Teeth which have suffered extrusive luxation (Fig. 15.3c) should be gently reinserted into their sockets and generally require only 2 weeks of splinting for the torn attachment apparatus to be restored.

Lateral luxation (Fig. 15.3a) may often require the tooth to be disengaged with forceps before gentle repositioning into its original location. Healing here involves more than just the repair of torn periodontal fibers, and splinting is routinely extended to 4 weeks in order to support the tooth until bony and periodontal healing are sufficient to make the tooth comfortable and secure in gentle function. Supplementary occlusal adjustments may also be necessary to promote comfort and limit functional trauma while healing takes place.

Intrusive luxations (Fig. 15.3b) are likely to have a devastating impact on the neurovascular supply to the pulp. Immature teeth may have some prospect of recovery, but the chances will be reduced greatly if any attempt is made to suddenly reposition the intruded tooth. The tooth should be allowed to extrude naturally, or with some orthodontic assistance if there has been no movement within 3 weeks. In the case of mature teeth, the pulp is almost certainly non-vital (Table 15.2) and no further harm will be done by surgical repositioning and splinting for 2–4 weeks, or by rapid extrusion with a fixed orthodontic appliance (20).

The need for general mouthcare and for careful long-term monitoring must be made clear to all patients who have suffered dental trauma. Follow-up appointments with clinical and radiographic examination should be arranged between 2 and 4 weeks after the injury (depending on the needs for splint removal and pulpectomy), at 6–8 weeks, 6 months, 1 year and annually up to 5 years. Minor concussion or subluxation injuries may only require follow-up at 4 weeks, 6–8 weeks and 1 year (20).

Each recall appointment should be informed by a structured template (Fig. 15.12) and include an assessment of symptoms, tooth position and stability, percussion note and pulp sensibility (see later section on Diagnostic quandaries). Radiographs should be inspected carefully to monitor periodontal healing, and identify early signs of periapical inflammation or root resorption.

Avulsion

The potential for periodontal healing and the recovery of vital pulp functions after tooth avulsion (Figs 15.3d and 15.11) warrants special consideration.

Teeth should generally be reimplanted as soon as possible after avulsion and supported by a flexible splint for just 2 weeks while the periodontal ligament is restored. Whether a periodontal ligament will re-establish over the entire root surface will depend on the degree of root surface injury. Key factors are the "extraoral dry time" and the way the tooth was handled. Teeth with an extraoral dry time of less than 1 hour, which have not been scrubbed, and have been maintained in conditions compatible with cell survival on the root surface (in the socket, the mouth, in milk or in tissue culture media such as Hank's Balanced Salt Solution) have the best chance of periodontal regeneration. Consideration should be given to the prescription of tetracyclines, with their proven anticollagenolytic activity to actively promote periodontal regeneration (12). This should not be carried out in young patients as tetracyclines bind to the mineralized component of developing teeth, causing discoloration.

Teeth with an extraoral dry time of greater than 1 hour, or which have been scrubbed or stored in nonphysiological solutions, are likely to have extensive root surface damage, and periodontal healing is not expected (21). In this case, the best healing response which can be anticipated is dentoalveolar ankylosis. While this will re-establish the tooth in a firm position, it will inevitably be followed by progressive replacement root resorption, resulting ultimately in tooth loss. Complications along the way may include communication of the resorptive lesion with the gingival crevice, which may promote troublesome periodontal infection and breakdown. Another undesirable complication is infraocclusion, where the ankylosed tooth remains in position as dentoalveolar growth moves adjacent teeth to mature positions. In short, dentoalveolar ankylosis and replacement resorption are undesirable outcomes, and should be prevented wherever possible.

In reality, clinicians faced with a tooth displaying signs of significant periodontal damage may have little choice but to reimplant it under optimal conditions and hope that the tooth will provide trouble-free service for as long as possible. In this situation, it is recommended that necrotic periodontal tissues are removed from the root surface with gauze before reimplantation (21), since failure to do so will result in breakdown of the surface tissues, periradicular inflammation and an increased risk that the tooth will not heal in place. Animal studies continue on the potential of attenuating such risks with local or systemic steroids (11), though these measures are not formally established in clinical practice. An additional step is to soak the root in 2% sodium fluoride solution for 20 min before reimplantation in order to increase its resistance to any form of resorption. Bony union with the root takes longer than periodontal healing, and the tooth is usually splinted for 4 rather than 2 weeks (21).

Pulp survival is dictated by the maturity of the root end and by the length of the time the tooth was out of its socket: "extra-alveolar time". There is no realistic prospect of vital pulp functions returning in avulsed teeth with mature root apices. In teeth with immature root apices and an extra-alveolar time of less than 45 min, there is a reasonable expectation that the neurovascular supply may be re-established.

As for other luxation-type injuries, root canal treatment is seldom commenced at the emergency visit; the focus is generally on reimplanting and stabilizing the tooth. One exception is the tooth with an extraoral dry time of greater than 60 min, where a decision has been made to remove the remaining periodontal tissues from the root surface before reimplantation. Here, the added extraoral time needed to commence or even complete root canal treatment will have no significant impact on outcome and may be considered.

In all other teeth with mature apices, root canal treatment is usually performed after stabilization of the tooth for 7–10 days, and the norm has been to medicate canals for up to 1 month with calcium hydroxide before root canal filling and review (see below). Alternative intracanal medicaments include steroid/antibiotic preparations, which may have some role in modulating cellular responses, promoting healing and reducing the risks of early resorptive change. If there is a risk of ankylosis followed by replacement root resorption, there may be merit in considering a root filling material which could resorb with the root, such as one of the commercially available polycaprolactone-based systems (19).

Clinical and radiographic examination should be planned weekly during the first month, at 3, 6 and 12 month intervals for the first year, and annually thereafter (21). Unfavorable outcomes would include the development of symptoms, unacceptable mobility or loss of the tooth, signs of inflammatory root resorption and, in some cases, the development of ankylosis and replacement resorption (see Clinical concept 15.2). In the case of immature teeth where pulp revascularization occurs, mineralized obliteration of the pulp is to be expected. Additional adverse outcomes for immature teeth would include arrested root formation (see earlier section on Arrest of dental development) and fracture of the tooth.

Alveolar fractures

Fractures of the alveolar process are frequently associated with complex dentoalveolar injuries, which may include a range of problems including gingival lacerations, tooth fractures and luxations. Alveolar fractures are best assessed by extraoral, panoramic or three-dimensional imaging techniques. Segmental fractures may displace groups of teeth *en masse* and may be repositioned during an emergency attendance and stabilized by splinting the teeth to their neighbors, typically for 4 weeks (20). Detailed discussion of bone injuries is beyond the scope of this chapter, and if there is any suspicion of a complex fracture, or if the practitioner is in any doubt, patients are best referred for specialist oral and maxillofacial care. It should be borne in mind that further dental injury may

272 Diagnostic Considerations and Clinical Decision Making

> **Clinical procedure 15.2   Management of teeth found to be undergoing replacement resorption**
>
> There is currently no effective treatment to arrest replacement resorption. Though the tooth may give effective service for many years, it is likely to be lost or need replacement at some stage in the future. Complications such as esthetic compromise due to infraocclusion, or periodontal infections following communication with the gingival crevice may necessitate intervention before the tooth itself fails. Following full discussion with the patient and their parent/guardian as appropriate, the decision may be made to:
>
> (1) Preserve the tooth for as long as possible with periodic clinical and radiographic monitoring.
> (2) Preserve the root for as long as possible to preserve the height and width of the alveolus for later placement of an implant fixture. This is often a good option for anterior teeth in infraocclusion, and requires decoronation of the tooth 2 mm below alveolar crest level and removal of any root filling materials, allowing the root canal space to fill with blood. The buried root is then covered by a mucoperiosteal flap (28). The resultant gap can be restored with an interim removable prosthesis or, better, resin-bonded bridgework.
> (3) Extract the tooth and close the space orthodontically.
> (4) Extract the tooth and restore the gap by autotransplantation of a premolar (48) or by conventional restorative means.

occur during the application of screw-retained fracture fixation plates to the jaws (26). Teeth involved in alveolar fractures should be monitored clinically and radiographically for evidence of vital pulp functions and for signs of periapical inflammation or resorptive change. A suggested follow-up schedule would be 4 weeks for splint removal, followed by monitoring at 6–8 weeks, 4 months, 6 months, 1 year and 5 years (20).

Diagnostic quandaries – to remove or review the pulp after trauma?

It could be argued that mature teeth do not need the support of a functioning pulp. Countless millions of successfully root canal treated teeth worldwide provide evidence that mature teeth can be preserved in a functional state and restored to satisfactory esthetics by standard contemporary methods. But that is not to say that pulp extirpation should be undertaken lightly, or that all traumatized teeth should be root canal treated. The pulp may retain helpful functions throughout the life of the tooth (see Chapter 4), and its unnecessary loss may have costs, financial and otherwise.

In immature teeth, the consequences of unnecessary pulpectomy are of greater immediate consequence to tooth survival. Here, the loss of functional pulp tissue

will arrest dental development, resulting in a short and fragile root which is vulnerable to fracture, and a tooth which presents considerable challenges for successful root canal treatment and long-term restoration.

On the other hand, it must be recognized that the pulps of both mature and immature teeth are at risk of breakdown and infection after trauma and that pulp extirpation and root canal treatment may be essential if the tooth is to be spared the ravages of inflammatory root resorption. Indecision can again be costly.

Therein lies one of the great challenges at the heart of trauma management: how can the condition of the pulp be diagnosed with certainty, and when is root canal treatment justified?

Pulp diagnosis is crude at the best of times, and the consequences of trauma may cloud the picture further. Diagnostic methods such as crown surface temperature assessment, laser–Doppler flowmetry, pulse oximetry and dual-wavelength spectrophotometry (35, 41), which may have potential to monitor vascular integrity and healthy perfusion of the pulp (43), are not yet sufficiently refined for everyday use in routine dental practice. Clinicians are therefore forced to rely on a careful history, clinical and radiographic examination and the application of thermal and electronic sensibility tests to build a picture of pulp status.

The neurovascular supply to the pulps of mature teeth cannot be expected to recover after avulsion or intrusive luxation, and root canal treatment should be commenced as soon as the tooth is stable (usually within 7–10 days). In all other situations, diagnostic information at the emergency attendance (Fig. 15.12) should form a baseline for monitoring the return or otherwise of vital pulp functions.

Electronic pulp testing remains the single most useful diagnostic test (8), particularly if the device has an analog output, which can be monitored over time. Consistent positioning of the pulp tester probe as close to the incisal edge of the tooth as possible assists reproducibility over time (41). Cautious clinicians should be mindful that reversibly damaged pulps may give negative responses for months after injury (see Key literature 15.3), especially if sensory nerves must regrow from the damaged apical region or from a deep horizontal fracture line into the crown. They should also be aware that immature teeth with incomplete sensory innervation and teeth whose pulps are becoming obliterated with mineralized tissue may also fail to respond.

Diagnostic uncertainty may be compounded by clinical features such as transient reddening or graying of the crown, caused by hemorrhage into dentin (38), yellowing of the crown associated with mineralized obliteration of the pulp and by transient radiographic periapical apical breakdown which may accompany traumatic injuries (2). No one test can provide conclusive evidence

Key literature 15.3

In a classical experimental study, Öhman (32) examined the extent of pulp tissue healing, regeneration of nerve fibers and restitution of pulp sensitivity in young human teeth following total severance of their neurovascular supply. The experimental teeth ($n = 85$) were to be removed for orthodontic reasons. Neurovascular injury was caused by extraction and the teeth were immediately reimplanted for periods of between 1 and 360 days. Electronic pulp sensitivity was recorded at the start and end points of the study. After the final electronic pulp sensitivity assessment, and without local anesthesia, a cavity was carefully prepared through the crown of each tooth. In the absence of pain on pulp entry, a root canal instrument was slowly introduced until pain was evoked. The histological extent of pulp tissue healing was correlated with the degree of root development and the time from initial extraction, with more severe pulp damage and slower pulp tissue regeneration in teeth with a narrow apical foramen. Some teeth had developed total pulp necrosis. Regenerating nerve fibers were not consistently observed until 2 months after injury. Although vital pulp tissue may have formed to the roof of the pulp chamber at earlier time points, no tooth responded to electronic provocation before 35 days after injury. Cavity preparation through the crown elicited no response in any tooth before the point of pulp exposure. From a clinical point of view, it was concluded that progressive reduction in the size and shape of the pulp cavity was more informative of pulp status in young traumatized teeth than the registration of pulp sensitivity by electronic testing alone.

Pulp regeneration – the dawn of a new era?

Traumatic injuries continue to endanger pulps, but established endodontic and restorative procedures have an impressive track record for the preservation of traumatized teeth. That said, contemporary restorative materials can seldom match the properties of the tissues they replace. Fragile, immature teeth serve as an example, where even the best MTA root canal filling and bonded restoration is unlikely to safeguard the future of the tooth as well as a functioning pulp which survives to complete root formation.

Recent clinical reports have described pulp regeneration in immature teeth with apical periodontitis after canal disinfection for several weeks with a cocktail of antibiotics, followed by deliberate overinstrumentation to induce bleeding into the canal. It has also been suggested that similar approaches may be applicable to avulsed mature teeth following deliberate opening of the apical foramen to at least 1.1 mm diameter. Techniques for pulp repair and regeneration ranging from gene therapy to stem cell implantation are the focus of considerable research activity and may open radically new prospects for the rehabilitation of traumatized teeth in years to come (31). The dawn of an exciting new era? Future editions will no doubt tell.

of pulp status and the need for pulpectomy. Rather, the decision should be made with due caution and integrity, and on the cumulative evidence of clinical and radiographic information.

Positive indications for pulp extirpation include the development of pulpitic symptoms (particularly lingering thermal or spontaneous pulpal pain), or evidence of apical periodontitis or of infection-related root resorption (internal or external inflammatory root resorption). In the case of root-fractured teeth, inflammation will likely present at the fracture line following breakdown and infection of the coronal pulp only.

In the case of immature teeth, evidence that root formation has arrested for 6 or more months may be an indication to intervene, though, in the absence of other adverse signs and symptoms, careful monitoring may be indicated.

Without good evidence to the contrary, tissues should be given the best opportunity to heal after trauma, though the danger of complications must be spelled out to patients, highlighting the need for long-term review and the willingness of the clinician to review them at any time if they have concerns or if worrying symptoms emerge.

References

1. Amir FA, Gutmann JL, Witherspoon DE. Calcific metamorphosis: a challenge in endodontic diagnosis and treatment. *Quintessence Int.* 2001; 32: 447–55.
2. Andreasen FM. Transient root resorption after dental trauma: the clinician's dilemma. *J. Esthet. Restor. Dent.* 2003; 15: 80–92.
3. Andreasen JO, Hjørting-Hansen E. Intraalveolar root fractures: radiographic and histologic studies of 50 cases. *J. Oral Surg.* 1967; 25: 414–26.
4. Andreasen JO, Farik B, Munksgaard EC. Long-term calcium hydroxide as a root canal dressing may increase risk of root fracture. *Dent. Traumatol.* 2002; 18: 134–7.
5. Andreasen JO, Andreasen FM, Mejàre I, Cvek M. Healing of 400 intra-alveolar root fractures. 1. Effect of pre-injury and injury factors such as sex, age, stage of root development, fracture type, location of fracture and severity of dislocation. *Dent. Traumatol.* 2004; 20: 192–202.
6. Andreasen JO, Andreasen FM, Mejàre I, Cvek M. Healing of 400 intra-alveolar root fractures. 2. Effect of treatment factors such as treatment delay, repositioning, splinting type and period and antibiotics. *Dent. Traumatol.* 2004; 20: 203–11.
7. Andreasen J, Andreasen F, Andersson L. *Textbook and Colour Atlas of Traumatic Injuries to the Teeth*, 4th edn. Oxford: Blackwell Publishing, 2007.

The definitive textbook of traumatic injuries to the teeth and their clinical management.

8. Bakland LK, Andreasen JO. Dental traumatology: essential diagnosis and treatment planning. *Endod. Topics* 2004; 7: 14–34.

9. Bergenholtz, G. Microorganisms from necrotic pulp of traumatized teeth. *Odontol. Revy* 1974; 25: 347–58.

10. Bonfante G, Kaizer OB, Pegoraro LF, do Valle LA. Fracture strength of teeth with flared root canals restored with glass fibre posts. *Int. Dent. J.* 2007; 57: 153–60.

11. Bryson EC, Levin L, Banchs F, Abbott PV, Trope M. Effect of immediate intracanal placement of Ledermix Paste® on healing of replanted dog teeth after extended dry times. *Dent. Traumatol.* 2002; 18: 316–21.

12. Chappuis V, von Arx T. Replantation of 45 avulsed permanent teeth: a 1 year follow-up study. *Dent. Traumatol.* 2005; 21: 289–96.

   Thirty-four patients with 45 avulsed and reimplanted permanent teeth were followed for 1 year. All were soaked in tetracycline before replantation. Semi-rigid splinting was limited to 7–10 days. All patients were given tetracyclines systemically for 10 days. Normal periodontal healing was observed in 58% of teeth; more favorable than previous studies. High success rates were attributed to factors including ideal tooth storage prior to reimplantation and the use of local and systemic tetracyclines.

13. Cohenca N, Simon JH, Mathur A, Malfaz JM. Clinical indications for digital imaging in dento-alveolar trauma. Part 2: root resorption. *Dent. Traumatol.* 2007; 23: 105–13.

14. Cvek M. Treatment of non-vital permanent incisors with calcium hydroxide. II. Effect on external root resorption in luxated teeth compared with effect of root filling with gutta-percha. A follow-up. *Odontol. Revy* 1973; 24: 343–54.

15. Cvek M. A clinical report on partial pulpotomy and capping with calcium hydroxide in permanent incisors with complicated crown fracture. *J. Endod.* 1978; 4: 232–7.

16. Cvek M, Granath L, Lundberg M. Failures and healing in endodontically treated non-vital anterior teeth with post-traumatically reduced pulpal lumen. *Acta Odontol. Scand.* 1982; 40: 223–8.

17. Cvek M. Prognosis of luxated non-vital maxillary incisors treated with calcium hydroxide and filled with gutta-percha. A retrospective clinical study. *Endod. Dent. Traumatol.* 1992; 8: 45–55.

   A retrospective radiographic study of 885 luxated permanent incisors with non-vital pulps. Evaluations for inflammatory root resorption, ankylosis and cervical root fracture were made 4 years after root canal treatment which included calcium hydroxide dressing and filling with gutta-percha and sealer. Periapical healing had occurred in 91% of the teeth. Inflammatory root resorption healed in 192 of 197 teeth (97%). Ankylosis occurred in 13 teeth, all of which had suffered intrusive luxation. The frequency of cervical root fracture was markedly higher in immature than mature teeth. Immature teeth with resorption in the cervical area were especially susceptible to fracture.

18. Cvek M, Mejare I, Andreasen JO. Conservative endodontic treatment of teeth fractured in the middle or apical part of the root. *Dent. Traumatol.* 2004; 20: 261–9.

   A clinical trial in root-fractured teeth to compare gutta-percha root canal filling of the coronal fragment only, gutta-percha root canal filling across the fracture line to the apex of the tooth, gutta-percha root canal filling of the coronal fragment with surgical removal of the apical fragment, and calcium hydroxide treatment of the coronal fragment before gutta-percha root filling. It was concluded that root canal filling of the coronal fragment only, with or without removal of the apical fragment, could be successful in selected cases. Pretreatment of the coronal fragment with calcium hydroxide appeared at that time to be the treatment of choice.

19. Elzubair A, Elias CN, Suarez JC, Lopes HP, Vieira MV. The physical characterization of a thermoplastic polymer for endodontic obturation. *Dent. Mater.* 2006; 34: 784–9.

20. Flores MT, Andersson L, Andreasen JO, Bakland LK, Malmgren B, Barnett F, *et al.*; International Association of Dental Traumatology. Guidelines for the management of traumatic dental injuries. I. Fractures and luxations of permanent teeth. *Dent. Traumatol.* 2007; 23: 66–71.

   The first part of a consensus statement after review of the current dental literature and expert group discussions on the management of trauma to permanent teeth.

21. Flores MT, Andersson L, Andreasen JO, Bakland LK, Malmgren B, Barnett F, *et al.*; International Association of Dental Traumatology. Guidelines for the management of traumatic dental injuries. II. Avulsion of permanent teeth. *Dent. Traumatol.* 2007; 23: 130–6.

   The second part of a consensus statement after review of the current dental literature and expert group discussions on the management of trauma to permanent teeth.

22. Goncalves LA, Vansan LP, Paulino SM, Sousa Neto MD. Fracture resistance of weakened roots restored with a trans-illuminating post and adhesive restorative materials. *J. Prosthet. Dent.* 2006; 96: 339–44.

23. Heithersay G. Invasive cervical resorption. *Endod. Topics* 2004; 7: 73–92.

24. Jacobsen I, Kerekes K. Long term prognosis of traumatized permanent anterior teeth showing calcifying processes in the pulp cavity. *Scand. J. Dent. Res.* 1977; 85: 588–98.

25. Katebzadeh N, Dalton BC, Trope M. Strengthening immature teeth during and after apexification. *J. Endod.* 1998; 24: 256–9.

26. Kocaelli HA, Kaptan F, Kayahan B, Haznedaroglu F. Management of the perforations due to miniplate application. *J. Endod.* 2006; 32: 482–5. Erratum in: *J. Endod.* 2006; 32: 905.

27. Love RM. Bacterial penetration of the root canal of intact incisor teeth after a simulated traumatic injury. *Endod. Dent. Traumatol.* 1996; 12: 289–93.

28. Malmgren B, Cvek M, Lundberg M, Frykholm A. Surgical treatment of ankylosed and infrapositioned reimplanted incisors in adolescents. *Scand. J. Dent. Res.* 1984; 92: 391–9.

29. Mandel U, Viidik A. Effect of splinting on the mechanical and histological properties of the healing periodontal ligament after experimental extrusive luxation in the monkey. *Arch. Oral Biol.* 1989; 34: 209–17.

30. Meltzer RS, Montgomery S. The effectiveness of ultrasonics and calcium hydroxide for the debridement of human mandibular molars. *J. Endod.* 1989; 15: 373–8.

31. Murray PE, Garcia-Godoy F, Hargreaves KM. Regenerative endodontics: a review of current status and a call for action. *J. Endod.* 2007; 33: 377–90.

32. Öhman A. Healing and sensitivity to pain in young replanted human teeth. An experimental, clinical and histological study (Thesis). *Odontol. Tidskr*. 1965; 73: 166–227.

33. Patel S, Dawood A, Pitt Ford TR, Whaites E. The potential applications of cone beam computed tomography in the management of endodontic problems. *Int. Endod. J.* 2007; 40: 818–30.

34. Pene JR, Nicholls JI, Harrington GW. Evaluation of fiber-composite laminate in the restoration of immature, nonvital maxillary central incisors. *J. Endod.* 2001; 27: 18–22.

35. Pitt-Ford TR, Patel S. Technical equipment for assessment of dental pulp status. *Endod. Topics* 2004; 7: 2–13.

36. Robertson A, Andreansen FM, Bergenholtz G, Andreasen JO, Norén JG. Incidence of pulp necrosis subsequent to pulp canal obliteration from trauma of permanent incisors. *J. Endod.* 1996; 22: 557–60.

37. Robinson HBG, Boling LR. The anachoretic effect in pulpitis. I. Bacteriologic studies. *J. Am. Dent. Assoc.* 1941; 28: 268–82.

38. Roy R, Chandler NP. Tooth discolouration following dental trauma. *ENDO – Endod. Prac. Today* 2007; 1: 181–7.

39. Schiøtt M, Andreasen JO. Emdogain does not prevent progressive root resorption after reimplantation of avulsed teeth: a clinical study. *Dent. Traumatol.* 2005; 21: 46–50.

40. Schwartz RS, Mauger M, Clement DJ, Walker WA III. Mineral trioxide aggregate: a new material for endodontics. *J. Am. Dent. Assoc.* 1999; 130: 967–75 (Review).

41. Sigurdsson A. Pulpal diagnosis. *Endod. Topics* 2003; 5: 12–25.

42. Simon S, Rilliard F, Berdal A, Machtou P. The use of mineral trioxide aggregate in one-visit apexification treatment: a prospective study. *Int. Endod. J.* 2007; 40: 186–97.

   Fifty-seven teeth with open apices in 50 patients received one-appointment apexification with MTA. Postoperative radiographs were assessed independently against the Periapical Index at 6 and 12 months, and annually thereafter. Forty-three patients were followed up for at least 12 months. Periapical healing occurred in 81% of cases. It was concluded that apexification in one step with an apical plug of MTA can be considered a predictable treatment and may be an alternative to the use of calcium hydroxide.

43. Strobl H, Haas M, Norer B, Gerhard S, Emshoff R. Evaluation of pulpal blood flow after tooth splinting of luxated permanent maxillary incisors. *Dent. Traumatol.* 2004; 20: 36–41.

44. Sundqvist G. *Bacteriological Studies of Necrotic Dental Pulps*. Odontological Dissertation No. 7, University of Umeå, 1976.

45. Tay FR, Pashley DH. Monoblocks in root canals: a hypothetical or tangible goal. *J. Endod.* 2007; 33: 391–8.

46. Tronstad L. Root resorption – etiology, terminology and clinical manifestations. *Endod. Dent. Traumatol.* 1988; 4: 241–52.

47. Trope M. Root resorption due to trauma. *Endod. Topics* 2002; 1: 79–100.

48. Tsukiboshi M. Autotransplantation of teeth: requirements for predictable success. *Dent. Traumatol.* 2002; 18: 157–80 (Review).

49. Von Arx T, Filippi A, Lussi A. Comparison of a new dental trauma splint device (TTS) with three commonly used splinting techniques. *Dent. Traumatol.* 2001; 17: 266–74.

50. Wedenberg C, Lindskog S. Experimental internal resorption in monkey teeth. *Endod. Dent. Traumatol.* 1985; 1: 221–7.

51. Wedenberg C, Zetterqvist L. Internal resorption in human teeth – a histological, scanning electron microscopic, and enzyme histochemical study. *J. Endod.* 1987; 13: 255–9.

52. Welbury R, Kinirons MJ, Day P, Humphreys K, Gregg TA. Outcomes for root-fractured permanent incisors: a retrospective study. *Pediatr. Dent.* 2002; 24: 98–102.

53. Welbury RR, Gregg T. *Managing Dental Trauma in Practice*. London: Quintessence, 2006.

54. Witherspoon DE, Small JC, Harris GZ. Mineral trioxide aggregate pulpotomies: a case series outcomes assessment. *J. Am. Dent. Assoc.* 2006; 137: 610–18.

Chapter 16
The multidimensional nature of pain

Ilana Eli and Peter Svensson

Introduction

Dental treatment is closely associated with pain. Pain is often the primary motivator for patients to seek dental care, most dental patients expect to experience some degree of pain during dental treatment and self-reports of pain serve as a common tool to locate possible pathology and to arrive at conclusions regarding diagnosis and treatment, e.g. the use of tooth pulp stimulation as a diagnostic test for pulp vitality (Chapter 14). However, pain is an unreliable indicator of pathology. In fact, little correlation exists between the amount of tissue destruction and the reported presence or absence of pain, whether derived from the tooth pulp, periodontal ligament or periapical region (65).

This chapter describes the fundamental nature of pain and the multitude of mechanisms that are associated with patients' perception of pain.

Definition of pain

Pain is defined as "an unpleasant and emotional experience associated with actual or potential tissue damage, or described in terms of such damage" (40). It is a complex experience of a multidimensional nature, and is always subjective and associated with emotional and cognitive factors. Today it is widely accepted that pain is much more than the mere activity in the nociceptor and nociceptive pathways of the nervous system elicited by a noxious stimulus. Pain is invariably a psychological state and can be reported in the absence of tissue damage or any likely pathophysiological causes.

The neuromatrix theory

According to Melzack (55), pain is a multidimensional experience produced by characteristic "neurosignature" patterns of nerve impulses generated by a widely distributed neural network in the brain. This neurosignature for pain experience is determined by the synaptic architecture of the neuromatrix, which is shaped by both genetic and sensory influences and modulated by sensory inputs and cognitive events, such as psychological stress. Disruption of the neuromatrix homeostasis by a stressor, either physical or psychological, activates programs of neural, hormonal and behavioral activity aimed at restoring homeostasis. Occasionally, when failure in the homeostasis regulation occurs, the neuromatrix produces the dysfunctional conditions that may cause chronic pain conditions, which are often resistant to treatment procedures developed for acute pain conditions. The particular activated programs are selected from a genetically determined repertoire of programs that have been modified by events, such as earlier exposure to stress, and are influenced by the extent and severity of the perceived stress.

The significance of the neuromatrix theory is that it guides us away from the concept of pain as just a simple sensation produced by injury, inflammation or other tissue pathology, and promotes the concept as a multidimensional experience shaped by multiple influences, e.g. stress, anxiety, expectation, focus of attention, gender and culture (Core concept 16.1).

Acute versus chronic pain

Although this overall view of pain as a multidimensional experience is attractive and prudent, it should be emphasized that there is an immense difference between acute and chronic types of pain. Acute pain is necessary for the organism to survive. It serves as a warning or alert sign for appropriate action to be taken and healing and restoration of function to occur. Chronic pain does not serve a biological purpose and is often closely associated with an

---

Core concept 16.1

Pain is often reported in the absence of visible tissue damage or any likely pathophysiological cause. In the clinic, there is no way to distinguish this experience from that of tissue damage and it therefore should be accepted as pain. Activity induced in the nociceptor and nociceptive pathways by a noxious stimulus is not equal to pain, which is always a psychological state.

impaired quality of life, distress and a negative impact on personal, social and work relationships. Pain associated with acute tissue damage, disease or intervention can be viewed as a symptom, whereas chronic pain, in addition to the psychological aspects, may resemble neurodegenerative conditions and can be classified as a disease in its own right. The arbitrary time point of 6 months is a realistic way to distinguish between acute and chronic pain. However, it is more reasonable to talk about chronic or persistent pain, if the pain lasts longer than expected after a normal healing period.

The neurobiological and psychological factors that affect the pain experience are summarized in the following paragraphs and their importance in dental treatment is indicated.

Neurobiological factors affecting the pain experience

Overview of pain mechanisms

In the field of pain, there is ongoing discussion as to what extent is it possible to classify pain according to the current knowledge of the mechanisms involved (71). The proposed mechanism-based classification has four main categories (Core concept 16.2).

Transient or nociceptive pain may be the easiest type of pain to understand, although recent advances in molecular biology have shown the complex nature of even "simple" processing of pain. The nociceptor is the basic receptor on primary afferent nerve fibers innervating the orofacial tissues. On the peripheral terminals, a multitude of transducing receptors and ion channels have been identified, e.g. acid-sensing ion channels (ASIC), a family of transient receptor potentials receptors (TRPV1-8), P2X3 receptors. These receptors are unique in that they detect and respond to specific high-intensity stimuli (heat, cold, mechanical, chemical stimuli), potentially associated with tissue damage and therefore serve as a warning system. It has been suggested that there is a nociceptor specialization (64) in that sophisticated "sensors" in the peripheral tissue, including tooth pulp and periodontium, can be activated unintentionally during numerous dental procedures (procedural types of pain). Besides the psychological aspects (described

below), there is a strong neurobiological rationale to prevent pain experience during dental procedures, including endodontics, by the appropriate use of local anesthetics.

Overt tissue damage, e.g. by trauma and surgical procedures, is commonly associated with pain. In most cases pain in this context can be viewed as part of the classical cardinal signs of inflammation: dolor (pain), tumor (swelling), rubor (redness), calor (heat sensation) and loss of function. However, significant progress has been made in terms of understanding the neurobiological changes in the nociceptive system in these conditions. One important aspect is that the nociceptor can initiate spontaneous activity without a peripheral stimulus leading to spontaneous pain (64). Another is "sensitization", where the threshold for activation of the nociceptor is reduced and the responses are longer and stronger (39). Additionally, previously silent nociceptors can be awakened and further contribute to pain (see also Chapter 3). There is also evidence that functional shifts occur in the number and activity of receptors and ion channels on the nociceptor, e.g. receptors for nerve growth factor (NGF), bradykinin (BK) and prostaglandins (PGE) are activated, increasing membrane excitability. Second-order neurons in the trigeminal sensory nucleus complex react to the increased trafficking of action potentials from the nociceptor and sensitization of the neurons in the central nervous system occurs (64). A multitude of biological responses takes place involving phosphorylation of NMDA receptors and activation of neurokinin and neurotrophic receptors (71). The understanding of the intracellular pathways is fairly advanced as they include alterations in gene expression of neurotransmitters and neuromodulators. Although the phenomenon of peripheral and central sensitization can develop within minutes, usually these processes are completely reversible in conditions with inflammatory types of pain.

Nervous system injury pain (neuropathic pain) can occur if the peripheral nerve fibers are damaged (71), for example, due to surgery (third molar surgery, orthognathic surgery on the maxilla and mandible, insertion of implants, etc.) or to disease, such as postherpetic neuralgia or diabetic neuropathy and even pulpitis. Neuropathic pain may also develop following injury to the central somatosensory system, e.g. by stroke, multiple sclerosis and spinal cord injuries. The consequences of these lesions are spontaneous pain and hypersensitivity to painful stimuli (64). Thus, the primary afferent nerve fiber can initiate spontaneous discharges due to ectopic neural activity near the peripheral nerve lesion. Phenotypic changes and alterations in the expression and distribution of ion channels can occur, which contribute to an increase in membrane excitability (71). Thus, it is easy to understand that sensitized nerve fibers play an important role in neuropathic pain.

Core concept 16.2

Main categories of pain:

- Transient (nociceptive) pain
- Tissue injury (inflammatory) pain
- Nervous system injury (neuropathic) pain
- Functional pain

Unfortunately, the neurobiological mechanisms underlying neuropathic pain are irreversible and resistant to current pharmacological therapy. The central nervous system also plays a significant role in these conditions. For example, one response at the second-order neuron is the loss of normal inhibitory mechanisms mediated by the neurotransmitter GABA and glycine (71). There is evidence that 1 week after nerve injury, signs of apoptosis appear in the dorsal horn neurons. Therefore, there is strong interest in developing therapies that will prevent activation of such changes to avoid disturbances in the delicate balance between inhibitory and excitatory pathways (Core concept 16.3).

The concept of functional pain is an evolving one. There appears to be nothing wrong in the peripheral tissues, but it is believed that for some unknown reasons there is an abnormal amplification and processing of peripheral stimuli in the central parts of the somatosensory system (71). Fibromyalgia, irritable bowel syndrome and possibly tension-type headaches are examples of this disorder. In contrast to the inflammatory and neuropathic types of pain in which there is local hypersensitivity to painful stimuli, in the functional types of pain this hypersensitivity is widespread and generalized. Comprehensive pain analysis and careful elucidation of the psychosocial aspects should be used to assess the somatosensory function in the painful and non-painful parts of the body (15). Simple tests of somatosensory function can easily be performed in the dental office and more elaborate tests (quantitative sensory tests – QST) are normally available at university clinics (64).

Distinguishing neuropathic pain from other pain conditions

From a management perspective it will be important to differentiate between the different types of pain. Neuropathic pain is a distinct condition and requires a careful clinical examination combined with confirmatory tests. To establish a definite diagnosis the following are required:

Core concept 16.3

A key message regarding neuropathic pain is that the underlying neurobiological events cannot be detected by normal clinical inspection or radiology of the painful region. Even in the absence of visible signs of structural damage, the somatosensory system may have undergone pathological changes which can explain many of the peculiar manifestations of neuropathic pain. For example, gentle brushing or touching of the painful region can often elicit strong pain that lasts longer than the stimulus – a situation referred to as allodynia (71).

- occurrence of pain with a distinct neuroanatomically plausible distribution;
- a history suggestive of a prior relevant lesion or disease affecting the peripheral or central somatosensory system;
- demonstration of the distinct neuroanatomical distribution by at least one confirmatory test (e.g. QST); and
- demonstration of the relevant lesion or disease by at least one confirmatory test (e.g. magnetic resonance imaging or recording of electrophysiological abnormalities).

Nevertheless, there will still be gray areas where the clinical manifestations of a nociceptive type of tooth pain may overlap with a neuropathic or functional type of pain. A diagnostic filter starting with exclusion of transient, nociceptive pain and neuropathic pain will lead to relatively few patients ending up in the functional pain category (5).

Pain genetics

In the field of pain, one of the most intriguing discoveries is the association between certain types of genes and pain expression. It is common knowledge from the dental office that some patients are more susceptible to stimulation of the orofacial region, i.e. patients reporting very high levels of pain even in the absence of a strong nociceptive input via the primary afferent nerve fibers. And vice versa, there are patients who are much more "pain resistant". Notwithstanding the significance of the psychosocial aspects of pain, several genetic markers of "pain-sensitive" and "pain-resistant" patients have recently been identified. One of these markers is based on the polymorphism of the cathecol-O-methyltransferase (COMT) gene. COMT is an enzyme that metabolizes catecholamines and is critically involved in pain perception, cognitive function and affective mood with a strong impact on the efficacy of the endogenous pain modulatory systems (75). Polymorphism of the adrenergic-receptor-beta-2 gene has been linked with differences in pain sensitivity. It is likely that there are many more gene candidates that may contribute to individual differences in the expression of pain and to analgesia. The significance of this new emerging knowledge is that there is a key to open some of the "black boxes" in understanding why pain is experienced differently.

Relevance for tooth-related pain

Dentists are usually good at understanding acute pain related to teeth. For most patients, stimulation of the tooth pulp, either by accident (trauma), drilling (procedural), caries (disease) or endodontic treatment, will be associated with a painful experience. There are numerous techniques that can be used (the psychological aspects will be covered below) to prevent or relieve transient and inflammatory pain. However, neuropathic and functional types of pain related to the teeth are less well understood and the underlying mechanisms are different (described above). Additionally, the nociceptive pathways are influenced by sex and sex hormones and are genetically controlled. Therefore, it is important for the dentist to establish the type of tooth-related pain suffered by the patient and to remember that neurobiological factors also cause the clinical presentation of pain.

Psychological factors affecting the pain experience

Affective factors

Impact of stress, fear and anxiety

It is widely believed that anxiety is associated with increased pain report (14). A tense and anxious patient is more inclined to report pain during treatment than a relaxed one, since anxiety creates expectancy for future pain. An anxious patient who arrives for treatment with former pain memory is likely to expect pain during treatment. This causes the patient to selectively filter any information given prior to treatment and to focus on stimuli which can resemble, or be associated with, pain. For example, the slightest pressure on the tooth can be interpreted as pain and initiate a pain reaction. Arousal caused by anxiety may also lead to increased sympathetic activity and muscle tension, which may cause additional pain.

Dental anxiety is a prevalent obstacle which affects human behavior in the dental setting (24). Among all dental situations, oral surgical procedures and endodontic therapies cause the highest levels of stress and anxiety (9, 26). According to Arntz *et al.* (4), anxiety experienced during dental treatment plays a role in maintaining the problem of inaccurate expectations of fear of treatment. For example, pain experienced by patients in oral surgery is best predicted by their anxiety at each time point (28).

There is a high probability that patients who arrive for endodontic treatment are anxious and expect to experience some degree of pain during treatment. This can cause patients to report pain during treatment even when there is no rationale (e.g. drilling in a tooth with non-vital pulp). Occasionally, proper local anesthesia is extremely difficult to achieve and the patient continues to complain of pain in spite of several attempts. These situations are closely associated with the patient's fear of dental treatment (41) (Key literature 16.1).

> ### Key literature 16.1
>
> In an extensive review on pain and anxiety in dental procedures, Litt (51) found that in acute pain situations, anxiety and pain may be indistinguishable. Anxiety not only lowers the pain threshold, but may actually lead to the perception that normally non-painful stimuli are painful (e.g. vibration of the drill felt on an anesthetized tooth).

By definition, pain is always subjective. In the clinic, there is no way to distinguish between pain due to psychological reasons and pain originating from actual tissue stimulation. In both, it is regarded and reported by the patient as pain and should be accepted and referred to as such.

Impact of mood

Mood, especially depression, influences pain perception and pain tolerance. There is a close relationship between chronic pain states and depression (63). It has been hypothesized that chronic pain and depression are closely related owing to similar neurochemical mechanisms involved in both disorders. Another reason for the depressed mood is the way in which chronic pain interferes with important areas of functioning, e.g. decline in social activities and social rewards (61).

Mood can also affect pain perception in short-term acute pain situations, e.g. dental treatment. For example, acute pain perception can be affected by a film-induced mood condition (69). Subjects who watched a humorous film prior to a painful stimulus tolerated the pain challenge better than other subjects. This suggests that psychological approaches could have a significant effect on the sensory dimensions of pain and that pain tolerance in patients can be substantially increased with simple measures, including the showing of humorous films in the waiting room.

Cognitive factors

One of the most potent forms of stress is pain. The pain experience includes actual confrontation with harm, which can be physical (e.g. injury), psychological (e.g. loss of control) or interpersonal (e.g. shame). As such, it is affected by both the potency of the stimulus and the individual's ability to cope with the stressful event (60).

Attention versus distraction

Almost any situation that attracts a sufficient degree of intense, prolonged attention (e.g. sports, battle) can provide conditions for other stimulation to go unnoticed, including wounds that would cause considerable suffering under normal circumstances. Broadly defined, distraction is directing one's attention from the sensations or emotional reactions produced by a noxious stimulus. Generally, distraction reduces pain compared to undistracted conditions (54).

Dentists can apply distraction techniques while treating their patients, e.g. using background music and talking to the patient. Several advanced methods have been described as effective in the dental clinic, such as mounting a television monitor near the ceiling, or asking the patient to play a video game "against the house" (13). While distraction techniques that require attentional capacity are effective in reducing pain-related distress, even the simplest distraction technique is beneficial in reducing the patient's stress and pain perception. Studies have shown that the use of video glasses during dental scaling and restorations had no or only minor effects on the perceived pain. However, a striking finding was that most patients would still like to use the video glasses and reported a positive effect of this "distraction" technique (7).

Control

Control affects stress, coping mechanisms and reaction to pain (50). People in pain usually search for information to give meaning to the experience. Therefore, anxiety and pain levels associated with dental procedures can be reduced by providing the patient with updated information on the forthcoming procedures and the description of the likely sensations. For example, patients provided with detailed information on how N_2O analgesia works showed higher pain tolerance thresholds to tooth pulp stimulation than patients without this information (22). Since the fear of uncontrolled, sudden, acute pain is a primary concern for most patients (48), continuous information regarding ongoing procedures is an important way to provide patients with some sense of control or involvement (Core concept 16.4).

Pain beliefs and expectations

Reaction to a stimulus, whether acute or chronic, is always affected by its meaning to the individual. For example, the patient can interpret an episode of an unexpected, unexplained pain during treatment as a sign of the dentist's insufficient professional skills. This, in turn,

can develop mistrust in the dentist and cause the patient to interpret any further minor stimulus as a threat and evoke a pain reaction. Conversely, when mutual trust exists, the patient's belief in the necessity of the treatment makes these incidences bearable and less traumatic.

In one experiment (3), subjects were requested to touch a vibrating surface for 1 second. Some were led to believe that the surface would cause pain, others that it would produce pleasure and the remainder had no hint on what vibrations would entail. As predicted, the "pain subjects" usually reported vibrations to be painful, the "pleasure subjects" as pleasurable and the "control subjects" as neutral sensations. This shows that expectation of pain to occur during dental treatment increases the likelihood of pain to be perceived. Thus, dentists should be aware of their potential to evoke negative "nocebo" responses and to make prudent use of the positive "placebo" responses (Core concept 16.5).

In stressful situations, behavior, thoughts and emotional reactions are influenced by the stimulus and by the individual's perception of "self-efficacy", which means one's belief in possession of relevant and necessary coping skills (6). Patients who believe they can successfully cope with the anticipated pain, increase the perception of pain tolerance and vice versa. Generally, people who avoid dental care because of fear and anxiety perceive themselves less able to tolerate pain. They often claim to have an "exceptionally low pain threshold" or report themselves as "completely unable to endure pain". A low self-efficacy further lowers their pain tolerance level during treatment and increases the probability that pain will be experienced (43) (Key literature 16.2).

Core concept 16.5

A patient's expectation of a given clinical situation influences a final interpretation of a stimulus as painful or non-painful. An ambiguous sensation can be perceived as either pleasurable or painful based on individual cognitions and expectations.

Key literature 16.2

In a study by Dworkin and Chen (21), subjects served as their own control when tooth pulp shock by an electronic pulp tester was delivered in either a laboratory or clinical setting. A substantial decrease in the subjects' thresholds for sensation and pain and in pain tolerance was found when patients were challenged in the clinical setting. From this study, it can be concluded that the patient's anticipation of threat and associated anxiety are potent cognitive mediators of pain behavior in the dental office. Thus, response to pain changes according to the situational context in which pain is experienced.

Core concept 16.4

Providing patients with control over pain stimulation reduces pain and increases tolerance. A sense of control can be achieved for example by providing information regarding the anticipated and ongoing treatment.

Pain prediction and memory

Usually, memory for the general intensity of pain is good. However, the level of pain remembered by patients regarding their dental treatment is more closely associated with their expectations of pain rather than their real experience (42). Furthermore, mood and affective states influence the memory of pain (29).

Memory of past pain experience also depends on the intensity of present pain. When present pain intensity is high, patients remember the levels of their prior pain as more severe than originally recorded (23). This situation is occasionally seen among patients who experience postoperative pain after their first session of endodontic therapy. Postoperative pain causes patients to remember former treatment as more painful than originally experienced. This, in turn, leads to higher stress, higher pain expectations and lower pain tolerance in the next appointment with the dentist.

Environmental factors

Direct and indirect learning

Part of our behavior results from life experiences. The concepts and coping strategies of various life events (including pain) are continually affected by learning processes. For a learned behavior to develop, exposure to the stimulus in question must occur, resulting in a response pattern (conditioning). Further reinforcement of the response pattern (positive or negative) leads to the acquisition of new behaviors.

Unfortunately, the dental situation provides numerous opportunities for negative conditioning and acquired maladaptive behaviors. The most common stimulus is pain. Although acute pain can be avoided during dental treatment in most cases, there are still many adults who have had past experiences. Numerous learned behaviors associated with pain are based on negative reinforcement – something uncomfortable or fearful that should be avoided. This type of learning includes escape and avoidance (to avoid or prevent the unpleasant situation before it occurs), e.g. patients who react with symptoms of pallor, nausea, sweating, dizziness or even fainting during administration of local anesthesia. In many instances, symptoms originate in the patient's fear of pain rather than pathophysiological reasons. The situation can cause significant stress to the dentist who occasionally chooses to postpone treatment to the next appointment. Once the symptoms have served the patient as an adequate means to avoid the stressful situation, it may serve as a reinforcement to increase the probability of recurrence during subsequent confrontations. Patients develop a "fainting-prone" behavior that "protects" them from the need to face treatment. The negative pattern is further reinforced by the dentist's reluctance to treat patients with this medical history.

Patients do not have to have direct experience for learning to take place. It can be the result of vicarious learning, i.e. observing what happens to another individual and assuming that one's own fate would be similar in the same kind of situation. Indeed, observing others respond to painful stimulation could provoke or reduce the pain response of the observer (57).

Social and cultural factors

The influence of social environmental factors and the level of approval given by different societies for the public expression of pain have a significant impact on pain behavior. For example, while the Irish tend to deny their problems and complain less, the Italians are more dramatic, with more symptoms and bodily dysfunctions (73). Americans of Jewish and Italian origin prefer company while in pain, whereas those from "Old American" and Irish origin tend to withdraw socially. "Old American" and Irish are usually non-expressive, whereas Jewish and Italians make no effort to control their emotional reactions to pain (72). There are also notable ethnic differences in the description of dental pain and the demand for local anesthesia, e.g. the Chinese seldom express the need for local anesthesia, whereas a minority of Americans will accept tooth drilling without local anesthesia; Scandinavians place themselves between these two groups (56). The acceptance of pain does not mean that the feeling quality of the sensation has changed. The sensation is always unpleasant, but the unpleasantness is tolerated when cultural traditions call for its acceptance.

While ethnic groups differ regarding factors that influence responses to pain, similarities exist in their reporting of the responses. For example, in facial pain patients, responses, attitudes and descriptions are relatively similar in Black, Irish, Italian, Jewish and Puerto Rican. Most items in which interethnic differences were found concern emotions (stoicism vs expressiveness) in response to pain, and interference in daily functioning attributed to pain (49).

Further evidence exists that some pain dimensions (time, intensity, location, quality, cause and curability) are universal, while others are culture specific.

Gender and pain

The literature is controversial regarding gender differences in response to pain perception. Some reports claim that women exhibit greater sensitivity to noxious stimuli than men (30), but other studies show only a few gender differences in ratings of chronic and experimental pain,

pain-related illness behavior and personality (11). A recently published consensus report summarizes the experimental studies of sex differences in pain and analgesia, the clinical and psychosocial studies of sex and gender differences in pain and analgesia, and the translational research in this area. The report concludes that although the evidence is not strong enough to warrant sex-specific pain interventions in most situations, including sex as a factor in clinical trials and reporting any differences in outcomes are paramount in addressing the lack of research in this area (33).

A neurobiological perspective on sex-related differences in pain experience

There are many differences in the way women and men experience and report pain, including pain from the orofacial region. Some of these differences may be related to the multidimensional nature of pain in which gender expectations, societal influence on pain behavior and other factors play important roles. Recently, studies have also shown that there can be neurobiological differences in the transmission and processing of nociceptive inputs (12).

Neurophysiological studies have provided strong evidence that primary afferent nerve fibers in female rats are much more sensitive to nociceptive inputs from the jaw muscles and temporomandibular joint (TMJ) than those in male rats. Thus, a greater afferent barrage is evoked by a painful stimulus applied to the masseter muscle or TMJ, based on the differences in expression of NMDA-receptor subtypes. Animal studies cannot be directly extrapolated to the clinical situation, but human parallel studies have shown greater sensory-discriminative pain scores in women than in men (12).

Studies have also demonstrated that the responsiveness of the second-order neuron in trigeminal sensory nucleus complex following painful stimulation of the orofacial region is significantly greater in women than in men. In terms of responsiveness to analgesics, such as opioids, there is now favorable evidence for sex-related differences, at both the peripheral and central levels in the nociceptive pathways (12).

Finally, brain imaging techniques have been used to demonstrate that activation of endogenous pain inhibitory pathways following painful stimulation of the orofacial region differs between men and women, with women having much less inhibition (74). Several other studies are in accordance with this suggestion based on psychophysical examinations of the diffuse noxious inhibitory control phenomena (62).

Overall, men and women are likely to have a number of significant functional differences in their nociceptive pathways that could contribute to different expressions of pain often encountered in the dental office (Core concept 16.7).

A psychosocial perspective on sex-related differences in pain experience

In a review regarding gender variations in clinical pain experience, Unruh (66) reports that women are more likely to experience a variety of recurrent pains than men. Women report more severe levels of pain, more frequent pain and pain of longer duration than men. Women may be at greater risk for pain-related disability than men, but women also respond more aggressively to pain through health-related activities. Men may be more embarrassed by pain than women and the meaning of pain may be affected by sociocultural factors and the perceived position of men and women in society. Embarrassment may cause men to minimize pain unless it increases in severity and interferes with work. Minimization of pain may be consistent with social and cultural norms that accept insensitivity to pain and pain endurance as measures of virility.

There are considerable differences between types of clinical pain (35). Experimental pain, produced under controlled conditions by brief, noxious stimuli, differs from procedural and postsurgical pain. These kinds of pain have different meanings and make the study of pain more complex.

Both men and women make different assessments of procedural pain and thus may be affected differently by the experience (25). In a study regarding clinical pain in the dental office (27), it was shown that men expect to experience more pain preoperatively than women but remember less pain postoperatively. It was concluded that in clinical situations cognitive pain perception differs between genders, a fact which may originate in psychosocial factors, such as expected sex roles.

Core concept 16.6

As in any other "stressor", pain experience is also influenced by individual learned responses. Respondent and operant conditioning, indirect learning through modeling and suggestions, and social learning have a significant impact on the pain experience (10).

Core concept 16.7

Men and women differ in:
- Primary afferent fiber excitability
- Degree of sensitization in second-order neurons
- Efficiency of endogenous pain modulatory pathways

Sensory focus and control are other factors closely related to the experience of acute pain. Focusing on pain helps men, but not women, to cope successfully with experimental pain (44). In a dental setting, sensory focus reduces sensory pain intensity among patients classified as having a high desire for control and a low perceived control (52). Since men and women differ in their pattern of cognitive competencies, including psychological control mechanisms (32), these differences may significantly affect their report of pain.

Unfortunately, pain is not a physical sign that can be measured directly. Clinical pain relies on the patient to detect the sensation, label it as pain, express it and seek treatment. Despite the progress that has been made during the past decades, stereotypes concerning how boys and girls should behave and what they should feel are still deeply incorporated in our societies. Both genders receive different clues from their environment regarding how to label their physiological arousal. Thus, girls could develop a greater tendency to label vague physiological states as painful (47). This cognitive appraisal may be less important when there is an obvious causal factor for the pain. However, it may be of greater importance when environmental clues are more equivocal.

A review of the literature on gender and clinical pain reveals a disproportionate representation of women receiving treatment for many pain conditions and suggest that women report more severe pain, more frequent pain and pain of longer duration than men. Dao and LeResche (16) summarized gender differences with regard to orofacial pain conditions. There is basic agreement that fluctuations of hormonal states affect the pain experience in women and that factors, such as the structural organization and function of the sympathetic nervous system and intrinsic descending pain inhibitory systems, differ in men and women (see above). The higher prevalence of chronic orofacial pain in women is due to sex differences in generic pain mechanisms and to as-yet unidentified factors unique to the craniofacial system (16).

Apparently, men and women differ in their appraisal of clinical pain. Interference of pain has a greater impact of threat appraisal of pain in women, which in turn, is associated with women's health care utilization (67). The higher use of specific health care services in women compared to men is partially explained by psychological need and meaning (68).

Women also report a greater number of female pain models (mother, sister, grandmother, aunt) than male pain models while no such difference is apparent for men (46). Thus, women may learn to observe their own gender and other people's pain and health status more through modeling their behavior to that of their female significant others and through rewards from the social environment.

Special populations

Effect of psychiatric illness and of cognitive impairment on the pain experience

The issue of pain perception and reaction in patients with psychiatric illness and with cognitive impairment is still controversial, with the general tendency to label these subjects as relatively "insensitive" to pain. Since the early 1990s, the literature has included studies that evaluate pain perception in various psychiatric disorders, such as borderline personality disorder, major depression and schizophrenia (2, 8, 19, 34, 58).

Reports indicate that relative to healthy subjects, individuals with schizophrenia are insensitive to physical pain associated with illness and injury. In one study, patients with schizophrenia had a significantly poorer sensory discrimination of painful thermal stimuli than control subjects, but did not differ from controls with respect to their response criterion for reports of pain (19). It was suggested that the pain insensitivity in schizophrenia may reflect affective and sensory abnormalities. Another study showed that the leg flexion nociceptive reflex threshold (claimed to correlate with the pain threshold) in patients with schizophrenia did not differ from that recorded in the control population (34). This result was contradicted by Blumensohn *et al.* (8), who showed that with electronic tooth pulp stimulation, sensation threshold, pain threshold and pain tolerance were significantly higher in patients with schizophrenia compared to age- and gender-matched healthy controls. A recent meta-analysis on hypoalgesia in schizophrenia substantiates the hypothesis of a diminished pain response in patients with schizophrenia and suggests that the hypoalgesic effect cannot be solely explained by the effects of antipsychotic drugs and that it may not be a pain-specific blunted response (58).

The clinical observation that different conditions may affect subjects' sensory abilities has gained increasing interest in the professional community. For example, individuals with Down syndrome express pain or discomfort more slowly and less precisely than the general population (36), and individuals with cognitive impairment (CI) are at an increased risk of experiencing pain. Nonetheless, they are often prescribed significantly less analgesic medication compared with cognitively intact individuals. These individuals may also experience delayed diagnosis and management of painful medical conditions, setbacks in hospitalization and increased death rates. This injustice might result from the tendency of individuals with CI not to report pain in potentially harmful situations and from the difficulty in assessing pain owing to their poor communication skills. Consequently, these individuals are regarded as less sensitive to pain than their cognitively intact peers.

Individuals with severe-to-profound CI exhibit high rates of "freezing reaction" (stillness) during injection, which could be misinterpreted as not experiencing pain (17). Lack of bodily manifestation among CI patients does not necessarily mean that pain does not exist. Facial reactions alone, as a representative of pain, often provide a false impression that individuals with severe profound CI are insensitive to pain (due to freezing).

These studies draw our attention to individuals whose ability to communicate their sensations and feelings may be severely impaired. Since pain is a subjective experience, mostly evaluated according to subject's reactions and report, the absence of reaction or report is sometimes interpreted as lack of pain. Thus, care should be taken that these patients are not underdiagnosed and/or undertreated with regard to pain problems. The usual definition of pain and pain-related behavior, such as moaning, withdrawal reflexes and mimic responses indicative of pain, should be remembered when treating CI patients.

Management and treatment of pain

Dentists should be aware of the important distinction between "management" and "treatment" of pain. Treatment implies that the cause can be identified and cured, e.g. pain due to pulpitis (inflammatory pain) can be efficiently treated by pulpectomy. However, neuropathic and functional types of pain, e.g. "atypical odontalgia", can rarely be cured because the underlying pain mechanisms are only partially understood. The goal in these cases is to relieve the pain and improve function, i.e. to manage the pain.

Systematic attempts to manage pain have been closely aligned with how pain is conceptualized and evaluated. Traditionally, the focus in medicine (and dentistry) was on the cause of the reported pain, with the assumption that there was a physical basis for the pain and once it was identified the source could be blocked by medical or operative intervention. In the absence of a physical basis, the situation was labeled as "psychogenic pain".

Today, it is widely accepted that this dichotomous view of the pain experience is incomplete and inadequate. There is no question that physical factors contribute to pain symptoms, or that psychological factors play a part in pain reporting of patients. Therefore, in acute and chronic pain management, both aspects should be incorporated.

Targeting the neurobiological factors

It is beyond the scope of this chapter to review all approaches that interfere with the neurobiological aspects of orofacial pain. The reader is referred to other

textbooks on this issue. The pharmacological strategies that can be considered in neuropathic and functional types of orofacial pain will be mentioned. The transient and inflammatory types of pain are covered elsewhere in this book.

There is general agreement that analgesic effective drugs used for transient and inflammatory types of pain (e.g. acetaminophen, acetylsalicylic acid and non-steroidal anti-inflammatory drugs) have little use in the management of neuropathic pain. The current guidelines recommend the use of low doses of tricyclic antidepressants (TCA), such as nortriptyline and desipramine (20), selective serotonin and norepinephrine reuptake inhibitors (SSNRIs), such as duloxentine and venlafaxine, calcium channel alpha$_2$-delta ligand compounds (e.g. gabapentin and pregabalin) have proven efficacy in various neuropathic pain conditions, as well as topical lidocaine and opioid agonists. Less effective and thus not first-line medications are tramadol (weak mu-opioid agonist and inhibitor of reuptake of norepinephrine and serotonin), NMDA-receptor antagonists and topical capsaicin. These compounds interfere with one or more of the ion channels and receptors that are activated in the somatosensory pathways in conditions with neuropathic pain. In patients with functional types of pain, TCA and SSNRIs have been suggested (5). It should be emphasized that pharmacology is only one way to manage pain and should be accompanied by appropriate techniques to deal with the psychosocial issues (64).

Targeting the psychological factors

Treatment of acute pain includes strategies based on information, distraction, relaxation and hypnosis (31). Generally, preparing the patient with coping skills, such as information, distraction and relaxation, helps to reduce the discomfort of potentially painful dental procedures. Patients properly prepared show less anxiety and report lower pain. Non-pharmacological strategies facilitate acute pain management and are relatively easy to learn and perform. They should be part of the professional training of every general and specialized dentist, especially endodontists.

Effective treatment strategies for management of prolonged chronic pain conditions (e.g. temporomandibular disorder pain) include operant conditioning, cognitive–behavioral therapy, psychodynamic therapy, group therapy, biofeedback, relaxation and hypnosis (Core concept 16.8).

Role of hypnosis as a mode for pain management in dental care

In spite of its ancient roots, hypnosis has been accepted only recently as a scientific and medical tool. Hypnosis

Core concept 16.8

Hypnosis has numerous potential applications in dentistry, including treatment of patients who suffer from dental fear, anxiety and phobia, excessive gagging reflex, managing acute and chronic pain, increasing patient compliance with dental hygiene, and enhancing patient adaptation to dentures.

has been surrounded by myths and mystery for so long that even today popular misconceptions exist. There is no doubt that it is a powerful therapeutic tool. The constantly increasing number of reports on hypnosis appearing in the scientific literature indicate an enduring willingness on the part of the scientific community to accept it as a legitimate topic for clinical and research investigation.

Hypnosis has been described in the dental literature as having a dramatic effect when used as a sole anesthetic. Under hypnosis, procedures, such as extractions, pulpotomies and pulpectomies, have been performed without other anesthetic agents (37).

In endodontic treatment and in other dental procedures, hypnosis is used to enable treatment without stress or pain. For example, hypnosis can reduce both the strength and unpleasantness of electrical tooth pulp stimulation (38). The use of hypnosis to induce local anesthesia is especially effective for medically compromised patients (53), for patients with specific fears (e.g. dental syringe, needle or injections) and in treating patients with true (or suspected) hypersensitivity to local anesthetic agents. Additionally, hypnosis can be used as an effective tool in the treatment of myofascial pain, especially with some of the subjective pain parameters (70).

Although it was previously shown that both pain effect and pain sensation are reduced in hypnosis, it has been suggested that hypnosis may exert a more powerful reduction of pain effect than pain sensation (59). A significant effect has been shown when hypnosis was used on patients with persistent idiopathic types of orofacial pain (functional pain) (1). According to pain diaries, there was consistent and clinical significant pain relief over the course of five sessions with hypnosis. Ongoing studies are also addressing the neurobiological mechanisms responsible for the pain-relieving effects of hypnosis, e.g. role of the forebrain and brain stem and genetic profiles.

Case study

Generally, anxiety increases the perception of noxious events as painful. Fear and anxiety are often encountered in the dental situation. Therefore, it could have a major effect on the patient's report of pain and concomitantly on the diagnosis (and treatment) of various dental pathologies, including endodontic lesions.

A 16-year-old girl suffering from dental phobia arrived at a dental clinic for a routine examination. Owing to high dental anxiety, the patient had previously received treatment under general anesthesia. On entering the clinic, she manifested a high degree of apprehension but agreed (with apparent stress) to undergo "initial" examination.

Examination revealed a radiolucent lesion between the roots of teeth 12 and 13. Sensibility tests performed on the teeth adjacent to the lesion evoked a clear pain response, suggesting a non-endodontic etiology. To avoid possible misdiagnosis, the tests were repeated several times by two independent dentists with identical result. Contralateral teeth reacted in a similar manner. The patient was referred for further consultation to an oral surgery clinic. The outcome of sensibility tests was consistent with previous results. Each time a cold or electrical stimulus was applied to the teeth in question, the patient reacted with pain coupled with apprehension.

It was decided to perform an excision biopsy of the lesion under general anesthesia. Owing to the proximity of the lesion to the apex of tooth 12, it was assumed that following the biopsy a possible devitalization of the tooth would occur. To avoid this complication and further trauma, preventive endodontic treatment was suggested prior to biopsy.

When the pulp of tooth 12 was opened, a non-vital, necrotic tissue was revealed. The canal was cleaned and sealed without further intervention. Six months later the lesion had resolved and no further treatment was necessary.

Comment: Pain is often a poor indicator of the cause of a condition. In this particular case, patient anxiety, stress and anticipation of pain may have led to subjective interpretation of the applied stimuli as pain and to a clinical reaction that suggested the presence of a vital pulp. In the diagnosis of endodontic pathology, pain often serves as an important parameter of evaluation. The high incidence of fear and anxiety among dental patients, and the influence of anxiety on the pain experience, call for a reserved frame of mind to individuals' report of pain.

Adverse reaction to local anesthesia

Occasionally, a patient presents a history of hypersensitivity to local anesthetic agents. Symptoms usually include immediate reactions to the injection procedure (dizziness, shortness of breath, tachycardia, etc.). Although the true incidence of local anesthetic allergy is low, this type of history often involves the patient's and dentist's anxiety regarding the use of the drug in question. Hypnosis can play a major role in controlling pain and the associated distress. In many cases, adverse reactions to local anesthetic are psychogenic in nature. Fear of injection, or of dental treatment in general, could lead to some of the most frightening "allergic" reactions – tachycardia and vasodepressor syncope. Even patients with a former diagnosis of allergy may not be allergic (18). Patients correctly or incorrectly labeled as "allergic" tend to postpone routine treatment until pain is intolerable, resulting in deterioration of their dental condition. Again, hypnosis may be used as an efficient tool to induce analgesia/anesthesia and to enable routine dental care. Generally, the hypnotic response is easily achieved because of the patient's high motivation and because the method is only used to achieve analgesia. Consequently, patients do not expect any "psychological" intervention and, therefore, have less need to mobilize psychological defenses (45).

Concluding remarks

This chapter has reviewed the current knowledge related to the many and often complex dimensions of pain. It is important for dentists working with endodontics that they have a good understanding of the neurobiological pain mechanisms underlying tooth-related pain conditions, as well as the influence of psychosocial aspects. Most often, pain is neither just a neurobiological phenomenon nor a pure psychological construct and this needs to be acknowledged in the diagnosis and intervention strategies. In the endodontic clinic, treating and managing pain from a multidimensional perspective is an important challenge.

References

1. Abrahamsen R, Baad-Hansen L, Svensson P. Hypnosis in the management of persistent idiopathic orofacial pain – clinical and psychosocial findings. *Pain* 2008; 136: 44–52.
2. Adler G, Gattaz WF. Pain perception threshold in major depression. *Biol. Psychiatry* 1993; 34: 687–9.
3. Anderson DB, Pennebaker JW. Pain and pleasure: alternative interpretations for identical stimulation. *Eur. J. Soc. Psychol.* 1980; 10: 207–12.
4. Arntz A, Van Eck M, Heumans M. Predictions of dental pain: the fear of any expected evil is worse than the evil itself. *Behav. Res. Ther.* 1990; 38: 29–41.
5. Baad-Hansen L. Atypical odontalgia – pathophysiology and clinical management. *J. Oral Rehabil.* 2008; 35: 1–11.
6. Bandura A. Self-efficacy. Toward a unifying theory of behavior change. *Psychol. Rev.* 1977; 84: 191–215.
7. Bentsen B, Svensson P, Wenzel A. Evaluation of effect of 3D video glasses on perceived pain and unpleasantness induced by restorative dental treatment. *Eur. J. Pain* 2001; 5: 373–8.
8. Blumenshon R, Ringler D, Eli I. Pain perception in patients with schizophrenia. *J. Nerv. Ment. Dis.* 2002; 190: 481–3.
9. Brand HS, Gortzak RATh, Palmer-Bouva CCR, Abraham RE, Abraham-Inpijn L. Cardiovascular and neuroendocrine responses during acute stress induced by different types of dental treatment. *Int. Dent. J.* 1995; 45: 45–8.
10. Burdette BH, Gale EN. Pain as a learned response: a review of behavioral factors in chronic pain. *J. Am. Dent. Assoc.* 1988; 116: 881.
11. Bush FM, Harkins SW, Harrington WG, Price DD. Analysis of gender effects on pain perception and symptom presentation in temporomandibular pain. *Pain* 1993; 53: 73–80.
12. Cairns BE. The influence of gender and sex steroids on craniofacial nociception. *Headache* 2007; 74: 319–24.
13. Corah NL, Gale EN, Illing SJ. Psychological stress reduction during dental procedures. *J. Dent. Res.* 1979; 58: 1347–51.
14. Craig KD. Emotional aspects of pain. In: *Textbook of Pain*, 2nd edn (Wall PD, Melzack R, eds). London: Churchill Livingstone, 1989.
15. Cruccu G, Anand P, Attal N, Garcia-Larrea L, Haanpää M, Jørum E, et al. EFNS guidelines on neuropathic pain assessment. *Eur. J. Neurol.* 2004; 11: 153–62.
16. Dao TTT, LeResche L. Gender differences in pain. *J. Orofac. Pain* 2000; 7: 169–84.
17. Defrin R, Lotan M, Pick CG. The evaluation of acute pain in individuals with cognitive impairment: a different effect of the level of impairment. *Pain* 2006; 124: 312–20.
18. deShazo RD, Nelson HS. An approach to the patient with a history of local anesthetic hypersensitivity: experience with 90 patients. *J. Allergy Clin. Immunol.* 1979; 63: 387–94.
19. Dworkin RH, Clark WC, Lipsitz JD, Amador XF, Kaufmann CA, Opler LA, et al. Affective deficits and pain insensitivity in schizophrenia. *Motivation Emotion* 1993; 17: 245–76.
20. Dworkin RH, O'Connor AB, Backonja M, Farrar JT, Finnerup NB, Jensen TS, et al. Pharmacologic management of neuropathic pain: evidence-based recommendations. *Pain* 2007; 132: 237–51.
21. Dworkin SF, Chen AC. Pain in clinical and laboratory contexts. *J. Dent. Res.* 1982; 61: 772–4.
22. Dworkin SF, Chen ACN, Schubert MM, Clark DW. Cognitive modification of pain: information in combination with N_2O. *Pain* 1984; 19: 339–51.
23. Eich E, Reeves JL, Jaeger B, Graff-Radford SB. Memory of pain: relation between past and present pain intensity. *Pain* 1985; 23: 375–9.
24. Eli I. *Psychophysiology: Stress, Pain and Behavior in Dental Care*. Boca Raton, FL: CRC Press, 1992.
25. Eli I, Bar-Tal Y, Fuss Z, Korff E. Effect of biological sex differences on the perception of acute pain stimulation in the dental setting. *Pain Res. Manage.* 1996; 1: 201–6.

26. Eli I, Bar-Tal Y, Fuss Z, Silberg A. Effect of intended treatment on anxiety and on reaction to electric pulp stimulation in dental patients. *J. Endod.* 1997; 23: 694–7.

27. Eli I, Baht R, Kozlovsky A, Simon H. Effect of gender on acute pain prediction and memory in periodontal surgery. *Eur. J. Oral Sci.* 2000; 108: 99–103.

28. Eli I, Schwartz-Arad D, Baht R, Ben-Tuvim H. Effect of anxiety on the experience of pain in implant insertion. *Clin. Oral Implant Res.* 2003; 14: 115–18.

29. Erskine A, Morley S, Pearce S. Memory for pain: a review. *Pain* 1990; 41: 255–65.

30. Fillingim RB, Maixner W. Gender differences in the responses to noxious stimuli. *Pain Forum* 1995; 4: 209–21.

31. Gatchel RJ, Turk DC (eds). *Psychological Approaches to Pain Management.* New York: The Guilford Press, 1996.

32. Geary DC. *Male, Female – The Evolution of Human Sex Differences.* Washington, DC: American Psychological Association, 1998.

33. Greenspan JD, Craft RM, LeResche L, Arendt-Nielsen L, Berkley KJ, Fillingim RB, *et al.* Studying sex and gender differences in pain and analgesia: a consensus report. *Pain* 2007; 132: S26–45.

34. Guieu R, Samuelian JC, Coulouvrat H. Objective evaluation of pain perception in patients with schizophrenia. *Br. J. Psychiatry* 1994; 164: 253–5.

35. Harkins SW. Discussion on "Long term memory of acute post-surgical pain" by Sisk AL, *et al*. *J. Oral Maxillofac. Surg.* 1991; 49: 358–9.

36. Hennequin M, Morin C, Feine JS. Pain expression and stimulus localisation in individuals with Down's syndrome. *The Lancet* 2000; 356: 1882–7.

37. Hilgard ER, Hilgard JR. *Hypnosis in the Relief of Pain.* Los Altos, CA: William Kaufmann, 1975.

38. Houle M, McGrath PA, Moran G, Garret OJ. The efficacy of hypnosis and relaxation-induced analgesia on two dimensions of pain for cold pressor and electric tooth pulp stimulation. *Pain* 1988; 33: 241–51.
    Twenty-eight subjects were submitted to tooth pulp stimulation and cold pressor stimulation of the forearm according to a specified protocol. Treatment conditions included progressive muscle relaxation and hypnotic induction with suggestions for analgesia. Both hypnosis and relaxation significantly reduced the strength and unpleasantness of tooth pulp stimulation, but only the unpleasantness dimension of cold pressor pain. Authors conclude that the quality of the cognitive-based therapies used varied according to subject's characteristics, the efficacy of the intervention and according to the nature of the noxious stimuli.

39. Hucho T, Levine JD. Signaling pathways in sensitization: toward a nociceptor cell biology. *Neuron* 2007; 55: 365–76.

40. IASP Subcommittee on Taxonomy. Pain terms: a list with definitions and notes on usage. *Pain* 1979; 6: 249–52.

41. Kaufman E, Weinstein P, Milgrom P. Difficulties in achieving local anesthesia. *J. Am. Dent. Assoc.* 1984; 108: 205–8.

42. Kent G. Memory of dental pain. *Pain* 1985; 21: 187–94.
    The possibility that patient memory for acute pain is reconstructed over time was tested by comparing the degree of pain remembered 3 months after a dental appointment with both expected and experienced pain, as reported immediately before and after the appointment. There was a closer association between remembered and expected pain than between remembered and experienced pain, particularly for patients with high dental anxiety.

43. Kent G. Self-efficacious control over reported physiological, cognitive and behavioural symptoms of dental anxiety. *Behav. Res. Ther.* 1987; 25: 341.

44. Keogh E, Hatton K, Ellery D. Avoidance versus focused attention and the perception of pain: differential effects for men and women. *Pain* 2000; 85: 225–30.

45. Kleinhauz M, Eli I. When pharmacologic anasthesia is precluded – the value of hypnosis as a slow anesthetic agent in dentistry. *Spec. Care Dent.* 1993; 13: 15–18.

46. Koutantji M, Pearce SA, Oakley DA. The relationship between gender and family history of pain with current pain experience and awareness of pain in others. *Pain* 1998; 77: 25–31.

47. Kupers R. Sex differences in pain: and now for something completely different. *Behav. Brain Sci.* 1997; 20: 455–6.

48. Lindsay SJE, Humphris G, Barnby GJ. Expectations and preferences for routine dentistry in anxious adult patients. *Br. Dent. J.* 1987; 163: 120.

49. Lipton JA, Marbach JJ. Ethnicity and the pain experience. *Soc. Sci. Med.* 1984; 19: 1279–98.

50. Litt MD. Self efficacy and perceived control: cognitive mediators of pain tolerance. *J. Pers. Soc. Psychol.* 1988; 54: 149–60.

51. Litt MD. A model of pain and anxiety associated with acute stressors: distress in dental procedures. *Behav. Res. Ther.* 1996; 34: 459–76.

52. Logan HL, Baron RS, Kohout F. Sensory focus as therapeutic treatments for acute pain. *Psychosom. Med.* 1995; 57: 475–484.

53. Lu DP, Lu GP. Hypnosis and pharmacological sedation for medically compromised patients. *Compend. Contin. Educ. Dent.* 1996; 17: 32–40.

54. McCaul KD, Malott JM. Distraction and coping with pain. *Psychol. Bull.* 1984; 95: 516–33.

55. Melzack R. Pain and stress: a new perspective. In: *Psychosocial Factors in Pain* (Gatchel RJ, Turk DC, eds). New York: The Guilford Press, 1999: 89–106.

56. Moore R, Brødsgaard I, Mao TK, Miller ML, Dworkin SF. Perceived need for local anesthesia in tooth drilling among Anglo-Americans, Chinese, and Scandinavians. *Anesth. Prog.* 1998; 45: 22–8.

57. Neufeld RWJ, Davidson PO. The effects of vicarious and cognitive rehearsal on pain tolerance. *J. Psychosom. Res.* 1971; 15: 329.

58. Potvin S, Marchand S. Hypoalgesia in schizophrenia is independent of antipsychotic drugs: a systematic quantitative review of experimental studies. *Pain* 2008; 138: 70–8.

59. Price DD. Psychological mechanisms of pain and analgesia. *Progress in Pain and Management*, Vol. 15. Seattle, WA: IASP Press, 1999: 183–204.

60. Roskies E, Lazarus RS. Coping theory and the teaching of coping skills. In: *Behavioral Medicine: Changing Health Lifestyles* (Davidson PO, Davidson SM, eds). New York: Brunner/Mazel, 1980: 38.

61. Rudy TE, Kerns RD, Turk DC. Chronic pain and depression: toward a cognitive–behavioral mediation model. *Pain* 1988; 35: 129–40.

62. Staud R, Robinson ME, Vierck CJ Jr, Price DD. Diffuse noxious inhibitory controls (DNIC) attenuate temporal summation of second pain in normal males but not in normal females or fibromyalgia patients. *Pain* 2003; 101: 167–74.

63. Sternbach RA. *Pain Patients, Traits and Treatment.* New York: Academic Press, 1974.

64. Svensson P, Sessle BJ. Orofacial pain. In: *Clinical Oral Physiology* (Miles TS, Nauntofte B, Svensson P, eds). Carol Stream, IL: Quintessence, 2004: 93–139.

65. Taintor JF, Langeland K, Valle GF, Krasny RM. Pain: a poor parameter of evaluation in dentistry. *Oral Surg. Oral Med. Oral Pathol.* 1981; 52: 299–303.

66. Unruh AM. Gender variations in clinical pain experience. *Pain* 1996; 65: 123–67.

67. Unruh AM, Ritchie J, Merskey H. Does gender affect appraisal of pain and pain coping strategies? *Clin. J. Pain* 1999; 15: 31–40.

68. Weir R, Browne G, Tunks E, Gafni A, Roberts J. Gender differences in psychosocial adjustment to chronic pain and pain and expenditures for health care services used. *Clin. J. Pain* 1996; 12: 277–90.

69. Weisenberg M, Raz T, Hener T. The influence of film-induced mood on pain perception. *Pain* 1998; 76: 365–75.

70. Winocur E, Gavish A, Emodi-Perlman A, Halachmi M, Eli I. Hypno-relaxation as treatment for myofacial pain disorder: a comparative study. *Oral Surg. Oral Med. Oral Pathol. Oral Radiol. Endod.* 2002; 93: 429–34.

71. Woolf CJ. Pain: moving from symptom control toward mechanism-specific pharmacologic management. *Ann. Intern. Med.* 2004; 140: 441–51.

72. Zborowski M. *People in Pain.* San Francisco, CA: Jossey-Bass, 1969.

73. Zola K. Culture and symptoms: an analysis of patient presenting complaints. *Am. Sociol. Rev.* 1966; 66: 615–30.

74. Zubieta JK, Smith YR, Bueller JA, Xu Y, Kilbourn MR, Jewett DM, *et al.* Mu-opioid receptor-mediated antinociceptive responses differ in men and women. *J. Neurosci.* 2002; 22: 5100–7.

75. Zubieta JK, Heitzeg MM, Smith YR, Bueller JA, Xu K, Xu Y, *et al.* COMT val158met genotype affects mu-opioid neurotransmitter responses to a pain stressor. *Science* 2003; 299: 1240–3.

Chapter 17
Clinical epidemiology

Claes Reit and Lise-Lotte Kirkevang

Introduction

A case scenario

A 48-year-old male visits your dental clinic because of mild pain from the right lower jaw. The patient has recently moved to your city. He tells you that he had two porcelain crowns made about 2 years ago. Approximately 6 months after the crowns were placed he began to feel some diffuse discomfort. Now he wants to see if anything can be done about his problem. At the clinical examination you find crowns on the first and second right lower molars. There is no tenderness to percussion or palpation. You tell the patient that it is necessary to perform a radiographic examination, and he accepts. In the radiographic image you detect signs of periapical bone destruction in relation to both the mesial and the distal root of the first molar. You tell the patient that you must test the vitality of the tooth, but probably the pulp is dead and microbes have invaded the root canals and caused an inflammatory response in the tissues surrounding the root tips. You probably will have to perform root canal treatment. In this situation a keen patient, besides the cost of the treatment, is likely to have many questions:

- How sure can you be of the diagnosis?
- What caused the pulp necrosis?
- Is periapical inflammation a common finding?
- What factors are associated with an increased risk?
- What is the probability that the suggested treatment will cure the disease?
- Will my general health be compromised if the tooth is not treated?
- How long can a root filled tooth be retained?

To answer these questions and predict what will happen in this specific case you have to rely on various sources of information: basically on the dental scientific literature, but also on your own experiences and information and advice of colleagues. In this chapter you will find an overview of relevant data found in the scientific literature.

Clinical epidemiology

From a conceptual point of view endodontic treatment might be regarded as a set of procedures used to either prevent or treat apical periodontitis (AP) (58). Thus, the treatment of a case with pulpitis is considered to be successful if the treatment prevents AP from developing. Accordingly, the treatment of a case with an infected necrotic pulp and periapical inflammation is considered successful if, after a healing period there are no clinical or radiographic signs of AP.

With this conceptual model in mind it becomes important to study the prevalence, incidence and healing of AP in various populations, and to identify factors that influence these parameters. Such studies enable us to make predictions about individual patients. The science based on studies of groups of patients to ensure that the predictions are valid is called *clinical epidemiology* (26). Clinical epidemiology seeks to answer important clinical questions using methods developed by epidemiologists (Core concept 17.1).

Epidemiological methods

Epidemiology is the study of factors affecting the health and illness of populations and is of fundamental importance when interventions are to be made in the interest of public health and preventive medicine. It is considered a basic methodology of public health research and is highly regarded in evidence-based medicine for identifying risk factors for disease. Furthermore, epidemiology is essential to establish optimal treatment approaches in clinical practice. Epidemiological studies are generally based on samples of populations. Populations are large numbers of people in a defined setting (e.g. Denmark or the county of Västra Götaland in Sweden) or with a certain trait or characteristic (e.g. AP or root filled teeth). For practical reasons it is usually impossible to examine every individual in the population, therefore a sample or a subset of the population is selected. In the selection of the material and registration of data the investigator has

Core concept 17.1 Definition of common concepts used in epidemiological research

Population:	Large group of people in a defined setting
Sample:	Subset of a population
Bias:	A process at any stage of inference tending to produce results that depart systematically from the true values (selection, measurement, confounding)
Exposure:	Any agent or factor that is thought to cause disease
Outcome:	The measure of disease occurrence
Prevalence:	The total number of present cases at a given point of time
Incidence:	The number of new cases that appear over a given period of time
Risk:	The probability of some untoward event (the outcome)
Risk factors:	Characteristics that are associated with an increased risk of becoming diseased
Prognosis:	Prediction of the future course of disease
Prognostic factors:	Conditions that are associated with a given outcome of the disease
Odds:	Ratio between two probabilities
Odds ratio:	Ratio of disease when exposed relative to ratio of disease when unexposed
Relative risk:	Risk of disease when exposed relative to risk of disease when unexposed

to control for bias. Bias is defined as "a process at any stage of inference tending to produce results that depart systematically from the true values" (52). Bias in relation to selection of patients is called selection bias and bias in relation to collection and registration of data is called information bias.

Another problem that may appear in epidemiological research is confounding. A confounding variable is associated with both the probable cause and the outcome, but is not included in the chain of cause and effect. For example it is known that smoking may cause larynx cancer, and it is known that smoking is frequent among individuals with heavy consumption of alcohol. If we want to estimate the effect of alcohol on larynx cancer, of course we then have to adjust for the confounding variable "smoking".

Epidemiologists use different types of study designs with varying levels of evidence. In dentistry the most frequently used are case series, which also represent the lowest level of evidence, followed by cross-sectional studies, case–control studies, cohort studies and eventually experimental studies (randomized controlled trials) which represent the highest level of evidence.

In a *case series* study a number of cases are collected in an *ad hoc* manner and the experience of a group of patients with a similar diagnosis or treatment is described. The sample is not necessarily drawn from a well-defined population. For example, teeth treated for pulpectomy in a certain clinic are followed over a period of time (often 2–4 years). At the end of the period the number of "successful" treatments (no symptoms or signs of AP) and number of "failures" (signs of AP) are registered. This type of study is rather common in endodontology. The classic study published by Strindberg (75) is a good example of a case series. Case series are mostly used to generate hypotheses that can be explored in other study models, since generalization is seldom justified.

In *cross-sectional studies* the prevalence (person-level) and frequency (tooth-level) of AP may be estimated, and risk indicators associated with the presence of AP may be identified. In this study design a sample of a well-defined population is examined at a specific moment in time. To assess the magnitude of a problem in a population, all individuals may be examined one by one, or a representative sample of the total population may be drawn. Often the latter is chosen because it is the most cost-efficient method to retrieve an estimate of the disease prevalence. The possibility of generalizing from the results therefore depends on how representative the study population is. During the last 20 years several cross-sectional studies addressing endodontic status in various countries have been performed (for an overview see Ref. 30). Sometimes cross-sectional studies are repeated, like the examinations of 35-year-olds living in Oslo, Norway. The investigation was originally carried out in 1973 and then repeated in 1984, 1993 and 2003 (73). Obviously each sample consists of different individuals and such a study design allows researchers to monitor population trends.

In a *case–control study* cases are selected according to outcome and within a well-defined population. Controls are individuals who could have been cases if they had developed the disease. Thus they should be selected from the same population as the cases, during the same time period and independent of exposure status. Case–control studies are an efficient way of retrieving estimates on the risk of different exposures, but are vulnerable to information bias since participants must remember past exposures. This study design has infrequently been used in endodontic research.

In a *cohort study* or longitudinal study, a well-defined group of people sharing a common experience or condition is followed over time. The group may include both healthy and diseased individuals. Since it is the same individuals who are examined repeatedly, a cohort study could be used to estimate both incidence and healing rate of a disease. Furthermore, risk factors can be identified and quantified (22, 30, 42, 43, 59).

Randomized controlled trials (RCTs) are studies in which subjects are assigned on a random basis to participate in one group receiving one treatment or another group receiving another treatment. The study design ensures that known and unknown confounding factors are evenly distributed between treatment groups by random allocation of subjects. RCTs are considered the most reliable form of scientific evidence in health care, because they eliminate spurious causality and bias.

In the following we will try to find answers to the clinically important questions mentioned earlier. The approach is inspired by Fletcher and Fletcher (26).

Diagnosis

Question: How sure can you be of the diagnosis of AP?

Since AP is infrequently associated with clinical symptoms, most epidemiological studies are based on data obtained from radiographic images. As in all diagnostic systems the accuracy is not perfect and the unavoidable presence of false-positive and/or false-negative diagnoses must be carefully considered and a strategy chosen (see Chapter 14). In radiographically based surveys the presence or absence of AP is often related to the occurrence of carious lesions, the quality of the coronal restoration and various technical aspects of the root filling. However, the two-dimensional nature of conventionally obtained radiographic images may not reveal minor occlusal, buccal or oral carious lesions, and approximal caries may be detectable only when a certain degree of demineralization has occurred (32, 63). There are similar limitations when the quality of restorations is evaluated in the radiograph. On the other hand, approximal defects may be more readily detected radiographically than clinically.

When the technical quality of root fillings is classified, the seal against the canal wall and the distance from the end of the root filling to the radiographic apex of the tooth are usually assessed and measured. Several studies have pointed out the difficulties in defining and maintaining radiographic criteria for the quality of seal resulting in substantial intra- and interobserver variation. Forsberg (27) found that when the distance between the root filling and the apex was measured the paralleling technique was superior to the bisecting-angle method.

Many epidemiological investigations just report on the presence or not of AP (or more exactly, the presence or not of periapical radiolucencies). Strindberg (75) based a very influential system for evaluating the outcome of endodontic therapy on this idea. Ørstavik *et al.* (57) did a more detailed interpretation of the radiographic image and proposed a five-step score (from a healthy periapical bone to severe AP), the "periapical index" (PAI). The PAI is based on original studies by Brynolf (11) in which she compared histology and radiography of periapical biopsy specimens (Key literature 17.1) Whatever system

is used for radiographic diagnosis of AP there are obvious problems with the accuracy and a substantial body of studies has been concerned with observer variation, calibration and observer strategy. The theoretical background to observer variation and how such problems could be handled are discussed in more detail in Chapter 14.

The short answer: *No diagnostic method is perfect and the risk of false-positive and false-negative diagnoses cannot be completely eliminated. However, in the clinical situation various diagnostic tests are combined and if radiographic signs of AP are found in combination with, for example, a negative pulp vitality test, the accuracy of the diagnosis is very good.*

Cause

Question: What caused the pulp necrosis?

Pulp necrosis is most frequently preceded by pulpal inflammation and caries generally is regarded as the main etiological reason for pulpal injury and endodontic treatment (see Chapter 2). This notion was supported by data from a study by Bjørndal *et al.* (8), who sent a questionnaire to 600 randomly selected Danish general dental practitioners. The practitioners were asked to recall the reason for doing their last root filling. Caries in teeth with vital pulps were given as the reason for performing root canal treatment in 55% of the cases. Kirkevang *et al.* (43) performed a cohort study including 473 individuals with 12443 teeth and found that teeth with primary caries had an increased risk of developing AP during a 5-year period (odds ratio = 2.9).

If the pulp resists a caries attack and survives there are several potential threats in the subsequent restoration of the crown. The use of rotary cutting instruments, leakage of bacterial elements along the margins of restorations and toxic effects of medicaments and materials used to restore cavities and cement crown and inlays may provoke pulpal inflammation and initiate processes that will lead to necrosis (see Chapter 2). Bergenholtz and Nyman (5) studied the effect prosthetic interventions might have on the pulp. They compared 255 abutment teeth and 417 non-abutment teeth in 52 patients treated for advanced periodontal disease. All pulps were initially diagnosed as vital and the observation period varied from 4 to 13 years (mean = 8.7 years). Pulpal necrosis (including periapical lesions) developed more frequently in abutment teeth than in non-abutment teeth (15% vs 3%). This finding was supported by a Danish cohort study where the presence of a filling as well as a crown increased the risk of developing AP, odds ratios being 2.8 and 7.9, respectively (43). Thus, pulp necrosis may be the result of repeated injuries that affect the pulp unfavorably.

Key literature 17.1   Systems for radiographic evaluation of the periapical tissues

Strindberg's (75) radiographic criteria for root canal treatment outcome were:

- **"Success"** when (a) the contours, width and structure of the periodontal margin were normal, and (b) the periodontal contours were widened mainly around the excess filling.
- **"Failure"** when there was (a) a decrease in the periradicular rarefaction, (b) unchanged periradicular rarefaction, and (c) an appearance of new rarefaction or an increase in the initial.
- **"Uncertain"** when (a) there were ambiguous or technically unsatisfactory control radiographs which could not for some reason be repeated, or (b) the tooth was extracted prior to the 3-year follow-up owing to unsuccessful treatment of another root of the tooth.

The periapical index (PAI)

Ørstavik et al. (57) used the results from a study by Brynolf (11) to develop an index for registration of AP, the periapical index (PAI). The index consists of five categories, each representing a step on an ordinal scale from sound periapical bone to severe apical periodontitis.

The visual references of the periapical index (PAI) (57)

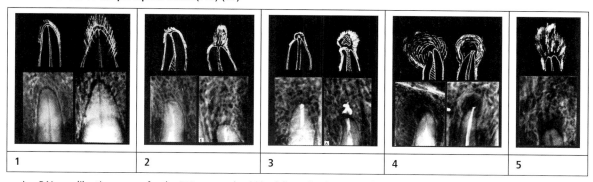

|1|2|3|4|5|

Before using PAI, a calibration course for the PAI system should be followed. When a tooth is to be scored, the observer should find the reference radiograph, by visual comparison, in which the periapical area is most similar to the periapical area of the tooth under evaluation. The corresponding score should then be assigned to the tooth. If the tooth is multirooted the highest score given to a root should be assigned to the tooth. If in doubt the higher score should be chosen.

The short answer: Necrosis often is the result of several accumulated injuries to the pulp. Even the most meticulous practitioner must expect some treated teeth to become necrotic.

Prevalence, frequency and incidence

Question: Is periapical inflammation a common finding?
Epidemiological studies on samples drawn from various populations demonstrate that AP is very common in adults. In the body of published data the prevalence of AP varies between 22 and 80% of the investigated individuals (Fig. 17.1), and the frequency of AP at tooth level is reported to be between 1 and 14% (Fig. 17.2).

Root fillings are frequently performed in Western countries and cross-sectional studies find 25–75% of individuals in various populations to have at least one root-filled tooth (30). Bjørndal and Reit (9) observed, despite the decreased caries prevalence, an increased number of endodontic treatments performed in Denmark between 1977 and 2003. At the same time a drastic reduction in tooth extractions was observed indicating a change in treatment attitude. To a greater extent molars were kept

and root filled instead of being extracted. Kirkevang et al. (40) compared two Danish subpopulations sampled in 1974–5 and 1997–8 and found that molars had become the most frequently root filled tooth group. Ridell et al. (66) found that endodontic treatment also is prevalent in younger age groups, and recorded in a sample of 19-year-olds in the city of Malmö, Sweden, that 9% had at least one root filled tooth.

In cross-sectional studies AP is often observed in root-filled teeth and frequencies between 25 and 50% have been reported (Fig. 17.3). In contrast, pulpectomy and root canal treatment were shown in many clinical studies to be highly successful procedures when carried out under optimal conditions. Studies (mostly designed as case series) generally demonstrate "failure" rates in only 5% (pulpectomy) to 15% (treatment of non-vital pulps in teeth with AP) when treatments are performed by specialists or students under supervision (38, 72, 75). The obvious difference between what is possible to achieve (as found in case series or RCTs) and what is observed in the general population (as found in cross-sectional studies) is of great concern for the profession. It is, however, important to realize that cross-sectional studies do

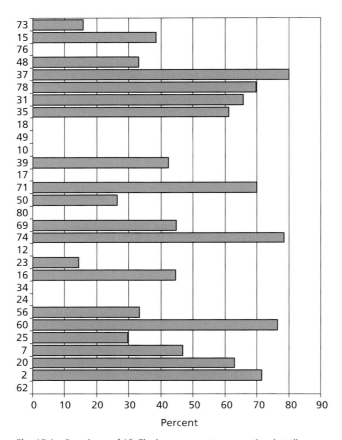

Fig. 17.1 Prevalence of AP. The bars represent cross-sectional studies numbered according to the reference list and arranged after publication year (newest on top). The studies report on the proportion of *individuals* in which at least one tooth is associated with radiographic signs of AP.

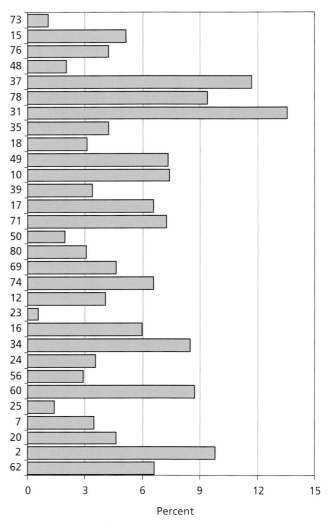

Fig. 17.2 Frequency of AP. The bars represent cross-sectional studies numbered according to the reference list and arranged after publication year (newest on top). The studies report on the proportion of *teeth* associated with radiographic signs of AP.

not include the time dimension and are therefore not suitable to investigate treatment success or failure.

Hypothetically the observed decreasing caries prevalence should lead to a decrease in the prevalence of AP over time. This hypothesis was confirmed in three repeated cross-sectional studies (23, 28, 59) but refuted in one (71). In the latter, which is the most recent and most comprehensive repeated cross-sectional study, it was demonstrated that the proportion of individuals with root fillings and the proportion of individuals with AP decreased over a 30-year time period. The overall presence of AP in teeth was almost stable, however the proportion of AP in root filled teeth had increased.

When we want to measure the *incidence* of AP in a population it is insufficient to only record the number of cases or the proportion of cases that are affected. A periapical inflammatory lesion might heal or persist and a new one might appear and therefore it is necessary to take the time dimension into account. The endodontic literature includes only a limited number of longitudinal observational studies that could give us information on the incidence and healing of AP (22, 28, 42, 61).

Frisk and Hakeberg (28) studied middle-aged and elderly women in Göteborg and, in relation to aging, found: a significant loss of teeth; that the ratio of root filled teeth increased; and that the number of teeth with AP tended to decrease. Eckerbom *et al.* (22) found no improvement in periapical health during a 20-year observation period; on the contrary, the number of root filled teeth and teeth with AP increased.

Data from two longitudinal studies, one Swedish (61) and one Danish (42), allow for a more detailed comparison. Both studies found that over an observation period of 5–10 years less than 5% of initially "healthy" teeth showed signs of pulpal or periapical disease. The proportion of root filled teeth with AP that remained diseased was higher in the Danish study, whereas the proportion of diseased root filled teeth that were

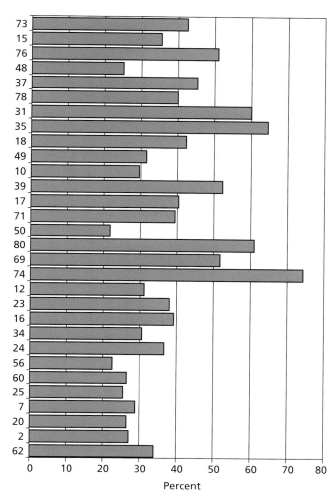

Fig. 17.3 Frequency of AP in root filled teeth. The bars represent cross-sectional studies numbered according to the reference list and arranged after publication year (newest on top). The studies report on the proportion of *root filled teeth* associated with radiographic signs of AP.

extracted was higher in the Swedish study. The healing proportion for the teeth that had received endodontic treatment in the Swedish study was higher than in the Danish study, but the observation period was longer. Comparing teeth with AP at baseline in the Danish study and in the Swedish study it seems as if teeth with AP, teeth that may be difficult to treat, or perhaps have other dental problems, were more likely to be extracted 20 years ago than today (61, 42). This observation corresponds well with the findings of Bjørndal and Reit (9), who found that in the adult Danish population more root fillings have been performed, especially in 40–60-year-old individuals, and the number of tooth extractions has more than halved from 1977 to 2003.

The short answer: *Teeth with AP and root filled teeth are very common in all investigated populations. AP is not only observed in teeth with infected necrotic pulps but is most frequently found in root filled teeth.*

Risk for apical periodontitis

Question: What factors are associated with an increased risk for AP?

Several cross-sectional studies have tried to identify risk indicators associated with the presence of AP. Such factors may indicate a risk for a certain person (person level) or for a certain tooth (tooth level) of having AP. Only a few studies have placed the individual in focus. Aleksejuniene *et al.* (1) found that regular visits to the dentist and high numbers of decayed and filled teeth were associated with AP in a Lithuanian population. The strong association between dental work/caries and AP was confirmed in a Danish study by Kirkevang and Wenzel (44), who also found smoking to be a risk indicator for having AP. However, smoking was not found to be associated with AP in a Swedish study by Bergström *et al.* (6).

Most endodontic epidemiological studies have tried to identify risk indicators at tooth level. In most cross-sectional studies the mere presence and also the technical quality of a root filling were associated with presence of AP (2, 7, 10, 12, 15–18, 20, 23–25, 31, 34, 35, 37, 39, 48–50, 56, 60, 62, 69, 71, 73, 74, 76, 78, 80).

Several studies have found an association between the quality of the coronal restoration and the presence or not of AP. Hypothetically microorganisms might invade the root canal via defective margins of fillings and crowns. Ray and Trope (64) found that the quality of the coronal restoration was of greater importance than the quality of the root filling for periapical health status, while others observed that if the root filling was adequate the coronal restoration was of less importance (41, 65, 69, 70, 71, 77).

If we want to assess risk factors associated with development of AP we must turn to longitudinal cohort studies (19, 22, 28, 43, 61). In a study by Petersson (59) it was found that periapical lesions that persisted or developed during the observation period were related to incomplete root canal obturation. In other longitudinal cohort studies the association between the quality of the root filling and AP was less clear (22, 43). Eckerbom *et al.* (22) found that the quality of root fillings improved over time, but the frequency of root filled teeth with AP increased. In a study by Kirkevang *et al.* (43) the interdependence of several potential risk factors related to the incidence of AP was investigated. Data suggested that smoking and reduced marginal bone level indicate an environment in the mouth that favors disease development. Furthermore the amount and quality of previous dental work could indicate whether a person was at high or low risk of developing AP. In teeth, the most decisive risk factors for developing AP were crowns and coronal fillings, especially inadequate ones. Presence of a root filling increased the risk of developing AP, whereas the quality of a root filling was insignificant. However, in relation to the healing of AP the quality of a root filling was of importance. Other dental diseases such as carious lesions and reduced marginal bone level also increased the risk of developing AP (Figs 17.4 and 17.5).

Thus, to lower the incidence of AP in the general population it seems that focus should be on improving the quality of restorative dental work, especially coronal restorations, and to diagnose and control the progression of carious lesions. Furthermore, to facilitate healing of AP the procedures by which root canals are cleaned, shaped, disinfected and filled should be optimal.

The short answer: AP develops as a result of microbial colonization of the root canal. Accordingly, factors that increase the potential for microorganisms to invade the canal (carious

lesions, pulp necrosis, defective root fillings and restorations) also increase the risk of AP. Risk factors at a personal level are not well understood at present.

Treatment

Question: What is the probability that the suggested treatment will cure the disease?
From a conceptual point of view there are three basic methodologies for endodontic treatment of teeth with apical periodontitis: (1) primary root canal treatment (the pulp is necrotic and the canal untreated); (2) non-surgical retreatment (the root filling is removed and the canal retreated); and (3) surgical retreatment (the apical area of a root filled tooth is approached surgically). The outcome of primary root canal treatment has been studied and reported on in more than 100 original scientific papers and several systematic literature reviews (for example 45, 47, 54, 55, 68). The key theory, of course, is that treatment should be directed towards combating the intracanal microbiota, and if this is successfully done and the canal is not re-infected, the lesion will heal. However, owing to substantial variations amongst studies in terms of case selection, study design, healing criteria, follow-up period, treatment methodology, etc., the basic data do not permit strong clinical conclusions. Nevertheless the studies indicate that if canals are cleaned and filled to within 2 mm of the apex and the seal is adequate, healing of AP can be expected with a probability of 0.85. This probability will decrease if the filling is short, the canal is overfilled or the seal is inadequate. Investigators have also found that the quality of the coronal restoration (risk of reinfection) of the tooth has a significant influence on the outcome. The significance of procedural parameters such as size, taper and extent of canal preparation, irrigation/medication regime and root filling material and technique still has to be further researched (55). When a tooth has to be surgically or non-surgically retreated the probability of healing will decrease (for a detailed discussion of prognosis and prognostic factors see Chapter 18), but with modern technique and instruments retreatment can also be performed with a very good prognosis.

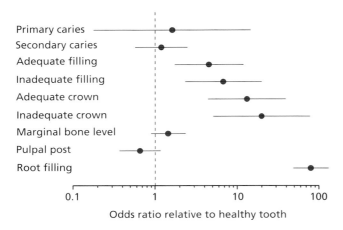

Fig. 17.4 Association between tooth-specific risk indicators and the presence of AP. The dots represent the risk estimates and the lines the 95% confidence intervals. The estimate is statistically significant if the confidence interval does not include 1. Odds ratio relative to a healthy tooth. All estimates are mutually adjusted (43).

The short answer: Good quality root canal treatment can be expected to heal AP in about 85 cases out of 100. If the primary treatment fails additional surgical or non-surgical retreatment leaves very few cases incurable.

Prognosis

Question: What are the effects of AP on general health?
The consequences, in terms of health risks, for a patient with AP are not well understood. It is widely documented that AP in an acute phase may be associated with local

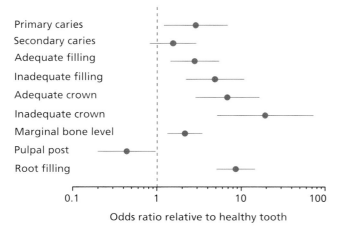

Fig. 17.5 Association between tooth-specific risk factors and incidence of AP. The dots represent the risk estimates and the lines the 95% confidence intervals. The estimate is statistically significant if the confidence interval does not include 1. Odds ratio relative to a healthy tooth. All estimates are mutually adjusted (43).

(e.g. swelling) as well as systemic (fever, intense pain, feeling of illness) reactions. Also, microorganisms from the root canal may disseminate to nearby regions and cause severe infections in, for example, the maxillary sinus and the deep regions of the throat (see Chapter 8). However, the potential of AP to cause disease in other bodily parts has been proposed as well as rejected over the years. Introduced by William Hunter (33) and based on the notion that microorganisms, or their associated toxins, could spread in the body and cause a range of diseases, the so-called focal infection theory, attracted many researchers in the first half of the 20th century. The theory was supported by clinicians and vast numbers of teeth with AP were extracted, primarily in order to prevent other more serious diseases. However, by the 1940s scientific data had discredited the theory and it lost its popularity (53).

In recent years a connection between chronic periodontal disease and an adverse systemic health condition like coronary heart disease (CHD) has been proposed (4). If the association is causal is not known but, broadly, the explanation could be that the regional inflammatory response to microorganisms releases cytokines systemically which in turn provoke deleterious vascular effects (4). The untreated root canal infection is rather similar to the microbiota isolated in periodontal disease and therefore a few investigators have studied a possible association between AP and CHD.

Frisk et al. (29) conducted a cross-sectional study of 1056 Swedish women aged 34–84 years. The material was examined clinically and radiographically. Number of root filled teeth and number of teeth with AP were registered as 0, 1, 2 or >2. AP was classified as either present or not. In a multivariate statistical analysis the authors found no association between CHD and any of the endodontic variables. Joshipura et al. (36) studied a sample of 34683 male health professionals. Data were collected by a questionnaire in which the participants had to report the number of root filled teeth and when treatments were carried out. By using this method it was not possible to get information on the presence or not of AP and the root filled tooth acted as a surrogate. The authors found a significant association between history of root canal treatment and incidence of CHD (relative risk = 1.38). However, the association was limited to the dentists in the investigated group. Caplan et al. (14) reported on 708 male participants who were examined every 3 years for a median follow-up time of 24 years. Teeth were classified as having an endodontic lesion if a periapical radiolucency was >2mm wide. The main exposure variable was "lesion-years", which was supposed to estimate the cumulative burden of of chronic apical inflammation experienced by each subject (for example, one tooth with an apical lesion for 3 years added 3 lesion-years to the participant-level total). The

main outcome variable was "time to first diagnosis of CHD". In a multivariate analysis the authors found an association between lesion-years and CHD risk among participants younger than 40 years.

The studies referred to show great variation, in terms of study design, case definition and the estimation of the burden of apical inflammation, which renders any definite conclusion about the connection between AP and CHD impossible to make at present. Future prospective studies are much needed since any general health risks (even if small) will make dentists and patients reconsider present treatment strategies (14).

The short answer: *At present there are no data that show a connection between AP and adverse general health conditions with any certainty. There might be an association between AP and CHD, but if such a relation exists it is not known if it is causal.*

Longevity of root filled teeth

Question: How long can a root filled tooth be retained?
Before starting on a root canal treatment most patients want to know whether a non-vital tooth will function equally well as a vital one. They want to know if the tooth's life span will be limited and the tooth extracted earlier than if it was not pulpally injured. This very central question has not been addressed by as many authors as would be expected. Caplan et al. (13) reported a matched cohort study in 202 subjects, each of whom had one tooth endodontically treated in 1987–88 and a similar contralateral tooth that was not root filled at that time. Teeth were followed up to 8 years (median = 6.7). Root filled teeth had significantly worse survival rate than their counterparts which were not root filled. Molars were more often extracted than non-molars. Adjusted hazard ratios for loss of root filled versus non-root filled molars and non-molars were 7.7 and 1.8, respectively. The authors concluded that endodontic therapy may prolong tooth survival but pulpal involvement may hasten tooth loss.

Lazarski et al. (46) and Salehrabi and Rotstein (67) investigated the databases of large US insurance companies. The former were able to record the outcome of 44163 cases and found that 94.4% of non-surgical root canal treated teeth remained functional over an average follow-up time of 3.5 years. In the Salehrabi and Rotstein (67) study the outcome of almost 1.5 million teeth was assessed. Overall, 97% of teeth were retained in the dental arch 8 years after initial non-surgical endodontic treatment. Substantially lower figures for the survival of endodontically treated teeth were reported by Meeuwissen and Eschen (51). In a study of 845 Dutch military servicemen they found that only 55% of root filled teeth had survived for 17 years.

Few investigators have been concerned with the reasons for extractions of root filled teeth. Potentially there are several reasons, for example, crown fracture, root fracture, marginal periodontitis, apical periodontitis and root resorption. In an attempt to analyze the reasons for extractions, Vire (79) collected all endodontically treated teeth that were removed over a 1-year period in a group practice. Of the 116 teeth, 59.4% were judged to be prosthetic failures primarily due to crown fracture. Periodontal failures constituted 32% of the material and only 8.6% of the extractions were due to endodontic causes. This study indicates that probably the most important step to prolong the survival of the tooth after the endodontic treatment is to consider its restoration. Accordingly several authors have proposed that crown placement may improve the longevity of root filled teeth. Aquilino and Caplan (3) followed a random sample of 400 teeth endodontically treated between 1985 and 1996. The authors found that root filled teeth not crowned after obturation were lost at a 6.0 times greater rate than teeth crowned after obturation.

The short answer: *Present knowledge indicates that non-vital root filled teeth are at greater risk of being extracted than teeth with a vital pulp. However, if the root canal treatment is of good quality and the crown properly restored the risks are lowered to what is an acceptable level for most people.*

Back to the case

Above we have reviewed literature that might help a clinician to answer questions put forward by patients in a situation like the one presented in the introductory case scenario. Based on this information and the clinical examination, the patient is informed that the tooth has developed apical periodontitis and that the diagnosis is very accurate. It should be explained to the patient that there is always a risk of pulp injury when enamel and dentin are removed to create space for a crown. The patient is informed that most often apical periodontitis is asymptomatic but symptoms like swelling and pain might develop. If the tooth is not treated the periapical bone destruction might increase. To eliminate the tooth as a health hazard and keep it functional, root canal treatment should be performed. There is a high probability that such a treatment will cure the disease.

It is obvious that information obtained in epidemiological studies is general in character and often refers to means of populations and often only can be expressed in the form of probabilities. Moreover, data tell of other patients treated by other dentists. Clinical knowledge is personal, which means that it is influenced by the armamentarium and the skill of the dentist. Therefore the best advice and answers to patients' questions are given if information from scientific studies is combined and compared with information from systematic recordings of the outcome of treatments provided by the individual dentist.

References

1. Aleksejuniene J, Eriksen H, Sidaravicius B, Haapasalo M. Apical periodontitis and related factors in an adult Lithuanian population. *Oral Surg. Oral Med. Oral Pathol. Oral Radiol. Endod.* 2000; 90: 95–101.
2. Allard U, Palmqvist S. A radiographic survey of periapical conditions in elderly people in a Swedish country population. *Endod. Dent. Traumatol.* 1986; 2: 103–8.
3. Aquilino SA, Caplan DJ. Relationship between crown placement and the survival of endodontically treated teeth. *J. Prosthet. Dent.* 2002; 67: 256–63.
4. Beck J, Garcia R, Heiss G, Vokonas PS, Offenbacher S. Periodontal disease and cardiovascular disease. *J. Periodontol.* 1996; 67: 1123–37.
5. Bergenholtz G, Nyman S. Endodontic complications following periodontal and prosthetic treatment of patients with advanced periodontal disease. *J. Periodontol.* 1984; 55: 63–8.
6. Bergström J, Babcan J, Eliasson S. Tobacco smoking and dental periapical condition. *Eur. J. Oral Sci.* 2004; 112: 115–20.
7. Bergström J, Eliasson S, Ahlberg KF. Periapical status in subjects with regular dental care habits. *Community Dent. Oral Epidemiol.* 1987; 15: 236–9.
8. Bjørndal L, Laustsen MH, Reit C. Root canal treatment in Denmark is most often carried out in carious vital molar teeth and retreatments are rare. *Int. Endod. J.* 2006; 39: 785–90.
9. Bjørndal L, Reit C. The annual frequency of root fillings, tooth extractions and pulp-related procedures in Danish adults during 1977–2003. *Int. Endod. J.* 2004; 38: 52–8.
10. Boucher Y, Matossian L, Rilliard F, Machtou P. Radiographic evaluation of the prevalence and technical quality of root canal treatment in a French population. *Int. Endod. J.* 2002; 35: 229–38.
11. Brynolf I. A histological and roentgenological study of the periapical region of human upper incisors (Thesis). *Odontol. Revy* 1967; 18 (Suppl. 11).
    A classic text in which the author investigated the correlation between radiographic and histological examination of the periapical tissues. The analyses were based on 320 human upper incisors (autopsy material) including 119 root filled and 201 unfilled teeth. The author compared bone structure, width and shape of radiolucency around the apex/foramen and width and shape of adjacent radiopacity as found in the radiographs with the histological appearances. She found it possible to distinguish different groups with well-defined pathological changes of different severity.
12. Buckley M, Spångberg LSW. The prevalence and technical quality of endodontic treatment in an American subpopulation. *Oral Surg. Oral Med. Oral Pathol.* 1995; 79: 92–100.
13. Caplan DJ, Cai J, Yin G, White BA. Root canal filled versus non-root canal filled teeth: a retrospective comparison of survival times. *J. Public Health Dent.* 2005; 65: 90–6.

14. Caplan DJ, Chasen JB, Krall EA, Cai J, Kang S, Garcia RI, *et al.* Lesions of endodontic origin and risk of coronary heart disease. *J. Dent. Res.* 2006; 85: 996–1000.

15. Chen CY, Hasselgren G, Serman N, Elkind MS, Desvarieux M, Engebretson SP. Prevalence and quality of endodontic treatment in the Northern Manhattan elderly. *J. Endod.* 2007; 33: 230–4.

16. De Cleen MJH, Schuurs AHB, Wesselink PR, Wu MK. Periapical status and prevalence of endodontic treatment in an adult Dutch population. *Int. Endod. J.* 1993: 26; 112–19.

17. De Moor RJG, Hommez GMG, De Boever JG, Delmé KIM, Martens GEI. Periapical health related to the quality of root canal treatment in a Belgian population. *Int. Endod. J.* 2000; 33: 113–20.

18. Dugas NN, Lawrence HP, Teplitsky PE, Pharoah MJ, Friedman S. Periapical health and treatment quality assessment of root filled teeth in two Canadian populations. *Int. Endod. J.* 2003; 36: 181–92.

19. Eckerbom M. *Prevalence and technical standard of endodontic treatment in a Swedish population.* Thesis, Stockholm, 1993.

20. Eckerbom M, Andersson J-E, Magnusson T. Frequency and technical standard of endodontic treatment in a Swedish population. *Endod. Dent. Traumatol.* 1987; 3: 245–8.

21. Eckerbom M, Andersson J-E, Magnusson T. A longitudinal study of changes in frequency and technical standard of endodontic treatment in a Swedish population. *Endod. Dent. Traumatol.* 1989; 5: 27–31.

22. Eckerbom M, Flygare L, Magnusson T. A 20-year follow-up study of endodontic variables and periapical status in a Swedish population. *Int. Endod. J.* 2007; 40: 940–8.

23. Eriksen HM, Berset GP, Hansen BF, Bjertness E. Changes in endodontic status 1973–1993 among 35-year-olds in Oslo, Norway. *Int. Endod. J.* 1995; 28: 129–32.

24. Eriksen HM, Bjertness E. Prevalence of apical periodontitis and results of endodontic treatment in middle-aged adults in Norway. *Endod. Dent. Traumatol.* 1991; 7: 1–4.

25. Eriksen HM, Bjertness E, Ørstavik D. Prevalence and quality of endodontic treatment in an urban adult population in Norway. *Endod. Dent. Traumatol.* 1988; 4: 122–6.

26. Fletcher RW, Fletcher SW. *Clinical Epidemiology: The Essentials.* Baltimore: Williams & Wilkins, 2005.

27. Forsberg J. *Radiographic distortion in endodontics.* Thesis, Univesity of Bergen, 1999.

28. Frisk F, Hakeberg M. A 24-year follow-up of rootfilled teeth and periapical health amongst middle aged and elderly women in Göteborg, Sweden. *Int. Endod. J.* 2005; 38: 246–54.

29. Frisk F, Hakeberg M, Ahlqwist M, Bengtsson C. Endodontic variables and coronary heart disease. *Acta Odontol. Scand.* 2003; 61: 257–62.

30. Frisk F. *Epidemiological aspects on apical periodontitis.* Thesis, Göteborg University, 2007.

31. Georgopoulou MK, Spanaki-Voreadi AP, Pantazis N, Kontakiotis EG. Frequency and distribution of root filled teeth and apical periodontitis in a Greek population. *Int. Endod. J.* 2005; 38: 105–11.

32. Gwinnett AJ. A comparison of proximal carious lesions as seen by clinical radiography, contact microradiography, and light microscopy. *J. Am. Dent. Assoc.* 1971; 83: 1078–80.

33. Hunter W. Oral sepsis as a cause of disease. *Br. Med. J.* 1900; 2: 215–16.

34. Imfeld TN. Prevalence and quality of endodontic treatment in an elderly urban population of Switzerland. *J. Endod.* 1991; 17: 604–7.

35. Jiménez-Pinzón A, Segura-Egea JJ, Poyato-Ferrera M, Velasco-Ortega E, Ríos-Santos JV. Prevalence of apical periodontitis and frequency of root filled teeth in an adult Spanish population. *Int. Endod. J.* 2004; 37: 167–73.

36. Joshipura KJ, Pitiphat W, Hung HC, Willett WC, Colditz GA, Douglass CW. Pulpal inflammation and incidence of coronary heart disease. *J. Endod.* 2006; 32: 99–103.

37. Kabak Y, Abbott PV. Prevalence of apical periodontitis and the quality of endodontic treatment in an adult Belarusian population. *Int. Endod. J.* 2005; 38: 238–45.

38. Kerekes K, Tronstad L. Long-term results of endodontic treatment performed with a standardized technique. *J. Endod.* 1979; 5: 83–90.

39. Kirkevang L-L, Hørsted-Bindslev P, Ørstavik D, Wenzel A. Frequency and distribution of endodontically treated teeth and apical periodontitis in an urban Danish population. *Int. Endod. J.* 2001; 34: 198–205.

40. Kirkevang L-L, Hørsted-Bindslev P, Ørstavik D, Wenzel A. A comparison of the quality of root canal treatment in two Danish subpopulations examined 1974–75 and 1997–98. *Int. Endod. J.* 2001; 34: 607–12.

41. Kirkevang L-L, Ørstavik D, Hørsted-Bindslev P, Wenzel A. Periapical status and quality of root fillings and coronal restorations in a Danish population. *Int. Endod. J.* 2000; 33: 509–15.

42. Kirkevang L-L, Væth M, Hørsted-Bindslev P, Wenzel A. Longitudinal study of periapical and endodontic status in a Danish population. *Int. Endod. J.* 2006; 39: 100–7.

43. Kirkevang L-L, Væth M, Hørsted-Bindslev P, Bahrami G, Wenzel A. Risk factors for developing apical periodontitis in a general population. *Int. Endod. J.* 2007; 40: 290–9.

44. Kirkevang L-L, Wenzel A. Risk indicators for apical periodontitis. *Community Dent. Oral Epidemiol.* 2003; 31; 59–67.

45. Kojima K, Inamoto K, Nagamatsu K, Hara A, Nakata K, Morita I, *et al.* Success rate of endodontic treatment of teeth with vital and nonvital pulps. A meta-analysis. *Oral Surg. Oral Med. Oral Pathol. Oral Radiol. Endod.* 2004; 97: 95–9.

46. Lazarski MP, Walker WA III, Flores CM, Schindler WG, Hargreaves KM. Epidemiological evaluation of the outcome of nonsurgical root canal treatment in a large cohort of insured dental patients. *J. Endod.* 2001; 27: 791–6.

47. Lewsey DJ, Gilthorp MS, Gulabivala K. An introduction to meta-analysis within the framework of multilevel modelling using the probability of success of root canal treatment as an illustration. *Community Dent. Health.* 2001; 18: 131–7.

48. Loftus JJ, Keating AP, McCartan BE. Periapical status and quality of endodontic treatment in an adult Irish population. *Int. Endod. J.* 2005; 38: 81–6.

49. Lupi-Pegurier L, Bertrand MF, Muller-Bolla M, Rocca JP, Bolla M. Periapical status, prevalence and quality of endodontic treatment in an adult French population. *Int. Endod. J.* 2002; 35: 690–7.

50. Marques MD, Moreira B, Eriksen HM. Prevalence of apical periodontitis and results of endodontic treatment in an adult, Portuguese population. *Int. Endod. J.* 1998; 31: 161–5.

51. Meeuwissen R, Eschen S. Twenty years of endodontic treatment. *J. Endod.* 1983; 9: 390–3.

52. Murphy EA. *The Logic of Medicine*. Baltimore: Johns Hopkins University Press, 1976.

53. Murray CA, Saunders WP. Root canal treatment and general health: a review of the literature. *Int. Endod. J.* 2000; 33: 1–18.

54. Ng YL, Mann V, Rahbaran S, Lewsey J, Gulabivala K. Outcome of primary root canal treatment: systematic review of the literature – Part 1. Effects of study characteristics on probability of success. *Int. Endod. J.* 2007; 40: 921–39.

55. Ng YL, Mann V, Rahbaran S, Lewsey J, Gulabivala K. Outcome of primary root canal treatment: systematic review of the literature – Part 2. Influence of clinical factors. *Int. Endod. J.* 2008; 41: 6–31.

56. Ödesjö B, Helldén L, Salonen L, Langeland K. Prevalence of previous endodontic treatment, technical standard and occurrence of periapical lesions in a randomly selected adult, general population. *Endod. Dent. Traumatol.* 1990; 6: 265–72.

57. Ørstavik D, Kerekes K, Eriksen HM. The periapical index: a scoring system for radiographic assessment of apical periodontitis. *Endod. Dent. Traumatol.* 1986; 2: 20–34.

58. Ørstavik D, Pitt Ford T. *Essential Endodontology*. Oxford: Blackwell Munksgaard, 2008.

59. Petersson K. Endodontic status of mandibular premolars and molars in an adult Swedish population. A longitudinal study 1974–1985. *Endod. Dent. Traumatol.* 1993; 9: 13–18.

60. Petersson K, Lewin B, Håkansson J, Olsson B, Wennberg A. Endodontic status and suggested treatment in a population requiring substantial dental care. *Endod. Dent. Traumatol.* 1989; 5: 153–8.

61. Petersson K, Håkansson R, Håkansson J, Olsson B, Wennberg A. Follow-up study of endodontic status in an adult Swedish population. *Endod. Dent. Traumatol.* 1991; 7: 221–5.

62. Petersson K, Petersson A, Olsson B, Håkansson J, Wennberg A. Technical quality of root fillings in an adult Swedish population. *Endod. Dent. Traumatol.* 1986; 2: 99–102.

63. Purdell-Lewis DJ, Groeneveld A, Pot TJ, Kwant W. Proximal carious lesions. A comparison of visual, radiographical and microradiographical appearance. *Neth. Dent. J.* 1974; 81: 6–15.

64. Ray HA, Trope M. Periapical status of endodontically treated teeth in relation to the technical quality of the root filling and the coronal restoration. *Int. Endod. J.* 1995; 28: 12–18.

65. Riccuci D, Gröndahl K, Bergenholtz G. Periapical status of root filled teeth exposed to the oral environment by loss of restoration or caries. *Oral Surg. Oral Med. Oral Pathol. Oral Radiol. Endod.* 2000; 90: 354–9.

66. Ridell K, Sundin B, Matsson L. Endodontic treatment during childhood and adolescence. A survey of 19-year-olds living in the city of Malmö, Sweden. *Swed. Dent. J.* 2003; 27: 83–9.

67. Salehrabi R, Rotstein I. Endodontic treatment outcomes in a large patient population in the USA: an epidemiological study. *J. Endod.* 2004; 30: 846–50.

68. Sathorn S, Parashos P, Messer HH. Effectiveness of single- versus multiple-visit endodontic treatment of teeth with apical periodontitis: a systematic review and meta-analysis. *Int. Endod. J.* 2005; 38: 347–55.

69. Saunders WP, Saunders EM, Sadiq J, Cruickshank E. Technical standard of root canal treatment in an adult Scottish sub-population. *Br. Dent. J.* 1997; 182: 382–6.

70. Segura-Egea JJ, Jiménez-Pinzón A, Poyato-Ferrera M, Velasco-Ortega E, Ríos-Santos JV. Periapical status and quality of root fillings and coronal restorations in an adult Spanish population. *Int. Endod. J.* 2004; 37: 525–30.

71. Sidaravicius B, Aleksejuniene J, Eriksen HM. Endodontic treatment and prevalence of apical periodontitis in an adult population of Vilnius, Lithuania. *Endod. Dent. Traumatol.* 1999; 15: 210–15.

72. Sjögren U, Hägglund B, Sundqvist G, Wing K. Factors affecting the long-term results of endodontic treatment. *J. Endod.* 1990; 16: 498–504.

73. Skudutyte-Rysstad R, Eriksen HM. Endodontic status amongst 35-year-old Oslo citizens and changes over a 30-year period. *Int. Endod. J.* 2006; 39: 637–42.

74. Soikkonen KT. Endodontically treated teeth and periapical findings in the elderly. *Int. Endod. J.* 1995; 28: 200–3.

75. Strindberg LZ. The dependence of the results of pulp therapy on certain factors. An analytic study based on radiographic and clinical follow-up examinations (Thesis). *Acta Odontol. Scand.* 1956; 14: Suppl. 21.

76. Sunay H, Tanalp J, Dikbas I, Bayirli G. Cross-sectional evaluation of the periapical status and quality of root canal treatment in a selected population of urban Turkish adults. *Int. Endod. J.* 2007; 40: 139–45.

77. Tronstad L, Asbjörnsen K, Døving L, Pedersen I, Eriksen HM. Influence of coronal restorations on the periapical health of endodontically treated teeth. *Endod. Dent. Traumatol.* 2000; 16: 218–21.

78. Tsuneishi M, Yamamoto T, Yamanaka R, Tamaki N, Sakamoto T, Tsuji K, Watanabe T. Radiographic evaluation of periapical status and prevalence of endodontic treatment in an adult Japanese population. *Oral Surg. Oral Med. Oral Pathol. Oral Radiol. Endod.* 2005; 100: 631–5.

79. Vire DE. Failure of endodontically treated teeth: classification and evaluation. *J. Endod.* 1991; 17: 338–42.

80. Weiger R, Hitzler S, Hermle G, Löst C. Periapical status, quality of root canal fillings and estimated endodontic treatment needs in an urban German population. *Endod. Dent. Traumatol.* 1997; 13: 69–74.

Chapter 18
Endodontic decision making

Claes Reit

The outcome of endodontic treatment

Essentially, endodontic treatment is concerned with the removal of diseased or infected pulp tissue, instrumentation and medication of the root canal system and, finally, the placement of a root filling. The ultimate objective is to protect the individual from a potentially painful and harmful infection and, at the same time, to preserve the affected tooth in the long term. The disease processes usually take place in body compartments hidden from direct inspection and therefore methods of evaluating the biological outcome of the treatment are limited to observation of clinical symptoms, signs in radiographs and microscopic findings in periapical biopsy specimens. Because clinical symptoms occur infrequently and periapical biopsies are difficult to obtain, the continuation of pathological alterations is largely determined by radiographic observations.

Evaluation of the outcome of endodontic therapy has a long tradition and numerous investigations based on radiographic examination have been published. Strindberg published a study with great impact on subsequent research in 1956 (68). He launched a system of criteria based on the absence or presence of radiographic rarefactions around the apex of the evaluated root. Basically, Strindberg held that a periapical radiolucency diagnosed at the end of a predetermined healing period should be considered a sign of biological treatment "failure". Although Strindberg found that complete periapical healing sometimes did not occur until 10 years after treatment, he recommended a 4-year follow-up period as a cut-off before a final classification be made. The system provided a simple distinction between healthy and diseased roots and has been widely used ever since as a tool to assess the general outcome of endodontic treatment but also to investigate the factors that might influence postoperative healing (Fig. 18.1).

A more detailed system for radiographic diagnosis of the periapical tissues was launched by Ørstavik *et al.* in 1986 (47). Based on a study by Brynolf (11) in which the histological and radiographic pictures of periapical

biopsy specimens were compared, a five-level score was constructed. The score is intended to represent a disease progression from normal periapical structures (score 1) to severe apical periodontitis with exacerbating features (score 5). In recent years the so-called periapical index (PAI) has often been used as an alternative to the Strindberg type of classification.

Investigations assessing the outcome of endodontic therapy often are designed as so-called follow-up studies. In these studies a cohort of patients is treated and followed clinically and radiographically for a certain period of time. Ideally such studies should be made prospectively and factors of interest randomized, but for ethical and practical reasons a retrospective (looking back in files and records) non-randomized approach has more often been used. However, this scientific strategy might bias the data produced and limit the confidence in conclusions made.

A substantial body of data has been collected from follow-up studies through the years. The accumulation of knowledge is impeded by the large variation among the investigations concerning factors such as case selection, sample size, treatment procedures, recall rate, length of observation period and radiographic interpretation. Regardless of the limitations, the studies clearly demonstrate that endodontic treatment can be a highly successful procedure. When teeth without apical periodontitis (irrespective of the pulp being vital or necrotic) are treated *lege artis*, a successful outcome might be expected in as many as 95% of cases. When treatment "fails", i.e. periapical inflammation develops, it is most often caused by microorganisms contaminating the root canal during treatment or postoperatively via defective margins of fillings and crowns.

Compared with vital pulp cases, teeth with necrotic pulp and apical periodontitis are associated with less probability of treatment success. In such cases microorganisms are present initially that, owing to the complexity of the root canal system, may not invariably be combated successfully. However, thorough cleaning, medication and obturation of the canal will produce periapical healing in 80–85% of cases.

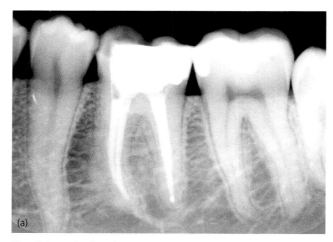 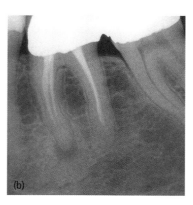

Fig. 18.1 Evaluation of treatment outcome according to Strindberg (68). (a) A 4-year follow-up of a first lower molar. The patient has no clinical symptoms and no signs of pathology are visible in the radiograph. The case is classified as a "success". (b) This tooth was treated 5 years ago for apical periodontitis. The periapical lesion has decreased but is still visible on the radiograph. The case is classified as a "failure".

Factors influencing treatment outcome

Although endodontic treatment is usually successful, some cases will fail and it is the responsibility of the individual clinician to minimize this number. Therefore, knowledge of the various factors that will influence treatment outcome is of supreme importance. Such "prognostic" factors might be found in the situation that precedes endodontic treatment (*preoperative* factors) or might be associated with the treatment *per se* (*operative* factors). Also, elements of the *postoperative* situation might exert influence on the long-term outcome (Core concept 18.1, Key literature 18.1).

Preoperative factors

In most studies general factors such as age, gender and health have not been demonstrated to influence the treatment outcome significantly. When local factors have been considered some investigators reported that certain teeth appeared to be more favorable than others, but a systematic pattern among the studies and teeth has not been found. The only preoperative factor that consistently has proven to influence significantly the treatment result is the diagnosis of apical periodontitis. Studies have reported a 10–25% lower healing rate when radiographic signs of periapical disease are present compared with when they are not.

Operative factors

The apical extent of the root canal preparation is one of the major prognostic factors. The instrumentation ideally should be terminated at the constriction of the canal,

> **Core concept 18.1   Factors influencing treatment outcome**
>
> **Preoperative factors**
> - Apical periodontitis
>
> **Operative factors**
> - Extent of canal preparation
> - Quality of seal
> - Procedural error
>
> **Postoperative factors**
> - Coronal leakage
> - Post preparation

which is normally located 1–2mm from the root apex. Sjögren *et al.* (65) reported periapical health to be restored in 94% of teeth with apical periodontitis when the preparation and root filling ended within 0–2mm of the radiographic apex. On the other hand, when preparations were made to a shorter distance from the apex, only 68% healed.

Over-instrumentation of the root canal should be avoided. When the instrument passes through the apical foramen it may induce displacement of infected dentin into the periapical tissues. Attached to dentin chips, microorganisms are protected from the defense mechanisms of the host and may therefore survive and impair the potential for healing (76). More importantly, repeated overinstrumentation may enlarge the apical foramen and alter its original anatomy. Consequently, the root canal preparation will lose its apical resistance form, which will often result in overfill combined with an inadequate apical seal of the canal (Fig. 18.2).

Key literature 18.1 Dependence of the results of pulp therapy on certain factors

In his influential thesis published in 1956, Strindberg (68) performed an analytical study of endodontic treatment results based on radiographic and clinical follow-up examinations. The case material consisted of 254 patients with 529 teeth and 775 roots treated by the author during a 6-year period. The root canals were instrumented by the use of Kerr files and Hedström files. Vital cases were mostly completed in two sessions. When a devitalizing agent was used (arsenic or paraformaldehyde paste) the treatment was extended to three appointments. The non-vital pulps were often treated in four or more sessions. The intracanal medicaments that were used varied considerably. Five percent chloramine solution was usually employed in vital cases. In non-vital cases rotation of the medicament (e.g. tricresol formalin, iodine preparations, oil of cloves, creosote) was preferred to prevent the bacteria from acquiring resistance to any one substance. The canals were filled with gutta-percha and either Alytit or an 8% solution of resin in chloroform as a binding agent. Although Strindberg's treatment methodology to a large extent must be regarded as obsolete, his scientific approach still is commendable.

Follow-ups were carried out over a period of 6 months to 10 years. The results of the therapy for a particular root were assessed at the radiographic examinations as a "success" when the contours, width and structure of the periodontal margin were normal and the periodontal contours were widened mainly around the excess filling, and as a "failure" when there was a decrease in the periradicular rarefaction, unchanged periradicular rarefaction and a new or an increase in the initial rarefaction.

After a follow-up period of 4 years, Strindberg found that 95% of cases without an initial rarefaction and 71% with an initial rarefaction could be classified as "successes". If the period was extended to include those observations that he had made beyond the 4-year point, the healing rate among the latter increased to 85%.

Strindberg's main idea was to study the impact of certain factors on periapical healing. He found that components such as *age, health status, number of interappointment dressings, treatment flare-up* and *root filling material* did not exert any significant influence on the therapeutic result. Among the statistically significant factors he reported *periradicular status, number of roots, canal preparation* and *type of root filling*. Healing was found less frequently among cases with an initial periapical radiolucency. Successful operations were carried out more often in three-rooted than in two-rooted teeth, which in turn displayed better results than single-rooted teeth. Where the apical part of the canal was mechanically widened only to a diameter corresponding to Hedström file no. 1, a higher proportion of success was obtained than when wider files were used. Negative influences were found if canals were prepared to or beyond the radiographic apex and if the root filling showed poor adaptation to the root canal or was forced through the apical foramen.

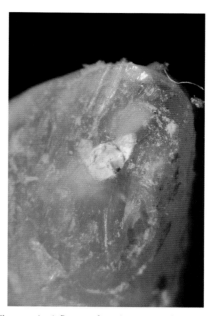

Fig. 18.2 The negative influence of overinstrumentation. A repeated instrumentation through the apical foramen will result in a "tear-drop" anatomy and hinder a good-quality root filling seal.

seal will allow tissue fluids to leak into the root canal and supply microorganisms with substrate, and also let bacterial products seep out into the periapical tissues. On the other hand, a defective coronal seal might provide the oral microorganisms with an avenue for a postoperative infection of the root canal, resulting in "late" or sustained periapical inflammation.

If negative prognostic factors accumulate, the chance of success will decrease substantially (19). For example, if an apical periodontitis case is overinstrumented and provided with a defective seal, the probability of healing will be low. In an epidemiological study Bergenholtz *et al.* (8) found that 55% of overfilled roots with defective seals were associated with periapical radiolucency. On the other hand, when root fillings ended within 2 mm of the apex and were assessed as adequate, only 12% demonstrated periapical radiolucency.

Procedural errors such as perforations, broken instruments and ledge formations will not directly impede periapical healing. However, the prognosis of the treatment is decreased if the complication obstructs the cleaning of an infected canal.

Postoperative factors

Data from recent studies indicate that the quality of the restoration of the tooth might exert an influence on the outcome of endodontic treatments (52). Microorganisms may enter via defective margins and colonize a poorly sealed root canal (60) (Fig. 18.3). Furthermore, leaking saliva may dissolve the sealer and break the resistance

Overfill of the root canal has been found to be associated with a decreased healing rate in teeth with apical periodontitis. The sustained lesion is probably caused not so much by the material itself (gutta-percha is well tolerated by the tissues) but more by intracanal microbes. Numerous outcome studies have proven the significance of the quality of the root filling seal. An inadequate apical

against reinfection (63). However, provided that instrumentation and root fillings are carefully performed, the problem of coronal leakage may not be of great clinical importance (58).

The placement of a post in the root canal does not influence the outcome of endodontic treatment *per se*. However, the post preparation might break the root filling seal either by disturbing the adaptation of the material to the dentinal walls or by leaving too little gutta-percha remaining. Studies have shown that not less than 3 mm should remain in the apical part of the canal (35).

Prevalence of endodontic "failures"

Assessment of the technical quality and the outcome of endodontic treatment at a population level has a long tradition in the Scandinavian countries. Studies have reported a relatively high frequency of defective root fillings. It has been reported consistently that 25–35% of endodontically treated teeth are associated with periapical radiolucencies (8, 17, 21, 50). Similar findings during recent years have been reported from other areas of Europe and North America as well as in Asia (12, 14, 15, 26, 39, 61, 62, 74) (see also Chapter 17). The most frequently adopted study design, the cross-sectional survey, does not disclose the dynamics of the periapical reactions and therefore does not provide direct information on the frequency of "failed" treatments. However, in a follow-up study, Petersson *et al.* (48) found about equal numbers of healing and developing periapical radiolucencies in a cohort followed over a period of 11 years. Obviously there is a contradiction between what is possible with

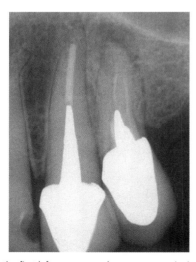

Fig. 18.3 In the first left upper premolar, an acute periapical lesion developed 1 year after placement of the post and crown. The root filling seal is defective and microorganisms probably have entered the canals either via microleakage or during the restorative procedures.

endodontic therapy (85–90% success) and what is actually obtained (60–70% success). It is an important task for the profession to try to close this gap.

At present the number of potential retreatment cases is huge; in Sweden (9 million inhabitants) it can be estimated to be about 2.5 million. However, the attitude to the clinical management of such cases has been found to vary substantially among clinicians (5, 25, 49, 54, 55, 66).

Variation in the management of periapical lesions in endodontically treated teeth

Variation in health care procedures was recognized early, at the beginning of the 20th century. In a classical study (4) of 1000 11-year-old schoolchildren in New York City it was found that 650 children had undergone tonsillectomy. The remaining 350 children were sent to a group of physicians. A total of 158 children were selected for tonsillectomy. Those rejected (182) were sent to another group of physicians and 88 of them were then suggested for tonsillectomy. After that, the remaining children were examined by a third group of physicians, and then only 65 children remained for whom tonsillectomy had not been suggested. At that point the study was interrupted owing to a shortage of physicians to consult. This report inspired investigators to challenge the clinical consensus of a variety of medical (and dental) procedures. Troubled over the results of these studies, Eddy (18) concluded:

> "Uncertainty creeps into medical practice through every pore. Whether a physician is defining a disease, making a diagnosis, selecting a procedure, observing outcomes, assessing probabilities, assigning preferences, or putting it all together, he is walking on a very slippery terrain. It is difficult for nonphysicians, and for many physicians, to appreciate how complex these tasks are, how poorly we understand them, and how easy it is for honest people to come to different conclusions."

The large variation among clinicians when suggesting the treatment or retreatment of endodontic cases was first demonstrated by Smith *et al.* (66). Several reports have confirmed that the mere diagnosis of a persistent periapical radiolucency in an endodontically treated tooth does not consistently result in suggestions for retreatment among clinicians (48, 49, 54) (Key literature 18.2). For example, Reit and Gröndahl (55) found that only 39% of persistent periapical lesions diagnosed by practitioners were followed by a retreatment decision.

Owing to their complexity, clinical decision problems have attracted interdisciplinary attention. In addition to interest from health professionals, philosophers, psy-

Key literature 18.2   Variation in management of
endodontic "failures"

Reit and Gröndahl (54) showed 35 dental officers from the Public
Dental Health Organization in Sweden 33 endodontically treated
teeth showing periapical radiolucencies of various sizes. The cases
were presented with radiographs and the same clinical history: "The
actual patient, aged 45, is in good general health and presents with
no clinical symptoms from his teeth or oral soft tissues. The present
radiographs were taken at a routine examination. Root fillings are
more than four years old. This is your first examination of the patient,
who has no other dental problems and no further dental treatment is
being considered." For each case the clinicians made a choice among
five options: no therapy indicated, wait 12 months, non-surgical
retreatment, surgical retreatment or extraction.

In the figure each bar represents one case. In no case was the same
option suggested unanimously by all examiners. In eight teeth all five
options were suggested, and in 15 cases four of the alternatives. The
number of teeth selected for therapy (surgical or non-surgical retreatment or extraction) had an interexaminer range of 7–26 teeth.

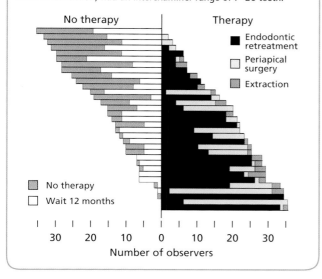

chologists and economists have also contributed (16).
Two main areas of research and thinking can be identified: descriptive and prescriptive. Descriptive projects
aim at mapping out and explaining how clinicians reason
and make decisions. Prescriptive, or normative, projects,
on the other hand, are concerned with how decisions
should or ought to be made.

Clinical decision making: descriptive projects

In studies of clinical reasoning several models have been
suggested and used (16). Some investigators have
focused on the artistic, or intuitive, aspects of clinical
practice (51). In the tradition of "judgment analysis",
researchers have tried to reveal the pieces of information
or "cues" used at conscious or unconscious levels that

influence a person's decision-making policy. This
approach has been applied in several domains (10),
including judgments of third molar removal (29). In a
series of innovative investigations Kahneman *et al.* (28)
explored a proposition that people most often rely on a
small number of heuristic principles to make decisions.

Attempts have been made to explain the observed
variation in the management of periapical lesions in
endodontically treated teeth. Because several studies
have demonstrated large interindividual variation in
radiographic interpretation of the periapical area (see
Chapter 14), it has been hypothesized that variation in
retreatment decisions might be regarded as a function of
diagnostic variation. However, studies of general practitioners have not supported this idea (55). The influence
of components, including risk assessment (56), clinical
context (5, 66), cognitive factors (56) and overall dental
treatment plans (49), has been explored. However, the
complexity and multiplicity of factors present in each
study have rendered interpretation of the results difficult. Kvist and Reit have proposed a model to explain
endodontic retreatment behavior (33, 34, 57). In the
"praxis concept" (Advanced concept 18.1) it is suggested
that dentists perceive periapical lesions of varying sizes
as different stages on a continuous health scale, based on
their radiographic appearance. Interindividual variation
then could be regarded as the result of different cut-off
points on the continuum for prescribing retreatment.

Kvist *et al.* (30) examined endodontic retreatment
concepts among 157 general dental practitioners from a
Swedish county. In the study it was possible to distinguish

Advanced concept 18.1   The praxis concept

This theory hypothesizes that dentists conceive of periapical health
and disease not as either/or situations but as states on a continuous
scale. On this scale a major lesion represents a more serious condition
than a smaller one. Variation between decision makers then could be
regarded as the result of the individual's selection of differing cut-off
points on the scale for prescribing retreatment. Placement of the cut-
off point is dependent on value but also is influenced by factors such
as costs, quality of seal and accessibility to the root canal.

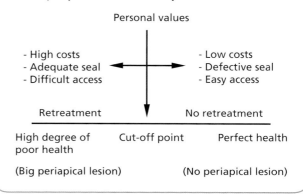

between two main types of strategies used by the practitioners: (i) disease-focused and (ii) illness-focused. The first group included three subgroups. (ia) The mere sign of periapical disease consistently implied retreatment. (ib) Signs of disease had to reach a higher level to elicit retreatment. (ic) Signs of disease were combined with non-disease factors, which modified the final retreatment decision (corresponding to the praxis concept). (ii) Focus on illness; as long as the patient did not complain or showed any clinical symptoms of periapical disease the treatment result was accepted. Among the observed strategies it was the one derived from the praxis concept that attracted most general dental practitioners.

Åkerblom Rawski et al. (1) used a qualitative approach and interviewed 20 Swedish endodontists and 20 general practitioners. They found that the endodontists seemed to mainly think in terms of strategy (ia) while the general practitioners reasoned in line with the praxis concept. The explanatory potential of the praxis concept was also supported in a study of endodontic retreatment decision making among 172 dental students in Saudi Arabia (2).

Endodontic retreatment decision making: a normative approach

Probably the most highly developed normative decision-making model is the "expected utility theory" (EUT) (for a review, see Ref. 23). The philosophical foundation is to be found in classical utilitarianism, whereas its mathematical origins are even older. The advent of modern EUT is associated with the influential work of von Neumann and Morgenstern (45), which made some of the psychological assumptions of utilitarianism redundant. The theory was introduced to medicine by Ledley and Lusted (37) and, under the concept of "clinical decision analysis", discussed in detail by Lusted (38) and Weinstein and Fineberg (75). Over the last 30 years clinical decision analysis has received increasing attention in medicine as well as dentistry (59).

Clinical decision analysis prescribes that the problem should be structured as a "decision tree", which logically displays the available actions and their possible consequences. Then the listed outcomes are assessed regarding probabilities and values ("utilities"). After this, the weighed sum (expected utility) of each strategy is computed and the action with the highest sum is chosen.

Reit and Gröndahl (54) approached the management of periapical lesions in endodontically treated teeth from a decision analysis point of view. The problem was structured graphically (54) and later probabilities and utilities were produced and "best" actions were calculated (53, 56). However, large parts of the critical information needed for calculations are very uncertain, therefore in the present context the decision tree will be used only as a rational basis for clinical deliberations, with no explicit calculations being made.

The structure of the decision problem

The structure of the decision-making problem is logically and temporally displayed in Fig. 18.4. Before retreatment of a root filled tooth with apical periodontitis is actually allowed to start, there are basically three clinical questions that have to be answered and three choices that have to be made. When a periapical radiolucency is detected the clinician first has to question whether the corresponding lesion might be expected to heal or not. If there is a chance of healing, the case should be followed for an additional period of time. If it is thought that the patient will not benefit from further observation, the second question will be raised: should the case be retreated or not? The choice is between accepting the situation as it is or trying to improve on it. This is the most difficult and complex of the choices that have to be made and no simple answers are available. If retreatment is favored there will be a question of which clinical procedure to use. Personal skills, knowledge of prognosis and cost-effectiveness estimations will influence this decision.

Choice 1: Decide now/wait and see

As mentioned above, endodontic treatment of teeth with apical periodontitis has a good prognosis. The majority of the cases that will succeed show complete periapical healing within the first 2 years of root canal treatment. By extending the observation period, the healing frequency will increase and single cases have been reported not to completely resolve until 10 years postoperatively (68). However, most investigators recommend the placement of a cut-off of 4 years postoperatively, a time during which the healing curve flattens out. Thus, from a clinical point of view, a case initially treated for apical periodontitis might be observed for up to 4 years. If the lesion still persists, a decision has to be made between performing additional treatment or accepting the situation as it is (Fig. 18.5).

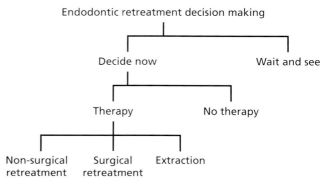

Fig. 18.4   The structure of the retreatment decision-making problem.

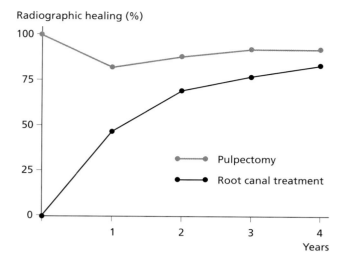

Fig. 18.5 Healing dynamics of the periapical tissues following treatment of vital and non-vital cases.

As a result of microbial contamination during intra-canal treatment procedures, roots without preoperative signs of apical periodontitis may develop disease. Most such cases may be detected within 1 year of the original treatment (46). "Late failures" are most often due to coronal leakage of microbes allowed to invade a defectively sealed root canal. Consequently, the diagnosis of a new periapical lesion in an endodontically treated root is normally regarded as a sign of root canal infection. Spontaneous healing is not expected to occur and therefore an extension of the observation period is not meaningful. Together with the patient, the clinician has to decide whether retreatment is indicated.

Occasionally transient apical radiolucencies develop around the apices of root filled teeth (68). Periapical inflammatory reactions with subsequent bone resorption might be elicited as responses to toxic components of antimicrobial medicaments and root filling materials. Toxicity usually decreases over time and inflammation resolves. Clinically this possibility should be considered if the radiolucency is associated with an overfill or is diagnosed within the first months of completed root canal treatment.

Choice 2: Therapy/no therapy

If a periapical lesion is not expected to heal, several factors have to be considered when choosing between retreating the root or not. For example, what is the probability that the detected periapical radiolucency represents disease? What are the general and local risks that have to be taken if the periapical disease is not treated? If retreatment is carried out, what are the risks of complications? What is the opinion of the patient; does he or she have any preferences? Are there any moral implications to be considered? See Core concept 18.2.

Core concept 18.2   To retreat or not?

Factors to consider:
- Probability of disease
- Risks of untreated disease
- Risks of retreatment procedures
- Personal preferences
- Ethical principles

Core concept 18.3   Basic retreatment decision-making principles

First principle
A periapical lesion in a root filled tooth that is not expected to heal should be retreated.

Second principle
If the first principle is not followed, reference must be made to respect for patient autonomy, retreatment risks or retreatment monetary costs.

To decide whether retreatment should be carried out or not is complex and each case can be the subject of counterproductive overdone deliberation. In the everyday situation the best consequences usually arise if a few simple principles are followed (Core concept 18.3).

It is assumed that the best overall consequences are obtained if dentists' primary suggestions to patients are to perform endodontic retreatment. The persistent lesion is an expression of a root canal infection and people benefit from having their infection treated. For the medically uncompromised patient the general health hazard is probably low and therefore false-positive diagnoses should be avoided. There is no solid scientific evidence available to distinguish among grades of periapical disease.

This first principle in Core concept 18.3 is quite dogmatic and leaves no room for deliberation: if retreatment is suggested and accepted no specific arguments are needed. However, if a persistent lesion is diagnosed and retreatment is not selected, then specific arguments have to be put forward. These are found in the second principle.

Respecting patient autonomy implies that the patient is fully informed regarding the situation but does not want retreatment. Attitudes to periapical disease vary among persons and subjectivity and personal values must be allowed to influence the decision-making process.

On an individual basis, potential risks associated with a retreatment procedure (e.g. root fracture following post removal, or nerve injury as a result of periapical surgery) might be judged to be too high. The objectively assessed risks (the probability of a certain event) should be weighed against the subjectively evaluated benefit of retreatment. When the patient's costs for retreatment are considered (treatment fee, drugs, loss of income, suffering), the cost/benefit ratio might be too low to be accepted.

Probability of disease

Biopsy specimens obtained from periapical areas showing radiolucencies have demonstrated the presence of pathologically altered tissue (granulomas, cysts) in about 95% of investigated cases (9, 67). It has been demonstrated convincingly that these reactions are mainly caused by microbial irritants present either in the root canal (36, 40, 43, 70) or in the periapical tissue (69, 73).

Risks of untreated disease

The risks of leaving a root with chronic periapical disease untreated are not well investigated. The infected root canal as a potential threat to systemic health is discussed in detail elsewhere in this book. The topic has been argued since Hunter in 1901 suggested that oral microorganisms could disseminate throughout the system and cause disease in other body compartments. Currently the evidence base is weak, but a connection between chronic periapical disease and coronary heart disease has been suggested (13, 27).

From a local point of view Eriksen (20) estimated the incidence of possible exacerbations per year to be less than 5%. The composition of the intracanal microbial flora of the root filled tooth generally varies from that of the necrotic pulp. It is not known if this difference influences the risk.

Risks of retreatment procedures

Clinical procedures may injure the tooth or the surrounding tissues. In order to re-enter the root canal tooth substance, crowns or posts often must be removed, with the risks of weakening the tooth structure or of causing direct fractures. Surgical retreatment might, for example, lead to mandibular nerve injury or to a visible retraction of the marginal gingiva. These risks have to be presented to the patient, included in the decision-making process and accepted before retreatment starts.

Personal preferences

Personal values will influence the decision-making process. As mentioned above, given identical information and similar diagnostic findings, patients (and doctors) will not choose the same clinical management of a certain disease. For example, some persons will be eager to have a bacteria-caused periapical inflammation in a root filled tooth treated, whereas others will be more reluctant.

The concept of value is multidimensional but it seems reasonable to suppose that there is a close connection between an individual's values and his or her value judgments. It has been suggested that one may apprehend values in acts of preferring (23, 45). This means that when faced with a choice, the values of an individual are reflected in his or her preference behavior. To measure preferences, various rating scales or the so-called "standard gamble" technique (Advanced concept 18.2) have been used (71, 72).

Reit and Kvist (57) transformed the standard gamble technique to suit an endodontic retreatment situation and investigated the subjective value of periapical health and disease among dental students as well as endodontic specialists (33). Substantial interindividual variations were registered in the evaluation of symptomless peri-

---

Advanced concept 18.2   The standard gamble

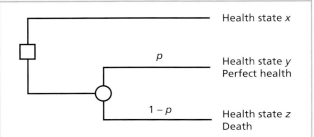

The subject is given a choice between two alternative courses of action. The options available are to continue living in the state of health described in a scenario (health state x) or to take a "gamble". The gamble is most often some type of treatment, e.g. surgery, that may lead to the restoration of health (health state y) but risks are involved and the patient might die (health state z). The probability (p) of attaining the best outcome of the gamble is systematically varied until the subject is indifferent between continuing to stay in health state x and taking the gamble. In this situation the value or "utility" of the two alternative actions is the same. This means that the utility of health state x (Ux) equals the relative sum of the utilities of state y (Uy) and state z (Uz). The formal expression will be:

$$Ux = (p)(Uy) + (1 - p)(Uz)$$

If perfect health is given a utility of 1 and death is given a utility of 0, then $Ux = (p) (1) + (1 - p) (0)$, i.e. $Ux = p$.

An example will make it easier to understand the method. Imagine that you have become blind and have not been able to see for a couple of years. A new surgical method is very promising and is offered to you. The problem is that there is a risk that you might die as a result of the surgical procedure. In the standard gamble the chance of survival or risk of dying is varied to find the frequency when you are indifferent between staying blind or being treated. Using the formula above, a person who is indifferent when there is a 10% risk of dying values the state of being blind to 0.90 on a scale from 1 to 0. Another person will perhaps be indifferent when there is only a 1% risk of dying, resulting in a utility value of 0.99.

apical lesions in root filled teeth. It was found that, at a subjective level, some persons will benefit much more from endodontic retreatment than others.

Ethical principles

Ethical reflection is a fundamental component of medical decision making. The utilitarian idea that it is the consequences, and only the consequences, of an action that will determine its moral value has been a central thought in Western moral philosophy, but it is still a controversial one. Traditionally, dentists and physicians have had a paternalistic approach to clinical practice. Today, however, patient autonomy is widely regarded as the primary ethical principle, emphasizing the importance of determining patient values. Besides respect for autonomy, the principles of beneficence (doing good to patients), non-maleficence (avoiding doing harm) and justice are often stressed in biomedical ethics (6).

Choice 3: Non-surgical versus surgical retreatment

The root filled tooth can be retreated using either an orthograde or a retrograde approach to the canal. In the orthograde or *non-surgical retreatment* the tooth is re-entered through the crown, the root filling removed and the canal once again negotiated before it is reobturated (Fig. 18.6). The main objective of the non-surgical retreatment is to eradicate potential intracanal microorganisms, thus allowing the periapical tissue to heal.

As an alternative to the orthograde approach, root canals might be retreated from a retrograde direction. A *surgical retreatment* will include removal of the periapical soft-tissue lesion, resection of the root tip and placement of a retrofill (Fig. 18.7). Using this method, complete eradication of intracanal microflora must not be expected. Rather, if the retrofill is effective, remaining microbes will be entombed in the root canal and shut off from periapical communication.

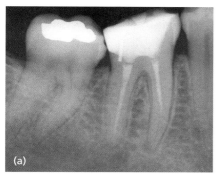 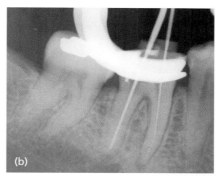 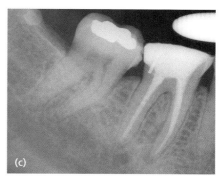

Fig. 18.6   Non-surgical endodontic retreatment. (a) The first lower molar was treated for pulpitis. (b) A periapical radiolucency developed 2 years postoperatively in the mesial root, signaling the presence of an intracanal infection. (c) The root canals were re-entered and subjected to antimicrobial procedures before they were refilled.

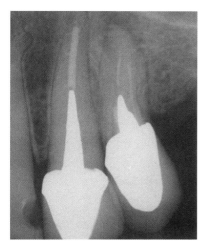 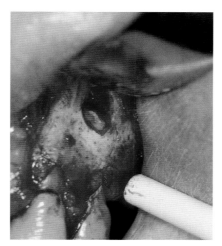 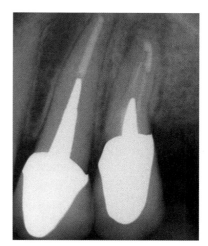

Fig. 18.7   Surgical endodontic retreatment. Following the placement of a post and crown, the second upper premolar developed periapical pathosis. The case was retreated surgically with removal of the soft-tissue lesion, apicoectomy, preparation of the apical portion of the canal with ultrasonic instruments and placement of a SuperEBA retrofill.

Several factors must influence the choice between non-surgical and surgical retreatment of a case, and aspects of biological outcome, costs and risks have to be deliberated.

Data on the outcome of non-surgical retreatment are most often available as part of general follow-up studies (for a review, see Ref. 24). Reported success rates in these investigations vary between 56% and 88%. The issue has been addressed specifically only by a few authors. After 2 years of observation, Bergenholtz *et al.* (7) found, in a prospective study, complete resolution of apical radiolucencies in 48% of 234 retreated roots. Decreased size of the radiolucency was observed in a further 30%. After a follow-up period of 5 years, Sundqvist *et al.* (70) reported complete resolution in 74% of 54 retreated teeth. Information on the outcome of surgical retreatment is abundant. Many methods have been adopted and reported success rates vary between 30% and 90% (24). In a comprehensive review of the literature, Hepworth and Friedman (24) tried to estimate the success rate of retreatment by means of a weighted average calculation, reporting 59% and 66% for surgical and non-surgical approaches, respectively.

Outcome studies have focused almost exclusively on either surgical *or* non-surgical retreatment procedures. However, Allen *et al.* (3), in a retrospective analysis of 633 cases where either of the two methods was used, found no difference. These observations were corroborated in a prospective, randomized investigation by Kvist and Reit (31, Key literature 18.3), who failed to show any systematic difference in the outcome of surgical and non-surgical endodontic retreatment.

Scientific data do not support the notion of a systematic difference in healing potential between surgical and non-surgical retreatment. However, whether the recent rapid development in technology (e.g. nickel–titanium instruments, rotary systems, surgical microscopes, ultrasonic retrotips, new retrofilling materials) will change this situation remains to be seen.

Because there seems to be no evidence for a systematic preference for one retreatment approach over the other, the choice has to be based on individual case-related factors (Core concept 18.4).

Core concept 18.4   Case-related factors influencing retreatment choice

- Etiology of the lesion
- Access to the root canal
- Monetary costs
- Quality of original treatment
- Position of the tooth
- Personal skills

Etiology of the lesion

In the majority of endodontic "failures" the periapical radiolucency is caused by an intracanal infection. However, in some cases the causative agent might be found in the periapical tissue, demanding a surgical retreatment approach. Bacteria such as *Actinomyces israelii* and *Propionibacterium propionicum* have been found to be able to prevail outside the root canal (22, 64). Additional strains have been observed (69, 73) but the prevalence of extraradicular microbes in chronic apical periodontitis is controversial (see also Chapters 6 and 7).

Key literature 18.3   Surgical versus non-surgical retreatment procedures

Kvist and Reit (31, 32) randomized 95 incisors and canines, classified as "failures" according to the Strindberg (68) criteria, to surgical or non-surgical retreatment. Three randomization factors were considered: size of the periapical radiolucency, the apical position and the technical quality of the root filling. Clinical and radiographic follow-ups were made at 6, 12, 24 and 48 months postoperatively. To obtain identical radiographs at consecutive intervals, an impression was obtained of the patient's dental arch. The impression was attached to a modified Eggen device. The observers used a strict definition of periapical disease. Disputed cases were subject to joint evaluation.

At the 12-month follow-up a statistically significantly higher healing rate was found in favor of surgical (●) over non-surgical (■) retreatment (*). At the final 48-month examination no such difference between groups was registered. Four surgically retreated cases classified as healed did show a relapse of the apical radiolucency, or presented with clinical symptoms at later follow-up. In one non-surgically retreated tooth the periapical radiolucency did recur.

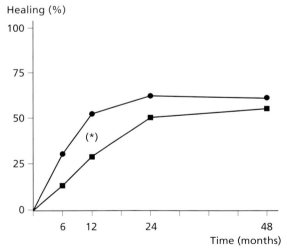

Significantly more patients reported discomfort (pain, swelling) after surgical retreatment than after non-surgical procedures. Analgesics were consumed significantly more often after surgery. Patients reported absence from work, mainly due to swelling and discoloration of the skin. Surgical retreatment tended to bring about greater indirect costs than non-surgical retreatment.

Periapical lesions in endodontically treated teeth may be associated with non-microbial agents, such as foreign body reactions to root filling materials (42) and the development of apical cysts. As described in Chapter 7 apical cysts are classified as "pocket" cysts and "true" cysts. The pocket cyst has an epithelial-lined cavity open to the root canal and might be expected to heal after conventional endodontic treatment (41). The cavity of the true cyst is completely enclosed by epithelial lining, which might make the dynamics of the cyst independent of any intra-canal treatment measures. Thus, traditionally it has been supposed that true cysts have to be enucleated surgically in order to heal. Yet, clinically it is not possible to differentiate between the various presentations of the periapical inflammatory reactions. No accurate tests are available but cysts are expected to be more prevalent among large lesions (44).

Access to the root canal

Endodontically treated teeth are often restored. In order to re-enter the root canal for retreatment, crowns sometimes have to be penetrated and posts removed. Such procedures will increase monetary costs and the risks for loosened crowns and root fractures. Therefore, the more complex the restoration, the more attractive the choice of surgical intervention.

Quality of original treatment

There is a strong correlation between the quality of the treatment (as reflected in the technical quality of the root filling) and the treatment outcome. In a canal with a defective seal (substantially short of apex, apical and lateral voids), non-surgical retreatment should be the first choice. Consequently, if the chances to improve the filling quality are small then surgical procedures should be considered.

Position of the tooth

Inaccessibility of the surgical site may be a contra-indication for surgical retreatment. The proximity of neurovascular bundles or the presence of thick alveolar bone might severely obstruct the possibility to cut, clean and seal the apical portion of the root.

Personal skills

Surgical and non-surgical retreatment procedures are often technically difficult and the results that can be achieved are highly dependent on the personal skills of the dentist. Therefore, complicated cases might benefit from being referred to a specialist or an experienced colleague.

Concluding remarks

Whether endodontic retreatment should be performed in a given case is a complex decision situation and many factors have to be considered. For the clinician it is important to appreciate the microbiology and pathology of the non-healing periapical lesion, as well as the technical potentials and limitations to resolve it. As important as professional knowledge and skill might be, it must be emphasized that the final decision is in the hands of the informed patient. Remember that the patient is the expert on which symptoms are tolerable, which economic costs are acceptable and which risks are worth taking.

References

1. Åkerblom Rawski A, Brehmer B, Knutsson K, Petersson K, Reit C, Rohlin M. The major factors that influence endodontic retreatment decisions. *Swed. Dent. J.* 2003; 27: 23–9.
2. Al-Ali K, Marghalani H, Al-Yahya, Omar R. An assessment of endodontic re-treatment decision-making in an educational setting. *Int. Endod. J.* 2005; 38: 470–6.
3. Allen RK, Newton CW, Beoen CE. A statistical analysis of surgical and nonsurgical retreatment cases. *J. Endod.* 1989; 15: 261–6.
4. American Child Health Association. *Physical Defects: The Pathway to Correction*. American Child Health Association, 1934; 80–96.
5. Aryanpour S, van Niewenhuysen J-P, D'Hoore W. Endodontic retreatment decisions. *Int. Endod. J.* 2000; 33: 208–18.
6. Beauchamp TL, Childress FF. *Principles of Biomedical Ethics.* New York: Oxford University Press, 1984.
   A most important text on medical ethics. The authors offer a detailed examination of theories and methods and present four basic groups of principles – respect for autonomy, non-maleficence, beneficence, and justice.
7. Bergenholtz G, Lekholm U, Milthon R, Heden G, Ödesjö B, Engström B. Retreatment of endodontic fillings. *Scand. J. Dent. Res.* 1979; 87: 217–24.
8. Bergenholtz G, Malmcrona E, Milthon R. Röntgenologisk bedömning av rotfyllningens kvalitet ställd i relation till förekomst av periapikala destruktioner (Summary in English). *Tandläkartidningen* 1973; 65: 269–79.
9. Bhaskar SN. Periapical lesions, types, incidence, and clinical features. *Oral Surg.* 1966; 21: 657–71.
10. Brehmer B, Joyce CRB. *Human Judgement. The SJT View.* Amsterdam: Elsevier Science Publishers, 1988.
11. Brynolf I. A histological and roentgenological study of the periapical region of human upper incisors. *Odontol. Revy* 1967; 18: Suppl. 11.
12. Buckley M, Spångberg LS. The prevalence and technical quality of endodontic treatment in an American subpopulation. *Oral Surg. Oral Med. Oral Pathol. Oral Radiol. Endod.* 1995; 79: 92–100.
13. Caplan DJ, Cai J, Yin G, White BA. Root canal filled versus non-root canal filled teeth: a retrospective comparison of survival times. *J. Public Health Dent.* 2005; 65: 90–6.

14. De Cleen MJH, Schuurs AHB, Wesselink PR, Wu M-K. Periapical status and prevalence of endodontic treatment in an adult Dutch population. *Int. Endod. J.* 1993; 26: 112–19.

15. De Moor RJG, Hommez GMG, De Boever JG, Delme KIM, Martens GEI. Periapical health related to the quality of root canal treatment in a Belgian population. *Int. Endod. J.* 2000; 33: 113–20.

16. Dowie J, Elstein A. *Professional Judgement. A Reader in Clinical Decision Making.* Cambridge: Cambridge University Press, 1988.

17. Eckerbom M, Andersson J-E, Magnusson T. A longitudinal study of changes in frequency and technical standard of endodontic treatment in a Swedish population. *Endod. Dent. Traumatol.* 1989; 5: 27–31.

18. Eddy DM. Variations in physician practice: the role of uncertainty. *Health Aff.* 1984; 5: 74–89.

19. Engström B. *Bacteriologic cultures in root canal therapy.* Thesis, Umeå, Sweden: University of Umeå, 1964.

20. Eriksen H. Epidemiology of apical periodontitis. In: *Essential Endodontology* (Ørstavik D, Pitt Ford TR, eds). Oxford: Blackwell Science, 1998.

21. Eriksen H, Bjertness E. Prevalence of apical periodontitis and results of endodontic treatment in middle-aged adults in Norway. *Endod. Dent. Traumatol.* 1991; 7: 1–4.

22. Happonen RP. Periapical actinomycosis: a follow-up study of 16 surgically treated cases. *Endod. Dent. Traumatol.* 1986; 2: 205–9.

23. Hargreaves Heap S, Hollis M, Lyons B, Sugden R, Weale A. *The Theory of Choice. A Critical Guide.* Oxford: Blackwell Publishing, 1992.

24. Hepworth MJ, Friedman S. Treatment outcome of surgical and non-surgical management of endodontic failures. *J. Can. Dent. Assoc.* 1997; 63: 364–71.

25. Hülsmann M. Retreatment decision making by a group of general dental practitioners in Germany. *Int. Endod. J.* 1994; 27: 125–32.

26. Imfeld TN. Prevalence and quality of endodontic treatment in an elderly urban population of Switzerland. *J. Endod.* 1991; 17: 604–7.

27. Joshipura KJ, Pitiphat W, Hung H-C, Willett WC, Colditz GA, Douglass CW. Pulpal inflammation and incidence of coronary heart disease. *J. Endod.* 2006; 32: 99–103.

28. Kahneman D, Slovic P, Tversky A. *Judgement under Uncertainty: Heuristics and Biases.* Cambridge: Cambridge University Press, 1982.

29. Knutsson K, Brehmer B, Lysell L, Rohlin M. Judgement of removal of asymptomatic mandibular molars: influence of position, degree of impaction, and patient's age. *Acta Odontol. Scand.* 1996; 54: 348–54.

30. Kvist T, Heden G, Reit C. Endodontic retreatment strategies used by general dental practitioners. *Oral Surg. Oral Med. Oral Pathol. Oral Radiol. Endod.* 2004; 97: 502–7.

31. Kvist T, Reit C. Results of endodontic retreatment: a randomised clinical study comparing surgical and nonsurgical procedures. *J. Endod.* 1999; 25; 814–17.

32. Kvist T, Reit C. Postoperative discomfort associated with surgical and nonsurgical endodontic retreatment. *Endod. Dent. Traumatol.* 2000; 16: 71–4.

33. Kvist T, Reit C. The perceived benefit of endodontic retreatment. *Int. Endod. J.* 2002; 35: 359–65.

34. Kvist T, Reit C, Esposito M, Mileman P, Bianchi S, Petersson K, Andersson C. Prescribing endodontic retreatment: towards a theory of dentist behaviour. *Int. Endod. J.* 1994; 27: 285–90.

35. Kvist T, Rydin E, Reit C. The relative frequency of periapical lesions in teeth with root canal-retained posts. *J. Endod.* 1989; 15: 578–80.

36. Langeland K, Block RM, Grossman LI. A histobacteriologic study of 35 periapical endodontic surgical specimens. *J. Endod.* 1977; 3: 8–23.

37. Ledley RS, Lusted LB. Reasoning foundations of medical diagnosis. *Science* 1959; 130: 9–21.

38. Lusted LB. *Introduction to Medical Decision Making.* Springfield, IL: Charles C. Thomas, 1968.

39. Marques MD, Moreira B, Eriksen HM. Prevalence of apical periodontitis and results of endodontic treatment in an adult, Portuguese population. *Int. Endod. J.* 1998; 31: 161–5.

40. Molander A, Reit C, Dahlén G, Kvist T. Microbiologic status of root filled teeth with apical periodontitis. *Int. Endod. J.* 1998; 31: 1–7.

41. Nair PNR, Pajarola G, Schroeder HE. Types and incidence of human periapical lesions obtained with extracted teeth. *Oral Surg. Oral Med. Oral Pathol. Oral Radiol. Endod.* 1996; 81: 93–102.

42. Nair PNR, Sjögren U, Krey G, Sundqvist G. Therapy-resistant foreign body giant cell granuloma at the periapex of a root filled human tooth. *J. Endod.* 1990; 16: 53–9.

43. Nair PNR, Sjögren U, Krey G, Kahnberg K-E, Sundqvist G. Intraradicular bacteria and fungi in root filled, asymptomatic human teeth with therapy-resistant periapical lesions: a long-term light and electron microscopic follow-up study. *J. Endod.* 1990; 16: 41–9.

44. Natkin E, Oswald RJ, Carnes LI. The relationship of lesion size to diagnosis, incidence, and treatment of periapical cysts and granulomas. *Oral Surg.* 1984; 57: 82–94.

45. von Neumann J, Morgenstern O. *Theory of Games and Economic Behaviour.* Princeton, NJ: Princeton University Press, 1947.

46. Ørstavik D. Time-course and risk analyses of the development and healing of chronic apical periodontitis in man. *Int. Endod. J.* 1996; 29: 150–5.

47. Ørstavik D, Kerekes K, Eriksen HM. The periapical index: a scoring system for radiographic assessment of apical periodontitis. *Endod. Dent. Traumatol.* 1986; 2: 20–34.

48. Petersson K, Håkansson R, Håkansson J, Olsson B, Wennberg A. Follow-up study of endodontic status in an adult Swedish population. *Endod. Dent. Traumatol.* 1991; 7: 221–5.

49. Petersson K, Lewin B, Håkansson J, Olsson B, Wennberg A. Endodontic status and suggested treatment in a population requiring substantial dental care. *Endod. Dent. Traumatol.* 1989; 5: 153–8.

50. Petersson K, Petersson A, Olsson B, Håkansson J, Wennberg A. Technical quality of root fillings in an adult Swedish population. *Endod. Dent. Traumatol.* 1986; 2: 99–102.

51. Politser P. Decision analysis and clinical judgement. *Med. Decis. Making* 1981; 1: 361–89.

52. Ray HA, Trope M. Periapical status of endodontically treated teeth in relation to the technical quality of the root

filling and the coronal restoration. *Int. Endod. J.* 1995; 28: 12–18.

53. Reit C. Decision strategies in endodontics: on the design of a recall program. *Endod. Dent. Traumatol.* 1987; 3: 233–9.
54. Reit C, Gröndahl H-G. Management of periapical lesions in endodontically treated teeth: a study on clinical decision making. *Swed. Dent. J.* 1984; 8: 1–7.
55. Reit C, Gröndahl H-G. Endodontic retreatment decision making among a group of general practitioners. *Scand. J. Dent. Res.* 1988; 96: 112–17.
56. Reit C, Gröndahl H-G, Engström B. Endodontic treatment decisions: a study of the clinical decision-making process. *Endod. Dent. Traumatol.* 1985; 1: 102–7.
57. Reit C, Kvist T. Endodontic retreatment behaviour: the influence of disease concepts and personal values. *Int. Endod. J.* 1998; 31: 358–63.

    This study presents a conceptual analysis of the terms "success" and "failure", often used in describing the outcome of endodontic therapy. The study also analyzes concepts like "value" and "value judgments" and uses a method (the standard gamble) to measure value judgments and incorporate them in the decision-making process.
58. Ricucci D, Gröndahl K, Bergenholtz G. Periapical status of root filled teeth exposed to the oral environment by loss of restoration or caries. *Oral Surg.* 2000; 90: 354–9.
59. Rohlin M, Mileman PA. Decision analysis in dentistry – the last 30 years. *J. Dent.* 2000; 28: 453–68.
60. Saunders WP, Saunders EM. Coronal leakage as a cause of failure in root canal therapy: a review. *Endod. Dent. Traumatol.* 1994; 10: 105–8.
61. Saunders WP, Saunders EM, Sadio J, Cruickshank E. Technical standard of root canal treatment in an adult Scottish sub-population. *Br. Dent. J.* 1997; 182: 382–6.
62. Sidaravicius B, Aleksejuniene J, Eriksen HM. Endodontic treatment and prevalence of apical periodontitis in adult population of Vilnius, Lithuania. *Endod. Dent. Traumatol.* 1999; 15: 210–15.
63. Siqueira JF Jr, Rocas IN, Lopes HP, Uzeda M. Coronal leakage of two root canal sealers containing calcium hydroxide after exposure to human saliva. *J. Endod.* 1999; 25: 14–16.
64. Sjögren U, Happonen RP, Kahnberg K-E, Sundqvist G. Survival of *Arachnia propionica* in periapical tissue. *Int. Endod. J.* 1988; 21: 277–82.
65. Sjögren U, Hägglund B, Sundqvist G, Wing K. Factors affecting the long-term results of endodontic treatment. *J. Endod.* 1990; 16: 31–7.
66. Smith J, Crisp J, Torney D. A survey: controversies in endodontic treatment and re-treatment. *J. Endod.* 1981; 7: 477–83.
67. Spatafore CM, Griffin JA, Keyes GG, Wearden S, Skidmore AE. Periapical biopsy report: an analysis over a 10-year period. *J. Endod.* 1990; 16: 239–41.
68. Strindberg LZ. The dependence of the results of pulp therapy on certain factors. *Acta Odontol. Scand.* 1956; 14 (Suppl. 21).
69. Sunde PT, Olsen I, Lind PO, Tronstad L. Extraradicular infection: a methodological study. *Endod. Dent. Traumatol.* 2000; 16: 84–90.
70. Sundqvist G, Figdor D, Persson S, Sjögren U. Microbiologic analysis of teeth with failed endodontic treatment and the outcome of conservative retreatment. *Oral Surg. Oral Med. Oral Pathol. Oral Radiol. Endod.* 1998; 85: 86–93.
71. Tengs TO, Wallace A. One thousand health-related quality-of-life estimates. *Med. Care* 2000; 38: 583–637.
72. Torrance GW. Measurements of health state utilities for economic appraisal. *J. Health Econ.* 1986; 5: 1–30.
73. Tronstad L, Barnett F, Riso K, Slots J. Extraradicular endodontic infections. *Endod. Dent. Traumatol.* 1987; 3: 86–90.
74. Tsuneishi M, Yamamoto T, Yamanaka R, Tamaki N, Sakamoto T, Tsuji K, Watanabe T. Radiographic evaluation of periapical status and prevalence of endodontic treatment in an adult Japanese population. *Oral Surg. Oral Med. Oral Pathol. Oral Radiol. Endod.* 2005; 100: 631–5.
75. Weinstein MC, Fineberg HV. *Clinical Decision Analysis.* Philadelphia, PA: WB Saunders, 1980.
76. Yusuf H. The significance of the presence of foreign material periapically as a cause of failure of root treatment. *Oral Surg. Oral Med. Oral Pathol.* 1982; 54: 566–74.

Part 5
The Root Filled Tooth

Chapter 19
The root filled tooth in prosthodontic reconstruction

Eckehard Kostka

Introduction

After endodontic therapy a tooth must be restored to functional and esthetic demands. Teeth which are to be used as abutments in prosthodontic reconstructions must be judged especially carefully regarding their ability to withstand a higher load than a single tooth normally is exposed to (Core concept 19.1). An important consideration is that in most cases the remaining tooth structure will often be substantially less than that in intact teeth because of caries or other causes. Additionally, further loss of tooth structure takes place during the preparation of the access cavity and the root canal. The amount of coronal tooth structure that remains is the most important factor in the decision for the kind of reconstruction to be made as it affects the retention of the restoration and the fracture susceptibility of the tooth. When the remaining tooth structure does not provide enough retention for a core build-up, the root canal can provide enhanced retention by the use of a post. Thus, in a single-rooted tooth with substantial loss of coronal tooth structure, a post and core are often needed.

There is experimental evidence that there are changes in receptor properties in teeth with non-vital pulps leading to higher bite forces than in teeth with vital pulps (Key literature 19.1) (49). This must be considered at the planning stage by estimating the fracture susceptibility of a root filled tooth, especially in a prosthodontic reconstruction substituting more than one tooth.

Problems associated with root filled teeth as abutments

In order to achieve long-term clinical success with prosthodontic restoration of root filled teeth it is essential to know the reasons for clinical failures. Some of these reasons, such as recurrent caries or periodontal breakdown, are the same as in non-root filled teeth. A major difference is the absence of a vital pulp with its potential to respond with specific pain symptoms that may act as an alarm for the patient. To minimize the development of new caries and periodontal disease, an individually adapted regimen of preventive care has to be established including an appropriate recall schedule.

The loss of retention of a crown is possible in non-vital as well as in vital abutment teeth, but in the latter case early symptoms warn the patient. The specific issues associated with prosthodontic reconstruction of root filled teeth are now discussed.

Loss of retention

Retention loss is a failure of the connection between two parts of the restoration or between the restoration and the tooth. A fracture within one of the materials may also result clinically in a loss of retention, but the cause must be differentiated.

When the retention is lost in one abutment, either the complete prosthodontic reconstruction will feel loose, causing only minor symptoms in a tooth with non-vital pulp, like malodor, or it will still be functioning satisfactorily and the failure may remain undetected by the patient. In these cases the diagnosis is difficult but nevertheless important. The continuous gap between crown and tooth gives access to bacteria, possibly causing caries, gingival inflammation, pulpal complications and apical periodontitis, depending on the location of the gap and the seal of the remaining barrier between the gap and the apex. Furthermore, the forces acting on the remaining reconstruction are higher, with an increased risk of fracture or subsequent loss of retention of the other abutments. Therefore, at each recall examination, it is of supreme importance to check the fit of every single abutment in a prosthodontic reconstruction.

The marginal fit is checked visually using loupes and with a suitable fine explorer by trying to penetrate between the tooth and the restoration margin from an apical direction. If a gap cannot be felt, a rocking and a push–pull motion with the fingers may disclose movement of the restoration. In the case of a loose restoration, passage of saliva along the cavosurface margin may be observed.

Core concept 19.1 Parts of prosthodontic reconstruction compared with chain links

From a mechanical point of view, in a restored abutment tooth, all parts of the prosthodontic reconstruction and their connections must resist the forces that act upon them. The strength of the complete reconstruction can be compared with a chain in which every link is one of the separate parts of the reconstruction, of the biological structures and their connections. Each chain is only as strong as its weakest link. In the case of two parallel chains, the overall strength is as high as the sum of the strengths of both chains, so when one is strong enough there is no need for the other one.

The term "strength" means both the internal (tensile) strength of part of the reconstruction and the retentive (bond) strength between two parts.

The links of the chains in an abutment tooth restored with a post and core are as shown below.

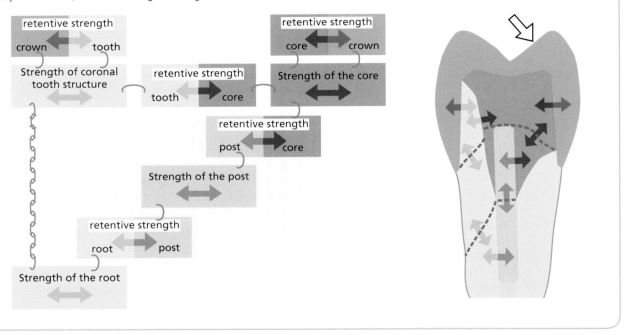

Key literature 19.1 Changes in perception

Randow and Glantz (49) carried out a clinical experiment of exceptional design: they cemented crowns with temporary extension bars at the buccal aspect on matched pairs of neighboring (contralateral) teeth in test people; one tooth was vital and one root filled, supported with an individual cast post and core. Weights were applied at different lever arm positions until the test persons experienced pain. The pain loading level of the pulpless teeth was more than twice as high as in teeth with vital pulps. The experiment was repeated under local anesthesia but terminated at a loading level exceeding 125% of the root filled tooth without anesthesia. Under these conditions no difference in the reaction levels within the pair of teeth was observed. In one root filled tooth a coronal dentin fracture occurred and the cemented post lost its retention.

These results show that pulpless teeth behave differently than teeth with vital pulps with regard to their tactile reactivity.

Factors influencing retention

Retention of a core build-up

Assuming that the retention for the crown is sufficient and appropriate to the prosthodontic reconstruction, the retention of the core build-up is the next link in the chain of retention. The more the retention of the crown relies on the build-up, the more important is the retention at the tooth structure. The build-up is attached to the tooth mechanically and may also be adhesively (micro-mechanically) attached, depending on the material used. A plastic filling material can be condensed or syringed into undercuts, retention grooves or the canal orifices. Additionally, it can be fixed by means of intradentinal pins or a post.

Retention of a post

The retention of a post depends on:

- its design (tapered, parallel, individual);
- insertion depth;
- macroretentions (thread, serrations);
- surface characteristics (composition, roughness, surface energy);
- cementing agent in combination with pretreatment of the dentin surface.

Fractures

Cohesive failure within a material occurs as a fracture.

Fractures of the superstructure

A fracture within the superstructure of a prosthesis does not depend on the endodontic treatment *per se* and can happen in a vital abutment tooth as well. The only difference is that the reflex control of bite forces is reduced (49) owing to the loss of receptors in the pulp or a change in the mechanoreceptor function in the periodontal membrane.

Core/post fractures

Core: The fracture susceptibility of a core build-up depends mostly on its dimensions, the material's strength and the forces acting upon it. Regarding these forces, there are major differences between anterior and posterior teeth in the amount and direction of force, the ratio between length and diameter and the area of the bonded surface. When a post is used, its coronal end can weaken the core build-up and exert stress, depending on its size and shape.

Post: A post often is the most retentive link in the chain of retention. In the case of overload either it breaks or it fractures the root, depending on which is the strongest component. The fracture susceptibility of a post depends on its diameter and the material from which it is fabricated.

Tooth fractures – factors influencing fracture risk

- *Mechanical characteristics of non-vital dentin:* For a long time endodontically treated teeth were thought to be more brittle owing to a loss of moisture content. Several studies have investigated the mechanical properties of dentin in vital versus non-vital teeth (Key literature 19.2) (see also overview in Ref. 32). Although the moisture content did vary significantly, the compression strength and tensile strength did not show any significant difference (28). Thus, factors other than dentin characteristics may be more important in the increased fracture susceptibility of endodontically treated teeth.
- *Amount of remaining tooth structure:* The loss of tooth structure in an endodontically treated tooth is much more responsible for its higher susceptibility to fracture than changes in its mechanical properties. Posterior teeth with intact marginal ridges and only a small access preparation are most resistant to fracture and are not significantly weaker than intact teeth without any preparation (51, 64). From a prosthodontic

---

> ### Key literature 19.2   Brittleness of dentin
>
> Sedgley and Messer (57) investigated the dentin in vital versus root filled teeth: 23 matched pairs of contralateral teeth freshly extracted for prosthodontic reasons were subjected to different mechanical tests. One of the corresponding teeth was vital and the other had been endodontically treated 1–25 years before (mean 10.1 years). Holes of 1 mm diameter were punched by a universal testing machine into two slices of dentin 0.3 mm thick cut from the necks of the teeth, and the shear strength and toughness were calculated from the stress–strain curve. Additionally, in one of the slices the Vickers hardness was determined midway between the root canal and the periphery. The coronal root canal openings of the remaining roots were prepared as a seat for a cone-shaped steel rod, followed by loading the teeth until fracture occurred in an axial direction.
>
> Neither the punch shear strength or toughness nor the load to fracture differed significantly between vital and root filled teeth. The hardness of the cervical dentin was 3.5% lower in endodontically treated teeth.
>
> These findings indicate that teeth do not become more brittle following endodontic treatment.

point of view, a maximum of internal tooth structure should be preserved to minimize the fracture risk. Thus, ideally, the access would be minimal, i.e. just large enough to gain access to the canal. From this point of view the preparation of the canal, especially in the cervical area, should be as small as possible. This prosthodontic desire is in conflict with modern concepts for root canal preparation in endodontic therapy where direct straight-line access to the canal with a wide access opening for good overview is a general requirement (see Chapter 11). Good cervical flaring is furthermore recommended to ensure an optimal apical preparation, especially in curved canals. In more demanding root canal treatments it might be necessary to sacrifice sound tooth structure, while in nearly straight canals the preservation of tooth structure can be the primary goal.

The prosthodontic reconstruction determines the forces acting on the tooth. The amount of tooth structure left after preparation determines its ability to carry loads. Which type of reconstruction is best suited for the remaining tooth structure needs to be judged at the very beginning of treatment.

When one or both of the proximal walls are lost, the tooth is substantially weakened as the support of the circumferential marginal ridges (and the roof of the pulp chamber) is lost and a horizontal force on a cusp acts over a long lever-arm on the weakest part in the cervical area, normally just above the alveolar crest. When a force acts on the oblique inner slopes of the cusps it will be divided into a vertical and a horizontal component, the latter exerting high stresses in the weak cervical portion (Fig. 19.1). Therefore an effective bonding or cuspal

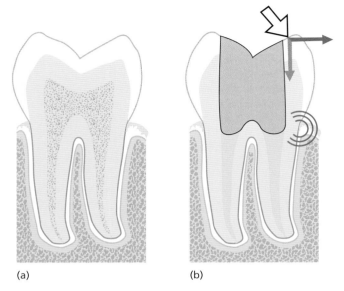

(a)   (b)

Fig. 19.1   (a) Intact tooth. (b) Forces acting on a root filled tooth and resulting stress peak.

coverage is necessary whenever a proximal wall is lost and the cusps are not flat owing to abrasion or anatomical form.

The (tensile) bond strength of any material to dentin is always weaker than the (tensile) strength of dentin. Therefore, the preservation of a maximum amount of dentinal bulk should be the aim in endodontic therapy of an abutment tooth.

- *Type of post:* A stiff material with a high modulus of elasticity may concentrate the forces onto a small area

at the end of the post, exerting more stress onto the root; a post material with a similar behavior to dentin could spread the forces, so they decrease towards the post's tip (Fig. 19.2). This seems to be more favorable with respect to fracture mode (2, 37). A stiff post may induce more damaging types of fractures (Fig. 19.3).

Tapered posts meet the shape of a canal prepared for root filling better than parallel posts which may need additional removal of tooth structure at the apical end. This leads to significant weakening of the root on a level where the thickness of the root is already decreasing naturally (36).

- *Length of post:* The longer a stiff post, the better the distribution of stresses, resulting in reduced stress at the apical end of the post because of leverage (63). Extending the length to two-thirds of the root length results in a superior fracture resistance compared with short posts (29, 55). The length of the post is not so significant for adhesively luted fiber posts (55).

There is a lack of clinical data regarding the length of posts in relation to the level of alveolar bone, but in the case of a metal post it seems more favorable to extend the post below the alveolar crest.

- *Post diameter:* The thicker a post, the thinner and weaker will the remaining tooth structure be, leading to increased risk of fracture. On the other hand, a post must be thick and stiff enough to transmit lateral forces to the root uniformly. Normally, depending on the diameter of the root, the post diameter should not exceed 1.5 mm at the cervical level and in small or fragile roots this is less. The removal of sound tooth structure for placing a post should be considered very carefully.

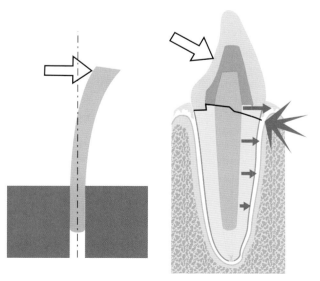
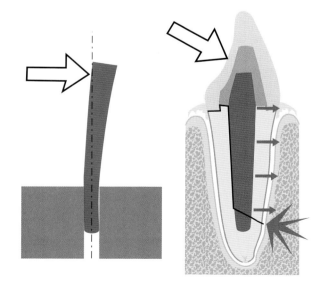

Fig. 19.2   Distribution of forces by posts with different stiffness.

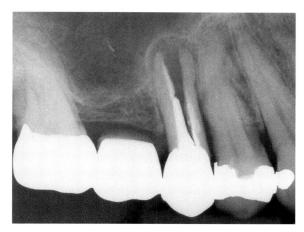

Fig. 19.3 Fracture of root filled tooth 15, probably due to forces from the metallic post. (Courtesy of Dr I.P. Sewerin.)

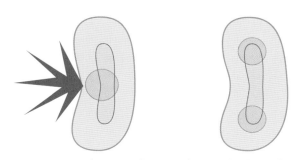

Fig. 19.4 Correct and incorrect placement of post in distal root of lower molar.

Perforations

Invaginations of the external root surface – stripping perforations

Roots are seldom round and often have curves, invaginations, flutes or other varieties in shape. The distal root of a mandibular molar is kidney-shaped in its cross-section, so care must be taken not to place the post preparation in the middle of the canal but in the bulkiest part of the root, i.e. the buccal or lingual edge (Fig. 19.4).

The mesial root of a lower molar and the mesiobuccal root of an upper molar are often curved in a distal direction. The most cervical parts of the canals go mostly in the mesial direction, so when this initial curve is not removed during the access preparation there is great danger of stripping perforation into the interradicular space or in the mesial direction (Fig. 19.5). Proper flaring and, especially, anticurvature filing are important not only to gain a straight-line access for the apical preparation of the canal but also for safe preparation of the post space (34).

Curvatures not perceptible in the radiograph

Even if the cervical part of the canal is straight, a more apical curvature may limit the length of a post. The most dangerous curvatures are in the plane not perceptible on the radiograph. Only knowledge of the anatomy of the root prevents perforation during preparation of a post space, e.g. the palatal roots of upper bicuspids and molars (75).

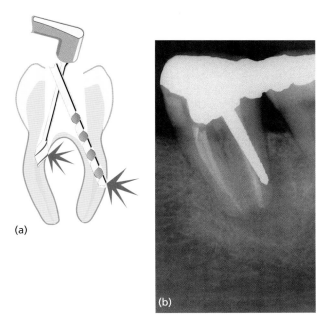

Fig. 19.5 (a) Danger of perforation in curved canals. (b) Perforation of the distal root by a post. (Courtesy of Dr I.P. Sewerin.)

Deviation of the prepared canal

Gates–Glidden drills as well as Peeso reamers and some specific drills for post systems have a non-cutting self-centering tip, which ensures that the preparation of the post space will not deviate from a guiding canal being enlarged concentrically. In the case of a root filled tooth, the center of the root filling is the guiding structure. When the root filling deviates from the original canal, the center of the root filling is no longer the center of the root. Enlarging a deviated canal preparation concentrically can therefore cause a lateral perforation, depending on the amounts of deviation, enlargement and dentinal bulk in that direction (24, 34).

Use of end-cutting drills

Special care must be taken when using the end-cutting drills provided with many post systems. Even when driven by hand, they can easily deviate from the canal (Fig. 19.5b). Therefore, removal of the root filling and preparation of the canal space should be done using drills with a non-cutting tip prior to use of the drills for these post systems (24).

Excessive length/diameter

When a post is longer than the straight portion of the canal, a perforation is likely to occur (Fig. 19.5). With increasing diameter of the post, not only the fracture risk but also the risk of perforation increases significantly, therefore a post should always be as thin as possible, i.e. just thick enough to gain some guidance and retention within the canal.

Reinfection/bacterial leakage

Microleakage of cemented posts

A major aim of the root filling is to seal the canal as tightly as possible to hinder bacterial leakage from the oral environment to the periapical tissues. Preparing the canal for receiving a post removes a substantial amount of the root filling and may disturb the seal of the remaining filling. The subsequent cementation of posts may again seal the canal and reduce the risk of infection. Adhesively luted posts leak less than conventionally cemented ones (4) but leakage increases after fatigue loading (53). However, leakage may occur during post space preparation. Immediate post space preparation is less likely to cause leakage than preparation after complete setting of the sealer (1); a root filling without a tight seal of the access cavity allows leakage of bacteria within a few weeks (5), so the post space preparation and the subsequent luting of the post should be established immediately. Aseptic conditions are imperative during post space preparation,

so a rubber dam should be used. If this is not possible, there must be adequate moisture control and the post space should be irrigated with antiseptic solutions such as sodium hypochlorite, chlorhexidine or alcohol.

There is clinical evidence that leaving at least 3 mm of apical root filling under posts decreases the probability of occurrence of periapical lesions (35). *In vitro* studies have shown that a remaining apical root filling of 5 or 7 mm prevents leakage better than one of 3 mm (41), therefore a residual root filling of 3 mm should be the absolute minimum.

Core build-ups

Core build-up without a post

If enough coronal tooth structure remains to yield retention to a core build-up, a post will not be necessary. The build-up will fill the access cavity and any substance loss from caries or other causes, and may increase the height of the abutment. It must be taken into account that during crown preparation the outside walls of the remaining tooth structure will be reduced in thickness or removed completely and so will not contribute to the final build-up retention. The retention of the build-up must be achieved with the tooth structure that will remain after the final preparation.

Modern dentin adhesives are able to retain composite fillings in cavities without any retentive form but they may be overrated in successfully bonding build-up and prosthodontic reconstruction alone. For build-ups, a mechanical retention in addition to dentin bonding should always be used to gain a maximum overall retention.

The possibilities for achieving mechanical retention are different between single- and multirooted teeth. The size of the pulp chamber (in width and depth) in multirooted teeth is of considerable advantage for achieving mechanical retention. Undercuts are a natural property of multirooted teeth, with divergent canal orifices providing excellent mechanical retention.

Because forces acting on all teeth are different and depend on the degree of destruction, further mechanical retention may be necessary via grooves (67) or posts. In anterior teeth the forces act in a more horizontal direction and their cross-sectional area is smaller than in posterior teeth. These unfavorable lever-arm relations necessitate the insertion of posts.

Whenever the remaining tooth structure and the pulpal space support sufficient retention for the build-up, a post will not be needed and should be avoided because the risks associated with the use of posts do not exceed the advantages in most cases (Core concept 19.2). Restorations without posts in premolar teeth with their

Core concept 19.2   Advantages of build-ups without posts

A build-up without a post offers some advantages:

- Additional weakening of the root is avoided.
- Danger of root perforation is minimized.
- Load transmission to the root is more uniform.
- Fracture mode is more favorable in case of failure.
- Salvaging of the tooth is more likely in case of failure.
- Non-surgical retreatment is facilitated.
- Costs for materials and treatment time are reduced.

clinical crowns removed resisted similar loads to those resisted by post-restored samples *in vitro* (10, 22, 65). In substantially decayed incisors, crowns without posts failed at significantly lower forces than teeth with post-retained build-ups did (70). Prospective clinical studies comparing root canal-treated teeth with or without insertion of posts found failure rates of the same level for both types of restorations in single crowns (19, 21, 54).

Post systems: cylindrical, tapered, screws

In general, prefabricated posts may be either cylindrical or conical in shape. A cylindrical post gains more retention than a tapered one even after the very first debonding, masking an initial failure. A slightly tapered post matches the shape of a prepared canal and in many cases the anatomy of the root, respectively. Selecting an appropriate size means that removal of tooth structure is minimized. In addition, a conical post is easier to put in place and leaves more space for the escape of the luting agent during insertion. Some metal posts are provided with a thread for better retention, which has to be tapped inside the root as well. This exerts more stress on the tooth and the clinical success rate is significantly lower (56).

Post materials

Metal cast post and core

Metal posts have been used for many decades and the fracture resistance of cast precious alloy post-and-core restorations served as the "gold standard" when new materials were introduced. There are two different methods for fabricating a cast post and core: the direct technique, where a special acrylic resin is used to form a core build-up directly in the mouth, and the indirect technique, making an impression and fabricating the post and core in the laboratory. The completely combustible resin can be used in combination either with a wrought precious alloy post, onto which the core part is cast, or with a burn-out acrylic post which is lost in the cast procedure.

Prefabricated metal post

The most important mechanical properties of a post material are its tensile strength, resulting in fracture strength against bending forces and Young's modulus resulting in stiffness. The mechanical properties of pre-fabricated metal posts are superior compared with completely cast ones (30).

Fiber-reinforced resins

In recent years, epoxy-based carbon-fiber posts were marketed, followed and widely displaced by quartz- and glass-fiber reinforced posts. They are luted adhesively and used in combination with a composite core material. *In vitro* studies have shown that the fracture resistance of such post-and-core restorations is lower compared with that of metal posts. The mode of failure is more likely to be a fracture of the post or cervical root fracture, which is re-restorable in contrast to the often much deeper root fractures of metal posts (40, 60). The fracture resistance of different brands of posts was found to show a direct correlation to their fiber content (58). In the case of a broken post or if retreatment of the root canal is needed, fiber posts are easy to remove (39).

Another common failure is debonding of the post, highlighting the issue of adhesion to the post as well as to the root dentin. Several procedures enhance bonding to the post, such as sandblasting or etching with different agents and subsequent silanization (8).

There are two other approaches to counter the problem of adhesion to the post, either using a special post containing an unpolymerized matrix (37) or using a woven band of high-molecular-weight polyethylene fibers that can be soaked with light- or dual-curing resin, folded and placed in wide post spaces (44, 48). Adhesively luting to the root dentin seems even more variable than to the post surface and is still a field of intensive research (9, 45, 74). Clinical long-term studies are still scarce and do not specify or standardize some clinical important factors, like amount of coronal tooth structure. Success rates of 65% (58) to 90% (18, 48) are reported after 7 years of service with no root fractures observed in the latter two studies.

Ceramics

Some years ago new high-strength ceramics came into clinical use as materials for full ceramic reconstructions, namely zirconium as prefabricated posts and glass-infiltrated aluminum oxide ceramics used for custom-made post and core construction. They offer high strength and their esthetic appearance is emphasized. Although a zirconium post is about as strong as a titanium post and has a higher stiffness (2), its use should be judged carefully. Microcracks can occur owing to aging or inadequate handling, weakening the post substantially (20). Bonding to zirconium is difficult and sensitive to fatigue (11). There are still no long-term clinical results but the removal of such a post in case of failure or if retreatment should become necessary might be impossible, or at least a very time-consuming procedure, leading to excessive dentin loss and a high risk of lateral root perforations.

Core build-up materials

Amalgam

Amalgam has been widely used for a long time as a plastic core material. It offers good mechanical and handling properties and has shown its suitability for core build-ups used with posts, pins or other retentive features (67). However, because of the debate about mercury toxicity, this material has gained a bad reputation in recent years and its use for that reason has been restricted in some countries.

Composites

Composite is the material of choice for a plastic core build-up. In combination with dentin adhesives it offers the possibility of superior bond strength to the tooth structure over the entire surface, leading to higher retentive strength. Its mechanical properties make it suitable even for substitution of more than half of the coronal tooth structure. Depending on the kind and amount of fillers, its hardness can be made similar to that of dentin, facilitating the final abutment preparation. Its modulus of elasticity should be equal to or higher than that of dentin, resulting in enhanced reinforcement. In anterior teeth it also has esthetic advantages when used in combination with all-ceramic reconstructions.

Ceramics

High-performance ceramics were introduced in the dental field for inlays, crowns and bridgework and are also used as core build-up materials, especially in anterior teeth. They have esthetic advantages and also superior strength. Using a surface pretreatment that depends on the kind of ceramic, they are cemented adhesively to the tooth, gaining a stabilizing effect. The fabrication of a ceramic post–core build-up is comparable to that of a cast metal post and core, not only because it is done in the laboratory but also because there is the option to use a ceramic pressed around a preformed ceramic post or to fabricate the post–core build-up in one material as glass-infiltrated alumina or by milling from an industrially prefabricated block of ceramic. As a third option, post and core can be separate parts bonded together during

insertion (23, 47). Because ceramic posts have to be used in combination with these build-ups the same problems apply to them.

Cements

Even cements with the highest compressive strength – the metal-reinforced glass ionomer cements – are not suitable as a core build-up material. Composite resin and amalgam performed much better than cements regarding fracture resistance (13).

Resin-modified glass ionomer cements and compomeres, respectively, achieve a fracture strength similar to that of composite, but they undergo a slow expansion with water absorption leading to cracks in overlying ceramic crowns (61). Thus, they are likely also to exert stress to other restorations and tooth structure.

Post and core systems

Prefabricated post/plastic core build-up

In contrast to a direct build-up with plastic material, an indirect one makes it necessary to remove undercuts, so that tooth structure, valuable for strength and retention, is removed. With a direct build-up the access cavity can be closed immediately after root filling. If this is done with a composite in combination with a suitable adhesive, the risk of bacterial leakage compared with a provisional closure is minimized. An adhesive build-up contributes more to the reinforcement of the tooth and minimizes the risk of fracture compared with a temporary material necessary during the period of manufacturing the laboratory-made post and core. These temporary materials do not bond to the tooth structure, they do not have the strength and it is necessary to remove them. A build-up with plastic material is preferred whenever it is possible (Core concept 19.3).

Indications for different kinds of core build-up

The kind of build-up that is best suited for the individual situation depends on:

- the remaining tooth structure;
- the burden of the superstructure.

The ratio of these two factors influences not only the choice of build-up but also the prognosis for long-term success.

In general, in all cases where sufficient retention can be gained without a post, a post should be avoided. Whether a post and core should be of plastic material or a cast one is still controversial. The plastic materials, especially composites, are increasingly preferred because their mechanical properties and the adhesive systems have been improved.

Core concept 19.3   Advantages of build-ups in plastic material with posts

The use of a prefabricated post in combination with a build-up in plastic material offers many advantages compared with a laboratory-made post:

- Saving of tooth structure:
  - undercuts can remain and serve for more retention.
- Immediate closure of the prepared canal:
  - less danger of bacterial leakage.
- No need for a provisional restoration:
  - no fracture risk during provisional restoration;
  - saves chairside time;
  - saves cost.

In the case of a composite build-up, additional advantages are:

- Improved esthetics
- Adhesive technique simply achievable
- Higher bond strength
- Decreased leakage

Clinical techniques

Bonding techniques for strengthening tooth structure

When a tooth with an open apex needs endodontic therapy, both the endodontic treatment procedures and the final restoration are a challenge. Because the walls of the root are thin, it is much more susceptible to fracture and therefore effective reinforcement is a major concern for long-term success. Effective reinforcement can be achieved by filling the post-carrying part of the root with light-curing composite using a transparent light-conducting post. After removal of that post, the apex is still accessible and a prefabricated post can be cemented (Clinical procedure 19.1), gaining a higher overall fracture resistance than a custom-made cast post and core, which is adapted to a weakened canal wall (25). By using light-transmitting posts, a curing depth up to 10 mm can be achieved, depending on the diameter of the post (73).

The risk of fracture increases from the beginning of endodontic therapy, so effective protection is necessary between appointments during a longer lasting endodontic treatment aiming at apexification of thin-walled roots. When apexification is not rapidly achieved with the use of calcium hydroxide or MTA, the above-described technique can also be used before finishing the endodontic treatment, allowing access to the apical part of the canal. The strengthening effect of an internal composite reinforcement up to 3 mm apical to the cemento-enamel junction has been verified (31).

Preparation techniques for posts

After finishing the endodontic treatment it is essential to take precautions so that the risk for bacterial leakage along the remaining root filling is avoided. The final

Clinical procedure 19.1   Strengthening a thin-walled root

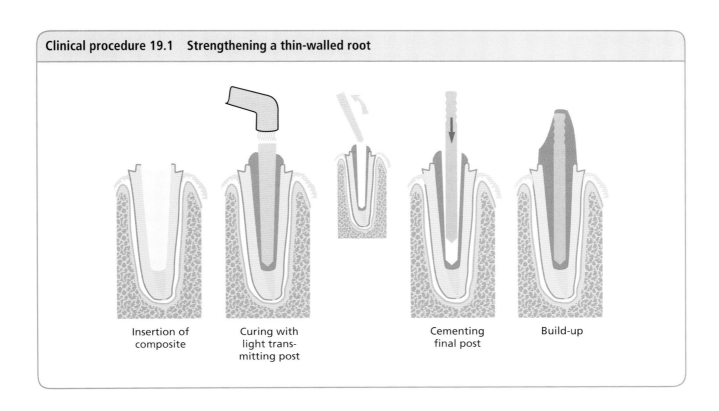

Insertion of composite

Curing with light trans-mitting post

Cementing final post

Build-up

Clinical procedure 19.2   Preparing and inserting a post

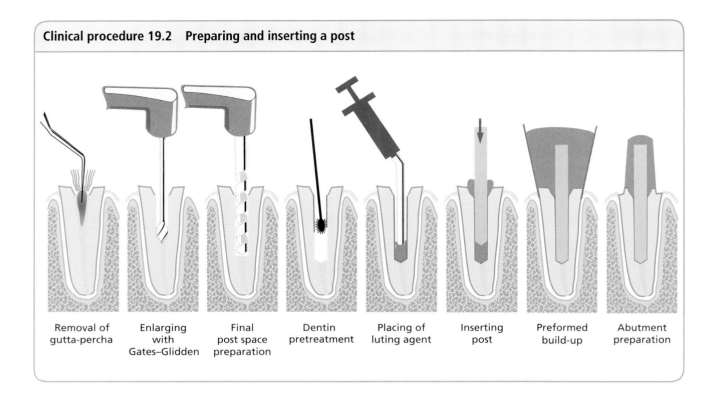

| Removal of gutta-percha | Enlarging with Gates–Glidden | Final post space preparation | Dentin pretreatment | Placing of luting agent | Inserting post | Preformed build-up | Abutment preparation |

---

restoration should therefore be established as soon as possible (5). Another reason for an immediate preparation of the post space is that the dentist is still familiar with the individual canal anatomy. In cases where an incremental vertical root filling technique is used a post may be inserted instead of backfilling the coronal part of the canal.

The safest method of removing the root filling material without leaving the canal is by using a heated instrument and this should be used always as a first step in achieving the post space preparation. A heat carrier is introduced into the canal, repeatedly softening and removing the gutta-percha until most of the final length is cleared. The next step in preparing the post space is the use of rotating instruments if the post's diameter will exceed the size of the root filling. It is safer to begin with instruments equipped with a non-cutting tip. In contrast to Gates–Glidden drills, Peeso reamers ensure a straight preparation. The drills are used in ascending diameters at low speed to avoid excessive heat. Orifice openers can also be used. The size of the last file gives information about the appropriate diameter for the post. As soon as the rotating instrument cuts into dentin over almost all of the circumference, the corresponding drill of the post system is used. These drills often have end-cutting tips so they must be used very carefully and only for the final preparation to avoid perforations. After completing the preparation, a radiograph should be taken with the post in place to ensure its proper positioning.

Length of posts

Post length is limited by the curvature of the root and the necessary root filling needed to prevent leakage. An absolute minimum of 3 mm of apical root filling should remain (41). The length of a cylindrical post may be limited owing to excessive weakening of the root at the apical end of the post.

Cementing posts

The retention of a metal post depends more on factors such as shape, length and surface roughness than on the cementing agent. The cementing agent has to fill the gap between post and dentin wall and to transduce the forces between both. The classical cementing agent for fixed restorations is zinc phosphate cement. It is still the material of choice for metal posts in a standard situation because it is not critical in handling and regarding dentin pretreatment (33). It is removable by ultrasonic instruments if retreatment is necessary. Resin cements are required for adhesive luting of fiber posts. They require an adequate dentin pretreatment for removing or modifying the smear layer that is always present on mechanically treated dentin surfaces. The manufacturer's instructions must be followed carefully when using dentin adhesives.

It is essential to ensure dry conditions in the cementing procedure. The post space is rinsed with water and dried with paper points. When using zinc phosphate cement, removing the smear layer with EDTA is recommended to clean the canal and enhance retention. The cement is mixed to a creamy consistency and applied with a lentulo spiral into the post preparation. The post is than seated carefully until it reaches the bottom of the preparation and the cement is left to harden undisturbed.

When using fast-setting resins the use of a lentulo spiral may be ill advised because premature setting may hinder complete positioning of the post. When using these materials only the post is coated with the cement. Materials with enough working time are applied with a syringe and a blunt hollow needle to reach the bottom of the post preparation (14).

Prosthodontic reconstruction

Single tooth

The simplest case of prosthodontic reconstruction is the restoration of a single tooth. Often a prosthodontic reconstruction can be substituted by a composite filling (Fig. 19.6). When the composite is bonded to etched enamel and dentin by use of a suitable adhesive, the fracture resistance is increased considerably (26, 42). As a temporary solution, an amalgam filling is also possible (Fig. 19.7). In the case of lost proximal ridges, cuspal coverage should be established to reduce the risk of fracture (27). Such an amalgam filling can last for some years and allow a proper observation period. Later on, the filling can remain as a core build-up and be prepared to receive the final restoration. This is also a cost benefit for the patient.

When the crown preparation is carried out, the margin of the preparation should end as high as possible occlusally in order not to weaken the cervical area, which is weakened from the inside during endodontic therapy (Fig. 19.8). For this reason a partial crown or an onlay (Fig. 19.9) with a maximum preservation of sound tooth structure is most desirable. With a metal onlay, even minimal embracing of a cusp ensures that occlusal forces cannot act in a horizontal direction (see detail in Fig. 19.9).

Where there are thin remaining walls of coronal tooth structure and esthetic demands, a full ceramic restoration (Fig. 19.10) offers the advantage of adhesive bonding throughout the entire surface (51, 53) and can be made as a core build-up and crown restoration in one piece (Fig. 19.11), which is desirable in the case of substantial loss of tooth structure (7).

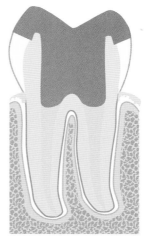

Fig. 19.7 Amalgam restoration.

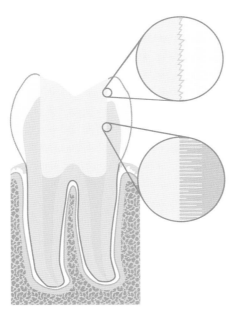

Fig. 19.6 Composite restoration.

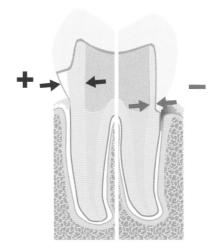

Fig. 19.8 Crown with different levels of preparation.

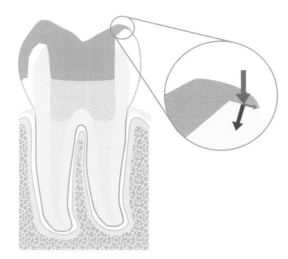

Fig. 19.9   Onlay.

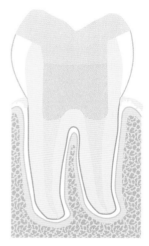

Fig. 19.10   Ceramic onlay.

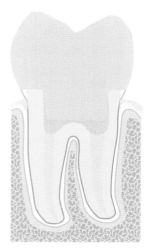

Fig. 19.11   Full ceramic "endo-crown".

Preparation principles

Saving of tooth structure

The reduction of internal tooth structure takes place in several steps during the endodontic and restorative treatment:

1. Access cavity.
2. Coronal flaring.
3. Preparing the root canal.
4. Preparing the post space (if needed).
5. Removing undercuts, if a custom cast post and core will be established.

Although sufficient access and proper flaring are necessary for the success of endodontic treatment, every loss of dentin weakens the tooth (27). Thus, when a tooth serving or going to be used as an abutment needs endodontic treatment, the preservation of tooth structure must be considered from the very beginning of the endodontic procedure. When a tooth is already provided with a crown, it is beneficial to detach the reconstruction before gaining access to the pulp chamber. This is done to achieve better orientation concerning two aspects: first, because the tooth has lost its natural shape, a deviation from the ideal straight-line access cavity is more likely to occur; and second, the amount of coronal dentin left is clearly visible. After endodontic treatment the decision for the kind of build-up is facilitated. Leaving the reconstruction in place makes the determination of the amount of coronal dentin impossible and allows only a blind estimation unless radiographic examination of the coronal tooth structure is possible, as in the case of some low radiopacity materials. When the crown preparation is done after endodontic treatment the circumferential cutback should be restricted to the minimally required reduction in order to save as much tooth structure as possible.

Ferrule design

Special care must be taken in the restoration of a tooth with a minimal amount of remaining coronal tooth structure, i.e. when the complete clinical crown is decayed and only the root remains. In this case a post will be necessary for sufficient retention. Generally, with decreasing root length the crown length will increase, resulting in an unfavorable ratio of leverage of crown versus root. Horizontal loads are supported and transferred by the post to the root, resulting in extreme tensile stress and thus dramatically increasing the risk of root fracture. A marginal preparation that embraces the root effectively participates in the transfer of horizontal forces onto the root and decreases the forces transferred by the post cervically on the opposite side (Fig. 19.12). Such an embracing collar is usually called a ferrule (Key literature 19.3).

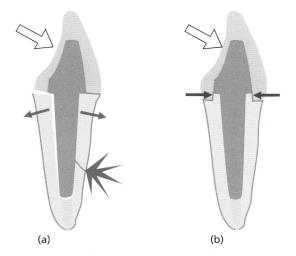

Fig. 19.12   (a) Risk of fracture without ferrule. (b) Effect of ferrule.

Key literature 19.3   Ferrule length in anterior teeth

Libman and Nicholls (38) prepared extracted human central incisors for complete cast crowns. Test teeth had cast dowel cores fabricated, with the ferrule height varying from 0.5 to 2.0 mm in 0.5 mm increments. The five control teeth did not have cast dowel cores. A 4.0 kg load was applied cyclically to each of the restored teeth at an angle of 135° to the long axis of each tooth at a rate of 72 cycles per minute. The load application point was predetermined by a waxing jig that was used to wax all crowns. An electrical resistance strain gauge was used to provide evidence of preliminary failure. Preliminary failure was defined here as the loss of the sealing cement layer between crown and tooth. The results of this study showed that the 0.5 mm and 1.0 mm ferrule lengths failed at a significantly lower number of cycles than the 1.5 mm and 2.0 mm ferrule lengths and control teeth.

In anterior teeth a prerequisite is the establishment of a ferrule of 1.5–2 mm (38, 66) whereas in premolars even a ferrule of 1 mm proved to be effective (3). If this ferrule length is not possible, a surgical crown lengthening procedure should be considered (Core concept 19.4).

Clinical outcome of crowns, bridges, prostheses

Clinical studies investigating the treatment outcome show that there are no significant differences between the long-term survival rate of vital and root filled teeth in single crowns (15, 69). As in laboratory studies the amount of coronal tooth structure plays a most important role for the success of restorations of root treated teeth (21).

Another significant factor for success of crowned root canal treated teeth is the presence of proximal contacts, since a tooth lacking the support of neighboring teeth is more prone to failure (12, 43).

In fixed partial dentures the long-term survival rate of endodontically treated teeth is somewhat lower compared to teeth with vital pulps, especially on the distal abutments (46) and in long-span bridges (16). A substantial decrease in survival rates of root filled teeth was found in cantilever bridges and again in the distal abutments (16, 71) leading to the recommendation to avoid this kind of restoration in pulpless teeth.

Very few studies deal with the outcome within removable partial dentures. In 1985 Sorensen and Martinoff found the success rate of root filled teeth as abutments within removable partial dentures to be lower than within bridges or single crowns, but looking only at post-supported teeth the outcome looked substantially better (62). Wegner *et al.* (72) reported a success rate half as good as that for fixed partial dentures after 5 years and found conical crown-retained partial dentures to be a major problem. In a recently published study a failure rate of 20% for pulpless telescopic retainer abutments compared to 5.7% for vital abutments was reported after 6 years in service (17). In contrast, Bergman *et al.* (6) presented clinical data of "carefully planned and designed" reconstructions with a strict maintenance regimen over 25 years where root filled teeth served as abutments as well as vital ones.

The conclusions to be drawn from these results are that the use of pulpless teeth for abutments of cantilever bridges, removable partial dentures and especially for double crown-retained dentures should be judged very carefully, maintained thoroughly and restricted to teeth with a maximum of tooth structure preserved.

Conversely, not only does root canal treatment affect the outcome of prosthodontic reconstructions but also the quality of the restoration may have an influence on the success of root filled teeth. When a restoration allows leakage of bacteria to the root filling there is no reliable seal of the access to the apex, thus increasing the risk of development or continuance of a periapical lesion. Tronstad *et al.* (68) and Ray and Trope (50) found a significant influence of an obviously poor restoration quality on the presence of periapical inflammation in radiographically examined teeth. The latter study showed that the quality of the restoration had a greater influence than the rating of the root filling.

Core concept 19.4   Indications for different build-ups

Indications for different kinds of build-ups for prosthodontic reconstruction in (a) anterior teeth and (b) premolar/molar teeth.

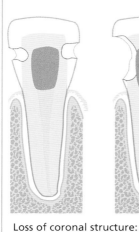 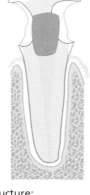 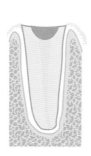 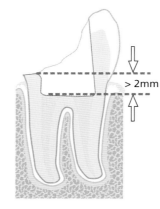 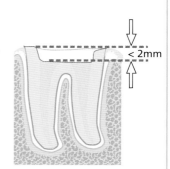

Loss of coronal structure:
– minimal   – moderate   – complete   – moderate   – complete

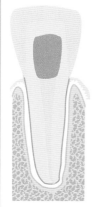 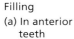 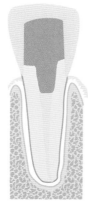 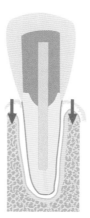 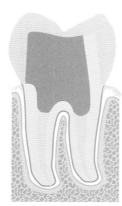 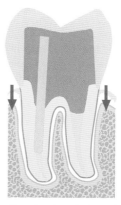

Filling
(a) In anterior teeth   Adhesive build-up   Post (and periodontal surgery)   Adhesive build-up
(b) In premolar / molar teeth   Post (and periodontal surgery)

Case study

Ceramic onlay with adhesive build-up

A 26-year-old woman with symptoms of acute pulpitis was referred for treatment of tooth 46. The present mod-composite filling was found to be suitable for being left for intermediate restoration until completion of the end-odontic therapy within two visits. Immediately after the root filling was performed using a warm vertical technique (a), the access cavity was closed with an adhesive composite build-up (b) extending some millimeters into the canals. Cuspal coverage with a full ceramic onlay was accomplished (c, d) to prevent fracture of the weakened cusps and due to esthetic demands.

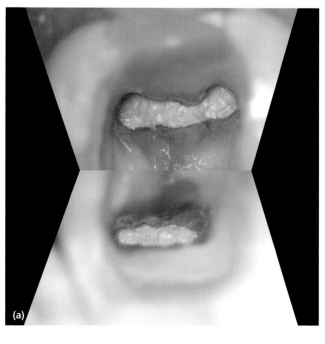

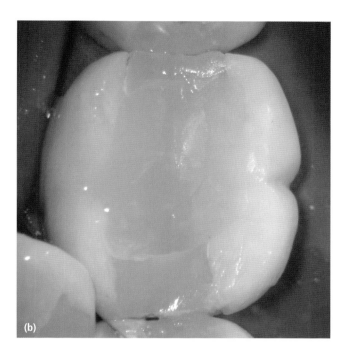

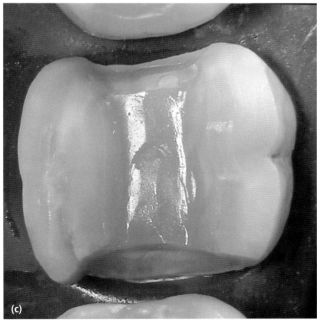

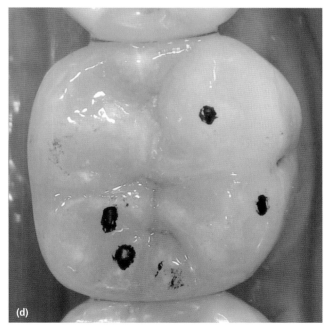

(Courtesy of Dr Jörg Schröder.)

References

1. Abramovitz I, Tagger M, Tamse A, Metzger Z. The effect of immediate vs. delayed post space preparation on the apical seal of a root canal filling: a study in an increased-sensitivity pressure-driven system. *J. Endod.* 2000; 26: 435–9.

2. Asmussen E, Peutzfeldt A, Heitmann T. Stiffness, elastic limit, and strength of newer types of endodontic posts. *J. Dent.* 1999; 27: 275–8.

3. Aykent F, Kalkan M, Yucel MT, Ozyesil AG. Effect of dentin bonding and ferrule preparation on the fracture strength of crowned teeth restored with dowels and amalgam cores. *J. Prosthet. Dent.* 2006; 95: 297–301.

4. Bachicha WS, DiFiore PM, Miller DA, Lautenschlager EP, Pashley DH. Microleakage of endodontically treated teeth restored with posts. *J. Endod.* 1998; 24: 703–8.

5. Barthel CR, Strobach A, Briedigkeit H, Göbel UB, Roulet JF. Leakage in roots coronally sealed with different temporary fillings. *J. Endod.* 1999; 25: 731–4.

6. Bergman B, Hugoson A, Olsson CO. A 25 year longitudinal study of patients treated with removable partial dentures. *J. Oral. Rehabil.* 1995; 22: 595–9.

7. Bindl A, Mörmann WH. Clinical evaluation of adhesively placed Cerec endo-crowns after 2 years – preliminary results. *J. Adhes. Dent.* 1999; 1: 255–65.

8. Bitter K, Kielbassa AM. Post-endodontic restorations with adhesively luted fiber-reinforced composite post systems: a review. *Am. J. Dent.* 2007; 20: 353–60.

9. Bitter K, Meyer-Lueckel H, Priehn K, Kanjuparambil JP, Neumann K, Kielbassa AM. Effects of luting agent and thermocycling on bond strengths to root canal dentine. *Int. Endod. J.* 2006; 39: 809–18.

10. Bolhuis HPB, De Gee AJ, Feilzer AJ, Davidson CL. Fracture strength of different core build-up designs. *Am. J. Dent.* 2001; 14: 286–90.

11. Bottino MA, Baldissara P, Valandro LF, Galhano GA, Scotti R. Effects of mechanical cycling on the bonding of zirconia and fiber posts to human root dentin. *J. Adhes. Dent.* 2007; 9: 327–31.

12. Caplan DJ, Kolker J, Rivera EM, Walton RE. Relationship between number of proximal contacts and survival of root canal treated teeth. *Int. Endod. J.* 2002; 35: 193–9.

13. Colak KM, Yanikoglu ND, Bayindir F. A comparison of the fracture resistance of core materials using different types of posts. *Quintessence Int.* 2007; 38: e511–16.

14. D'Arcangelo C, D'Amario M, Vadini M, Zazzeroni S, De Angelis F, Caputi S. An evaluation of luting agent application technique effect on fibre post retention. *J. Dent.* 2008; 36: 235–40.

15. De Backer H, Van Maele G, De Moor N, Van den Berghe L, De Boever J. An 18-year retrospective survival study of full crowns with or without posts. *Int. J. Prosthodont.* 2006; 19: 136–42.

16. De Backer H, Van Maele G, Decock V, Van den Berghe L. Long-term survival of complete crowns, fixed dental prostheses, and cantilever fixed dental prostheses with posts and cores on root canal-treated teeth. *Int. J. Prosthodont.* 2007; 20: 229–34.

There was no statistically significant difference in the long-term survival of crowns on vital teeth versus post-and-core complete crowns or in the survival of three-unit bridges on vital abutments versus those with at least one pulpless tooth. For bridges with more than three units and cantilever constructions, the use of a post-and-core abutment led to significantly more failures.

17. Dittmann B, Rammelsberg P. Survival of abutment teeth used for telescopic abutment retainers in removable partial dentures. *Int. J. Prosthodont.* 2008; 21: 319–21.

18. Ferrari M, Cagidiaco MC, Goracci C, Vichi A, Mason PN, Radovic I, Tay F. Long-term retrospective study of the clinical performance of fiber posts. *Am. J. Dent.* 2007; 20: 287–91.

A total of 985 carbon or quartz fiber posts were observed over 7–11 years. Four combinations of dentin adhesives/luting materials were used. A 7–11% failure rate was recorded for the three types of posts. Under the 79 failures were one root fracture, one post fracture and 21 failed due to post debonding. The mechanical failures were always related to a lack of coronal tooth structure.

19. Ferrari M, Cagidiaco MC, Grandini S, De Sanctis M, Goracci C. Post placement affects survival of endodontically treated premolars. *J. Dent. Res.* 2007; 86: 729–34.

In this prospective clinical study premolar teeth scheduled for single crown restorations were classified into six groups based on the number of remaining coronal walls (4–0) and also the capability to create a surrounding ferrule of 2 mm. Twenty teeth per group were randomly assigned to be built up with or without a quartz fiber post. Follow-up examinations at 2 years revealed similar failure rates when crown dislodgements were excluded. With one or less dentin wall remaining, up to 20% of the post-supported crowns failed due to debonding of the posts whereas nearly the same number of the restorations without posts showed root fractures mostly resulting in extraction.

20. Fischer H, Rentzsch W, Marx R. Elimination of low-quality ceramic posts by proof testing. *Dent. Mater.* 2002; 18: 570–5.

21. Fokkinga WA, Kreulen CM, Bronkhorst EM, Creugers NHJ. Up to 17-year controlled clinical study on post-and-cores and covering crowns. *J. Dent.* 2007; 35: 778–86.

In a clinical long-term follow-up for 15–17 years, 307 core restorations with single crowns done by 18 practitioners were included. Remaining tooth substance was categorized with well defined criteria as "substantial" or "minimal" dentin height. In teeth with "minimal" dentin support a cast post-and-core restoration or a prefabricated metal post with composite build-up was inserted, in teeth with "substantial" remaining dentin post-free restorations were also used. The type of post-and-core restoration had no influence on the survival probability. The 17-year survival rates at restoration level varied from 71% to 80%, and at tooth level from 83% to 92%.

22. Fokkinga WA, Le Bell AM, Kreulen CM, Lassila LVJ, Vallittu PK, Creugers NHJ. *Ex vivo* fracture resistance of direct resin composite complete crowns with and without posts on maxillary premolars. *Int. Endod. J.* 2005; 38: 230–7.

23. Friedel W, Kern M. Fracture strength of teeth restored with all-ceramic posts and cores. *Quintessence Int.* 2006; 37: 289–95.

24. Gegauff AG, Kerby RE, Rosenstiel SF. A comparative study of post preparation diameters and deviations using Para-Post and Gates Glidden drills. *J. Endod.* 1988; 14: 377–80.

25. Goncalves LA, Vansan LP, Paulino SM, Sousa Neto MD. Fracture resistance of weakened roots restored with a trans-

illuminating post and adhesive restorative materials. *J. Prosthet. Dent.* 2006; 96: 339–44.

26. Hansen EK, Asmussen E. *In vivo* fractures of endodontically treated posterior teeth restored with enamel-bonded resin. *Endod. Dent. Traumatol.* 1990; 6: 218–25.

27. Hansen EK, Asmussen E. Cusp fracture of endodontically treated posterior teeth restored with amalgam. Teeth restored in Denmark before 1975 versus after 1979. *Acta Odontol. Scand.* 1993; 51: 73–7.

    1584 teeth with class II amalgam fillings after endodontic treatment done by 91 Danish dentists were analyzed. They were divided into subgroups treated before 1975 or after 1979. In the latter period the frequency and severity of fractures increased significantly. It is suggested that weakening of the cervical part of the root due to the introduction of Gates–Glidden burs and the use of expanding high-copper amalgam may be the most important reasons.

28. Huang TJ, Schilder H, Nathanson D. Effects of moisture content and endodontic treatment on some mechanical properties of human dentin. *J. Endod.* 1992; 18: 209–15.

29. Isidor F, Brondum K, Ravnholt G. The influence of post length and crown ferrule length on the resistance to cyclic loading of bovine teeth with prefabricated titanium posts. *Int. J. Prosthodont.* 1999; 12: 78–82.

30. Kappert HF. Titan als Werkstoff für die zahnärztliche Prothetik und Implantologie. (Titanium as a material for dental prosthetics and implants.) *Dtsch. Zahnärztl. Z.* 1994; 49: 573–83.

31. Katebzadeh N, Dalton BC, Trope M. Strengthening immature teeth during and after apexification. *J. Endod.* 1998; 24: 256–9.

32. Kishen A. Mechanisms and risk factors for fracture predilection in endodontically treated teeth. *Endod.Topics* 2006; 13: 57–83.

33. Kostka EC, Roulet JF. Retention of posts luted with different materials after root filling with Eugenol containing sealer. *J. Dent. Res.* 1998; 77: 680.

34. Kuttler S, McLean A, Dorn S, Fischzang A. The impact of post space preparation with Gates–Glidden drills on residual dentin thickness in distal roots of mandibular molars. *J. Am. Dent. Assoc.* 2004; 135: 903–9.

35. Kvist T, Rydin E, Reit C. The relative frequency of periapical lesions in teeth with root canal-retained posts. *J. Endod.* 1989; 15: 578–80.

36. Lang H, Korkmaz Y, Schneider K, Raab WHM. Impact of endodontic treatments on the rigidity of the root. *J. Dent. Res.* 2006; 85: 364–8.

    Sound incisors were loaded, and deformations of the root were assessed by Laser Speckle interferometry. The teeth underwent access preparation, manual instrumentation (ISO-40, 60, 80, 110), tapered and parallel-sided post preparation with subsequent measurement of deformability. A significant destabilization was found after access and post preparation but not with the manual enlargement. A further weakening was found after conversion of the tapered post preparation to parallel-sided one.

37. Lassila LVJ, Tanner J, Le Bell A-M, Narva K, Vallittu PK. Flexural properties of fiber reinforced root canal posts. *Dent. Mater.* 2004; 20: 29–36.

38. Libman WJ, Nicholls JI. Load fatigue of teeth restored with cast posts and cores and complete crowns. *Int. J. Prosthodont.* 1995; 8: 155–61.

39. Lindemann M, Yaman P, Dennison JB, Herrero AA. Comparison of the efficiency and effectiveness of various techniques for removal of fiber posts. *J. Endod.* 2005; 31: 520–2.

40. Mannocci F, Ferrari M, Watson TF. Intermittent loading of teeth restored using quartz fiber, carbon-quartz fiber, and zirconium dioxide ceramic root canal posts. *J. Adhes. Dent.* 1999; 1: 153–8.

41. Metzger Z, Abramovitz R, Abramovitz L, Tagger M. Correlation between remaining length of root canal fillings after immediate post space preparation and coronal leakage. *J. Endod.* 2000; 26: 724–8.

42. Nagasiri R, Chitmongkolsuk S. Long-term survival of endodontically treated molars without crown coverage: a retrospective cohort study. *J. Prosthet. Dent.* 2005; 93: 164–70.

    In a population in Thailand the survival rate of 220 endodontically treated molars without crown coverage was evaluated under several aspects. Estimated overall survival rates at 1, 2 and 5 years were 96%, 88% and 36%, respectively. With at least 2 mm surrounding wall thickness the survival probability at 5 years increased to 78%. Composite restorations had a better survival rate than amalgam and reinforced zinc oxide–eugenol restorations.

43. Naumann M, Blankenstein F, Kiessling S, Dietrich T. Risk factors for failure of glass fiber-reinforced composite post restorations: a prospective observational clinical study. *Eur. J. Oral. Sci.* 2005; 113: 519–24.

    A total of 149 crowned teeth restored with glass fiber-reinforced posts and composite build-ups were followed-up for a mean time of 3.3 years. Higher failure rates were found for restorations of anterior teeth, for restorations in teeth with no proximal contacts compared with at least one proximal contact and for teeth restored with single crowns compared with fixed bridges. The maiority of failures were post fractures.

44. Newman MP, Yaman P, Dennison J, Rafter M, Billy E. Fracture resistance of endodontically treated teeth restored with composite posts. *J. Prosthet. Dent.* 2003; 89: 360–7.

45. Ohlmann B, Fickenscher F, Dreyhaupt J, Rammelsberg P, Gabbert O, Schmitter M. The effect of two luting agents, pretreatment of the post, and pretreatment of the canal dentin on the retention of fiber-reinforced composite posts. *J. Dent.* 2008; 36: 87–92.

46. Palmqvist S, Swartz B. Artificial crowns and fixed partial dentures 18 to 23 years after placement. *Int. J. Prosthodont.* 1993; 6: 279–85.

47. Paul SJ, Werder P. Clinical success of zirconium oxide posts with resin composite or glass–ceramic cores in endodontically treated teeth: a 4-year retrospective study. *Int. J. Prosthodont.* 2004; 17: 524–8.

48. Piovesan EM, Demarco FF, Cenci MS, Pereira-Cenci T. Survival rates of endodontically treated teeth restored with fiber-reinforced custom posts and cores: a 97-month study. *Int. J. Prosthodont.* 2007; 20: 633–9.

49. Randow K, Glantz PO. On cantilever loading of vital and non-vital teeth. An experimental clinical study. *Acta Odontol. Scand.* 1986; 44: 271–7.

50. Ray HA, Trope M. Periapical status of endodontically treated teeth in relation to the technical quality of the root filling and the coronal restoration. *Int. Endod. J.* 1995; 28: 12–18.

51. Reeh ES, Douglas WH, Messer HH. Stiffness of endodontically-treated teeth related to restoration technique. *J. Dent. Res.* 1989; 68: 1540–4.

 Strains generated by non-destructive occlusal loading were measured on extracted maxillary premolars after endodontic treatment and MOD restorations with amalgam, cast gold onlay, composite with enamel etch and with total etch, respectively. Cast gold onlay was the strongest restoration tested with a stiffness of 211% of the unaltered tooth, and amalgam was the weakest with 35% of the primarily value. Composite restoration with total etch was almost as strong as the unaltered tooth (87%), while enamel-etch-only yielded a stiffness of 51%.

52. Reid LC, Kazemi RB, Meiers JC. Effect of fatigue testing on core integrity and post microleakage of teeth restored with different post systems. *J. Endod.* 2003; 29: 125–31.

53. Roulet JF. Benefits and disadvantages of tooth-coloured alternatives to amalgam. *J. Dent.* 1997; 25: 459–73.

54. Salvi GE, Siegrist Guldener BE, Amstad T, Joss A, Lang NP. Clinical evaluation of root filled teeth restored with or without post-and-core systems in a specialist practice setting. *Int. Endod. J.* 2007; 40: 209–15.

55. Santos-Filho PCF, Castro CG, Silva GR, Campos RE, Soares CJ. Effects of post system and length on the strain and fracture resistance of root filled bovine teeth. *Int. Endod. J.* 2008; 41: 493–501.

56. Schmitter M, Rammelsberg P, Gabbert O, Ohlmann B. Influence of clinical baseline findings on the survival of 2 post systems: a randomized clinical trial. *Int. J. Prosthodont.* 2007; 20: 173–8.

57. Sedgley CM, Messer HH. Are endodontically treated teeth more brittle? *J. Endod.* 1992; 18: 332–5.

58. Seefeld F, Wenz H-J, Ludwig K, Kern M. Resistance to fracture and structural characteristics of different fiber reinforced post systems. *Dent. Mater.* 2007; 23: 265–71.

59. Segerström S, Astbäck J, Ekstrand KD. A retrospective long term study of teeth restored with prefabricated carbon fiber reinforced epoxy resin posts. *Swed. Dent. J.* 2006; 30: 1–8.

60. Sidoli GE, King PA, Setchell DJ. An *in vitro* evaluation of a carbon fiber-based post and core system. *J. Prosthet. Dent.* 1997; 78: 5–9.

61. Sindel J, Frankenberger R, Kramer N, Petschelt A. Crack formation of all-ceramic crowns dependent on different core build-up and luting materials. *J. Dent.* 1999; 27: 175–81.

62. Sorensen JA, Martinoff JT. Endodontically treated teeth as abutments. *J. Prosthet. Dent.* 1985; 53: 631–6.

63. Standlee JP, Caputo AA, Collard EW, Pollack MH. Analysis of stress distribution by endodontic posts. *Oral Surg. Oral Med. Oral Pathol.* 1972; 33: 952–60.

64. Steele A, Johnson BR. *In vitro* fracture strength of endodontically treated premolars. *J. Endod.* 1999; 25: 6–8.

65. Stricker EJ, Gohring TN. Influence of different posts and cores on marginal adaptation, fracture resistance, and fracture mode of composite resin crowns on human mandibular premolars. An *in vitro* study. *J. Dent.* 2006; 34: 326–35.

66. Tan PLB, Aquilino SA, Gratton DG, Stanford CM, Tan SC, Johnson WT, Dawson D. *In vitro* fracture resistance of endodontically treated central incisors with varying ferrule heights and configurations. *J. Prosthet. Dent.* 2005; 93: 331–6.

67. Tjan AH, Dunn JR, Lee JK. Fracture resistance of amalgam and composite resin cores retained by various intradential retentive features. *Quintessence. Int.* 1993; 24: 211–17.

68. Tronstad L, Asbjornsen K, Doving L, Pedersen I, Eriksen HM. Influence of coronal restorations on the periapical health of endodontically treated teeth. *Endod. Dent. Traumatol.* 2000; 16: 218–21.

69. Valderhaug J, Jokstad A, Ambjornsen E, Norheim PW. Assessment of the periapical and clinical status of crowned teeth over 25 years. *J. Dent.* 1997; 25: 97–105.

70. Varvara G, Perinetti G, Di Iorio D, Murmura G, Caputi S. *In vitro* evaluation of fracture resistance and failure mode of internally restored endodontically treated maxillary incisors with differing heights of residual dentin. *J. Prosthet. Dent.* 2007; 98: 365–72.

71. Walton TR. An up to 15-year longitudinal study of 515 metal–ceramic FPDs. Part 2. Modes of failure and influence of various clinical characteristics. *Int. J. Prosthodont.* 2003; 16: 177–82.

72. Wegner PK, Freitag S, Kern M. Survival rate of endodontically treated teeth with posts after prosthetic restoration. *J. Endod.* 2006; 32: 928–31.

73. Yoldas O, Alacam T. Microhardness of composites in simulated root canals cured with light transmitting posts and glass-fiber reinforced composite posts. *J. Endod.* 2005; 31: 104–6.

74. Zicari F, Couthino E, De Munck J, Poitevin A, Scotti R, Naert I, Van Meerbeek B. Bonding effectiveness and sealing ability of fiber-post bonding. *Dent. Mater.* 2008; 24: 967–77.

75. Zillich R, Yaman P. Effect of root curvature on post length in the restoration of endodontically treated premolars. *Endod. Dent. Traumatol.* 1985; 1: 135–7.

Chapter 20
Non-surgical retreatment

Pierre Machtou and Claes Reit

Introduction

Endodontic treatment is not always successful and periradicular inflammatory lesions might persist or develop postoperatively. Such "failures" are most often caused by microorganisms that have either survived the conventional treatment procedures or invaded the root canal system at later stages via coronal leakage. In order to combat the infection, the root canal has to be renegotiated using either an orthograde (non-surgical retreatment) or a retrograde (surgical retreatment) route of entry. It is the aim of this chapter to review non-surgical retreatment procedures.

In terms of treatment objectives there are no differences between the primary treatment of the infected root canal system and a retreatment, i.e. microorganisms should be eliminated and the space hermetically sealed with a biocompatible filling material. However, retreatment cases are often technically complicated and require high-level skills of the dentist. Because endodontically treated teeth are frequently prosthodontically restored, canals regularly have to be re-entered through crowns. The canals might be obstructed by posts, insoluble filling materials or separated instruments. Furthermore, during the previous treatment a variety of procedural errors such as canal blockage, ledging, apical transportation and root perforation may have occurred.

Indications

Clinical outcome studies have failed to show any systematic difference between a surgical and non-surgical approach to retreatment (1, 17). Consequently the selection of retreatment procedures primarily has to be based on case-specific factors such as the technical quality of the root filling and the personal evaluation of risks and monetary costs.

The typical indication for non-surgical retreatment is a case classified as a "failure" in which the canals are poorly sealed. As soon as it is possible to improve on the quality of the previous instrumentation and filling, the non-

surgical approach should be considered as the primary choice. However, an orthograde route may be contraindicated subjectively if the patient regards the costs or risks of the procedures to be unacceptably high. The monetary costs will increase if crowns, bridges and posts have to be removed and later replaced. In certain situations access openings through the crowns of abutment teeth and removal of posts might increase the risk of bridges loosening and roots fracturing.

Non-surgical retreatment might also be indicated for preventive reasons. In conjunction with the placement of new crowns or posts, the root filling seal inevitably will be challenged by oral microorganisms. A poor fill might not resist such provocation and thus allow microorganisms to invade the root canal. Therefore the replacement of defective root fillings should always be considered when new prosthodontic restorations are to be carried out.

Core concept 20.1 summarizes the critical steps in non-surgical retreatment, and these are discussed in more detail below.

Access to the root canal

Because defective restorations might allow oral microorganisms to invade the root canal system, amalgam and composite fillings frequently have to be removed completely prior to retreatment. Sometimes crowns and

---

Core concept 20.1   Critical steps in non-surgical retreatment

- Access to the root canal:
  - access opening through crowns
  - removal of crowns, bridges, posts
- Access to the apical area:
  - removal of root filling material
  - removal of separated instruments
- Reshaping the root canal
- Antimicrobial treatment

bridges have to be disassembled. Dismantling enables the clinician to assess the actual axis of the tooth and the remaining coronal structure, excavate recurrent or hidden caries and look for cracks, missed or additional canals. The decision to retain a restoration may be taken only when the latter is well fitting and fulfills esthetic, functional and periodontal requirements, and if the access preparation will not seriously damage it. In the case of an access cavity via a metallic restoration, care should be taken to make the occlusal outline wide enough at the start to allow for controlled manipulation of the endodontic instruments without interfering with or scraping the cavity walls. Metal chips may be shaved off the walls and forced into the canal to create irreversible blockage, especially in mandibular teeth. Owing to their own weight, the shavings will not stay in suspension in the irrigating solution (Fig. 20.1).

Removing crowns and bridges

Disassembling involves the use of a transmetal bur (Clinical procedure 20.1) to cut off the crown while preserving at best the underlying tooth structure, instead of using "tapping off" techniques with crown removers in order to break the luting cement (Advanced concept 20.1). The latter techniques are too aggressive and dangerous for the tooth structure. They are unpleasant and painful for the patient and a crown or tooth fracture may often ensue.

Clinical procedure 20.1   Crown removal technique

(1) With a transmetal bur, a slot is made on the buccal aspect of the crown to reach the tooth structure, starting at the gingival margin and stopping in the middle of the occlusal surface.
(2) An ultrasonic insert is then worked to disaggregate the cement bond and help the placement of an elevator to force apart the crown and then dislodge it. The procedure is safe, expedient and, if needed, the crown can be relined to be reused as a temporary one. For bridges, the abutments are separated and individually removed.

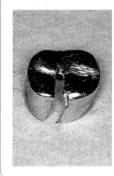
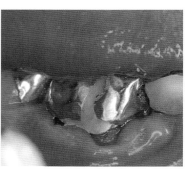

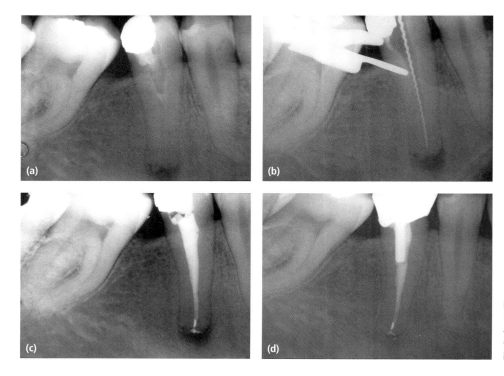

Fig. 20.1 (a) Access cavity was prepared through an amalgam filling. During instrumentation of the root canal (b) amalgam shavings were packed apically (c). (d) A 2-year follow-up radiograph indicates periapical healing.

Advanced concept 20.1   Alternative crown removal techniques

- The WAM Key technique is a safe and efficient way to remove both metallic and porcelain crowns. Step one: create a horizontal slot with a transmetal bur on the buccal aspect of the crown. If the crown is covered with porcelain a round diamond bur is used to perforate the porcelain. To protect the porcelain margins during crown removal the preparation should be tapered (a). Step two: inside the slot a transmetal bur is used to perforate the metal and create a trench. Step three: insert the WAM Key in the slot and gently rotate it to elevate the crown along its own axis (b, c).
- The Metalift Crown Removal System is recommended to gently remove individual crowns because the procedure is simple and highly efficient with minimal damage to the prosthetic crown (a tiny hole is created on the occlusal surface) and tooth structure. A self-tapping instrument threads the metal on the occlusal surface, pushes against the dentin, breaks the cement layer and results in a loosening and lifting of the restoration.

- Coronaflex forceps may be used when maintenance of the crown integrity is mandatory. The forceps are placed at the margins of the crown, then the Coronaflex handpiece is positioned against the forceps arch to ensure an axial pulling direction, and several impulses are delivered to lift off the crown.
- To remove permanently or temporarily cemented bridges without any damage, the parachute technique should always be used in conjunction with air-driven pneumatic crown removers such as the Kavo Coronaflex or the Easy Pneumatic Crown and Bridge Remover from Dentco. The technique allows the removal of bridges in an axial pulling direction. The parachute technique uses metallic wires placed through two or more embrasures of the bridge in order to create loops acting as a rest for a metal rod. The pneumatic handpiece delivers a lot of energy via a curved insert, in an axial pulling direction, that breaks the cement bond.

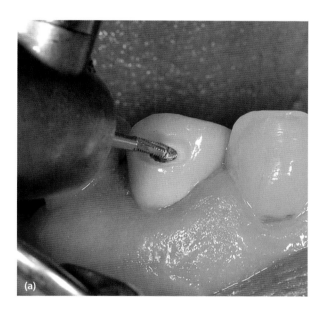

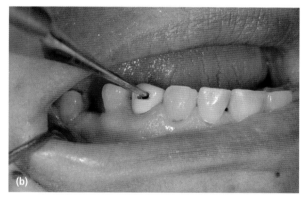

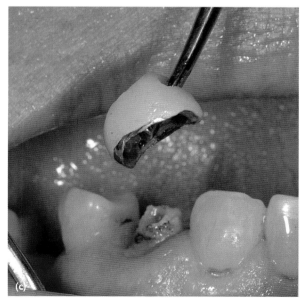

Removing cores and posts

Composite and amalgam cores are easily removed with a high-speed handpiece bur. When a post is present, care must be taken not to damage the protruding head in the pulp chamber. In the case of a composite core, the difference in color between the metallic post and the filling material acts as a guide and makes the procedure easy. Amalgam cores should be drilled in a concentric fashion, starting from the outline of the cavity and moving closer and closer to the post. In both cases, with good illumination and magnification, an ultrasonic tip placed in a piezoelectric ultrasonic unit is well suited to remove residual pieces of restorative material from around the post and the pulp chamber floor.

To remove a cast post and core in one piece from a single-rooted supporting tooth, the "parachute" technique works well (Fig. 20.2). First the metallic core has to be pierced right through with a transmetal bur. A metallic wire is then passed through the hole and tied with a knot to create a loop, acting as a rest for the Coronaflex or the Pneumatic Crown Remover (see Advanced concept 20.1). Depending upon the number of posts present, cast cores should be separated into two or more pieces with

transmetal burs to isolate each post. Utmost care is needed when reaching the pulp chamber floor, especially in the case of a very hard core such as those fabricated of NiCr. In many instances, the huge amount of vibration delivered during the drilling of the core, coupled with the use of ultrasonics, is sufficient to loosen the post.

When considering post removal it is essential to make a careful assessment of the root anatomy and the type, length and width of the post (Fig. 20.3). *Screw posts* or *threaded posts* should usually be unscrewed after sufficient ultrasonic vibration with a piezoelectric unit. A 10 min session of ultrasonics is considered to be the minimum amount of time needed to expect efficacy.

Passive conical or *parallel posts* along with *cast posts* are good indications for using a post-removal system. Either the Gonon or the Ruddle Post Removal System may be used. Both devices are safe, efficient and predictable. Their use is similar and based on the principle of a corkscrew: one force is applied on the tooth structure, providing the fulcrum, while the pulling force is placed on the post (21).

When a post is broken deep inside the canal, the Masserann kit should be the preferred post-removal device because it is more conservative for the root struc-

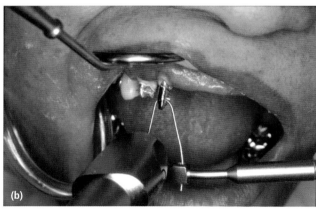

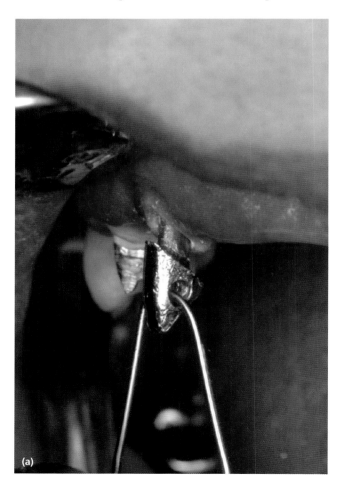

Fig. 20.2 The "parachute" technique may be used to remove a cast post and core in one piece.

ture. Alternately, the post may be troughed with one of the suborifice ultrasonic tips in a dry operating field. While grooving around the post, the ultrasonic energy will vibrate the post and loosen it. The surgical microscope (7), which provides coaxial light and magnification, has made these procedures easier and allows them to be conducted in a controlled manner (see Chapter 10).

After post removal, some residual luting cement may have been left in the canal beyond the apical tip of the post. This can be removed easily with the use of a suborifice tip or an ultrasonic file.

Access to the apical area

Before attempting to reach the apical portion of the canal, the material that obstructs the space has to be removed. In order to avoid the risk of definitive canal blockage or pushing and extruding debris into the periapical tissues, a pronounced crown-down instrumentation procedure should be used (see Chapter 11). As a complicating factor, root canal instruments might have fractured and been left in the canal; in a retreatment situation they have to be removed or at least passed.

Removing gutta-percha

Gutta-percha is quite easy to remove but an organic solvent is often a necessary adjunct, especially in the case of densely filled or curved canals. Chloroform is the best solvent for gutta-percha but great concern exists as to its potential carcinogenicity and mutagenicity. McDonald and Vire (22) reported that there were no negative health effects to the dentist or assistant and air vapor levels were well below mandated maximum levels when chloroform was used in common endodontic treatment procedures. The report concluded that with careful and controlled use, chloroform can be a useful adjunct in the practice of dentistry. Several alternatives to chloroform have been suggested, such as eucalyptol, methyl chloroform, halothane and rectified white turpentine, but all solvents are toxic and, whenever possible, retreatment should be carried out without using solvents (2).

When gutta-percha-filled canals demonstrate some degree of taper, a rotary nickel–titanium instrument is used at 1200 rpm. This will generate sufficient heat to soften the gutta-percha, which is evacuated in a coronal direction owing to the fluted design of the instrument (5). Care should be taken to use a light pecking motion

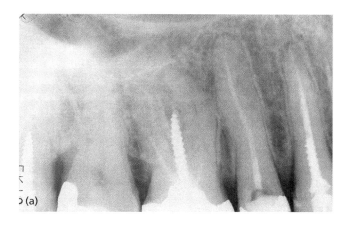
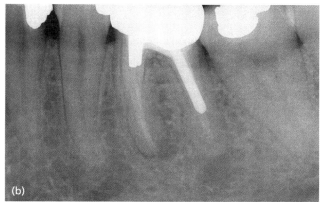
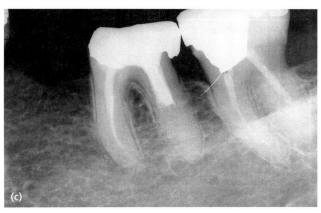
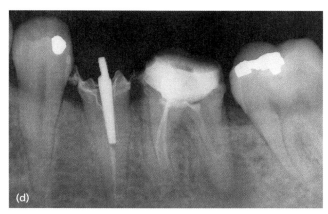

Fig. 20.3 Radiographs showing (a) screwposts, (b) cast posts, (c) Para post and (d) carbon-fiber post (distal canal in first molar).

with the instrument and always visualize the presence of the filling materials on the apical flutes. If resistance to progression is felt, go to hand H-files and proceed as described in Clinical procedure 20.2.

When a canal is small and curved it is safer to use chloroform to avoid creating a ledge or a perforation. The coronal portion of gutta-percha is removed with either a hot heat carrier or plugger or by using an appropriate sized Gates–Glidden drill or an orifice shaper (or similar) at 1200 rpm. Using a glass syringe, two or three drops of chloroform are introduced into the newly created reservoir inside the root canal. The softened gutta-percha then can be removed with Hedström files in an apical direction.

The "wicking technique" – flushing the canal with solvent followed by drying it with paper points – helps to remove any residual gutta-percha and sealer and gives the irrigation solution access to the canal walls during subsequent cleaning and shaping procedures (28) (see Advanced concept 20.2).

Removal of sealers, cements and pastes

It is critical that any residual sealer is eliminated from the canal walls because bacteria may be harbored in the interface (40). Moreover, successful removal will allow irrigation of the contaminated walls during the canal re-instrumentation (10). This step in the retreatment procedure is difficult and is often overlooked.

Removing silver cones

Silver cones were introduced in endodontics by Jasper (15) 75 years ago to simplify the obturation of curved and narrow canals. Their widespread use has led to numerous endodontic failures. Often canals with silver cones are underprepared and, with a defective seal, coronal

---

Clinical procedure 20.2   Removing soluble pastes

(1) The four-wall access cavity is flooded with the solvent and an explorer firmly probes the canal orifice, brings the solvent in contact with the paste and starts the first penetration.

(2) Select a 21 mm Hedström file whose size is adapted to the canal width. The H-file has a sharp tip and aggressive flutes on pulling, so the filling material can be removed laterally as the instrument penetrates into the paste. The material is removed in a coronal–apical direction, using smaller files as the apical portion of the canal is reached. Irrigate copiously with NaOCl to flush out debris and renew the solvent.

(3) It must be anticipated that a ledge is present at the terminus of the previous obturation. Therefore, if an obstruction or blockage is felt, the penetration should be stopped, a radiograph taken and specific measures implemented (see later).

Advanced concept 20.2   Removing Thermafil plastic carriers and paste fills

The Thermafil obturators were introduced about 10 years ago. First marketed with metallic carriers, they were later modified and plastic replaced the metal. Currently, the obturators are available with a special grooved plastic carrier designed to make retreatment easier.

Plastic carriers are easily removed initially using, for example, a D2 or D3 ProTaper rotary file placed at the groove location and rotated at 700 rpm with light pressure. The frictional heat melts the gutta-percha, which allows the instrument to advance apically. Owing to the greater taper, the instrument will bind between the plastic carrier and the dentin and exert an extracting force. In large canals the carrier is usually retrieved in one piece. As a last resort, an H-file can be used to engage the softened plastic carrier and lift it out (14). Once the carrier is removed, the wicking technique must be used to eliminate any residual gutta-percha before re-instrumentation.

In paste-filled teeth, generally some paste is present in the pulp chamber. During the access cavity preparation, the clinician has to clean out the pulp chamber floor with an ultrasonic tip and the amount of time taken indicates the type of paste that has been used. Most of the time it is a zinc oxide–eugenol paste that is removed easily. To dissolve the paste inside the root canals, a solvent must be used (Clinical procedure 20.2). Tetrachloroethylene is recommended but xylene, orange solvent, eucalyptol or eugenol is also efficient. A zinc oxide–eugenol paste that is easily dissolved with these solvents is N2.

For several pastes (epoxy resins, bakelites, glass ionomers, zinc phosphates) no efficient solvents are available (8). Currently, the best method is to use a piezoelectric ultrasonic unit with an ultrasonic tip. If the procedure can be monitored permanently under the surgical microscope, it can be more predictable. Of course, only straight parts of root canals can be managed in this way, but fortunately the densest portion of the paste is usually the coronal one and the apical portion is often not set.

---

and apical leakage will bring about metallic corrosion. Today, silver cones are considered outdated.

Various techniques have been described to retrieve silver cones (20) (Clinical procedure 20.3), but their removal depends mainly on two factors: being able to grab them; and the canal morphology, i.e. whether it is possible to bypass them with a K-file (33).

Removing broken instruments

It is not uncommon to find broken instruments left inside the root canal system. An instrument usually fractures when an overaggressive manipulation has tightly locked its tip in the root dentin. One should realize that the broken instrument itself is not a direct cause of treatment failure but rather an indirect one, because it may have prevented cleaning, shaping and filling of the apical portion of the root canal. Therefore, the therapeutic goal is either to retrieve the fractured instrument or to bypass it

Clinical procedure 20.3   Removing silver cones

(1) A preoperative radiograph gives information about length and fitting of the cone, and whether the coronal head is protruding into the pulp chamber. If there is a crown, a second radiograph must be taken after crown removal.

(2) The restorative material is carefully eliminated from the pulp chamber with an ultrasonic tip, being careful not to damage the fragile silver cone end. At this stage, no attempt should be made to pull out the cone, unless it is very loose.

(3) Flood the access cavity with Endosolv E and try to bypass the cone with a no. 08 or 10 K-file to dissolve and break up the sealer around the cone. Then enlarge this pathway to allow the placement of a no. 15 K-file.

(4) Work a no. 15 or larger ultrasonic file alongside the cone with a short amplitude and in-and-out movements under copious water irrigation to float out the cone. If unsuccessful, then:

(5) Grasp the coronal end of the cone with a modified Stieglitz forceps, whose beaks have been made thinner, and use the tooth structure as a fulcrum to pull out the cone. If resistance is felt, indirect ultrasonics is applied on the beaks of the pliers close to the cone, to help dislodge it.

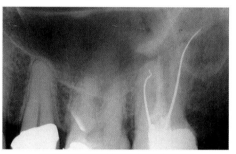

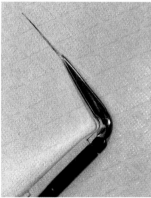

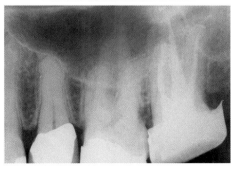

Clinical procedure 20.4   Removing stainless steel instruments

(1) If the fragment can be bypassed, use the technique described for floating out silver cones. If unsuccessful, do not persist and proceed to cleaning and shaping. Often, the fragment is eliminated during these procedures, but if not it will be entombed in the filling material.

(2) If the instrument cannot be bypassed, get a straight radicular access to it. This is done using a sequence of K-files from no. 10 to no. 35, followed by an ascending sequence of Gates–Glidden drills from no. 1 to no. 4, taking care not to damage the root structure. In curved canals, this step provides a relocation of the canal orifice.

(3) At this stage the instrument can be seen in the microscope. A staging platform is created to gain better lateral access to the fragment (28). This can be done with a no. 3 Gates–Glidden drill in which the working head has been cut at the largest cross-sectional diameter. Depending upon the depth of its location in the canal, select an appropriate ultrasonic suborifice tip to make a trench around it. Under vision control and with a permanent light stream of air given by the Stropko syringe, rotate the tip anticlockwise against the coronal end of the fragment to vibrate it, unwind it and then lift it out.

Clinical procedure 20.5   Removing fractured rotary NiTi instruments

Nickel–titanium alloys are brittle, so using ultrasonics may break the instrument if it is tightly locked. Therefore the "tube technique" is indicated in this situation. Radicular access is gained and a staging platform is created as described in Clinical procedure 20.4. Then a blunt needle slightly larger than the instrument is selected and mounted on a Centrix syringe. After the canal has been dried with pure alcohol and the Stropko, 1 ml of Core-Paste is loaded in the syringe and a small excess of material is extruded from the needle. The needle is removed from the syringe and wiped clean. The loaded needle is placed over the fractured instrument and the material is allowed to set for 5 min. The instrument is removed with a counter-clockwise twist. The Cancelier tubes in combination with super glue and its monomer accelerator may also be used. When the fragment is short (1 or 2 mm) it can be completely or partially disintegrated. In the latter situation the short fragment may then be bypassed.

in order to get access to the uncleaned portion of the canal (Core concept 20.2 and Clinical procedures 20.4 and 20.5).

New technological advances such as surgical microscopes, powerful piezoelectric ultrasonic units and refined ultrasonic instruments have significantly increased the possibilities for retrieval of separated instruments. Using this novel approach Suter *et al.* (36) succeeded in retrieving 84 of 97 instruments fractured in the root canal. As a rule, any broken instrument even partially located in the straight portion of the canal that can be visualized in the

---

Core concept 20.2   Clinical strategies in canals with fractured instruments

(1) Try to remove the fragment as described in Clinical procedure 20.4 or 20.5.

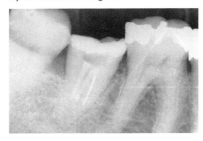 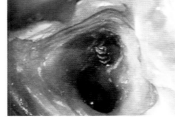 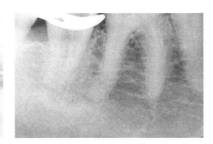

(2) If removal is not successful, attempt to bypass the instrument and incorporate it in the subsequent root filling.

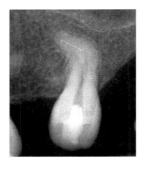 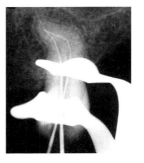 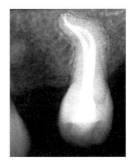

(3) If the instrument cannot be bypassed, clean the canal up to the fragment and seal the space. Observe the case for a period of time before apical surgery is conducted.

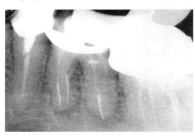 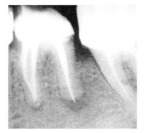 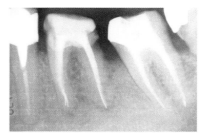

---

microscope should be removed. However, if the fragment is close to the foramen or protrudes beyond it, surgical endodontics is indicated.

Instrumentation of the root canal

Reshaping the root canal

Reshaping the root canal system may be done by hand or by rotary instrumentation. In any case, the crown-down and patency concepts should be used to allow passive apical progression of the endodontic instruments working in a progressively deeper intracanal reservoir of sodium hypochlorite. The constant use of the patency file will move the irrigating solution into the restricted apical area to clean it. The apical preparation is done last, keeping in mind that a sufficiently deep shape should be produced to enable copious renewal of irrigation during final flushing and to pack the canal three-dimensionally.

If Ni–Ti rotary instrumentation is elected, a smooth path guide to the canal terminus must be obtained beforehand for safe shaping of the root canal.

One should be aware that the requested reshaping of an already instrumented canal might create an overenlargement of the root canal space (41), therefore the danger zones of the root anatomy should have been assessed thoroughly before starting the retreatment. Avoiding canal deviation during reinstrumentation should be a permanent concern (27).

Apical obstructions

When canals have been underfilled, obstructive calcifications might be found in the apical unfilled portion. After coronal pre-enlargement and relocation of the canal orifice with Gates–Glidden drills, the coronal portion of the canal is copiously rinsed with sodium hypochlorite and then thoroughly dried with paper points and the

Stropko syringe (see Fig. 10.8, Chapter 10). At this stage, and if possible, the intracanal anatomy should be inspected carefully under the microscope to get information about the obstruction. Then, a small-size precurved K-file in association with a lubricating gel is worked with a slight pecking motion to try to find a catch. As long as a catch is felt at the tip of the K-file, apical progression should be continued and checked periodically with a radiograph until the canal terminus is reached (Fig. 20.4).

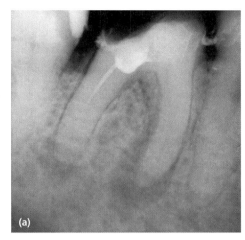
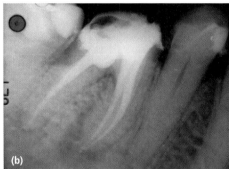
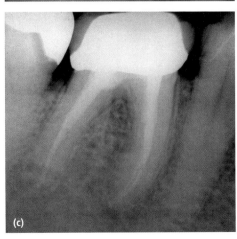

Fig. 20.4 Retreatment of a lower molar with apical periodontitis. (a) Originally the mesial root canals were not negotiated due to obstructive calcifications. (b) The canals were found, instrumented and filled. (c) Radiograph 1 year postoperatively.

Ledges

Often a ledge has been formed at the end of the previous filling of the canal. Most of the time a ledge is the result of an inadequate angle of access to the root canal and goes hand in hand with canal blockage. Preflaring the coronal portion of the canal with K-files and relocating the canal orifice with Gates–Glidden drills are preliminary steps to bypassing a ledge (Clinical procedure 20.6) and recovering patency.

If the ledge is located in the apical portion of the canal, the fitting of the gutta-percha cone may be frustrating and repeatedly unsuccessful. Once the canal has been negotiated with a no. 20 SS K-file, select a 0.06 GT hand file. *Prebend* the tip of the instrument to get a permanent

Clinical procedure 20.6   Bypassing a ledge

(1) Flood the canal with RC Prep or a similar product such as File-Eze or Glyde.
(2) Select a no. 10 SS K-file, place a sharp 1mm curvature at the tip and orientate the directional stop toward the file tip.
(3) Insert the file in the canal with the tip directed toward the canal curvature.
(4) Pick gently with very short strokes, searching for a catch. This procedure will move the irrigant and help to disintegrate the dentin mud. If unsuccessful, rebend the file tip and repeat the same procedure while slightly reorientating the tip.
(5) When a catch is felt, slightly wiggle the file back and forth while maintaining a light apical pressure.
(6) When the block is bypassed, move the file in an up-and-down motion to smooth the ledge. After obtaining a good glide path, copious irrigation with sodium hypochlorite should replace the lubricating gel.

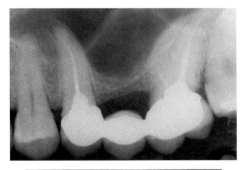
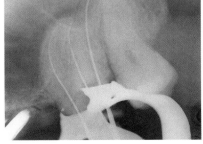

deformation. Insert the tip file beyond the ledge and move the GT file to length with the balanced force technique. Repeat the procedure with a 0.08 GT file. Owing to the greater taper of these files, the ledge is quickly smoothed and a perfect deep shape is obtained.

Missed canals

Sometimes missed canals can be seen overtly in well-positioned radiographs but often they must just be suspected, e.g. when a tooth is reacting to thermal stimuli or is sore after an apparently adequate treatment (37).

After the main canals have been completely cleaned and shaped, the pulp chamber floor should be examined thoroughly. At this stage in the treatment this area is well cleaned by the irrigating solution. A careful inspection of the floor anatomy is made under high magnification and with good illumination. Shifts in dentin color and anatomical grooves may lead to the orifice of an additional canal. An ultrasonic tip might be used on the pulpal floor to uncover hidden orifices and calcified canals. The MB2 orifice is usually located on the groove stretching from the MB1 to the palatal canal orifice. Flooding the pulp chamber with NaOCl may be helpful to locate a hidden canal. When the solution reacts with the underlying pulpal tissue in the hidden canal tiny bubbles are released.

Perforation repair

Furcal or root perforations might occur during root canal therapy, post space preparation or as a result of the extension of an internal resorptive defect. According to Ruddle (28), the four dimensions of a perforation that have to be analyzed are its *level*, *location*, *size* and the *time* that has elapsed since its occurrence.

At a coronal level the inflammatory process that evolves as a response to the perforation might communicate with the gingival pocket and establish a periodontal defect. It is therefore favorable to seal the perforation site at an early stage before any major bone resorption has taken place. A wide perforation will be more difficult to seal than a small one. The sites are mostly elliptical because an instrument usually perforates the canal wall at an oblique angle. Non-surgical repair is less affected by the location of the perforation than a surgical approach to treatment, which can be impossible in certain areas of the root.

Through the years numerous techniques and materials to repair perforations have been described. In this chapter two techniques are described (see Clinical procedures 20.7 and 20.8): the one-visit internal matrix technique using absorbable bovine collagen (Collacote) (18); and the two-visit technique using mineral trioxide aggregate (MTA) (38).

Clinical procedure 20.7   Perforation repair: the internal matrix technique

(1) After cleaning the perforation walls with 0.5% NaOCl, the working length is established using an apex locator and several paper points. The consistently wet portion of the paper point indicates the level of the perforation.
(2) Small pieces of Collacote are cut and sequentially packed with a prefitted plugger through the perforation site and into the bony lesion until a solid barrier is established at the borderline of the root defect.
(3) The perforation site is copiously rinsed with 2.5% NaOCl and then dried. Finally, the defect is covered with a restorative material such as glass ionomer or a composite.

Clinical procedure 20.8   Perforation repair: the MTA technique

First visit
(1) After cleaning the perforation site with 0.5% NaOCl, the working length is established using an apex locator and several paper points. The consistently wet portion of the paper points indicates the level of the perforation.
(2) The MTA is mixed with distilled water to a thick cement consistency. When a granulation tissue is present and can be visualized under the microscope, an aliquot of MTA is delivered (for example with the MTA gun) at the perforation orifice level. The material is gently packed with a big paper point. A second aliquot is delivered to provide a denser material and packed with a plugger. The material excess is removed with an explorer and is smoothed and covered with a wet cotton pellet. The access cavity is filled with a temporary filling and the patient is dismissed.

Second visit: 48 hours later
(1) After removal of the Cavit and the cotton pellet, the MTA hardness is probed with a sharp explorer. If found to be hard:
(2) The definitive obturation is made with the same restorative materials as used with the matrix technique.

Antimicrobial treatment

Microbiota of the root filled tooth

Compared with the microbiota of non-treated pulps, little is known about the flora associated with failed root canal treatments. In canals where major portions have been left unnegotiated, it is reasonable to assume that the flora is similar to that of the necrotic pulp (34). Consequently, in such cases the procedures recommended for primary treatment should be applied also in retreatment cases. However, when canals have been instrumented in their main parts, a strikingly different composition of the recovered microflora has been found (9, 23, 24, 26, 34).

Instead of polymicrobial microbiota, often only one or two strains are detected in failed cases. The microorganisms are predominantly Gram-positive with a slight dominance of facultative over obligate anaerobes (Core concept 20.3). *Enterococcus faecalis* is rarely found in primary samples of the necrotic pulp but has been recovered frequently in filled canals. Among culture-positive teeth, *E. faecalis* was found in 24% by Engström (9), in 47% by Molander *et al.* (23) and in 71% by Peciuliene *et al.* (26). Attention also has been attracted to such species as *Actinomyces* (12, 32, 35), *Candida* (30, 39) and enteric rods (11, 16, 19).

It must be observed that sampling of root filled canals is fraught with difficulties. Initially it has to be preceded by removal of the sealing material. This physical activity might influence the anaerobes more negatively because they are generally more vulnerable. Yet, the composition of the described flora is as would be expected, i.e. more robust and treatment-resistant microorganisms may remain after completion of root canal therapy. The intracanal antimicrobial treatment acts as a selection procedure, favoring a certain type of microbiota either resistant to applied antimicrobial measures or able to survive in such a restricted nutritional habitat.

Antimicrobial retreatment strategies

When treating the non-vital pulp, calcium hydroxide often is recommended as the routine interappointment dressing (Chapter 9). Few organisms will survive when directly exposed to calcium hydroxide, but several factors may impair its antimicrobial potency in the root canal. Complex anatomy will make it difficult to pack the whole canal system satisfactorily with paste (31). Also, calcium hydroxide lacks the potential to reach microbes colonizing the dentinal tubules (25). Furthermore, some species such as enterococci (6, 29) and yeasts (39) may resist high pH levels and thus show low sensitivity to calcium hydroxide. Therefore, in a retreatment situation other medicaments are likely to have greater antimicrobial potentials.

A *standardized retreatment strategy* (Clinical procedure 20.9) must include measures to combat a potential *E. faecalis* infection. It has been observed that enterococci are sensitive to iodine compounds. Safavi *et al.* (29) infected dentinal tubules of human teeth with *E. faecalis* and treated the canals with 2% iodine potassium iodide (IPI). A 10 min period of medicament–dentin contact was sufficient to prevent growth. The presence of a smear layer on the canal walls may delay the intratubular antibacterial activity of a medicament (25), therefore in a clinical situation the application of IPI should be preceded by a procedure to remove the smear layer. Owing to its vaporization, IPI has a long-distance bactericidal effect. However, its duration in the root canal has been shown to be very short (9, 24) and therefore it should not be left as an interappointment dressing. Instead, IPI in a mix with calcium hydroxide paste has been proposed (23).

Core concept 20.3   Features of the microbiota of the "failed" root canal

- Few strains (one or two)
- Gram-positive microorganisms predominate
- Dominance of facultatives over anaerobes
- *E. faecalis* frequently found

Clinical procedure 20.9   Standardized antimicrobial retreatment strategy

(1) Remove smear layer with citric acid or EDTA.
(2) Fill the root canal with 5% iodine potassium iodide or Churchill's solution for 10–15 min. Churchill's solution consists of iodine (16.5 g), potassium iodide (3.5 g), distilled water (20 g) and 90% ethanol (60 g).
(3) Prepare a mix of calcium hydroxide paste and the iodine compound used. Fill up the canal by means of a lentulo spiral.
(4) Make a recall appointment 1–2 weeks later. Repeat steps (1) and (2) and obturate the canal.

There are several reasons (microbial and non-microbial) why an endodontic treatment fails and a standardized retreatment protocol will not consider these various reasons. As an alternative, *individualized monitoring* of retreatment cases might be designed based on intracanal microbiological sampling (Advanced concept 20.3).

Advanced concept 20.3   Individualized strategy based on microbiological sampling

The microbiological situation will vary between cases and "individual" monitoring might be tried as an alternative to the standardized retreatment strategy. Such a strategy must be based on a microbiological diagnosis. After removal of the root filling (preferably without the use of chloroform) the canal is explored and an "initial" sample is obtained. When interpreting the test results, cases are assigned to one of four categories:

(1) "Specific microorganisms". The test results show the presence of enterococci, enteric rods, *Actinomyces* or *Candida*. Specific retreatment strategies are needed.
(2) "Typical residual flora". No "specific" microorganisms are isolated, but the flora are what otherwise might be expected to persist in root canals.
(3) "Atypical microflora". Microorganisms not expected in a "typical" retreatment case, e.g. a large number of species and bacterial cells with a mixture of anaerobes and facultatives. Such a test result indicates leakage due to loosening bridgework or a vertical root fracture, for example.
(4) No microorganisms detected. The cause of failure might be non-microbial (for example a persisting radicular cyst) or due to microorganisms not located within the root canal. Consider surgical retreatment.

Preventive retreatment

Intracanal microorganisms have been recovered in root filled teeth *without* apical periodontitis (9, 23). However, the lack of a visible periapical radiolucency does not necessarily imply the absence of periapical pathosis. Attention must be paid to the possibility of periapical healing, although microbes survive in the root canal. Consequently, when a canal is retreated on a preventive indication, the case should be regarded as potentially infected. Also, patency filing through the foramen should be avoided. As long as there is no pathway to the periapex, a periapical tissue response will not develop. If an avenue is opened up, nutritional supply will increase and an inflammatory lesion may be induced. Supportive clinical data have been presented showing that the development of periapical radiolucencies *after* retreatment is significantly associated with overinstrumentation and overfilling of the root canal (3). Bergenholtz *et al.* (4) diagnosed postoperative periapical radiolucencies in 3% of cases where the root fillings ended short of the apex, and in 18% when canals were overinstrumented and overfilled.

Prognosis

Data on the outcome of non-surgical retreatment are most often available as part of general endodontic follow-up studies (for a review, see Ref. 13). Reported success rates in these investigations vary between 56% and 88%. The issue has been addressed specifically only by a few authors. After 2 years of observation, Bergenholtz *et al.* (3) found, in a prospective study, complete resolution of apical radiolucencies in 48% of 234 retreated roots. Decreased size of the radiolucency was observed in a further 30%. After a follow-up period of 5 years, Sundqvist *et al.* (34) reported complete healing in 74% of 54 retreated teeth. In this study microbiological samples were obtained at the time of root filling and only in two of six "positive" cases did healing take place (33%). Three of the "failed" canals did contain *E. faecalis* and in one canal *Actinomyces israelii* was recovered. The samples were "negative" in 44 cases and 35 of these showed radiographic signs of healing (80%).

Based on the available data, the prognosis of retreatment seems not to be as good as that of initial treatment. However, three out of four cases retreated non-surgically might be expected to heal. When retreatment is conducted for preventive reasons, and procedures are kept within the canal, failure might be anticipated in very few cases.

References

1. Allen RK, Newton CW, Brown CE. A statistical analysis of surgical and non surgical retreatment cases. *J. Endod.* 1989; 15: 261–6.
2. Barbosa SV, Burkhard DH, Spangberg LSV. Cytotoxic effects of gutta-percha solvents. *J. Endod.* 1994; 20: 6–8.
3. Bergenholtz G, Lekholm U, Milthon R, Heden G, Ödesjö B, Engström B. Retreatment of endodontic fillings. *Scand. J. Dent. Res.* 1979; 87: 217–23.
4. Bergenholtz G, Lekholm U, Milthon R, Engström B. Influence of apical overinstrumentation and overfilling on re-treated root canals. *J. Endod.* 1979; 5: 310–14.
5. Bramante CM, Betti LV. Efficacy of Quantec rotary instruments for gutta-percha removal. *Int. Endod. J.* 2000; 33: 463–7.
6. Byström A, Claesson R, Sundqvist G. The antibacterial effect of camphorated paramonochlorophenol, camphorated phenol and calcium hydroxide in the treatment of infected root canals. *Endod. Dent. Traumatol.* 1985; 1: 170–5.
7. Carr GB. Microscopes in endodontics. *J. Calif. Dent. Assoc.* 1992; 20: 55–61.
8. Cohen AG. *The efficiency of different solvents used in the retreatment of paste-filled root canals.* Master Thesis, Boston University, 1986.
9. Engström B. The significance of enterococci in root canal treatment. *Odontol. Revy* 1964; 15: 87–106.
10. Friedman S. Treatment outcome and prognosis of endodontic therapy. In: *Essential Endodontology* (Ørstavik D, Pitt-Ford T, eds). Oxford: Blackwell Science, 1998.
11. Haapasalo M, Ranta H, Ranta K. Facultative Gram-negative enteric rods in persistent periapical infections. *Acta Odontol. Scand.* 1983; 41: 19–22.
12. Happonen R-P. Periapical actinomycosis: a follow-up study of 16 surgically treated cases. *Endod. Dent. Traumatol.* 1986; 2: 205–9.
13. Hepworth MJ, Friedman S. Treatment outcome of surgical and nonsurgical management of endodontic failures. *J. Can. Dent. Assoc.* 1997; 63: 364–71.
14. Ibarrola JL, Knowles KI, Ludlow MO. Retrievability of Thermafil plastic cores using organic solvents. *J. Endod.* 1993; 19: 417–19.
15. Jasper EA. Root canal therapy in modern dentistry. *Dent. Cosmos* 1933; 75: 823–9.
16. Kaufman A, Henig EF. The microbiologic approach in endodontics. *Oral Surg.* 1976; 42: 810–16.
17. Kvist T, Reit C. Results of endodontic retreatment: a randomized clinical study comparing surgical and nonsurgical procedures. *J. Endod.* 1999; 25: 814–17.
18. Lemon RR. Non surgical repair of perforation defects. Internal matrix concept. *Dent. Clin. North Am.* 1992; 36: 439–57.
19. Little JA. *Klebsiella pneumoniae* in endodontic therapy. *Oral Surg.* 1975; 40: 278–81.
20. Lovdahl PE, Gutmann JL. Problems in nonsurgical root canal retreatment. In: *Problem Solving in Endodontics*, 2nd edn (Gutmann JL, Dumsha TC, Lovdahl PE, Hovland EJ, eds). St Louis: Mosby Year Book, 1992.

21. Machtou P, Cohen A, Sarfati P. Post removal prior to retreatment. *J. Endod.* 1989; 15: 552–4.

22. McDonald MN, Vire DE. Chloroform in the endodontic operatory. *J. Endod.* 1992; 18: 301–3.

23. Molander A, Reit C, Dahlén G, Kvist T. Microbiological status of root filled teeth with apical periodontitis. *Int. Endodont. J.* 1998; 31: 1–7.

    Study examining the microbiological status of 100 root-filled teeth with apical periodontitis. In most cases one or two strains were found. Facultative anaerobic species predominated (69% of identified strains) and enterococci were the most frequently isolated genera. Also 20 teeth without signs of apical periodontitis were examined. In 11 of these cases microbes were recovered.

24. Möller ÅJR. Microbiological examination of root canals and periapical tissues of human teeth. *Odontol. Tidskr.* 1966; 74.

    A classic monograph in the endodontic literature. In numerous experiments the author covered almost all stages of microbiological sampling and culturing.

25. Ørstavik D, Haapasalo M. Disinfection by endodontic irrigants and dressings of experimentally infected dentinal tubules. *Endod. Dent. Traumatol.* 1990; 6: 142–9.

26. Peciuliene V, Reynaud AH, Balciuniene I, Haapasalo M. Isolation of yeasts and enteric bacteria in root filled teeth with chronic apical periodontitis. *Int. Endod. J.* 2001; 34: 429–34.

27. Peters O, Barbakow F. Apical transportation revisited or "Where did the file go?" *Int. Endod. J.* 1999; 32: 131–7.

28. Ruddle CJ. Nonsurgical endodontic retreatment. *J. Calif. Dent. Assoc.* 1997; 25: 769–99.

29. Safavi E, Spångberg L, Langeland K. Root canal dentinal tubule disinfection. *J. Endod.* 1990; 16: 207–10.

30. Se BH, Piskin B, Demirci D. Observation of bacteria and fungi in infected root canals and dentinal tubules by SEM. *Endod. Dent. Traumatol.* 1995; 11: 6–9.

31. Sigurdsson A, Stancill R, Madison S. Intracanal placement of Ca(OH)$_2$: a comparison of techniques. *J. Endod.* 1992; 18: 367–70.

32. Sjögren U, Happonen R-P, Kahnberg K-E, Sundqvist G. Survival of *Arachnia propionica* in periapical tissue. *Int. Endod. J.* 1988; 21: 277–82.

33. Stabholtz A, Friedman S, Tamse A. Endodontic failures and re-treatment. In: *Pathways of the Pulp*, 6th edn (Cohen S, Burns RC, eds). St Louis: Mosby Company, 1994.

34. Sundqvist G, Figdor D, Persson S. Microbiologic findings of teeth with failed endodontic treatment and the outcome of conservative re-treatment. *Oral Surg. Oral Med. Oral Pathol. Oral Radiol. Endod.* 1998; 85: 86–93.

35. Sundqvist G, Reuterving C-O. Isolation of *Actinomyces israelii* from periapical lesion. *J. Endod.* 1980; 6: 602–6.

36. Suter B, Lussi A, Sequeira P. Probability of removing fractured instruments from root canals. *Int. Endod. J.* 2005; 38: 112–23.

37. Tidwell E, Witherspoon DE, Gutmann JL, Vreeland DL, Sweet PM. Thermal sensitivity of endodontically treated teeth. *Int. Endod. J.* 1999; 32: 138–45.

38. Torabinejad M, Chivian N. Clinical applications of mineral trioxide aggregate. *J. Endod.* 1999; 25: 197–205.

39. Waltimo TMT, Sirén EK, Ørstavik D, Haapasalo MP. Susceptibility of oral *Candida* species to calcium hydroxide *in vitro*. *Int. Endod. J.* 1999; 32: 94–8.

40. Wilcox LR, Krell KV, Madison S, Rittman B. Endodontic retreatment: evaluation of gutta-percha and sealer removal and canal reinstrumentation. *J. Endod.* 1987; 13: 453–7.

41. Wilcox LR, Swift ML. Endodontic retreatment in small and large curved canals. *J. Endod.* 1991; 17: 313–15.

Chapter 21
Surgical endodontics

Peter Velvart

Introduction

Microorganisms lodging in root filled canals may cause endodontic treatment failure. In order to eradicate the microbes in such cases, the root canal system has to be renegotiated and retreated. If the canals are poorly filled and fairly easy to access, an orthograde route of re-entry is generally to be preferred (Chapter 20). However, in many cases non-surgical retreatment may not be feasible from technical as well as financial aspects. Furthermore, an endodontic treatment failure might be caused by factors located outside the root canal, such as microorganisms colonizing the periapical tissues, cysts and foreign body reactions (Chapter 7). In such cases a surgical approach to retreatment may be considered (Fig. 21.1).

Although extensively debated over the years, there is little evidence to suggest that cysts are unable to heal following conventional endodontic therapy. Nair (42) has drawn attention to the fact that some radicular cyst cavities do not connect directly with the root canal space. These so-called true radicular cysts are therefore thought to be autonomous processes and not likely to respond to conventional therapy. From a clinical point of view, however, there are no means by which the existence of such a pathological condition can be determined. Consequently, all radiolucent lesions associated with non-vital pulps, whether cyst or not, should be seen as treatable by conventional means and be subjected to surgery only if healing by orthograde root canal treatment cannot be attained.

In surgical endodontics the procedural objectives are to expose the root tip and the periapical tissues with the treatment aim to restrain a potential intracanal infection (usually the root tip is cut and the apical part of the canal is instrumented and sealed). Core concept 21.1 summarizes the typical indications for surgical retreatment.

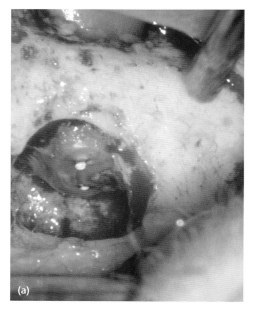
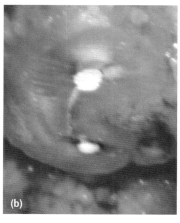

Fig. 21.1 (a) Clinical photograph showing access to the root tips of a lower first molar in an endodontic surgical procedure, at which a root tip resection was carried out. (b) High-power magnification of the resected surface showing the buccal and lingual canal with gutta-percha and isthmus between the canals.

Core concept 21.1   Typical indications for surgical retreatment

- Blocked root canal in an esthetically satisfactory post-supported crown restoration with a good marginal adaptation that could not be removed. The top-right radiograph was taken immediately postoperatively and the bottom radiograph, taken after 1 year of follow-up, shows apical healing.

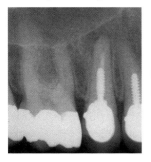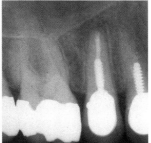

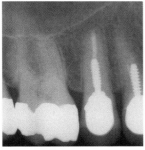

- Apical root canals blocked by ledge.

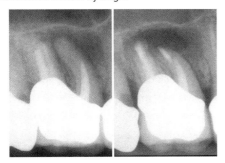

- Grossly overinstrumented and overfilled canal.

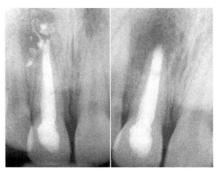

- Failed treatment in spite of adequate root filling. Persistence of a fistula.

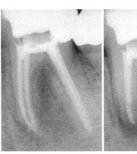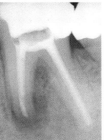

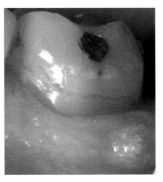

General outline of the procedure (Core concept 21.2)

Following local anesthesia (step 1) a mucoperiosteal flap is raised (step 2). If the periapical tissue response has not perforated the cortical bone plate, bone has to be removed (step 3) to provide access to the root tip. The soft-tissue lesion is then curetted (step 4) and the root tip is cut (step 5). A root-end preparation is made (step 6) and a filling (retrofill) is placed (step 7). The surgical procedure is finished with meticulous cleaning of the wound area and repositioning and suturing of the flap (step 8).

Local anesthesia

Proper pain control is required to perform surgical endodontics. Normally the procedure can be conducted under local anesthesia.

Choice of anesthetic agent

Anesthetic agents are most effective in a non-ionized form within a pH range near 7.4. In this state the drug can easily penetrate the nerve membranes and displace the calcium ions at the membrane receptor sites. The sodium channels are then blocked and upon nerve stimulation

---

Core concept 21.2   Critical steps in surgical endodontics

(1) Local anesthesia

(2) Raising a flap

(3) Bone removal

(4) Soft-tissue lesion curettage

(5) Root-end resection

(6) Root-end preparation

(7) Retrofill

(8) Suturing

---

the membrane will remain in a polarized state. In acutely inflamed tissue the pH is lowered. In such an environment the anesthetic may remain in ionized form. The result can be lesser penetration of the drug, leading to inadequate anesthesia. This is one possible explanation for the deficient pain control sometimes experienced when operating on acutely inflamed tissue. If possible, endodontic surgery should therefore not be performed in such instances. There are several anesthetics suitable for surgical pain control. Because allergic reactions to anesthetic drugs occur mainly to ester-based agents (such as procaine) (23), anesthetics based on amide groups are preferred. Good and profound anesthesia can generally be obtained with articaine, lidocaine and bupivacaine.

Vasoconstrictors

A vasoconstrictor added to local anesthetics reduces the blood flow at the injection site. This serves two important purposes:

- To retain the agent longer in the tissue, thereby extending the time for the anesthetic effect.
- To enhance hemostasis.

The reduced blood flow will also decrease absorption of the anesthetic and minimize systemic toxic effects.

The most widely used vasoconstrictor is epinephrine. This sympathomimetic agent causes vasoconstriction by stimulating specific membrane-bound receptors on the vascular smooth-muscle cells. The pharmacological action of epinephrine depends largely on the type of receptors present in the tissue. There are two types of adrenergic receptors: alpha vasoconstrictive and beta vasodilating receptors. Similar to mucosal and gingival tissues, alpha-adrenergic receptors predominate in the apical periodontium. Thus, upon its penetration to these tissue sites, the effect of epinephrine will be contraction of blood vessels. In skeletal muscles, on the other hand, vessels are controlled by beta-adrenergic vasodilating receptors (38). This means that injection of epinephrine to muscle tissue will result in increased blood flow and cause the opposite of the desired hemostatic effect (3). For this reason, the anesthetic should be administered to mucosal tissue only and close to the bone in the area in focus for the operation.

Concentrations of vasoconstrictor among anesthetic solutions vary between 1:50 000 and 1:200 000. The higher the concentration, the better the hemostatic effect. Most widely used is the concentration 1:100 000–200 000. Although this concentration is adequate for non-surgical needs (29), it will not produce sufficient hemostasis for surgical procedures. For this purpose, at least 1:80 000 or rather 1:50 000 is recommended. It has been found that

Core concept 21.3   Injection technique

To reduce pain and cardiovascular effects upon injecting an anesthetic solution containing epinephrine:

(1) Aspirate to prevent intravascular administration.
(2) Inject at a slow pace. Speed should not exceed 1–2 ml per minute.
(3) Anesthetize first with half the dose of the solution at a concentration of 1:100 000 epinephrine. Wait 3–5 min until initial vasoconstriction and then use 1:50 000 epinephrine.
(4) Use a pulse oximeter to monitor pulse rate.

the use of 1:50 000 epinephrine results in good visualization of the surgical site, reduced surgery time and decreased postoperative bleeding and blood loss (3). High concentrations of epinephrine may cause an undesirable increased heart rate, cardiac contractility and peripheral vascular resistance. These systemic effects can be reduced by using several measures (see Core concept 21.3).

It should be realized that sufficient hemostasis can be achieved only if the anesthetic has reached the tissue. Therefore, with inferior alveolar nerve blocks additional anesthetic must be administered to the surgical site to obtain adequate hemostasis, even though blood flow peripheral to such nerve blocks becomes reduced (27).

Raising the flap

The success of any surgical procedure depends largely upon the extent to which adequate access can be obtained. Endodontic surgery first requires exposure of the bone overlying the tip of the root(s) and then the root end(s) *per se* (Fig. 21.1). To access the bone, a full-thickness flap must be raised. This means a soft-tissue flap, which consists of gingival and mucosal tissue as well as periosteum. To mobilize the flap various modes of incision can be selected, including horizontal incisions (sulcular and submarginal) and vertical releasing incisions.

It is critical that incisions and flap elevations are carried out in a manner such that soft-tissue healing by primary intention is facilitated. This is secured by:

- complete and sharp incision of the tissues;
- avoiding tearing of the tissues during flap elevation;
- preventing drying of the tissue remnants on the root surface during the procedure (see further below).

Proper treatment of the soft tissues with adequate surgical techniques is also a challenge from an esthetic point of view. Incorrect manipulation of soft tissues in areas with restoration margins placed subgingivally for esthetic reasons can, for example, lead to exposure of these margins because of recession following the surgery. Therefore, the presence, type and quality of restorations, especially with regard to the position of the restoration margin in relation to the gingiva, must be carefully assessed prior to surgery, as they are critical to the esthetic outcome of the procedure.

Flap designs

Triangular flap: A horizontal incision extending one tooth distally and one tooth mesially to the involved area, combined with only one vertical releasing incision (Fig. 21.2), forms the triangular flap. The main advantage of this flap design is easy repositioning and minimal disruption of the vascular supply to the flap. It is indicated for correction of marginally located processes such as perforations, cervical root resorptions or resections of very short roots. If it turns out that the access is too limited, the triangular flap can be converted easily to a rectangular flap by placing an additional releasing incision at the distal end of the horizontal incision (see below).

Rectangular flap: The rectangular flap is formed by a horizontal incision with two vertical releasing incisions (Fig. 21.3) and is the most frequently used flap in endodontic surgery. The rectangular flap will give excellent surgical access to the apical area in any region. In esthetically critical areas with prosthetic restorations involving submarginally placed crown margins, a postoperative sequela can result in recession, leading to exposure of the crown margins. Using a proper atraumatic and gentle surgical technique with proper wound management minimizes such esthetic disadvantages.

(a)

(b)

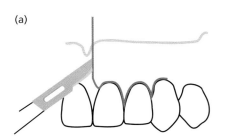
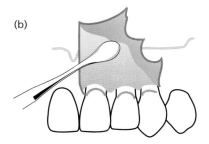

Fig. 21.2 (a) A triangular flap requires a sulcular incision, usually with mesial placement of the vertical releasing incision. (b) Flap reflected.

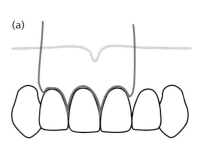

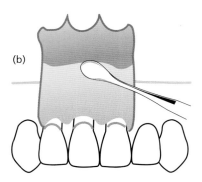

Fig. 21.3   (a) A rectangular flap involves two releasing incisions combined with a marginal sulcular incision. The releasing incisions are placed at least one tooth away from the tooth to be operated on, except in the area of the mental foramen, which should not be subjected to vertical incisions. (b) Flap reflected.

Submarginal flap according to Ochsenbein–Luebke: The submarginal flap is formed by a scalloped horizontal submarginal incision with two vertical releasing incisions (Fig. 21.4). The submarginal flap is only to be used when there is a broad attached gingiva and when the expected apical lesion or surgical bony access will not involve the incision margins. This flap design has the advantage of preserving the marginal gingiva and does not expose the marginal crestal bone.

As well as the risk of massive loss of marginal tissue due to a possible insufficient blood supply to the unreflected gingival tissue (see above), the risk of scarring is another disadvantage of this flap design. Owing to drying out of the tissue the flap tends to shrink during surgery, resulting in tension and difficulty in replacing and securing it by suturing.

Papilla-base flap: This flap consists of two releasing vertical incisions, connected by the papilla base incision and intrasulcular incision in the cervical area of the tooth. It was designed to prevent recession of the papilla. A microsurgical blade of a size not exceeding 2.5 mm in width should be used. Controlled and minute movement of the surgical blade within the small dimensions of the

interproximal space is crucial. The papilla base incision requires two different incisions at the base of the papilla. A first shallow incision severs the epithelium and connective tissue to the depth of 1.5 mm from the surface of the gingiva (Fig. 21.5, blue line). The path is a curved line, connecting one side of the papilla to the other. The incision begins and ends perpendicular to the gingival margin (Fig. 21.6). In the second step, the scalpel retraces the base of the previously created incision while inclined vertically, towards the crestal bone margin. The second incision results in a split-thickness flap in the apical third of the base of the papilla (Fig. 21.5). From this point on apically, a full-thickness mucoperiosteal flap is elevated (Fig. 21.7). Although the papilla base flap achieves predictable healing results, this technique requires a skilled surgeon. Atraumatic handling of the soft tissues is of utmost importance in order to obtain rapid healing through primary intention. The epithelium of the partial-thickness flap has to be supported by underlying connective tissue, otherwise it will break down and lead to scar formation. On the other hand, excessive thickness of the connective tissue layer of the split flap portion can jeopardize the survival of the buccal papilla left in place (59).

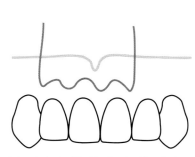

Fig. 21.4   An Ochsenbein–Luebke flap is raised by placing a scalloped horizontal incision within the attached gingiva, reflecting the gingival and mucosal tissues (37). For vertical incisions, the same rules apply as for the rectangular flaps.

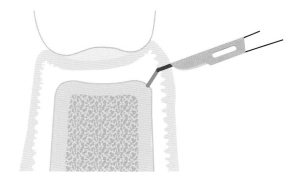

Fig. 21.5   Schematic drawing of incision type for the papilla base flap. The first shallow incision is placed at the lower end of the papilla in a slightly curved line, perpendicular to the gingival margin (blue line). A second incision is placed, directed to the crestal bone margin from the base of the previously created incision (green line). The result is a split-thickness flap on the base of the papilla.

Incisions

Sulcular incision: The scalpel size has to be small enough to allow free movement of the blade within the sulcus and to avoid cutting into the gingiva (Figs 21.8 and 21.9). The scalpel should be kept in constant contact with the

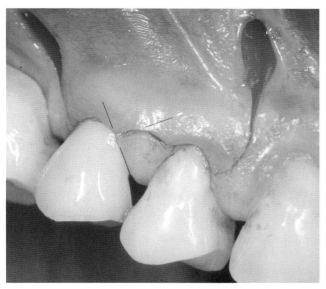

Fig. 21.6   Curved incision placed perpendicular to the gingival margin (lines). (Reprinted with permission from (60).)

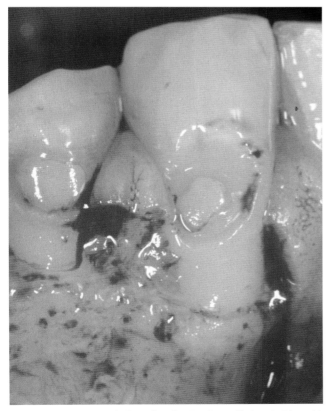

Fig. 21.7   Elevated spit-thickness flap showing the papilla base incision with the major part of the papilla unaltered. (Reprinted with permission from (60).)

tooth. Even so, the incision will sever sulcular epithelium and fibers of the gingival attachment, leaving epithelium and connective tissue at the root surface (Fig. 21.9). These tissue remnants are delicate and easily injured, which can result in impaired healing (16), and should not be allowed to dry out because they facilitate epithelial and gingival reattachment. Interproximally the tissue should be dissected in the middle of the papilla, to preserve its buccal and lingual aspects (Fig. 21.10).

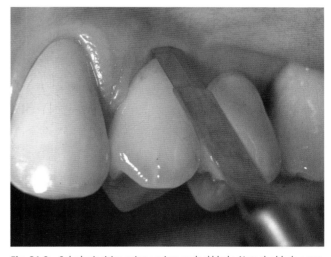

Fig. 21.8   Sulcular incision using a micro-scalpel blade. Note the blade entering the gingival tissue owing to a small root diameter in the cervical area of the root.

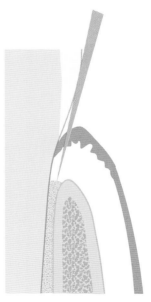

Fig. 21.9   Marginal incision leaves small amounts of gingival connective tissue and epithelium on the tooth surface, which should be kept moist and vital for reattachment at the preoperative attachment level.

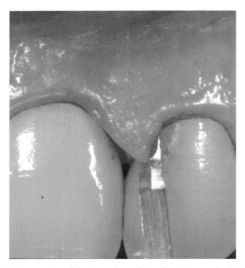

Fig. 21.10 Dissection of the buccal papilla with a micro-scalpel. Note complete separation from the lingual portion of the papilla and the preservation of the tissue in all its dimensions.

Submarginal incision: The submarginal incision to raise an Ochsenbein–Luebke flap is performed within the attached gingiva and should be at a level where the incision cuts well into the crestal bone (36). The cutting action is a continuous firm stroke with the blade, which separates the tissue all the way to the bone. For easy and precise repositioning of the flap, the incision should not be in a straight line, but scalloped and extending slightly in the interproximal direction. Thus, the contour of the incision should reflect the contour of the marginal gingiva (Fig. 21.11c). The submarginal incision should be at a level that is 2 mm apical to the base of the sulcus in order to avoid the risk of subsequent necrosis and recession of the unreflected marginal portion. To size up the width of the attached gingiva, the pocket probing depth has to be determined (Fig. 21.11a). The width of the attached gingiva is then calculated on the basis of the distance from the base of the sulcus to the *linea girlandiformis* (Fig. 21.11b).

In general, healing after this mode of incision is favorable because there is sufficient blood supply from vessels exiting at the crestal bone level and from anastomosing vessels deriving from the papilla.

Where there are deep periodontal pockets, this type of incision is contraindicated and a marginal incision should be performed instead. The incision also should not be used when there is danger of having the incision over the bone defect, which increases the risk of postoperative infection. Therefore, the selection of this type of incision requires thorough treatment planning. The main advantage is that the original level of the epithelial attachment can be maintained, which may not always be the case following sulcular incision. This is certainly an important esthetic consideration especially with full crowns, where healing after a sulcular incision can result in gingival recession to such an extent that the crown margins become visible.

Vertical incisions: At least one and usually two vertical incisions are needed in an endodontic surgical procedure to allow sufficient exposure of the root tip area. The incision should extend apically enough to prevent tension on the flap during retraction. When cutting in the apical area the blade often does not reach the bone owing to the thickness of the mucosa, therefore a second stroke has to be taken to completely separate the tissue through the periosteum.

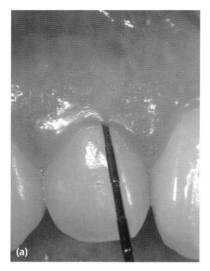 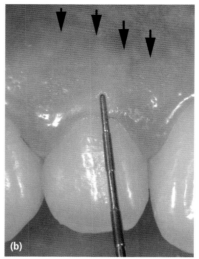 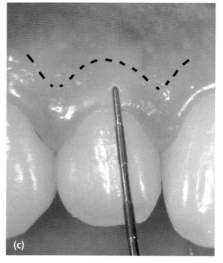

Fig. 21.11 (a) Measuring the pocket probing depth is necessary for calculation of the width of the attached gingiva in a submarginal incision procedure. (b) The probe is held on the buccal surface of the gingiva to visualize the base of the probing depth. The attached gingiva represents the distance from the tip of the probe to the linea girlandiformis (arrows). (c) The line represents the location for a submarginal incision.

The vertical releasing incision is placed usually one tooth laterally to the tooth to be operated on (Fig. 21.3). An exception to this rule is the lower premolar region, where a vertical cut can interfere with the nerve bundles exiting from the mental foramen and cause temporary or permanent paresthesia. In such cases the vertical incision is placed one tooth mesial to the mental foramen. In any case, it is important to determine radiographically the position of the foramen prior to surgery if it is going to be exposed by the flap.

The placement of the vertical incision should be such that the integrity of the papilla is maintained. Figure 21.12 illustrates the correct paramedian releasing incision to be used. Incisions mid-crown and incisions that split the papilla should be avoided because they may lead to necrosis of a large portion of the tissue and recessions.

Flap elevation and retraction

After the incision, lifting the tissue from the underlying bone should raise the flap. In the process, the periosteum should not be perforated or torn. To optimize the healing conditions, maintenance of an intact periosteum is essential because it will protect the surgical cavity from being in direct contact with the mucosal tissue, which otherwise can enter the cavity and prevent complete bone fill.

Flap elevation should begin from the releasing incision in an undermining action (Fig. 21.13). The elevating instrument then should be directed toward the marginal ridge. If the periosteum cannot be separated completely from the crestal bone, the flap will be freed

by carefully dissecting the unseparated tissue remnants with a scalpel.

Once the flap has been retracted, a small groove should be prepared in the bone with a small round bur. This groove serves as a rest for the retractor, to prevent crushing of the flap during the surgery (Fig. 21.14).

Bone removal

Once the flap has been retracted and held in place, bone usually needs to be removed to uncover the soft-tissue lesion and the apical area of the tooth. A sufficient amount of bone tissue must be eliminated to gain proper access.

It is important that the osseous tissue is managed with caution to prevent postoperative pain and to enhance healing. Heat generation is damaging and should be monitored by using rotating burs with light shaving motions while irrigating with copious amounts of sterile saline (13). Supplementary saline irrigation must be used

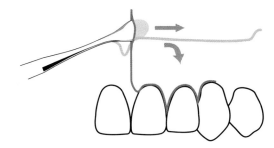

Fig. 21.13   Raising a flap from the releasing incision with a distal–coronal-directed motion, undermining the periosteum.

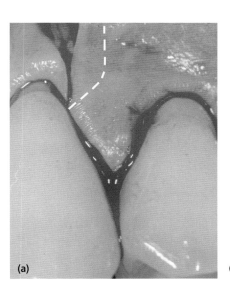
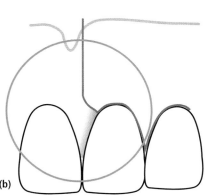
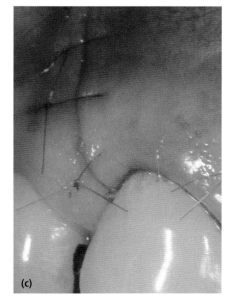

Fig. 21.12   Vertical releasing incision. (a) Incorrect straight vertical incision creates compromised tissue area with insufficient blood supply, which will eventually necrose. The dashed line indicates the desired incision course. (Reprinted with permission from (58).) (b) Correct vertical incision preserving the body of the papilla. (c) Clinical example of correctly placed incision after suture placement. (Reprinted with permission from (61).)

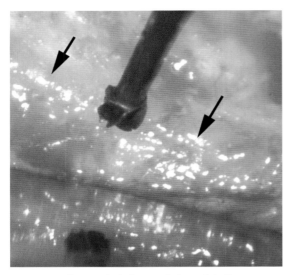

Fig. 21.14 A small groove in the bone at the base of the flap serves as a rest for the periosteal elevator, giving the assistant a safe position for it so that it will not slip and possibly crush the tissues.

when cutting deep to uncover, for example, palatal or lingual roots. Excessive pressure during drilling should be avoided at all times. The bone drill, in addition, should be sharp and clean. Diamond burs are inefficient and should not be used (2).

Curettage of the soft-tissue lesion

Because the soft-tissue lesion most often represents an inflammatory response to a root canal infection and/or to extruded root filling material, removal of this tissue is not essential *per se* but it needs be taken out for technical reasons to allow visibility and accessibility to the root tip for the management of the root canal system (Advanced concept 21.1). Therefore, curettage to remove the soft-tissue lesion has to be performed. This task is greatly facilitated by the use of sharp curettes, because fibrous tissue in the periphery of the lesion often is difficult to detach.

In case of a radicular cyst the cyst capsule can be released from the adjacent bone by careful dissection and removed in its entirety. If the blood supply of the adjacent tooth (teeth) or other vital structures, such as neurovascular bundles, is endangered, complete removal of the soft-tissue lesion should not be attempted.

Management of bleeding

Hemostasis during endodontic surgery is essential to ensure successful management of the root end. Hemorrhage control is not only required for visibility and assessment of the root structure but also necessary to allow insertion and setting of the retrograde root filling material in the absence of moisture. Several means, described here, can be undertaken to control bleeding.

> **Advanced concept 21.1   The importance of complete removal of the soft-tissue lesion**
>
> Over the years it has been debated extensively whether or not the removal of the soft-tissue lesion is a critical step in endodontic surgery. It has been held that the lesion represents a pathological process and therefore should be removed in its entirety. Given the fact that the soft-tissue lesion actually is a host tissue response to irritants associated with the tooth, most often to a root canal infection, complete curettage should not be necessary. In fact, in a publication comparing complete and incomplete removal of periradicular tissues during surgery, no difference in clinical outcome was found in terms of periradicular healing at clinical follow-up (34). It is therefore likely that any inflamed tissue left behind will be incorporated into the new granulation tissue that will form as part of the healing process. Even leaving some epithelial remnants should not jeopardize the healing process. It has been proposed that as long as the irritants of the root canal system are eliminated, the host's defense mechanisms will destroy and eliminate proliferated epithelial cells (52). An exception to this view is the case where bacteria are located within the lesion itself, e.g. *Actinomyces* species (see Chapter 7). These microorganisms appear in nests and can be observed macroscopically as yellow granules. As a lesion of this nature may be sustained by the organisms, it should be curetted carefully. Curettage of the soft-tissue lesion diminishes bleeding. Also, from this perspective it is essential to remove as much of the soft-tissue process as necessary to enhance the management of the root end, including preparation and retrofilling.

Proper local anesthesia: Hemorrhage reduction is achieved by local anesthesia using a sufficient concentration of the vasoconstrictor (see above). It should be recognized that, even though numbness is achieved soon after the injection, sufficient vasoconstriction takes several minutes to attain.

Proper operation technique: Proper handling of the soft tissue minimizes bleeding. Remember that most vessels run parallel to the long axis of the teeth. Therefore the releasing incision, for example, should be placed along the long axis of the root to limit the number of blood vessels that may be severed. Furthermore, gentle and atraumatic elevation of the full-thickness flap prevents perforation and tearing of the periosteum. This measure retains the microvasculature within the body of the flap and thus further reduces the risk of bleeding.

Suctioning: Suctioning controls localized bleeding. Injured vessels will normally constrict at the first stage of the hemostatic cascade, eventually to be blocked by a fibrin clot. Thus, bleeding ceases spontaneously with time.

Obstruction by mechanical means: Slight *hammering* of the bone with a dull object can mechanically obstruct localized hemorrhage from a vessel in the bone. By this measure, the bony space for the vessel is occluded. The procedure is most effective on bleeds from the cortical bone, whereas in loose cancellous bone the effect is less predictable.

Loading the bottom of the bone cavity with a material that mechanically obstructs the openings of the cancellous bone is useful. Two options are available: *bone wax* and *calcium sulfate*. Bone wax has been used for this purpose for many years (50). It has no effect on the clotting and essentially has only a blocking effect. Note that bone wax causes a foreign body reaction if left in the cavity after surgery (25), therefore it has to be curetted out completely. A thick mixture of calcium sulfate in sterile water (45) should be inserted by pressing the material against the cavity walls with a wet cotton pellet. The material sets within minutes. Calcium sulfate is used extensively in general surgery because it is biocompatible (22), resorbs completely and is reported to be osteoinductive (8).

Electrocoagulation: Electrocoagulation for hemorrhage control should use bipolar units. The monopolar units frequently used in dental practice for exposing preparation margins before impression are too traumatic owing to the massive heat these units generate. Bipolar units where the electric current flows only between the two electrodes (usually the branches of the pliers) are much less damaging to the collateral tissues. When monopolar was compared with bipolar electrosurgery, significantly more damage and elevation in lateral tissue temperature was observed (31). For a bipolar coagulation the vessel needs to be grabbed to be effective. Frequently the cut vessels contract and cannot be reached. In such instances, other hemostatic measures should be applied.

Chemicals: Small pieces of gauze fitting the bone cavity and saturated with vasoconstrictive agent, e.g. epinephrine, effectively control hemorrhage. The systemic effects are usually insignificant owing to the immediate vasoconstriction that is promoted (28). However, the amount of epinephrine given in conjunction with the local anesthetic should be assessed and if the maximum dose is reached then other means of hemorrhage control should be used.

Ferric sulfate at a concentration of 20%, also known as Monsel's solution, reacts with blood proteins to form a plug that occludes the capillary orifices. The pH is low and the chemical is clearly toxic, which will therefore severely delay healing and in some cases cause abscess formation if left after surgery (33). The dark stain often formed represents agglutinated blood on the bone surface and has to be curetted thoroughly and removed by saline rinses. The bone surface may be freshened with a round drill to remove any remaining coagulated material. Jeansonne *et al.* (26) reported that healing is normal with

only a mild foreign body reaction provided that the surgical wound is thoroughly cleansed prior to wound closure.

Aluminum chlorite was suggested to be effective in an animal experiment (62) and in clinical use. Although the bleeding control appeared effective, histological analysis demonstrated inflammatory and foreign body reaction after 3 and 12 weeks.

Resorbable agents: Collagen-based hemostatic materials applied directly to the bleeding area under pressure result in hemostasis within a few minutes (15). If left in the osseous defects there is minimal interference with the wound healing process and the foreign body reaction is minimal (9).

Surgicel is a substance for hemorrhage control prepared by the oxidation of oxycellulose. Initially it serves as a barrier and then transforms to a sticky mass that will act as an artificial coagulum. The material should be removed from the surgical site after completion of the operation because it can cause foreign body reaction and impair osseous regeneration (25).

Gelfoam consists of gelatin-based sponges, which promote the disintegration of platelets and cause subsequent release of thromboplastin. This in turn stimulates the formation of thrombin in the sponge spaces (29). If gelfoam is left *in situ*, it will slow down healing initially (2) but after a few months there are no negative effects (44).

Root-end resection

Following completion of the surgical access to the root end area, the tip of the root(s) normally has to be cut off at around 2–3 mm (14). This procedure is known under different terms, of which apicectomy or apicoectomy are the most common. The rationales for this measure are:

- To provide convenient access to the root canal(s) for the apical instrumentation (see below).
- To remove any bacterial organisms lodged in accessory and main canals of an apex delta and/or on the surface of the root tip.

The angle of the cut surface should be as square as possible to the long axis of the root to reduce the number of exposed dentinal tubules (Fig. 20.15), as dentinal tubules may serve as pathways for bacterial elements released from the infected root canal. This is especially important in cases when the root-end filling becomes short (12). Occasionally a slight bevel preparation is needed to allow proper access and visual observation of the resected tip (Advanced concept 21.2). Buccally inclined roots do not need a bevel, whereas roots inclined in the opposite direction and roots under a thick bone plate need beveling. When there is a post in the tooth, the resection

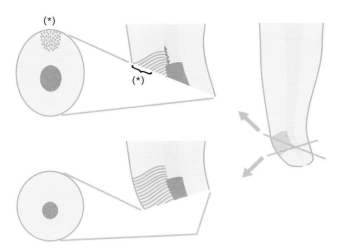

Fig. 21.15 Principle for root-end resection. Excessive bevel allows penetration of bacterial elements through dentinal tubules to the resection surface (*). Ideal angulation is perpendicular to the long axis of the root (bottom).

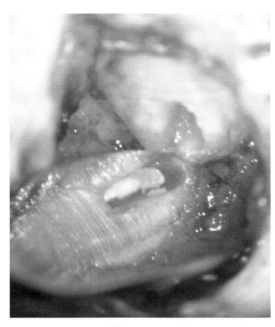

Fig. 21.16 Micro-mirror view following root-end resection and preparation.

should not be performed to the base of it, because of the risk of breaking the seal of the luting cement.

Following resection, the cut surface should be inspected for the presence of apical ramifications, isthmus formation and possible fracture lines. The inspection needs to be carried out with the use of magnification and if necessary with micro-mirrors (Fig. 21.16).

Root-end preparation

The root canal of the resected root tip needs to be cleaned and shaped to accommodate a retrograde root filling according to the same rationales as for conventional root canal therapy (Clinical procedure 21.1). Thus, the primary objective of this measure is to exclude the root canal as a source of microorganisms. The cleaning procedure can

be carried out with properly angled ultrasonic root-end tips (Fig. 21.17) and with hand-held root canal files or both. Preparation with a small round bur in a micro-handpiece was used for years. Often cavities that are too large and root canals that are insufficiently cleaned resulted from this technique. Also, the cavity frequently became extended to the palatal side of the root and in certain cases even perforations occurred. In small and fine roots, and frequently in fused roots where an isthmus has formed between them (Fig. 21.18), this technique is quite unsuitable because the diameter of the smallest bur size may exceed the width of the root (Advanced concept 21.3).

In recent years the use of ultrasonic devices has led to a significant improvement in apical instrumentation in endodontic surgery. Indeed retro-tips used with the surgical microscope have offset many of the drawbacks from the preparation with rotary instruments and made it possible to perform surgical treatment of virtually any tooth.

Advanced concept 21.2   Beveling of the root end

Gilheany *et al.* (12) demonstrated that there is no other basis for beveling the root end in endodontic surgery than to achieve convenient access to the root canal system. In fact, an acute bevel in combination with an inadequate root-end preparation and filling carries the risk for penetration of bacterial elements along the dentinal tubules or the root-end filling, or both, to the resected root surface. Using the hydraulic conductance method *in vitro*, these investigators evaluated the degree of apical leakage as a function of various depths of retrograde fillings and different cutting angles (0°, 30° and 45° to the long axis of the root). Findings were a significant increase of leakage with increased angulation and significantly decreased leakage with increasing depth of the retrograde filling, suggesting that both the permeability of the resected apical dentin and the length of the retrograde filling are significant factors in whether or not the procedure will succeed.

Clinical procedure 21.1   Retrograde hand file preparation

A procedure where the complete root canal is debrided, shaped and filled from the apical end was originally proposed by Nygaard-Östby (43) and later clinically tried and evaluated by Reit and Hirsch (47). Following a small resection of the root tip, the canal is cleaned and enlarged with Hedström files held in a hemostat. The canal is irrigated with 0.5% sodium hypochlorite and sealed with cold laterally condensed or injectable gutta-percha.

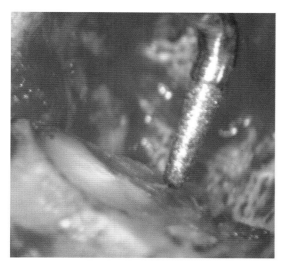

Fig. 21.17   Diamond-coated ultrasonic tip.

Advanced concept 21.3   Isthmuses

The anatomic complexity of the root canal system has been known for years (19), but it was not until recently that the importance of isthmuses in the endodontic surgery of certain teeth was recognized (7). Hsu and Kim (24) studied the resected surfaces of different teeth in the human dentition and observed that, in general, the chance of isthmus formation is higher when more of the root is resected. With the aid of proper magnification, anatomical structures, isthmuses and ramifications can be detected and effectively treated by the use of ultrasonic instrumentation (see Fig. 21.18).

The ultrasonic energy puts the tip into vibration, which will remove both hard- and soft-tissue elements in the root canal, including root filling material. A light touch has to be applied, because the vibration wave is only effective when the tip is not pressed to the surface during its operation. The methodology offers the following advantages:

- An ultrasonic tip is smaller and more delicate than a round bur in a micro-handpiece.
- About 3–4 mm of vertical space in the root can be instrumented.
- Preparation can be performed at the long axis of the tooth and thus can follow the true path of the root canal and thereby avoid perforation.

Ultrasonic preparation will result in cleaner, more parallel and deeper preparations than those with conventional preparation with a round bur (63). The drawback of ultrasonics is the reported risk of microcracks and fractures (32). The use of ultrasonically energized file tips has reduced the fracture risk. Powering files requires much lower energy than for the stiffer root-end tips. Files furthermore are resilient when tilted during the preparation, which minimizes the wedging forces. An additional advantage of the use of prebent files, commonly used for orthograde instrumentation, is the improved cleaning/shaping and extended preparation further up the canal (58).

Retrofill

The goal of the retrograde filling is to seal the prepared cavity to prevent leakage of tissue fluid to the remainder

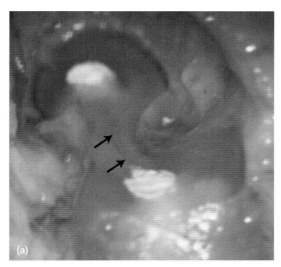
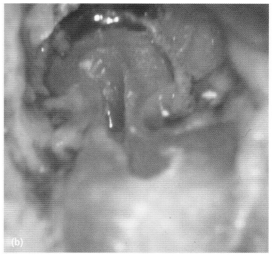

Fig. 21.18   (a) The tip of a resected upper premolar displays gutta-percha in the buccal and palatal canals. The fused roots in the connecting area have a fine line (arrowheads) – an isthmus – barely visible in 25× magnification. Failure to diagnose and treat this anatomical structure led to persistence of symptoms after the first surgical treatment. (b) The cleaned retrograde preparation with the isthmus area to be filled.

of the root canal space and the exchange of bacterial elements that may result from such leakage. The significance of the retrograde root filling for a successful outcome has been demonstrated in numerous clinical follow-up studies (11). Therefore an important feature of a retrograde root filling is to hermetically seal the apical portion of the root canal space. Furthermore, because the surface of the filling can be quite large, e.g. following cleaning of isthmuses, the material should resist disintegration in tissue fluids over time. As with all other root-filling materials important requirements are biological compatibility and that the material interferes minimally with the wound healing process.

Ideally a retrograde root filling should allow new formation of cementum on its surface into which periodontal ligament fibers can insert. Such a tissue response should ensure minimal dissolution of the material over time and thus ensure good long-term prognosis.

Various retrograde filling materials have been employed over the years. Over many years amalgam enjoyed great acceptance (11) but has lost popularity because:

- Sealing ability is questionable (25).
- Handling is difficult during the surgical procedure and amalgam remnants may be left behind in the surgical cavity.
- It corrodes, which, by release of metal ions into the surrounding tissues (39), may lead to discoloration and tattoos of the gingiva or mucosa in visible areas, causing non-esthetic disfigurations.
- It contains mercury, which is why amalgam is banned for clinical use in several countries.

The most salient problem with amalgam as a retrograde filling material is the poor clinical outcome obtained in several clinical follow-up studies with this material (7, 10).

Alternatives to amalgam are glass ionomer cements, resin composites in combination with dentin bonding (5, 48) and mineral trioxide aggregate (MTA) (53). Glass ionomers and composites seal the cavity quite well but are technique and moisture sensitive (46).

Excellent clinical results have been obtained with zinc oxide–eugenol (ZnOE)-based cements (7). The handling of these retrograde filling materials is good but their biological compatibility is questionable. Persistent release of eugenol by hydrolysis maintains toxic reactions and will prevent the development of a biological seal at the root end. The toxicity of eugenol depends on the amount of free eugenol in the cement (17). It can be reduced if the cement is mixed to a very dry consistency, leaving little free eugenol in the mix, which also improves its handling. The ZnOE-based cements set rapidly when exposed to moisture after condensation. The beveled root surface can be polished in a few minutes, and any excess filling material can be removed from the root-end surface.

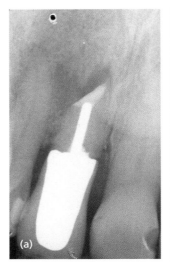 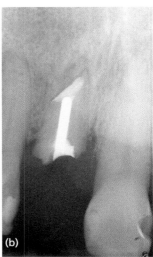

Fig. 21.19 (a) Retrograde filling with resin composite of an upper incisor that had extensive apical root resorption. Healing was uneventful except that the crown later fractured off from the root. (b) Complete bone fill at about 19 months of follow-up. (Courtesy of Dr G. Bergenholtz.)

MTA has gained popularity in recent years as a retrograde filling material (53–56). The hydrophilic powder is mixed with water to a creamy consistency, which sets to a hard mass. It seals well, it is reasonably biocompatible (56) and, owing to its hydrophilic properties, is probably the best material to use when moisture control is precarious (54). Because of its consistency, the material is difficult to handle.

Several authors (12, 51) have pointed out the potential pathway for leakage of bacterial elements at the resected root end along the dentinal tubules. Sealing the entire beveled surface with dentin bonding was therefore proposed and introduced by Rud *et al.* (48). The method includes preparing a slight concavity at the root end and applying a bonding agent, which is followed by the application of a chemically cured composite (Fig. 21.19). If properly managed, the healing potential is reported to be excellent (49).

Flap closure and suturing

Repositioning of the soft tissue to its original position, with the wound edges closely approximated by careful suturing, is normally sufficient for rapid healing. Although various techniques for suturing can be used, in endodontic surgery usually single sutures are applied to hold the flap in place during the initial healing phase. The sutures are placed in each proximal space and at the vertical releasing incisions.

Atraumatic needles should be used. Select sutures in sizes 6/0 and smaller. Although fine, the needle should still be rigid and have a 3/8 circle with sharp pointed triangular cross-section. The needle length can be a problem in papilla closure, because small suture sizes have rather short needles. The needle length for a comfortable interproximal suture should be at least 12 mm.

The suture material should be non-resorbable because the irritation is considerably less than with a resorbable suture material. They should have a smooth coating or be monofilamentous in sizes 7/0 and smaller. If wound healing is uneventful, sutures can usually be removed within 3 days, at which time an epithelial lining has developed (Fig. 21.20).

Various phases in the wound healing process after an endodontic surgical procedure include:

- clotting and inflammation;
- epithelial healing;
- connective tissue healing;
- maturation and remodeling of the soft and hard tissues.

These stages are not distinctly separated from each other. They overlap considerably and take place almost simultaneously. Because the original incision disrupted blood vessels, hemostasis has to take place first. Humoral and cellular mediators released cause clot formation that will connect the wound edges and form a pathway for the migration of inflammatory and repairing cells. If hemostasis is not complete, blood continues to flow into the wound site and a hematoma may develop. This will delay healing considerably and the coagulum must first be resorbed before connective tissue healing can proceed (20). Applying pressure with soft gauze to the flap for about 5 min after repositioning and suturing can reduce

clot and hematoma formation and thereby enhance the healing process.

Under optimal conditions the maturation and remodeling phase of both soft and hard tissue may begin within 5–7 days after surgery. The first step is the formation of an epithelial barrier to protect the underlying connective tissue from irritants of the oral cavity. Sutures can be removed as soon as the epithelial lining has formed, which is usually within 3 days.

Pain control after surgery

The use of an atraumatic operation technique is critical to lessen postsurgical discomfort in terms of pain and swelling. It also enhances the healing process. Additional measures to be taken are:

- Application of a cold compress to the surgical site for ca. 10 min every half hour on the day of surgery to reduce swelling.
- Prescription of an analgesic with swelling-reducing properties with a dose given prior to the cessation of the anesthetic effect.

Different drugs have varying degrees of analgesic and anti-inflammatory potential. Pain perception is elevated in the presence of prostaglandins and an analgesic that slows down the synthesis of prostaglandins will reduce the excitability of the pain receptors to normal levels at the same time as providing pain relief. Inhibition of prostaglandin synthesis will also produce an antiphlogistic effect.

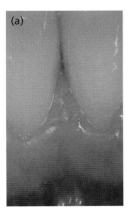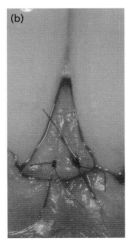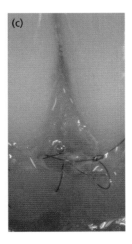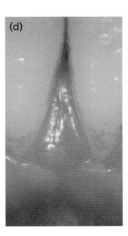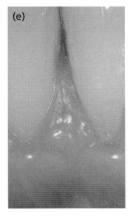

Fig. 21.20 Interproximal space in the lower incisal area treated with a papilla base incision. (a) Preoperative situation. (b) Wound closure using two interrupted sutures (polypropylene 7/0). (c) Healing view prior to suture removal after 3 days. (d) Healing view after 1 month; the incision line is slightly visible. (e) Healing view after 3 months displaying a virtually undetectable incision line. (Reprinted with permission from (62).)

Bone healing

Like orthograde endodontics, surgical endodontics aims to attain healthy periapical conditions. The extent to which the surgical defect becomes filled with bone is therefore an important outcome measure. It should be understood that complete bone healing only takes place if the etiology for the inflammatory lesion that led to the surgical procedure is eliminated, most often a root canal infection. If not, an inflammatory process will persist that may present itself as a persistent radiolucent bone lesion or recurring swelling or fistulous tract, or both. A successful case is characterized by regeneration of the missing structures (bone and cementum) and reorganization of the periodontal ligament at the periapex. Complete fill with bone in the surgical cavity may take 6–12 months to show in conventional radiographs (Fig. 21.21). Postsurgical follow-ups should therefore be scheduled accordingly (Core concept 21.4).

During the healing phase mucogingival connective tissue may enter the surgical cavity and result in incomplete bone healing, a so-called periapical scar (40) (Fig. 21.22). This is especially common in cases where the original lesion defect extended from the buccal to the oral side. Resorbable protective membranes may be placed to prevent this kind of rest defect, which is not to be considered a treatment failure *per se*.

Prognosis

Clinical follow-up studies on the outcome of endodontic surgery are abundant. Reported success rates vary between 30% and 90%. Varying inclusion criteria, length of follow-up periods, criteria for evaluation and observer variation render generalized conclusions difficult. It is to be expected that with the use of the surgical microscope and other modern technological aids, success rates will be at the higher end.

There seems to be no systematic outcome difference between a surgical and a non-surgical approach to

| Core concept 21.4 | Scheduling of postsurgical follow-ups |

- *3–5 days:* to check soft-tissue healing and remove sutures.
- *6 months–1 year:* to check extent of bone fill or clinical signs of persisting infection.

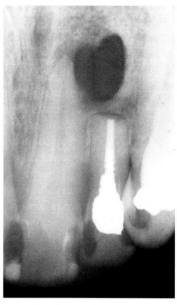

Fig. 21.22 Demonstration of a typical image suggesting scar tissue repair after endodontic surgery. Note the bone fill and periodontal ligament space at the tip of the resected lateral incisor. (Courtesy of Dr Johan Warfvinge.)

retreatment (1, 18, 30, for review see Ref. 6). As a rough guide three cases out of four might be expected to heal, but case selection and operator skill are among the factors that are likely to have a profound impact.

Several authors have emphasized that the presence of an initial good quality root filling is essential (21, 37, 41). Yet, the quality of the retroseal seems to be a most important factor. The choice of root-end filling material

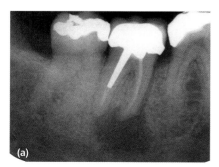 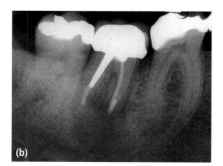 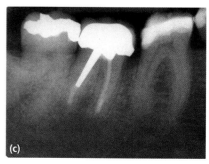

(a) (b) (c)

Fig. 21.21 Successful outcome of an endodontic surgery procedure of a lower second molar: (a) preoperative radiograph; (b) radiograph immediately postoperatively; (c) 1-year follow-up radiograph with complete bone fill in the previous surgical defect.

is nevertheless subject to debate and scientific investigations have not singled out one specific material as being superior.

The outcome of endodontic surgery is time dependent. Not only does it take time for bone to completely fill the surgical cavity but lesions may recur after some time: a so-called "late failure". Frank *et al.* (10) found that among 104 investigated healed cases 44 were classified 10 years later as failures. Similar relapses of periapical inflammatory lesions have been reported by others (e.g. Ref. 30). These findings indicate that cases treated by endodontic surgery should be subject to a long-term recall program.

Case study

Surgery as a primary choice of endodontic treatment

Often endodontic treatment has to be conducted through crowns. When canals are hard to find, substantial amounts of gold and dentin will have to be removed, jeopardizing the retention of the prosthodontic construction. In some situations the risks for such complications may be judged to be too high and a primary surgical approach to endodontic treatment may therefore be carried out.

In this case an acute apical periodontitis was diagnosed in the right upper canine. The patient had received a full mouth bridge, fixed on four abutments in the upper jaw several years ago. Before the bridge was placed, the canine pulp vitality was confirmed. Subsequent to the prosthetic treatment the pulp became necrotic and apical periodontitis developed (a). If a conventional endodontic treatment had been attempted, there would have been a high risk for the crown to lose its retention, upon or after accessing the pulp space for endodontic treatment. Instead, a flap was raised and the root canal cleaned with ultrasonically energized files in a retrograde direction. The canal was sealed with gutta-percha and an apical MTA plug (b). One-year follow-up showed complete apical bone healing (c).

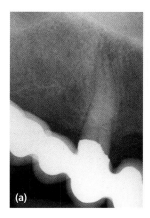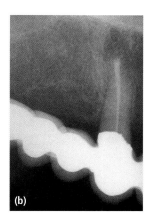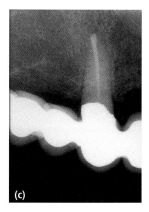

References

1. Allen RK, Newton CW, Brown CE. A statistical analysis of surgical and nonsurgical retreatment cases. *J. Endod.* 1989; 15: 261–6.

2. Boyes-Varley JG, Cleaton-Jones PE, Lownie JF. Effect of a topical drug combination on the early healing of extraction sockets in the vervet monkey. *Int. J. Oral Maxillofac. Surg.* 1988; 17: 138–41.

3. Buckley JA, Ciancio SG, McMullen JA. Efficacy of epineph-rine concentration in local anesthesia during periodontal surgery. *J. Periodontol.* 1984; 55: 653–7.

4. Cambruzzi JV, Marshall FJ. Molar endodontic surgery. *J. Can. Dent. Assoc.* 1983; 49: 61–5.

5. Chong BS, Pitt Ford TR, Watson TF, Wilson RF. Sealing abil-ity of potential retrograde root filling materials. *Endod. Dent. Traumatol.* 1995; 11: 264–9.

   The sealing ability of two potential retrograde root filling materials in extracted teeth – a light-cured glass ionomer cement (Vitrebond) and a reinforced zinc oxide–eugenol cement (Kalzinol) – was compared with that of amalgam. Bacterial leakage occurred in more teeth filled with amalgam compared with both Vitrebond and Kalzinol. Confocal microscopy showed that the size of the marginal gap was the largest with amalgam and smallest with Vitrebond.

6. Del Fabbro M, Taschieri S, Testori T, Francetti L, Weinstein RL. Surgical versus non-surgical endodontic re-treatment for periradicular lesions. *Cochrane Database Syst Rev.* 2007: CD005511.

7. Dorn SO, Gardner AH. Retrograde filling materials: a retro-spective success/failure study of amalgam, EBA and IRM. *J. Endod.* 1990; 16: 391–3.

8. Elkins AD, Jones LP. The effects of plaster of Paris and autogenous cancellous bone on the healing of cortical defects in femurs of dogs. *Vet. Surg.* 1988; 17: 71–6.

   Experimental study in dogs showing no difference in the degree of bone healing between autogenous cancellous bone, plaster of Paris and a mixture of plaster of Paris and autogenous cancel-lous bone. Bone healing was superior to the control with all implants.

9. Finn MD, Schow SR, Schneiderman ED. Osseous regenera-tion in the presence of four common hemostatic agents. *J. Oral Maxillofac. Surg.* 1992; 50: 608–12.

10. Frank AL, Glick DH, Patterson SS, Weine FS. Long term evaluation of surgically placed amalgam fillings. *J. Endod.* 1992; 18: 391–8.

11. Friedman S. Retrograde approaches in endodontic therapy. *Endod. Dent. Traumatol.* 1991; 7: 97–107.

12. Gilheany PA, Figdor D, Tyas M. Apical dentin permeability and microleakage associated with root end resection and retrograde filling. *J. Endod.* 1994; 20: 22–6.

13. Grunder U, Strub JR. Die Problematik der Temperaturerhöhung beim Bearbeiten des Knochens mit rotierenden Instrumenten – eine Literaturübersicht. *Schweiz. Monatsschr. Zahnmed.* 1986; 96: 965–9.

14. Gutmann JL, Harrison JW. *Surgical Endodontics.* Boston: Blackwell Scientific Publications, 1991; 213–14.

15. Haasch GC, Gerstein H, Austin BP. Effect of two hemostatic agents on osseous healing. *J. Endod.* 1989; 15: 310–14.

16. Harrison JW, Juroski KA. Wound healing in the tissues of the periodontium following periradicular surgery. I. The incisional wound. *J. Endod.* 1991; 17: 425–35.

   Little difference was found in the temporal and qualitative heal-ing responses to incisional wounds of two flap designs. The sub-marginal rectangular design showed less predictable results, with a greater intersample variation of wound healing responses in the earlier postsurgical evaluation periods. Vital connective tissue and epithelium, although not visible clinically, remained attached to the root surfaces following reflection of flaps, which included an intrasulcular incision. Preservation of these root-attached tissues seemed to prevent apical epithelial down-growth along the root surfaces and loss of soft-tissue attachment levels. Preventing dehydration preserved the vitality of root-attached tissues.

17. Hashimoto S, Uchiama K, Maeda M, Ishitsuka K, Furumoto K, Nakamura Y. *In vivo* and *in vitro* effects of zinc oxide-eugenol (ZOE) on biosynthesis of cyclo-oxygenase produc-tion in rat dental pulp. *J. Dent. Res.* 1988; 67: 1092–6.

18. Hepworth MJ, Friedman S. Treatment outcome of surgical and non-surgical management of endodontic failures. *J. Can. Dent. Assoc.* 1997; 63: 364–71.

19. Hess W. *Zur Wurzelkanalanatomie der Wurzelkanäle des men-schlichen Gebisses.* Zürich: Berichthaus Zürich, 1917; 38–42.

20. Hiatt WH, Stallard RE, Butler ED, Badget B. Repair follow-ing mucoperiosteal flap surgery with full gingival retention. *J. Periodontol.* 1968; 39: 11–16.

21. Hirsch J, Ahlström U, Henriksson P-Å, Heyden G, Peterson L-E. Periapical surgery. *Int. J. Oral Surg.* 1979; 8: 173–85.

22. Hogset O, Bredberg G. Plaster of Paris: thermal properties and biocompatibility. A study on an alternative implant material for ear surgery. *Acta Otolaryngol.* 1986; 101: 445–52.

23. Holroyd SV, Requa-Clark B. Local anesthetics. In: *Clinical Pharmacology in Dental Practice,* 4th edn (Holroyd SV, Wynn RL, Requa-Clark B, eds). St Louis: Mosby, 1988; 196–215.

24. Hsu YY, Kim S. The resected root surface. The issue of canal isthmuses. *Dent. Clin. North Am.* 1997; 41: 529–40.

25. Ibarrola JL, Bjorgenson JE, Austin BP, Gerstein H. Osseous reaction to three hemostatic agents. *J. Endod.* 1985; 11: 75–83.

26. Jeansonne BG, Steele PJ, Lemon RR. Ferric sulfate hemosta-sis. Effect on osseous wound healing: II. With curettage and irrigation. *J. Endod.* 1993; 19: 174–6.

27. Kim S, Edwall L, Trowbridge H, Chien S. Effects of local anesthetics on pulpal blood flow in dogs. *J. Dent. Res.* 1984; 63: 650–2.

28. Kim S, Rethnam S. Hemostasis in endodontic microsurgery. *Dent. Clin. North Am.* 1997; 41: 499–511.

29. Knöll-Köhler E, Förtsch G. Pulpal anesthesia dependent on epinephrine dose in 2% lidocaine. *Oral Surg. Oral Med. Oral Pathol.* 1992; 73: 537–40.

30. Kvist T, Reit C. Results of endodontic retreatment: a ran-domized clinical study comparing surgical and nonsurgical procedures. *J. Endod.* 1999; 25: 814–17.

31. Lantis JC II, Durville FM, Connolly R, Schwaitzberg SD. Comparison of coagulation modalities in surgery. *Laparoendosc. Surg. Tech. A* 1998; 8: 381–94.

32. Layton CA, Marshall JG, Morgan LA, Baumgartner JC. Evaluation of cracks associated with ultrasonic root-end preparation. *J. Endod.* 1996; 22: 157–60.

33. Lemon RR, Steele PJ, Jeansonne BG. Ferric sulfate hemostasis. Effect on osseous wound healing: I. Left *in situ* for maximum exposure. *J. Endod.* 1993; 19: 170–3.

34. Lin LM, Gängler P, Langeland K. Periradicular curettage. *Int. Endod. J.* 1996; 29: 220–7.

35. Lobene RR, Glickman I. The response of alveolar bone to grinding with rotary diamond stones. *J. Periodontol.* 1963; 34: 105–19.

36. Luebke RG. Surgical endodontics. *Dent. Clin. North Am.* 1974; 18: 379–91.

37. Lustmann J, Friedman S, Sharabany V. Relation of pre- and postoperative factors to prognosis of posterior apical surgery. *J. Endod.* 1991; 17: 239–41.

38. Milam SB, Giovannitti JA. Local anesthetics in dental practice. *Dent. Clin. North Am.* 1984; 28: 493–508.

39. Moberg LE. Electrochemical properties of corroded amalgams. *Scand. J. Dent. Res.* 1987; 95: 441–8.

40. Molven O, Halse A, Grung B. Incomplete healing (scar tissue) after periapical surgery – radiographic findings 8 to 12 years after treatment. *J. Endod.* 1996; 22: 264–8.

41. Molven O, Halse A, Grung B. Surgical management of endodontic failures: indications and treatment results. *Int. Dent. J.* 1991; 41: 33–42.

42. Nair PNR. New perspectives on radicular cysts: do they heal? *Int. Endod. J.* 1998; 31: 155–60.

43. Nygaard-Östby B. *Introduction to Endodontics.* Oslo: Universitetsforlaget, 1971; 74.

44. Olson RAJ, Roberts DL, Osbon DB. A comparative study of polylactic acid, Gelfoam and Surgicel in healing extraction sites. *Oral Surg. Oral Med. Oral Pathol.* 1982; 53: 441–9.

45. Pecora G, Baek SH, Rethnam S, Kim S. Barrier membrane techniques in endodontic microsurgery. *Dent. Clin. North Am.* 1997; 41: 585–602.

46. Powers JM, Finger WJ, Xie J. Bonding of composite resin to contaminated human enamel and dentin. *J. Prosthodont.* 1995; 4: 28–32.

47. Reit C, Hirsch J. Surgical endodontic retreatment. *Int. Endod. J.* 1986; 19: 107–12.

48. Rud J, Munksgaard EC, Andreasen JO, Rud V, Asmussen E. Retrograde root filling with composite and a dentin-bonding agent. *Endod. Dent. Traumatol.* 1991; 7: 118–25.

49. Rud J, Rud V, Munksgaard EC. Effect of root canal contents on healing of teeth with dentine-bonded resin composite retrograde seal. *J. Endod.* 1997; 23: 535–41.

   Presentation of healing results of 551 periapical surgery cases apically sealed with a dentin-bonded resin composite (Gluma-Retroplast). Success rates varied from 81% to 92%, depending on the root filling quality. Cases with no root filling were the least successful.

50. Selden HS. Bone wax as an effective hemostat in periapical surgery. *Oral Surg.* 1970; 29: 262–4.

51. Tidmarsh BG, Arrowsmith MG. Dentinal tubules at the root ends of apicected teeth: a scanning electron microscopic study. *Int. Endod. J.* 1989; 22: 184–9.

52. Torabinejad M. The role of immunological reactions in apical cyst formation and the fat of epithelial cells after root canal therapy: a theory. *Int. J. Oral Surg.* 1983; 12: 14–22.

53. Torabinejad M, Watson TF, Pitt Ford TR. The sealing ability of a mineral trioxide aggregate as a retrograde root filling material. *J. Endod.* 1993; 19: 591–5.

54. Torabinejad M, Higa RK, McKendry DJ, Pitt Ford TR. Effect of blood contamination of dry leakage of root-end filling materials. *J. Endod.* 1994; 20: 159–63.

55. Torabinejad M, Falah Rastegar A, Kettering JD, Pitt Ford TR. Bacterial leakage of mineral trioxide aggregate as a root end filling material. *J. Endod.* 1995; 21: 109–12.

56. Torabinejad M, Hong CU, Pitt Ford TR, Kettering JD. Cytotoxicity of four root end filling materials. *J. Endod.* 1995; 21: 483–92.

57. Velvart P. Das Operationsmikroskop in der Wurzelspitzenresektion. Teil I: Die Resektion. *Schweiz. Monatschr. Zahnmed.* 1997; 107: 507–21.

58. Velvart P. Das Operationsmikroskop in der Wurzelspitzenresektion. Teil II: Die retrograde Versorgung. *Schweiz. Monatschr. Zahnmed.* 1997; 107: 969–78.

59. Velvart P. Papilla base incision: a new approach to recession-free healing of the interdental papilla after endodontic surgery. *Int. Endod. J.* 2002; 35: 453–60.

60. Velvart P, Peters CI, Peters OA. Soft tissue management: flap design, incision, tissue elevation, and tissue retraction. *Endod. Topics* 2005: 11: 78–97.

61. Velvart P, Peters CI, Peters OA. Soft tissue management: suturing and wound healing. *Endod. Topics* 2005: 11: 179–95.

62. Von Arx T, Jensen SS, Hänni S, Schnek RK. Haemostatic agents used in periradicular surgery: an experimental study of efficacy and tissue reactions. *Int. Endod. J.* 39: 2006: 800–8.

63. Wuchenich G, Meadows D, Torabinejad M. A comparison between two root end preparation techniques in human cadavers. *J. Endod.* 1994; 20: 279–82.

   Twenty anterior teeth in human cadavers were instrumented and obturated with gutta-percha and sealer. After raising a full-thickness flap, the apices of the roots were exposed and beveled at a 45° angle. Half of the apical cavities were prepared with an appropriate-sized Carr alloy tip. The other half was prepared with an inverted cone bur in a slow-speed handpiece. The teeth were extracted, sectioned longitudinally and observed in a scanning electron microscope. The ultrasonic cavities produced more parallel walls and deeper depths for retention. In addition, the ultrasonic tips followed the direction of the canals more closely than those prepared by burs.

Failures after surgical endodontics

Thomas von Arx

Healing outcome after apical surgery can normally be determined clinically and radiographically at a recall 1 year after the procedure. A failure is defined when clinical signs (fistula, apicomarginal defect, swelling) or any other symptoms, such as pain, tooth tenderness to palpation and percussion, are present regardless of radiographic evidence of bone healing. Failure is also recognized when follow-up radiographs show no or only a minimal decrease of the former bone defect, or if there is recurrence of periapical lesion.

The likely cause of failure of surgical retreatment is an unsuccessful seal by the root-end filling of any potential pathway of communication between the root canal system and the surrounding tissues. Possible leakage routes for persistent infection include isthmuses, accessory or lateral canals, perforations, dentinal cracks and gap formation between the root canal filling and the canal wall. Other causes of surgical failure are an apicomarginal communication that persisted or developed following apical surgery, and a (micro)crack progressing into a root fracture.

Case study 1

A 43-year-old male patient was referred for apical surgery of the second premolar and the first molar in the left maxilla. The radiograph demonstrated apical lesions associated with the second premolar and the mesiobuccal root of the first molar (Fig. 1a). The patient refused conventional retreatment of both teeth. Following flap elevation, the mesiobuccal root of the first molar was resected because of complete loss of the facial bone wall. Apical surgery was performed on the second premolar with root-end resection about 3 mm from the apex. A rigid endoscope was used for intraoperative diagnostics showing an improperly filled buccal canal, an adequately obturated palatal canal and a curved hair-line isthmus connecting the two canals (Fig. 1b). Root-end cavity preparation was performed with sonic-driven microtips, and the outline of the cavity is depicted in Fig. 1c. Note the isthmus at the bottom of the cavity. For root-end filling, SuperEBA cement was placed, condensed and finished (Fig. 1d). A postoperative radiograph was taken 4 days after the surgery (Fig. 1e). At the 1-year recall, the patient was free of pain. Both teeth felt comfortable and were clinically inconspicuous. However, the radiograph presented with a persistent apical lesion at the second premolar (Fig. 1f). Subsequent re-examinations 2 and

3 years after surgery demonstrated no clinical changes, but the lesion at the second premolar persisted in size and shape.

Five years following surgery, the patient presented with pain located at the second premolar, and the tooth also had increased mobility. Besides the apical lesion, the radiograph showed an enlargement of the periodontal ligament space at both mesial and distal aspects of the root (Fig. 1g). The patient agreed to have the tooth extracted. Staining of the extracted tooth with methylene blue revealed no root fracture. However, the SuperEBA was washed out over the palatal canal (gutta-percha visible) (Fig. 1h). Inspection using the endoscope at 60× magnification showed gap formation between the gutta-percha and the palatal wall of the root canal (Fig. 1i, arrows). A histological section of the root end demonstrated that the root-end filling did not encompass the palatal canal (Fig. 1j). Comparison with Fig. 1c and d confirmed that the root-end cavity preparation was not significantly extended into the palatal canal during the surgical procedure. As a consequence, the root-end filling became too shallow in that area and was subsequently washed out, probably allowing continued leakage of bacterial elements along the palatal wall of the root canal.

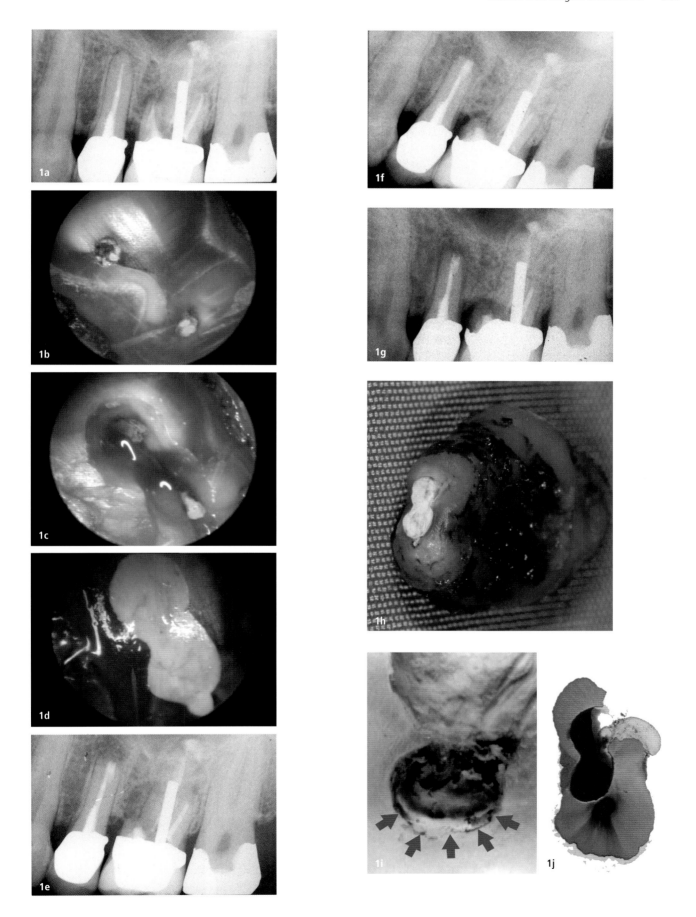

Case study 2

A 48-year-old female patient, presenting with recurrent pain and swelling in the right mandible, reported that apical surgery had been performed of the first molar about 10 years ago. The periapical radiograph of this tooth demonstrated root-end fillings in both roots with a diffuse, apical lesion at the mesial root extending into the interradicular area (Fig. 2a). The patient was offered re-surgery of the mesial root. The mesial root was surgically exposed and resected by 2 mm. Intraoperative inspection showed a buccal and a lingual canal, but no isthmus. Two root-end cavities were prepared in the mesial root using sonic microtips. Root-end filling was accomplished with mineral trioxide aggregate (MTA) (Fig. 2b). A post-operative infection was treated with drainage and antibiotics, and the patient was fully recovered within 10 days. At the 1-year follow-up, the patient had no pain but presented with a sinus tract on the buccal aspect of the right mandibular first molar (Fig. 2c). The 1-year radiograph showed a persistent lesion on the distal aspect of the mesial root, but with bone healing around the mesial aspect of the cut root face (Fig. 2d). The periodontal liga-

ment space on the mesial aspect of the mesial root also appeared slightly enlarged. Treatment options were discussed with the patient including tooth extraction, hemi-section or another attempt at apical surgery (second resurgery). The patient opted for the latter. Again, the mesial root was surgically located, and endoscopic inspection of the root revealed a lateral canal on the distal aspect of the mesial root (Fig. 2e). This lateral canal was subsequently instrumented using sonically driven, diamond-coated microtips, and a preparation was made perpendicular to the long axis of the tooth (Fig. 2f). The postoperative radiograph clearly shows the "new and transverse" root-end filling in the mesial root (Fig. 2g). This time, the initial healing course was uneventful, and the 1-year follow-up revealed healing of the former sinus tract (Fig. 2h) and also complete radiographic bone healing at the mesial root (Fig. 2i).

In summary, the failure of the first two surgeries must be attributed to the missed lateral canal in the mesial root, and only after instrumentation and obturation of this lateral canal was healing attainable after the third surgical procedure (i.e. second resurgery).

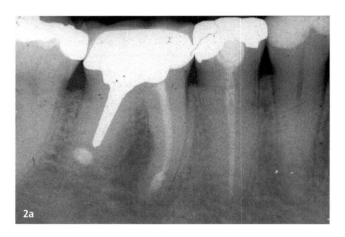

2a

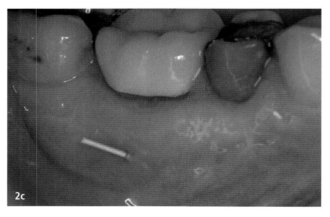

2c

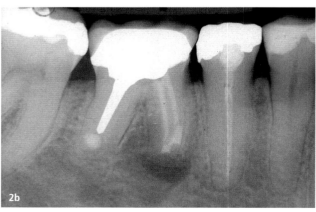

2b

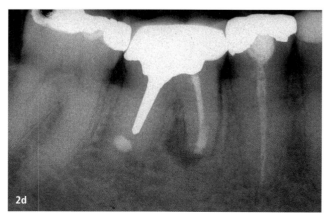

2d

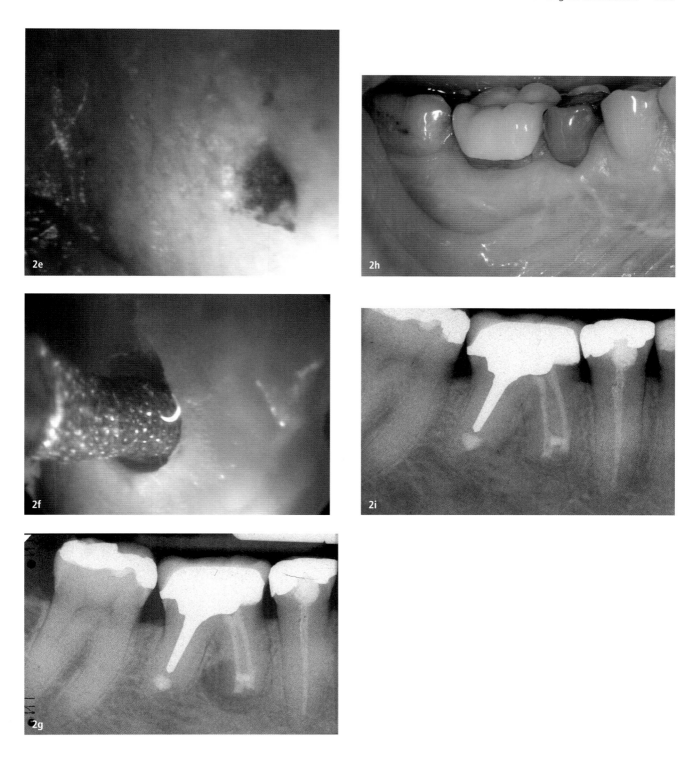

Index

Note: Locators in *italics* denote tables and figures (when outside locator ranges)

access opening, RCT 143, 175–6
access to the apical area, non-surgical retreatment 339–42
access to the root canal, non-surgical retreatment 335–9
acute apical abscess, apical periodontitis 124
acute periapical infections
    as origin of metastatic infections 128–35
    systemic complications 128–35
adverse reaction, local anesthesia 287
affective factors, pain 280
age, success factor, pulp capping/partial pulpotomy 54
AHA recommendations, antibiotic prophylaxis 133–5
allergic potential, root canal filling materials 196
allergic reaction, epoxy resin sealers 206–7
alveolar fractures, management 272–3
anesthesia
    see also local anesthesia
    adverse reaction 287
    pain 287
    pulpectomy 60–1
antibacterial effect, calcium hydroxide 150
antibiotic prophylaxis
    AHA recommendations 133–5
    bacteremia sequelae 133–5
    compromised hosts 134–5
    risk assessments 133
antibiotics
    irrigation 148
    RCT 155
antigen presentation, apical periodontitis 115
antigen-presenting cells (APCs), immune defense 17–18
antimicrobial resistance 103
antimicrobial retreatment strategies, non-surgical
    retreatment 345
antimicrobial treatment, non-surgical retreatment 344–5
APCs *see* antigen-presenting cells
apical abscess
    acute 124
    apical periodontitis 116, 124, 125
    chronic 125
apical configuration, root canal system anatomy 173–4
apical cyst, apical periodontitis 116–18
apical granuloma, apical periodontitis 114–16
apical obstructions, non-surgical retreatment 342–3
apical periodontitis 113–27
    acute apical abscess 124
    antigen presentation 115
    apical abscess 116, 124, 125
    apical cyst 116–18
    apical granuloma 114–16
    asymptomatic 114, 123–4, 248

bacterial elimination 118–19
bacterial front line 119–20
bone resorption 113–14, 120–1
cellulitis 126
chronic apical abscess 125
clinical manifestations 123–6
complement functions 119
condensing osteitis 126
dendritic cell function 115
diagnostic terminology 123–6
endodontic flare-up 122–3
equilibrium, bacteria/host 121–2
immunoglobulins 123
micro-organisms interaction 118–23
micro-organisms role 95–6
nature of 113–18
normal periapical conditions 123
sinus recess simulating apical periodontitis 249
sites, potential 113
symptomatic 124, 248
T-cells 120
apical radiolucencies in teeth with vital pulps 248
    case study 247
arrest of dental development, trauma 266–7
aseptic technique, pulpectomy 61–2
assessment
    antibiotic prophylaxis, risk assessments 133
    preoperative condition, vital pulp conditions 51–2
    RCT pre-assessment 174
    root filling quality, root filling techniques 229–30
asymptomatic apical periodontitis 114, 123–4, 248
avascular necrosis, luxation 259
avulsion, trauma 271–2

baceriological sampling, RCT 152
bacteremia 129–35
    see also micro-organisms; systemic complications
    antibiotic prevention of sequelae 133–5
    and endodontic treatment 129–30
    frequency 129
    infective endocarditis 130–3
    types of micro-organism 129–30
bacterial leakage
    dentin–pulp complex 28–9
    pulpal response 29
'balanced force motion', root canal instrumentation
    184
biofilms, root canals, micro-organisms 97–102
bleeding management, surgical endodontics 356–7
blockage, root canal instrumentation 188

blood flow
    see also vascular supply
    dentin–pulp complex 18–19, 22
    local control 18–19
    remote control 19
    vascular reactions 19
blood samples
    micro-organisms 129–31
    systemic complications 129–31
    testing 131
bone healing, surgical endodontics 362
bone removal, surgical endodontics 355–6
bone resorption
    apical periodontitis 113–14, 120–1
    regulation 121
bridge removal, non-surgical retreatment 336–7
bridges, clinical outcome 329
broken instrument removal, non-surgical retreatment
    340–2

calcium hydroxide
    antibacterial effect 150
    direct pulp capping 56–8
    pulpotomy 82
    RCT 150
    wound dressings 75–7
calcium hydroxide sealers 207–9
    anti-microbial properties 208–9
    biological properties 208–9
    composition 207–8
    handling properties 209
    leakage 208
    root-end closure 209
    technical properties 208
canals, missed, non-surgical retreatment 344
cardiac conditions, infective endocarditis 131–3
caries
    deep 25–8
    dentin–pulp complex 23–8
    neurovascular events 26–7
    nitric oxide 25
    periapical tissue 27
    primary dentin 23–5, 27
    pulp polyp 27–8
    responses to 23–8
    tissue changes in pulp 27
case–control studies, clinical epidemiology 291
case-related factors, decision making 310
case series studies, clinical epidemiology 291
case study
    condensing osteitis/sclerosing apical periodontitis 252
    discoloration, tooth 244
    formocresol (FC) 88
    granuloma/radicular cyst 251
    internal root resorption 244
    malignant tumor 253
    pain 286
    periapical healing with scar tissue 250
    primary teeth 87, 88
    prosthodontic reconstruction 331

pulp vitality 240
pulpitis 69
pulpotomy 88
radicular cyst/granuloma 251
radiolucencies in teeth with vital pulps 247
root filled tooth 331
sclerosing apical periodontitis/condensing osteitis 252
sinus recess simulating apical periodontitis 249
stepwise excavation 87
surgical endodontics 363, 366–9
systemic complications 137
tooth-related pain/swelling 241, 245–6
toxic medicaments 68
tumor, malignant 253
vital pulp conditions 68–9
CE sign, root canal filling materials 195
cellulitis, apical periodontitis 126
cement removal, non-surgical retreatment 340
central nervous system mechanisms
    dentin hypersensitivity 43
    pain 43
chemical disinfection, RCT 147–8
chlorhexidine, irrigation 148
chloroform-resin technique, root filling techniques 229
chronic apical abscess, apical periodontitis 125
chronic dental infections, systemic effects 135–8
chronic periapical infections, as origin of metastatic
    infections 135–8
clinical epidemiology 290–300
    case–control studies 291
    case scenario 290
    case series studies 291
    cause 292–3
    cohort studies 291
    concepts 291
    cross-sectional studies 291
    definitions 291
    diagnosis 292
    epidemiological methods 290–2
    frequency 293–5
    incidence 293–5
    longevity of root filled teeth 297–8
    longitudinal studies 291
    prevalence 293–5
    prognosis 296–7
    pulp necrosis 292–3
    RCTs 291–2
    risk 295–6
    treatment 296
clinical evaluation, periapical tissues, diagnosis 246
clinical examination, trauma 267
clinical manifestations
    apical periodontitis 123–6
    inflammation 238, *239*
clinical problems/solutions, endodontology 3–5
clinically healthy pulp, terms/expressions 247–8
cognitive factors, pain 280–2
cognitive impairment, pain 284–5
cohort studies, clinical epidemiology 291
complications, infection *see* systemic complications

condensing osteitis, apical periodontitis 126
condensing osteitis/sclerosing apical periodontitis, case
    study 252
continuous reaming motion, nickel–titanium rotary
    systems 185–6
contraindications, pulp treatment, primary teeth 85
core build-ups
    prosthodontic reconstruction 322–5, 330
    root filled tooth 322–5, 330
core carrier technique, root filling techniques 228
core removal, non-surgical retreatment 338–9
coronal restoration, root filling techniques 230
corticosteroids, wound dressings 78
cracked tooth, pain 242
cross-sectional studies, clinical epidemiology 291
'crown-down sequence', nickel–titanium rotary systems
    184–5
crown removal, non-surgical retreatment 336–7
crowns, clinical outcome 329
cultivation, micro-organisms 104–5
curettage, soft-tissue lesion, surgical endodontics 356–7
cyst, apical *see* apical cyst

DCs *see* dendritic cells
debris information, nickel–titanium rotary systems 185
decision making 301–13
    case-related factors 310
    descriptive projects 305–6
    EUT 306
    factors influencing treatment outcome 302–4
    failures prevalence 304
    normative approach 306–11
    operative factors 302–3
    outcome of treatment 301–2
    postoperative factors 303–4
    praxis concept 305–6
    preoperative factors 302
    standard gamble 308–9
    surgical vs non-surgical retreatment procedures 310
    variation, treatment management 304–5
deep carious lesions 80
dendritic cells (DCs)
    apical periodontitis 115
    immune defense 17–18
dental trauma *see* trauma
dental treatment procedures
    dentin–pulp complex 28–30
    endocarditis prophylaxis 131–3
    infective endocarditis 131–3
dentinal fluid, protective roles 20–1
dentinal pain 33–46
dentinal repair 13–14
dentinal tubules 11–12
dentin 11–12
dentin-adhesive materials, root filling techniques 223–4
dentin brittleness 319
dentin formation, odontoblasts 12–13
dentin hypersensitivity
    central nervous system mechanisms 43
    pain 42–4

dentin–pulp complex 11–32
    bacterial leakage 28–9
    basal maintenance 18–19
    blood flow 18–19, 22
    caries 23–8
    constituents 11–18
    dental treatment procedures 28–30
    destructive stimuli effects 23–30
    functions 11–18
    immune defense 17–18
    inflammatory cells migration 22–3
    lymphatics 16
    nerves 14–15
    neurovascular responses 22
    preparation trauma 28
    responses to external threats 19–23
    responses to non-destructive stimuli 19
    restorative materials effects 29
    restorative procedures 20–1, 29
    trauma 29–30
    vascular supply 15–16
dentin sensitivity
    dentin hypersensitivity 42–4
    hydrodynamic mechanism in pulpal A-fiber activation
        37–9
dentinogenesis 12, 13
    terms/expressions 13
descriptive projects, decision making 305–6
destructive stimuli effects, dentin–pulp complex 23–30
diagnosis 235–54
    accuracy 235–6
    classification 247–53
    clinical evaluation, periapical tissues 246
    collecting diagnostic information 238–47
    discoloration, tooth 243–5
    evaluation of diagnostic information 235–7
    granuloma/radicular cyst 251
    interpretation, periapical radiographs 245
    observer variation 235–6
    pain 241–3
    periapical disease 235–54
    pulp inflammation 73–4
    pulp vitality 239–41
    pulpal diagnosis and pain symptoms 43–4
    pulpal disease 235–54
    radicular cyst/granuloma 251
    radiographs interpretation 245
    strategy 237–8
    symptomless periapical inflammation 244–5
    terms/expressions 247–8
    variation 235–6
diagnostic dilemma, endodontology 5–6
diagnostic methodology, pain 241–3
diagnostic quandries
    pulpectomy 273–4
    trauma 273–4
diagnostic terminology, apical periodontitis 123–6
differential diagnosis
    granuloma/radicular cyst 251
    radicular cyst/granuloma 251

direct pulp capping 50, 52–9
  calcium hydroxide 56–8
  clinical procedure 54–5
  follow-up 59
  healing patterns 56–8
  historical perspectives 52–4
  materials 56–8
  postoperative recall 58–9
  primary teeth 81
  success factors 54–6
discoloration, tooth
  case study 244
  diagnosis 243–5
dressings, wound *see* wound dressings
drying canal, root filling techniques 229

ecological determinants, microbial growth in root canals
    98–103
EDTA *see* ethylenediaminetetraacetic acid
electrical test, pulp vitality 240–1
electronic apex locators, working length 179, *180*
electrophysiological methods, recording pulp nerve
    activity 36
emergency treatment
  pulpectomy 65–9
  pulpitis 66–7, 69
  pulpotomy 66–7
  RCT 153–5
  vital pulp conditions 65–9
endocarditis prophylaxis, dental treatment procedures
    131–3
endodontic flare-up
  apical periodontitis 122–3
  RCT 155–6
endodontic infections, systemic complications *see* systemic
    complications
endodontology
  clinical problems/solutions 3–5
  diagnostic dilemma 5–6
  episteme 1
  extraction/dental implant 6
  modern 2–3
  objective of endodontic treatment 3
  phronesis 2
  techne 1
  tools of treatment 6
environmental factors, pain 282
epidemiology, clinical *see* clinical epidemiology
episteme, endodontology 1
epoxy resin sealers 205–7
  allergic reaction 206–7
  biological properties 206–7
  composition 205–6
  handling properties 207
  leakage 206
  technical properties 206
ethylenediaminetetraacetic acid (EDTA), irrigation 147–8
EUT *see* expected utility theory
expected utility theory (EUT), decision making 306
extraction, primary teeth 82

extraction/dental implant, endodontology 6

factors influencing treatment outcome
    operative factors 302–3
    postoperative factors 303–4
    preoperative factors 302
failure, treatment *see* treatment failure
failures, surgical endodontics 366–9
failures prevalence, decision making 304
FC *see* formocresol (FC)
ferric sulfate (FS)
  pulpotomy 82
  wound dressings 78–9
ferrule design
  prosthodontic reconstruction 328–9
  root filled tooth 328–9
file manipulation, root canal instrumentation 183–4
flap closure/suturing, surgical endodontics 360–1
flap designs, surgical endodontics 351–2
flap raising, surgical endodontics 351–5
follow-up
  direct pulp capping 59
  primary teeth 83
  RCT 151–2
  surgical endodontics 362–3
formocresol (FC)
  case study 88
  concerns 80
  pulpotomy 82–3, 88
  wound dressings 77–8, 80
fracture, instrument, root canal instrumentation 187–8,
    190
fractures 255–8
  see also trauma
  alveolar fractures 272–3
  classification 256, 258
  clinical features 256, 258
  complications risk 256, 258
  consequences 259
  dentin brittleness 319
  factors influencing 319–20
  management 268–70
  prosthodontic reconstruction 319–21
  root filled tooth 319–21
frequency, clinical epidemiology 293–5
FS *see* ferric sulfate
future directions
  operative treatment procedures 85–6
  primary teeth 85–6
  pulp inflammation 85–6

GA *see* glutaraldehyde
gender, pain 282–4
genetics, pain 279
glutaraldehyde (GA)
  pulpotomy 83
  wound dressings 78
granuloma/radicular cyst
  case study 251
  differential diagnosis 251

gutta-percha
    root filling techniques 221–9
    sealers 222–9
    softened gutta-percha techniques 225–9
gutta-percha cones
    anti-microbial properties 201
    biological properties 200–1
    composition 198–9
    handling properties 201–2
    leakage 199–200
    root canal filling materials 198–202
    root filling techniques 221–9
    technical properties 199–200
gutta-percha removal, non-surgical retreatment 339–40

hydrodynamic mechanism in pulpal A-fiber activation,
        dentin sensitivity 37–9
hypnosis, pain 286

identification methods, micro-organisms 105–6
immune defense
    APCs 17–18
    DCs 17–18
    dentin–pulp complex 17–18
    odontoblasts 13
    pulpal immunity 13
immune responses, nerves 15
immunoglobulins
    apical periodontitis 123
    micro-organisms 123
    root canal bacteria, specificity 123
incidence, clinical epidemiology 293–5
indications
    non-surgical retreatment 335
    pulp treatment, primary teeth 85
    surgical endodontics 348–9
indirect pulp capping
    primary teeth 79–81
    stepwise excavation 79–81
    without further excavation 81
infection complications see systemic complications
infective endocarditis 130–3
    bacteremia 130–3
    cardiac conditions 131–3
    dental treatment procedures 131–3
    risk factors 131–3
inflammation
    see also pain
    clinical manifestations 238, 239
    mediators 40–1
    mediators of pulpal inflammation 23
    morphological versus functional changes of pulpal
        nerves 41–2
    nerves 39–42
    neurogenic vasodilation and inflammation 40
    pulp inflammation, primary teeth 73–5
    responses of intradental nerves to tissue injury and
        inflammation 39–42
    symptomless periapical inflammation 244–5
inflammatory cell migration, dentin–pulp complex 22–3

initial root canal preparation (coronal preflaring), RCT
        176–8
injection technique
    local anesthesia 351
    root filling techniques 227–8
instrumentation, root canal see root canal
        instrumentation
instruments, broken, removal 340–2
integrity of permanent restoration, success factor, pulp
        capping/partial pulpotomy 55–6
internal root resorption 83–4
    case study 244
interpretation, test results, pulp vitality 241
interradicular periodontitis 84
intracanal dressing, RCT 148–50
intracanal microbiota effects, RCT 153
irrigation
    antibiotics 148
    chlorhexidine 148
    complications 148
    EDTA 147–8
    photodynamic therapy 148
    RCT 147–8
    sodium hypochlorite 147

lateral compaction, root filling techniques 224–5
leakage
    gutta-percha cones 199–200
    leakage tests 226
leakage/sealing, root canal filling materials 197–8
ledges, non-surgical retreatment 343–4
ledging, root canal instrumentation 188–9
local anesthesia
    see also anesthesia
    adverse reaction 287
    choice of anesthetic agent 349–50
    injection technique 351
    pain 287
    surgical endodontics 349–51
    vasoconstrictors 351
longevity of root filled teeth, clinical epidemiology
        297–8
longitudinal studies, clinical epidemiology 291
luxation 255–60
    avascular necrosis 259
    classification 257
    clinical features 257
    complications risk 257
    consequences 259–60
    management 270–1
lymphatics, dentin–pulp complex 16

malignant tumor, case study 253
mandibular nerve injuries, root canal filling materials
        215–16
materials
    direct pulp capping 56–8
    root canal filling see root canal filling materials
mechanical tests, pulp vitality 240
medicaments, sealers 224

metastatic infections
    acute periapical infections as origin of 128–35
    chronic periapical infections as origin of 135–8
methacrylate-based sealers 209–12
    biological properties 211–12
    composition 210
    handling properties 212
    leakage 210–11
    technical properties 210–11
micro-organisms
    see also bacteremia; systemic complications
    antimicrobial resistance 103
    apical periodontitis interaction 118–23
    apical periodontitis role 95–6
    bacteremia 129–35
    bacterial elimination, apical periodontitis 118–19
    bacterial front line, apical periodontitis 119–20
    biofilms, root canals 97–102
    blood samples 129–31
    composition, endodontic microflora 106–9
    cultivation 104–5
    ecological determinants, microbial growth in root
        canals 98–103
    equilibrium, bacteria/host 121–2
    extra-oral micro-organisms in necrotic pulp 107–8
    extraradicular colonization 98
    identification methods 105–6
    immunoglobulins 123
    interactions, biofilms 102
    methods of study, root canal microflora 103–6
    microscopy 105
    modes of colonization 97–8
    nutrition 100–2
    oral micro-organisms in necrotic pulp 106–7
    pathways 95–7
    persisting after root canal treatment 105–8
    polymicrobial opportunistic infection 108–9
    RCT effects 153
    redox potential 102
    role, apical periodontitis 95–6
    routes of entry, pulpal space 96–7
    sampling 103–4
    signs/symptoms, specific bacteria 109–10
    spread 129–33
    virulence factors 108–9
microbiology, necrotic pulp 95–112
microbiota of the root filled tooth, non-surgical
    retreatment 344–5
microscopy
    see also surgical microscope
    micro-organisms 105
mineral trioxide aggregate (MTA) 212–13
    biological properties 212–13
    composition 212
    handling properties 213
    leakage 212
    replantation 214–15
    retrograde fillings 214–15
    root-end fillings 214–15
    technical properties 212

wound dressings 79
missed canals, non-surgical retreatment 344
modern endodontology 2–3
modified double flared approach, RCT 176–8, 183
morphology, intradental sensory innervation 33–6
MTA *see* mineral trioxide aggregate

necrotic pulp 4–5
    see also root canal therapy (RCT)
    biofilms, root canals 97–102
    composition, endodontic microflora 106–9
    extra-oral micro-organisms in necrotic pulp 107–8
    microbiology 95–112
    oral micro-organisms in necrotic pulp 106–7
    RCT 4–5, 140–59
    terms/expressions 248
    treatment 4–5, 140–59
nerve fibers classification, pain 33
nerves
    see also pain
    dentin–pulp complex 14–15
    dentin sensitivity 37–9
    electrophysiological methods, recording pulp nerve
        activity 36
    hydrodynamic mechanism in pulpal A-fiber activation
        37–9
    immune responses 15
    inflammation 39–42
    intradental sensory innervation, function 36–7
    intradental sensory innervation, morphology 33–6
    morphological versus functional changes of pulpal
        nerves in inflammation 41–2
    recording pulp nerve activity 36
    responses of intradental nerves to tissue injury and
        inflammation 39–42
neurobiological factors, pain 278–80, 283, 285
neurogenic vasodilation and inflammation 40
neuromatrix theory, pain 277
neuropathic pain 279
neurovascular events, caries 26–7
neurovascular responses, dentin–pulp complex 22
nickel–titanium rotary systems
    continuous reaming motion 185–6
    'crown-down sequence' 184–5
    cutting efficiency 183
    debris information 185
    'greater taper' 182–3
    root canal instrumentation 180, 181–3, 184–6
    vs stainless steel hand files 186–7
    treatment sequence 185
    variable tip variable taper sequence 185
nitric oxide, caries 25
non-surgical retreatment 335–47
    access to the apical area 339–42
    access to the root canal 335–9
    antimicrobial retreatment strategies 345
    antimicrobial treatment 344–5
    apical obstructions 342–3
    bridge removal 336–7
    broken instrument removal 340–2

canals, missed 344
cement removal 340
core removal 338–9
crown removal 336–7
gutta-percha removal 339–40
indications 335
instrumentation of the root canal 342–4
ledges 343–4
microbiota of the root filled tooth 344–5
missed canals 344
paste removal 340
perforation repair 344
post removal 338–9
preventive retreatment 346
prognosis 346
root canal reshaping 342
sealer removal 340
silver cone removal 340, *341*
steps 335
Thermafil plastic carrier removal 340
normal periapical tissue, terms/expressions 248
normative approach
    decision making 306–11
    EUT 306
nutrition, micro-organisms 100–2

objectives
    endodontic treatment 3
    pulp treatment 79
    pulpectomy 59–60
    root filling techniques 219
odontoblasts 11–14
    dentinal repair 13–14
    dentin formation 12–13
    multifunctional cell 12
    pulpal immunity 13
    as receptor cells 39
one-appointment endodontics, RCT 149
operative factors, influencing treatment outcome 302–3
operative treatment procedures
    future directions 85–6
    primary teeth 79–85
origin of metastatic infections
    acute periapical infections as 128–35
    chronic periapical infections as 135–8
overextension of the apical foramen, RCT 146

pain 33–46
    see also anesthesia; inflammation; local anesthesia;
        nerves
    acute vs chronic 277–8
    affective factors 280
    beliefs 281
    case study 241, 286
    categories 278
    central nervous system mechanisms 43
    chronic vs acute 277–8
    cognitive factors 280–2
    cognitive impairment 284–5
    control 146–7, 155–6, 281, 361

cracked tooth 242
cultural/social factors 282
defining 277
dentinal pain 33–46
dentin hypersensitivity 42–4
dentin sensitivity 37–9
diagnosis 241–3
diagnostic methodology 241–3
differential diagnosis 243
distraction 280–1
endodontic flare-up 122–3, 155–6
environmental factors 282
expectations 281
gender 282–4
genetics 279
hydrodynamic mechanism in pulpal A-fiber activation
    37–9
hypnosis 286
intradental sensory innervation, function 36–7
intradental sensory innervation, morphology 33–6
learning 282
management 285–7
mechanisms 278–9
memory 282
mood impact 280
multi-dimensional nature 277–89
nerve fibers classification 33
neurobiological factors 278–80, 283, 285
neuromatrix theory 277
neuropathic 279
pain symptoms and pulpal diagnosis 43–4
peripheral neural changes 39–40
postoperative 155–6
prediction 282
provocation/inhibition 243
psychiatric illness 284–5
psycho-social perspective 283–4
psychological factors 280–2, 285–6
pulpal inflammatory lesion symptoms 48
pulpal nociceptor activation 42
pulpal pain 33–46, 48
recording pulp nerve activity 36
responses of intradental nerves to tissue injury and
    inflammation 39–42
sensitivity, dentine 37–9
sex-related differences 282–4
social/cultural factors 282
symptoms, pulpal inflammatory lesion 48
tooth-related pain 241
treatment 285–7
pain control 281
    RCT 146–7, 155–6
    surgical endodontics 361
painful cases prior to RCT 153–5
paper point evaluation, working length 179–80
partial pulpotomy 52–9
    primary teeth 81, 82
    procedures 82
paste removal, non-surgical retreatment 340
pathways, micro-organisms 95–7

patient information/advice, RCT 156
perforation
    root canal instrumentation 189–90
    root filled tooth 321–2
perforation repair, non-surgical retreatment 344
periapical abscess, systemic complications 128–9
periapical disease, diagnosis 235–54
periapical healing with scar tissue, case study 250
periapical periodontitis 84
periapical radiography
    observer variation 235–6
    radiographic evaluation 293
    ROC analysis 236–7
periapical tissue, caries 27
periodontitis, apical *see* apical periodontitis
permanent molars, cf primary molars 74
photodynamic therapy, irrigation 148
phronesis, endodontology 2
polymicrobial opportunistic infection 108–9
post preparation, root filled tooth 325–7
post removal, non-surgical retreatment 338–9
postoperative factors, influencing treatment outcome
        303–4
postoperative pain, RCT 155–6
postoperative recall, direct pulp capping 58–9
praxis concept, decision making 305–6
premature exfoliation 85
preoperative factors, influencing treatment outcome 302
preparation trauma, dentin–pulp complex 28
prevalence
    clinical epidemiology 293–5
    failures 304
preventive retreatment, non-surgical retreatment 346
primary dentine, caries 23–5, 27
primary molars, cf permanent molars 74
primary teeth 73–91
    case study 87, 88
    contraindications, pulp treatment 85
    direct pulp capping 81
    endodontics 73–91
    extraction 82
    follow-up 83
    future directions 85–6
    indications, pulp treatment 85
    indirect pulp capping 79–81
    normal pulp 73
    objectives of pulp treatment 79
    operative treatment procedures 79–85
    partial pulpotomy 81, 82
    pulp inflammation 73–5
    pulpectomy 82
    pulpotomy 81–3
    root canal treatment 82
    stepwise excavation 79–81, 82, 87
    treatment failure 83–5
    wound dressings 75–9, 80
prognosis
    clinical epidemiology 296–7
    non-surgical retreatment 346
    surgical endodontics 362–3

prophylaxis
    antibiotic 133–5
    endocarditis, dental treatment procedures 131–3
prostheses, clinical outcome 329
prosthodontic reconstruction 317–34
    see also root filled tooth
    case study 331
    clinical techniques 325–7
    core build-ups 322–5, 330
    ferrule design 328–9
    fractures 319–21
    posts, preparation 325–7
    problems, abutment teeth 317–22
    single tooth 327–9
protective roles, dentinal fluid 20–1
psychiatric illness, pain 284–5
psycho-social perspective, pain 283–4
psychological factors, pain 280–2, 285–6
pulp, diagnostic quandries 273–4
pulp capping, direct *see* direct pulp capping
pulp chamber filling, root filling techniques 230
pulp inflammation
    see also pulpitis
    diagnosis 73–4
    future directions 85–6
    healing 75
    primary teeth 73–5
pulp necrosis
    cause 292–3
    clinical epidemiology 292–3
    RCT 155
pulp obliteration 85
pulp polyp, caries 27–8
pulp regeneration, trauma 274
pulp treatment
    contraindications, primary teeth 85
    indications, primary teeth 85
    objectives 79
pulp vitality
    case study 240
    diagnosis 239–41
    electrical test 240–1
    interpretation, test results 241
    mechanical tests 240
    thermal tests 240
pulpal diagnosis and pain symptoms 43–4
pulpal disease, diagnosis 235–54
pulpal immunity, odontoblasts 13
pulpal inflammatory lesion symptoms 48
pulpal nociceptor activation
    local control 42
    pain 42
pulpal pain 33–46, 48
pulpectomy 50–1, 59–65
    access 62
    anesthesia 60–1
    apical wound, location/management 62–3
    aseptic technique 61–2
    diagnostic quandries 273–4
    emergency treatment 65–9

objective 59–60
preparation 62
primary teeth 82
reasons 59
root filling 63–4
steps 60
wound healing 64–5
pulpitis
see also pulp inflammation
case study 69
clinical signs 74
emergency treatment 66–7, 69
symptomatic/asymptomatic 248
pulpotomy 48–59
calcium hydroxide 82
case study 88
clinical procedure 54–5
emergency treatment 66–7
ferric sulfate (FS) 82
formocresol (FC) 82–3, 88
glutaraldehyde (GA) 83
partial pulpotomy 52–9, 81
primary teeth 81–3
success factors 54–6

radicular cyst/granuloma
case study 251
differential diagnosis 251
radiographic evaluation, periapical radiography
293
radiographic examination, trauma 267–8
radiographic signs of failure 83–5
radiography, working length 179
radiolucencies in teeth with vital pulps 248
case study 247
randomized controlled trials (RCTs), clinical
epidemiology 291–2
RCT *see* root canal therapy
receiver operating characteristic (ROC) analysis
diagnosis 236–7
periapical radiography 236–7
receptor cells, odontoblasts as 39
redox potential, micro-organisms 102
replacement resorption, management 273
replantation, root canal filling materials 214–15
resin-based sealers, root filling techniques 223
resorption
apical periodontitis, bone resorption 113–14, 120–1
cervical resorption 263
inflammatory bone resorption 261
inflammatory root resorption 261–2
internal inflammatory root resorption 262–4
internal root resorption 83–4, 244
management 273
non-inflammatory root resorption 264–6
replacement resorption 273
restorative materials effects, dentin–pulp complex
29
restorative procedures, dentin–pulp complex 20–1,
29

retention loss, root filled tooth 317–18
retention of a core build-up, root filled tooth 318
retention of a post, root filled tooth 318
retreatment, non-surgical *see* non-surgical retreatment
retrograde fillings
root canal filling materials 214–15
surgical endodontics 360
risk, clinical epidemiology 295–6
ROC analysis *see* receiver operating characteristic
analysis
root canal bacteria, immunoglobulins specificity
123
root canal filling materials 193–218
allergic potential 196
biocompatibility 195–7
biological properties 194
CE sign 195
classification 193
gutta-percha cones 198–202
handling properties 194–5
ideal 194
leakage/sealing 197–8
limitations 193
mandibular nerve injuries 215–16
purpose 193
replantation 214–15
requirements 194–7, 219–21
retrograde fillings 214–15
root-end fillings 214–15
root filling techniques 219–21
sealers 202–13
sealing/leakage 197–8
selecting 193–4, 219–21
technical properties 194
root canal instrumentation 169–92
see also root canal therapy (RCT)
'balanced force motion' 184
blockage 188
endodontic instruments 180–3
file manipulation 183–4
fracture, instrument 187–8, 190
hand instrumentation 183–4
ledging 188–9
limitations 186–8
limited reach vs unwanted dentin removal 187
mishaps, preventing 188–90
modified double flared approach 176–8, 183
nickel–titanium rotary systems 180, 181–3, 184–7
nickel–titanium rotary systems vs stainless steel hand
files 186–7
non-surgical retreatment 342–4
perforation 189–90
principles 169–70
root canal system anatomy 170–4
stripping 188
techniques 183–6
traditional systems 180–1
'watch-winding' 184
zipping 189
root canal reshaping, non-surgical retreatment 342

root canal system anatomy
   apical configuration 173–4
   cross-sectional shape and diameter 171–3
   physiologically and pathologically induced changes
      174
   root canal curvature 170–1
   root canal instrumentation 170–4
   root canal(s) vs root canal system 170
root canal therapy (RCT)
   see also root canal instrumentation
   access opening 143, 175–6
   antibiotics 155
   aseptic technique 143
   bacteriological sampling 152
   calcium hydroxide 150
   chemical disinfection 147–8
   closing root canal system 151
   complex cases 152–3
   complications 146, 148
   considerations, complex cases 152–3
   considerations, routine cases 144–6
   dressing, interappointment 148–50
   emergency treatment 153–5
   endodontic flare-up 155–6
   evaluation criteria 152
   field isolation 174–5
   final canal preparation 180
   follow-up 151–2
   historical perspectives 141–2
   initial root canal preparation (coronal preflaring)
      176–8
   interappointment dressing 148–50
   intracanal dressing 148–50
   intracanal microbiota effects 153
   irrigation 147–8
   management aspects 156
   mechanical instrumentation 143–7
   modified double flared approach 176–8, 183
   necrotic pulp 4–5, 140–59
   objectives 140–2
   one-appointment endodontics 149
   overextension of the apical foramen 146
   pain control 146–7, 155–6
   painful cases prior to RCT 153–5
   patient information/advice 156
   postoperative pain 155–6
   pre-assessment 174
   procedural steps 174–80
   pulp necrosis 155
   root filling 151
   routine procedure 143–52
   strategies 140–2
   symptomatic lesions management 153–6
   withholding root filling 149
   working length 146, 179–80
root canal treatment, primary teeth 82
root-end closure, calcium hydroxide sealers 209
root-end fillings, root canal filling materials 214–15
root-end preparation
   beveling of the root end 358

   isthmuses 359
   retrograde hand file preparation 358
   surgical endodontics 358–60
root-end resection, surgical endodontics 357–8
root filled tooth 5
   bonding techniques 325
   bridges, clinical outcome 329
   case study 331
   clinical techniques 325–7
   core build-ups 322–5, 330
   crowns, clinical outcome 329
   ferrule design 328–9
   fractures 319–21
   perforation 321–2
   post preparation 325–7
   problems, abutment teeth 317–22
   prostheses, clinical outcome 329
   prosthodontic reconstruction 317–34
   pulpectomy 63–4
   RCT 149, 151
   reinfection/bacterial leakage 322
   retention loss 317–18
   retention of a core build-up 318
   retention of a post 318
   strengthening tooth structure 325
root filling techniques 219–32
   assessing root filling quality 229–30
   chloroform-resin technique 229
   core carrier technique 228
   core concept 224
   coronal restoration 230
   dentine-adhesive materials 223–4
   drying canal 229
   functions, root fillings 220
   gutta-percha 221–9
   gutta-percha cones 221–9
   injection technique 227–8
   lateral compaction 224–5
   leakage tests 226
   materials, selecting 219–21
   objectives 219
   procedures prior to root canal filling 229
   pulp chamber filling 230
   recommendations 230
   requirements, root fillings 219–21
   resin-based sealers 223
   root canal filling materials 219–21
   sealer placement 229
   sealers 222–9
   single cone 224–5
   smear layer removal 229
   softened gutta-percha techniques 225–9
   solid core techniques 224–5
   thermomechanical compaction 227
   warm gutta-percha techniques 228–9
   warm lateral compaction 225
   warm vertical compaction 225–7
   zinc oxide–eugenol (ZnOE) sealers 223
routes of entry, pulpal space, micro-organisms
   96–7

sampling, micro-organisms 103–4
sclerosing apical periodontitis/condensing osteitis, case study 252
sealer placement, root filling techniques 229
sealer removal, non-surgical retreatment 340
sealers
  calcium hydroxide sealers 207–9
  classification 202
  dentin-adhesive materials 223–4
  epoxy resin sealers 205–7
  gutta-percha 222–9
  medicaments 224
  methacrylate-based sealers 209–12
  mineral trioxide aggregate (MTA) 212–13
  properties 223
  resin-based sealers 223
  root canal filling materials 202–13
  silicones 213
  zinc oxide–eugenol (ZnOE) sealers 202–5, 223
sealing/leakage, root canal filling materials 197–8
sensitivity, dentin, hydrodynamic mechanism in pulpal A-fiber activation 37–9
sex-related differences, pain 282–4
silicones 213
  biological properties 213
  composition 213
  handling properties 213
  leakage 213
  technical properties 213
silver cone removal, non-surgical retreatment 340, *341*
single cone, root filling techniques 224–5
sinus recess simulating apical periodontitis, case study 249
size/location of pulp exposure, success factor, pulp capping/partial pulpotomy 54
smear layer removal, root filling techniques 229
sodium hypochlorite, irrigation 147
softened gutta-percha techniques, root filling techniques 225–9
solid core techniques, root filling techniques 224–5
stainless steel hand files, vs nickel–titanium rotary systems 186–7
standard gamble, decision making 308–9
stepwise excavation
  case study 87
  indirect pulp capping 79–81
  primary teeth 79–81, 82, 87
  procedures 82
stripping, root canal instrumentation 188
surgical endodontics 348–69
  bleeding management 356–7
  bone healing 362
  bone removal 355–6
  case study 363, 366–9
  curettage, soft-tissue lesion 356–7
  failures 366–9
  flap closure/suturing 360–1
  flap designs 351–2
  flap raising 351–5
  follow-up 362–3

incisions 353–5
indications 348–9
local anesthesia 349–51
pain control 361
procedure outline 349–61
prognosis 362–3
raising the flap 351–5
retrograde fillings 360
root-end preparation 358–60
root-end resection 357–8
steps 350
surgical microscope 163–8
  critical steps 167–8
  ergonomics 164–7
  illumination system 164
  mechanical system 163–4
  micro-instrumentation 167
  mirrors 164, 167, *168*
  optical system 163
  working positions 164–7
  working techniques 164–7
surgical vs non-surgical retreatment procedures, decision making 310
symptomatic apical periodontitis 124
symptomatic lesions management, RCT 153–6
systemic complications
  acute periapical infections 128–35
  bacteremia 129–35
  blood samples 129–31
  case study 137
  chronic periapical infections 135–8
  deliberations in recent years 136–8
  endodontic infections 128–39
  infective endocarditis 130–3
  periapical abscess 128–9
  potential mechanisms 136
  preventive measures 133–5
systemic effects, chronic dental infections 135–8

T-cells, apical periodontitis 120
techne, endodontology 1
techniques, root filling *see* root filling techniques
terms/expressions
  apical periodontitis: symptomatic/asymptomatic 248
  clinically healthy pulp 247–8
  dentinogenesis 13
  diagnosis 247–8
  disease conditions *4*
  necrotic pulp 248
  normal periapical tissue 248
  pulpitis: symptomatic/asymptomatic 248
  treatment procedures *4*
Thermafil plastic carrier removal, non-surgical retreatment 340
thermal tests, pulp vitality 240
thermomechanical compaction, root filling techniques 227
tools of treatment, endodontology 6
tooth-related pain/swelling, case study 241, 245–6
toxic medicaments, case study 68

trauma 255–76
  alveolar fractures 272–3
  arrest of dental development 266–7
  avulsion 271–2
  cervical resorption 263
  clinical examination 267
  common injuries 255–8
  complications 258–67
  consequences 255, 258–67
  dentin–pulp complex 29–30
  diagnostic quandries 273–4
  fractures 255–9, 268–70
  inflammatory bone resorption 261
  inflammatory root resorption 261–2
  internal inflammatory root resorption 262–4, 265
  luxation 255–60, 270–1
  management 267–73
  non-inflammatory root resorption 264–6
  obliteration of pulp space by mineralized tissue 260–1
  pulp regeneration 274
  pulpectomy, diagnostic quandries 273–4
  radiographic examination 267–8
treatment choice, factors influencing 50–2
treatment failure, primary teeth 83–5
tumor, malignant, case study 253
type of injury, success factor, pulp capping/partial
      pulpotomy 54

variable tip variable taper sequence, nickel–titanium rotary
      systems 185
variation, treatment management 304–5
vascular reactions, blood flow 19
vascular supply
  see also blood flow
  dentin–pulp complex 15–16
vasoconstrictors, local anesthesia 351
virulence factors, micro-organisms 108–9
vital pulp 3–4
vital pulp conditions
  assessment, preoperative condition 51–2
  case study 68–9
  clinical scenarios 47–8
  emergency treatment 65–9

treatment 47–72
treatment choice, factors influencing 50–2
treatment options 48–50

warm gutta-percha techniques, root filling techniques
      228–9
warm lateral compaction, root filling techniques 225
warm vertical compaction, root filling techniques
      225–7
'watch-winding', root canal instrumentation 184
working length
  electronic apex locators 179, 180
  paper point evaluation 179–80
  radiography 179
  RCT 146, 179–80
wound dressings
  calcium hydroxide 75–7
  characteristics 75–9
  clinical success rates 75–9
  corticosteroids 78
  ferric sulfate (FS) 78–9
  formocresol (FC) 77–8, 80
  glutaraldehyde (GA) 78
  mineral trioxide aggregate (MTA) 79
  modes of action 75–9
  primary teeth 75–9, 80
  zinc oxide-eugenol cement 78
wound healing, pulpectomy 64–5

zinc oxide–eugenol cement, wound dressings 78
zinc oxide–eugenol (ZnOE) sealers 202–5, 223
  anti-microbial properties 205
  biological properties 203–5
  composition 202–3
  handling properties 205
  leakage 203
  replantation 214–15
  retrograde fillings 214–15
  root-end fillings 214–15
  root filling techniques 223
  technical properties 203
zipping
  root canal instrumentation 189